Jane Hiscock

Frances Lovett

BEAUTY THERAPY

3rd edition

www.pearsonschoolsandfe.co.uk

✓ Free online support
✓ Useful weblinks
✓ 24 hour online ordering

0845 630 44 44

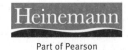

Heinemann

Part of Pearson

Heinemann is an imprint of Pearson Education Limited, a company incorporated in England and Wales, having its registered office at Edinburgh Gate, Harlow, Essex, CM20 2JE. Registered company number: 872828

www.pearsonschoolsandfecolleges.co.uk

Heinemann is a registered trademark of Pearson Education Limited

Text © Jane Hiscock, Frances Lovett, Fareham College, 2009

First published 2010

12 11 10
10 9 8 7 6 5 4 3 2 1

British Library Cataloguing in Publication Data
A catalogue record for this book is available from the British Library

ISBN 978 0 435 02657 8

Edited by Susan Ross
Designed by Wooden Ark
Typeset by Oxford Designers & Illustrators Ltd
Original illustrations © Pearson Education 2010
Illustrated by Hardlines, Oxford Designers & Illustrators Ltd
Cover design by Wooden Ark
Picture research by Susi Paz
Cover photo/illustration © Imagesource
Printed in Italy by Rotolito Lombarda S.p.A

Websites
The websites used in this book were correct and up-to-date at the time of publication. It is essential for tutors to preview each website before using it in class so as to ensure that the URL is still accurate, relevant and appropriate. We suggest that tutors bookmark useful websites and consider enabling students to access them through the school/college intranet.

Contents

Unit S1 Assist with spa operations is available on the Pearson Education website at www.pearsonfe.co.uk/BeautyTherapyLevel2UnitS1. Answers to the Check your knowledge quizzes are available on the Level 2 Tutor Resource Disk.

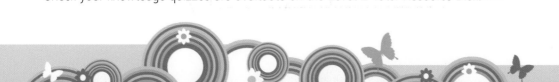

Acknowledgements

The authors and publisher would like to thank the following individuals and organisations for permission to reproduce photographs and realia:

Student book photos: Stockdisc/Getty Images p 14 (bottom); ShutterStock/Yuri Arcurs p 22; Dermalogica p 23, p 280, 282, 283, 284, 285, 287, 288; Cut2White p 34, p 94, p 117, p 167, p 183, p 212, p 218, p 275 (ingrowing hair), 343 (top), p 427, p 460 (manicure bowl); SCIENCE PHOTO LIBRARY p 36/200/470 (boil, wart), p 201 (ringworm), p 204/496 (chloasma), p 205 (strawberry naevus), p 275 (keloid scar), p 331 (bruising to the eye); DR P. MARAZZI/SCIENCE PHOTO LIBRARY p 36/200 (impetigo), p 37 (measles, oral thrush), p 200/331 (conjunctivitis), p 201 (blepharitis, bruise, scar tissue), p 202/331/496 (eczema, psoriasis, acne rosacea), p 204 (lentigo, haemangioma), p 205 (spider naevus), p 275 (papule), p 469, p 471, p 472 (finger biting, splinter haemorrhage), p 474 (spoon nail); ST BARTHOLOMEW'S HOSPITAL/SCIENCE PHOTO LIBRARY p 36/200 (cold sore), p 202 (dermatitis, acne vulgaris), p 275 (pustule); BIOPHOTO ASSOCIATES/SCIENCE PHOTO LIBRARY p 37 (chickenpox); Carlton Professional p 43; MediSwab p 42 (Medi-wipes); Valua Vitaly/ShutterStock p 71, p 348, p 258; ICP/Alamy p 79 (PAT testing); BeautyExpress.co.uk p 88, p 359, p 378, p 379 (mascara), p 384, p 385, p 402 (make-up), p 423, p 429, p 430; Foodfolio/Alamy p 95; Dmitry Goygel-Sokol/Alamy p 97; ShutterStock/Wessel du Plooy p 113; PhotoLibrary/John Warburton-Lee p 127; Renee Tillmann p 129; ShutterStock/Rui Vale de Sousa p 139; ShutterStock/Stephen Coburn p 150; Jonathan Tennant/Alamy p 151; Chris Cooper-Smith/Alamy p 154; Stephen Jakub/Alamy p 170; Najin/Shutterstock p 175; ShutterStock/Yuri Arcurs p 176 (top), p 186, p 211 (left); ShutterStock/Monkey Business Images p 176 (bottom); Photodisc/Cole Publishing Group/Keith Ovregaard p 178; ShutterStock/Rj Lerich p 192 (top); ShutterStock/János Gehring p 192 (bottom); Image Source Ltd/Nigel Riches p 193; ShutterStock/Omkar.a.v p 194; Skinlogic.co.uk p 196; ALAIN DEX/PUBLIPHOTO DIFFUSION/SCIENCE PHOTO LIBRARY p 200 (common cold); WESTERN OPHTHALMIC HOSPITAL/SCIENCE PHOTO LIBRARY p 200/331 (stye); JANE SHEMILT/SCIENCE PHOTO LIBRARY p 201 (cuts), p 473; Scott Camazine/PHOTOTAKE/Alamy p 202 (skin tag); DR H.C.ROBINSON / SCIENCE PHOTO LIBRARY p 203; JAMES STEVENSON/SCIENCE PHOTO LIBRARY p 204/496 (vitiligo); Moodboard/Alamy p 204 (freckles); Medical-on-Line/Alamy p 204 (dilated and split capillaries); JOHN RADCLIFFE HOSPITAL/SCIENCE PHOTO p 205 (port wine stain); Aramis p 208; Photodisc/Kevin Peterson p 210 (middle), p 371; ShutterStock/Archana Bhartia p 210 (right); ShutterStock/Martina Ebel p 211 (right); ShutterStock/Brenda Carson p 215; Shutterstock/Luba V Nel p 221; Shutterstock/Andresr p 222; Vlad Gaviloff/

Shutterstock p 261; Shutterstock/Serghei Starus p 262; Shutterstock/Photobank.ch p 273 (top); DR. CHRIS HALE / SCIENCE PHOTO LIBRARY p 274; Shutterstock/Tania Zbrodko p 289; BE&W Agencja Fotograficzna Sp.zo.o./Alamy p 315 (top); David Woolley/Getty Images p 327; ImageSource p 352; Beauty Archive/Shutterstock; p 357; Bruce Talbot/Getty Images p 377; Tasha Lavigne/Shutterstock p 379 (lipliner); Titov Andriy/Shutterstock p 379 (lipstick); Advertising Archives p 396; Peter Banos/Alamy p 402 (skincare); ShutterStock/R. Gino Santa Maria p 403; Image Source Ltd p 407; Shutterstock/Vladimir Kozieiev p 408; HadK/Shutterstock p 419; Jupiterimages/Getty Images p 455; Shutterstock/Ruslan Kudrin p 460 (polishes); Oleksii Abramov/Shutterstock p 468; MIKE DEVLIN/SCIENCE PHOTO LIBRARY p 470 (paronychia); DAVID PARKER/SCIENCE PHOTO LIBRARY p 470 (verruca); Shutterstock/Jason Stitt p 472 (Aisha); Mediscan p 472 (Beau's line); FRANCOISE SAUZE/SCIENCE PHOTO LIBRARY p 474 (bunion); BSIP, JOLYOT/SCIENCE PHOTO LIBRARY p 474 (corn); PRINCESS MARGARET ROSE ORTHOPAEDIC HOSPITAL/SCIENCE PHOTO LIBRARY p 474 (claw nail); Shutterstock/AVAVA p 475; Shutterstock/Ury p 482 (using a nail art brush); Ralf Nau/Getty Images p 495; Charles Fox p 496 (before and after shots); ShutterStock/Bartosz Ostrowski p 504; Andreas Kuehn/Getty Images p 506; Philippe Regard/Getty p 105; Jeffrey Blackler/Alamy p 106.

All other photos: Pearson Education Ltd/Mindstudio; Pearson Education Ltd/Image Source Ltd; Pearson Education Ltd/Gareth Boden; Pearson Education Ltd/ Studio 8/Clark Wiseman; Pearson Education Ltd/Lord and Leverett; Pearson Education Ltd/Jules Selmes; Pearson Education Ltd/Peter Morris; Pearson Education Ltd/Stuart Cox.

Unit S1 photos: Solovieva Ekaterina/Shutterstock p 1; Dale Saunas p 3, p 6, p 10, p 11 (laconium), p 19; Personalsaunas.co.uk p 11; Shutterstock/xJJx p 12; Shutterstock/Zsolt Nyulaszi p 14; Roger Bamber/Alamy p 23 (caldarium); Shutterstock/Egezilci p 23 (hammam); Jerko Grubisic/Shutterstock p 23 (spa pool); IMAGEMORE Co. Ltd./Alamy p 31; IMAND/Alamy p 32; Dead Sea Range p 33; Pevonia-UK p 34; Pat Behnke/Alamy p 36.

Realia: Dermalogica (Facial treatment record card, p 30 and Skin mapping diagram, p 31); Federation of Holistic Therapists www.fht.org.uk) for text reproduced on p 67.

Every effort has been made to contact copyright holders of material reproduced in this book. Any omissions will be rectified in subsequent printings if notice is given to the publishers.

Crown copyright material reproduced with permission of the Controller of Her Majesty's Stationery Office and the Queen's Printer for Scotland.

Introduction

Why choose a career in beauty therapy?

The world of beauty therapy is an exciting one, with close links to the fashion and hairdressing industries. It is varied and diverse, offering lots of opportunities to learn and develop skills in a range of different areas. Ultimately it is a service industry and its main, and most rewarding, aim is to help others to feel good about their appearance and be the very best they can be.

A career in beauty therapy offers you the opportunity to tailor a job most suited to your personal circumstances or passion, whether that be travelling, working in a spa, working for yourself or specialising in one particular field, such as make-up design. With a Diploma (NVQ/SVQ), you have a firm foundation.

My story

Hi, my name is Lauren and I work as a beauty therapist on board a cruise ship – I'm currently on a nine-month trip around the Caribbean! I signed up to do a Level 2 Diploma (NVQ/SVQ) when I was 23 after a couple of jobs that I didn't enjoy. I worked hard and within two years, I had my L2 and L3 qualifications. I also worked part-time in a local salon to really learn the trade. I'm glad I did because I think my salon experience gave me the edge when I applied to work on the cruise ship. I had to attend a nine week training course in London before starting the job to learn about the products we'd be using as well as health and safety procedures to make sure all the passengers on board were safe at all times. I would thoroughly recommend this career route to anyone who wants to see the world. You work hard and the hours are long but you get to see some amazing places and meet so many great people.

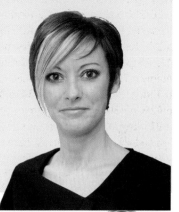

My story

Hi, I'm Zoe and I'm married with two small boys. I worked part-time in a supermarket for many years before finally plucking up the courage to sign up for a beauty therapy qualification at my local college. It was scary and I was worried about being the oldest in the class but it was the best thing I ever did. Because I did part-time evening classes, I was also able to carry on working and taking care of my boys. After a year, I qualified at Level 2 and decided to work from home in the spare room above our garage. Once I started letting people know, the word got round and now I have a thriving business with lots of regular clients. I can choose my own hours to best suit my family and I've been able to invest in some key pieces of equipment. It's so fulfilling to have a job that I love and I feel so much more confident.

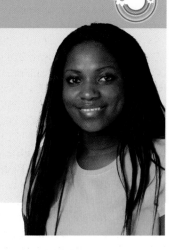

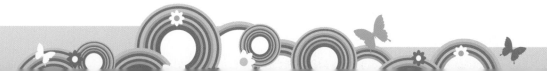

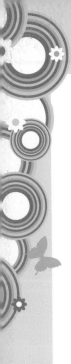

What is a Certificate/Diploma (NVQ/SVQ)?

If you are familiar with the Diploma (NVQ/SVQ) system and are confident about the background to this method of gaining a qualification, then skip this section, and move on! If you are new to the system, then read on.

NVQ = National Vocational Qualification
SVQ = Scottish Vocational Qualification

This is a different but highly successful method of gaining a qualification. You may not have used it before, for example if you have come straight from school, or if you have not been in a training situation for some time.

This is not an exam with a pass or fail outcome. NVQ/SVQ uses continual assessments, in each unit, building up to a qualification. It is a fairer option for those of us who freeze at the thought of an exam room!

There are several beauty therapy awarding bodies offering NVQs/SVQs. Your training establishment will be able to guide you through the particular one they use, but the standards do not vary too much, and the information within this book should cover all eventualities.

How do I gain a Certificate/Diploma (NVQ/SVQ)?

The qualification is gained by showing lots of **evidence** within each unit and is practically based, so each student gets a very good grounding in all the skill areas. This means that when you go into a salon, you have dealt with most client requests and have lots of confidence to perform the service that the client is paying for.

How do I get my evidence?

Many forms of evidence are acceptable and your trainer/lecturer will be able to guide you through the best options for your individual learning programme. Each of the different types of evidence is valid. These are:

- observed work
- witness statements
- assessment of prior learning and experience (APL)
- oral questions
- written questions and/or assignments
- other.

These will be recorded on **evidence sheets** provided and will form a **portfolio**. A portfolio is just a collection of all the evidence together. It should be indexed and easy to follow.

Why index?

An assessor will observe or guide you through the types of evidence listed above. This person will have had special training for a specific qualification designed to help you present your evidence in a format suitable for your awarding body.

For quality control and fairness across the subject areas, an internal verifier will check the assessor and the portfolio instruction. This will be performed within your section/school at your place of training and should happen on a regular basis.

The awarding body also has an external verifier who will visit your training establishment regularly and check that both assessors and internal verifiers are giving the correct information to you, the candidate. Then your portfolio can be accredited with a certificate. This can be achieved a unit at a time, or applied for all at once. It's essential that you keep your portfolio organised and present your work in an easy-to-view format.

What evidence do I need?

You should ask your assessor about the most suitable method for the work you are doing. Most portfolios have a mixture of evidence.

If you have previous experience (APL) — perhaps gained whilst working — or recent qualifications, they can also be counted. For example, if you work in a shop, part-time, and have experience using the till, dealing with customers and handling complaints, then a witness statement from your employer that is current, valid, signed and dated is very acceptable evidence.

This evidence would cover some of the reception units, as well as some communication units and the interpersonal skills required. It also covers some of the ranges required in your assessment books.

Other valid evidence could be photographs, project work, videotape or client record cards.

Standards

To give the overall picture we can look at what you are going to need to do. First, your training establishment will register you with its awarding body.

The awarding body will then issue you, the candidate, with your assessment book. Take care of it; it is very precious. It will become your only source of evidence for all your hard work.

Within your assessment book you will be given guidance on how to achieve each unit. There are conditions and terms that you must follow.

Performance criteria

You must perform these in the course of your assessed treatment. They are numbered and your assessor will tick them off as they are observed. For example, Unit B4 has performance criteria including 'using consultation techniques in a polite and friendly manner to determine the client's treatment plan'.

Ranges

These must be covered through the various methods of assessment previously discussed — observed performance, oral question or simulation, written question, project or through APL; for example, different skin types for Unit B4.

Beauty therapy pathway

The new Level 2 (NVQ/SVQ) Diploma in Beauty Therapy qualification has been designed to enhance the career path of those wishing to have an all-round qualification, or provide routes for those wishing to specialise in a make-up route.

The mandatory units are:

- ○ G20 Make sure your own actions reduce risks to health and safety
- ○ G18 Promote additional services or products to clients
- ○ G8 Develop and maintain your effectiveness at work

These are compulsory to all students, and cover all aspects of health and safety, product promotion and how to become a good team worker for your salon. You must take these three, and then choose one of the following routes:

- ○ Beauty Therapy General Route
- ○ Beauty Therapy Make-up Route

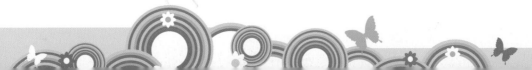

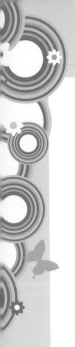

There are optional units as well, such as G4 Fulfil salon reception duties, B10 Enhance appearance using skin camouflage, and so on.

The object of the book is to support you by providing the units for all routes to the qualification. This will make you into a highly employable beauty therapist, as you will qualify in the units most useful to clients, salon owners and their managers. You may decide that the General route is preferable because specialising early on in your training may narrow your employability.

Those who gain a good grounding of all the units may wish to further their careers by going on to take a Level 3 qualification. You may find it helpful to refer to HABIA's Career Ladder for Beauty Therapy. This can be found on the HABIA website at the following link: http://www.habia.org/uploads/Beauty_Leaflet.pdf

How to use this book

This book has been designed with *you* in mind. It has a dual purpose:

1. To lead you through the Level 2 (NVQ/SVQ) Diploma in Beauty Therapy, providing background, technical guidance with suggested evidence collection and key skill information.

2. To provide a reference book that you will find useful to dip into, long after you have gained your qualification. The comprehensive cross-referencing within the individual chapters will guide you through the NVQ units and indicate where the information applies — and should prevent repetition!

Each of the practical units contains the same essentials — the **Professional basics**. This has been presented as a separate section that should be worked through and adapted to the unit you are taking, at the time. The anatomy and physiology required for each unit has also been separated so that it can be accessed and referred to easily. As the anatomy and physiology is a constant theme throughout the qualification, there is a mapping grid on page 223 showing what anatomy and physiology you will need in each unit. Remember that you only have to learn it once and apply the knowledge to the practical area you are working through.

Features to help your learning

The purpose of this book is to inform and guide you through your Level 2 (NVQ/SVQ) Diploma in Beauty Therapy. To reinforce your learning process and get you thinking, there are several features to help you.

Key terms
These highlight terms that are central to your understanding of the topic that you may not have come across before.

Think about it
These activities will get you to think about applying theory to a practical situation. They will give you an opportunity to stop and think about what you are doing when you are carrying out treatments to ensure that you are striving for and achieving best practice.

Salon Life
This is a full-page feature designed to look like the page of a magazine. It covers a key issue or problem, including an account of a therapist's experience in the salon and expert guidance on the issue or problem covered.

My Story
Appearing throughout the units and within the Salon life feature page, these are short, real-life accounts from people working within the industry with tips and

suggestions. They are designed to get you to think about the different things you may encounter and may need to think about in your day-to-day life as a beauty therapist.

Frequently asked questions

Expert advice and answers to some of the most commonly asked questions on each practical topic — questions that may come up as you work through the practical units.

Check your knowledge

This is a list of multiple choice and/or short-answer questions provided at the end of each unit to help you check your knowledge and understanding of that unit. Answers are provided on the Level 2 Beauty Therapy Tutor Resource Disk.

For your portfolio

These are tasks or activities which encourage learning through research and investigation. They are designed to help you to gather and generate evidence for your portfolio and key skills.

Getting ready for assessment

At the end of each unit you will find helpful information and advice about how that unit is assessed and guidance on what you will need to be able to demonstrate to your assessor in terms of skills and competencies.

SAKS

We are pleased that this book has been endorsed by SAKS. Saks Education is officially acknowledged as the UK's Best Training Provider, having been awarded Beacon Status by the Quality Improvement Agency and all grade ones by the Adult Learning Inspectorate for providing outstanding training. It is the only hair and beauty work-based learning provider to have been awarded both accolades.

Saks recognise that Education is the key to success! A good sound education can lead to numerous career opportunities within the beauty industry and the basis for that is NVQ Level 2.

About Hair and Beauty at Fareham College

The Hairdressing and Beauty Therapy Department at Fareham College is long established and has been innovative in the implementation and delivery of a wide range of successful courses.

On four consecutive occasions (1997, 2001, 2005 and 2008), the department achieved the Government Inspectorate's highest accolade of a Grade 1 for all-round provision in courses and teaching and learning. In 2006 they were awarded the prestigious Beacon Award by the Association of Colleges sponsored by City and Guilds.

Over the years the department has been a leader in developing new initiatives which have been recognised nationally; for example, teaching staff at Fareham College have been involved with HABIA, working on the Expert Working Group during the conception of the 14–19 Diplomas and are at the forefront of developing this educational initiative with local consortia as Network Leads. The new Diploma in Hair and Beauty studies has been delivered at Fareham College since September 2009. This is the biggest educational change for 50 years and is an exciting introduction to our sector for 14–19 learners, providing the opportunity for a variety of career paths.

Beverley Woolford
Head of Department for Beauty and Holistic Therapies

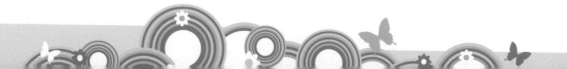

Section

1

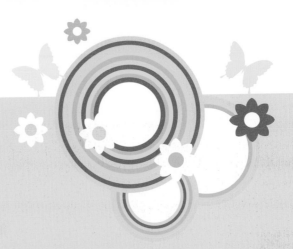

Professional skills

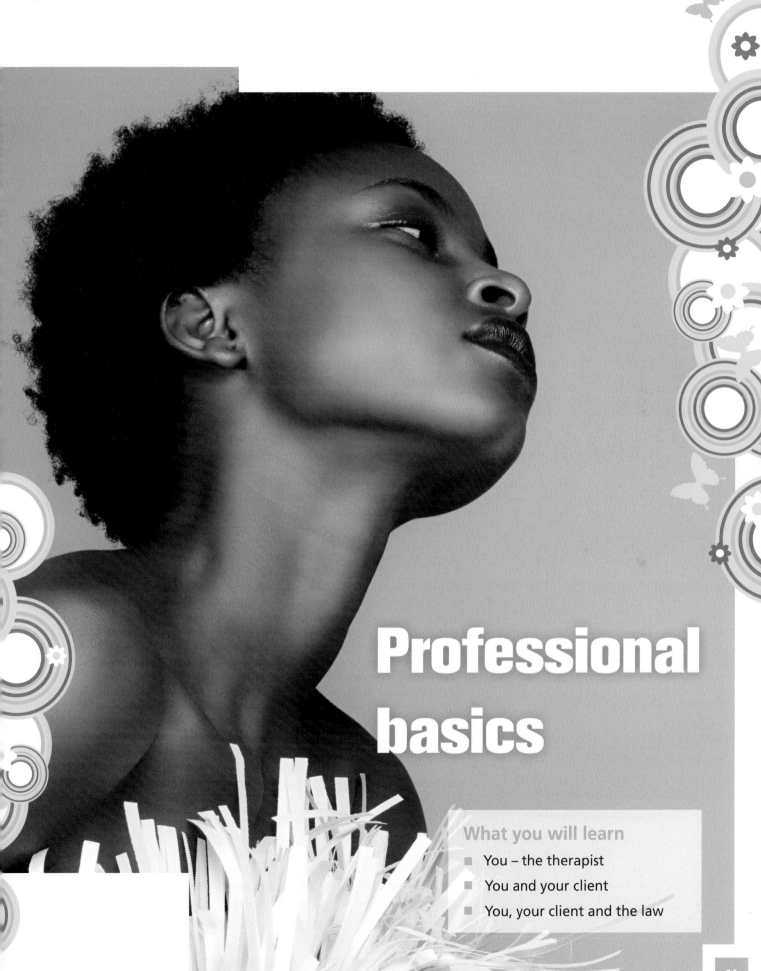

Professional basics

What you will learn

- You – the therapist
- You and your client
- You, your client and the law

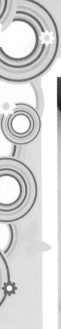

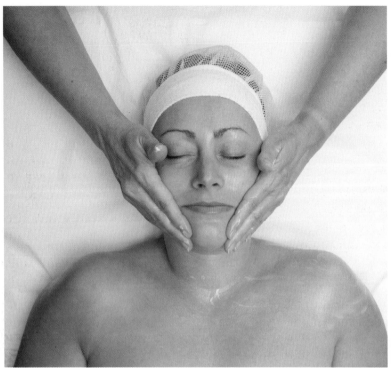

Introduction

The professional basics are literally everything that underpins the skills you will require to become a qualified beauty therapist.

Before you can decide upon the most suitable treatment for your client, or prepare **treatment plans**, you need to have a clear understanding of the basic underlying principles of what you are doing.

This section covers the basic knowledge you will need before you start working through any practical unit. You will need to refer back to this section each time you start a new practical unit.

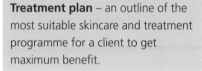

Key terms

Treatment plan – an outline of the most suitable skincare and treatment programme for a client to get maximum benefit.

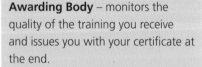

Key terms

Awarding Body – monitors the quality of the training you receive and issues you with your certificate at the end.

Hygiene – conditions and good practices that promote and preserve health by preventing cross-infection.

You – the therapist

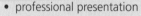

In this outcome you will learn about:

- professional presentation
- preparing to work
- effective communication
- salon services
- treatment planning and preparation
- effective teamwork and relationships
- record keeping.

Professional presentation

All **Awarding Bodies**, clients and employers will expect you to have a professional appearance, not only to achieve your assessments but also to set the standards within your working life as a fully qualified therapist.

A professional appearance helps you feel the part and gives the client confidence in your ability as a therapist. Your personal presentation includes the aspects described below.

Hair

Hair needs to be clean, tidy and professional looking. It should be tied back away from the face. Your hairstyle should not interfere with the treatment. It is very distracting for clients if you have to keep flicking hair out of your eyes, and they may find this irritating. Equally important, by constantly touching your hair you will be breaking hygiene rules. You'll read more about **hygiene** on pages 39–47.

Nails

Nails should be clean, short and unvarnished (unless the employer states that, as a nail technician, you can have varnish on). Clients may develop an allergy to varnish, and chipped nail varnish is not a good advert for your trade! Unvarnished nails can also be seen to be clean. Long nails may scratch the client's skin when performing massage. Rough cuticles, bitten or dirty nails set a poor example and will not inspire confidence in your skills.

Jewellery

Hygiene and professional ethics state that the only jewellery permitted is a plain wedding band and small unobtrusive earrings. Rings could scratch the client and carry germs. Remember that other body piercing may cause offence to some clients and does not reflect a professional image. It is also a good idea not to take precious jewellery to work – this will reduce the risk of losing it.

Uniforms

Most salons and training establishments require a professional uniform to be worn. This should be clean, pressed, and of a suitable length to work in. It is advisable to go up a size to allow free movement, or at least try it on with arm movements tested!

It is also advisable to have several uniforms in order to allow one to be in the wash, and to prevent one uniform getting too soiled. Regular washing is essential to prevent body odour build-up as this can give off an unpleasant stale smell to the client.

Your training establishment will probably have a uniform policy and tell you the recommended supplier to go to – you should receive a good discount for bulk purchase as you are in a college or training establishment. Wear your uniform with pride – it will help you to feel professional and look the part!

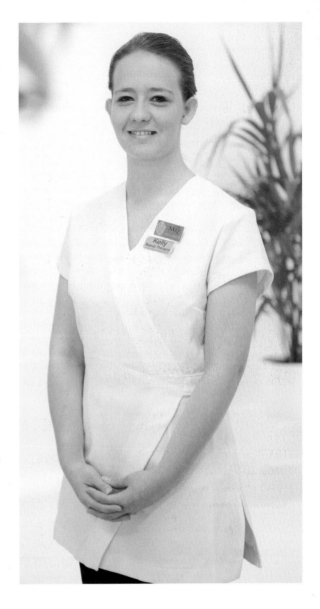

Make-up

Subtle make-up may be worn, but heavy make-up or stale-make-up (e.g. left over from last night) is not professional. If the skin is clear and the eyebrows tidy, the therapist may decide not to wear make-up at all – this is personal choice. The key should be how the therapist feels and looks on the day! Light make-up can hide minor blemishes and help tired eyes. If you need a 'pick me up', use it wisely.

Perfume

Remember that strong perfume may be as unpleasant to the client as body odour. Choose a light fragrance that does not overpower, and remember that stale perfume can be very off-putting.

Also bear in mind that perfume cannot hide body odour, so the use of anti-perspirants and deodorants is recommended, as well as daily bathing to prevent an accumulation of smells. An anti-perspirant will prevent perspiration building up, and a deodorant will help prevent odour. Most of the products available do both jobs.

Think about it

Personal presentation not only includes a professional appearance – good grooming and a smart uniform – but for Unit G20 Make sure your actions reduce risks to health and safety, it specifically covers personal hygiene, clothing and accessories suitable for the workplace and avoiding anything which has the potential for an accident, such as very high heels, or dangling jewellery.

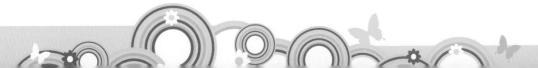

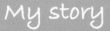

My story

Being aware of body odour

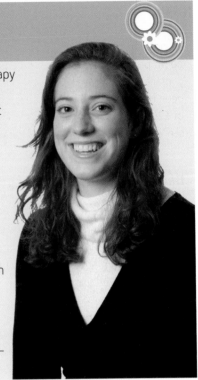

Hello. My name is Melissa, and I am coming to the end of my first term as a Beauty Therapy student at college. In my group, I occasionally have to work with a student who, although she always looks good, has a bad case of body odour. Everyone in the group had noticed it but felt too embarrassed to tell her. As I am slightly older than the rest of the group, they asked me if I would have a word.

I thought it through and realised that the tutor should tackle the problem. If it was me, I would want to know, but I didn't want to upset the student by mentioning it. So, our tutor spoke to the student. She hadn't realised it was such a strong smell, and was puzzled why she should have body odour since she washed and bathed regularly and changed her overall daily. She decided to see her GP to find out if anything was wrong.

It turned out she had overactive sweat glands under her arms and was producing too much sweat — it is called Bromohyperdrosis. She was given a special deodorant, which helped dry up the sweat, and she is having some Botox injections to freeze the glands and stop the problem.

She was slightly embarrassed when she rejoined the group, but we were all sympathetic — and it would not have been pleasant for clients. I would want to be told — wouldn't you?

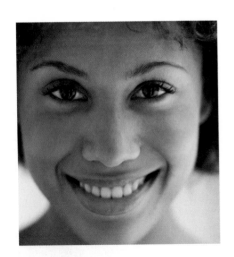

Shoes

Your shoes should be clean and comfortable for a full day's work. If your shoes do not fit securely, you could have or cause an accident.

Check with your training establishment about your footwear — commercial companies that supply uniforms often supply shoes too. Although in adverts for uniforms you may see the model wearing flip flops or open-toe shoes, they are not practical for all treatments. They would not provide protection if, say, hot wax were to be spilt on your feet.

Remember high heels are for going out in; they are not suitable for long working days and can damage your posture. Leather shoes allow the feet to breathe and are therefore more hygienic, preventing a build-up of bacteria, which may cause odour problems and lead to athlete's foot. All people in occupations that involve long periods of standing would benefit from support tights — even the young — as these can prevent varicose veins forming and stop the legs from aching!

Oral hygiene

Regular dental care will prevent tooth decay and keep gums healthy, so stopping bad breath forming. Regular brushing, mouth sprays, sugar-free mints and breath fresheners are also advisable to prevent stale breath being passed over the client. Remember that bad breath can be a sign of illness, so it may be worthwhile getting a dental or medical check-up if you think you may have a problem.

It is only polite and courteous to your client to avoid strongly flavoured foods, such as curry, garlic and onions, especially at lunchtime. Smoking can also cause odours that cling to the breath — a good excuse to give up smoking, even if only at work.

Think about it

It's not only on the breath that smoke lingers – it clings to clothing and hair, which can be off putting if you are delivering a treatment, say a facial, where you are in very close contact with your client. A mint cannot hide all of that! Smoking in public places has been banned since July 2007 so you will be liable to a heavy fine – £50 or a maximum of £200, if prosecuted – if you are found smoking in your workplace. For more on this, see You, your client and the law on page 55.

Benefits of professional presentation

For the therapist:

- Professional presentation helps you feel ready to take on a professional job role.
- It helps you feel part of a team as you all look the same.
- It encourages you to feel confident – you can take pride in looking proficient.
- It gives you self-assurance that you are meeting health and safety regulations.
- It gives you a self-belief and identity – you look as if you belong in the salon.
- It allows you to represent both yourself and the whole salon image.

For the client:

- A clean, tidy appearance gives a positive, lasting impression of both you as a therapist and the corporate image of the salon.
- Clients feel 'in safe hands' as you look competent and efficient.
- It gives clients encouragement with their treatments – clients often want to look like their therapist.
- It instils trust and a belief in you and your abilities because you look groomed and clients then realise that your treatments are effective.

Preparing to work

Personal presentation will take you only so far in your job role and dealing with clients – your attitude has to be right, too. Beauty therapy is a service industry. The general public are your clients and they pay for your service and expertise. Therefore they should also be entitled to your full attention and care.

It is not just the décor of a salon that creates atmosphere, it is the ambience created by the people within it. How the therapist mentally prepares for work goes a long way to producing the calm, relaxed feeling of a salon which allows the client to gain maximum benefit from the treatment.

Put on a smiling, caring expression when you are working – you may have lots of your own personal problems but passing them on to your client is not acceptable. Never gossip to your client about others: either staff or clients. Do not shout, swear or curse at work – you will develop the habit and not even realise when or to whom you are doing it.

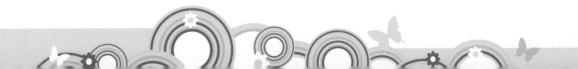

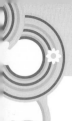

> **Think about it**
>
> Imagine going to a really grumpy therapist, who started late, rushed the consultation, didn't even remember your name and was generally rude. You just wouldn't go back again, would you?
>
> It is said that you get out of life what you put in – and that is also true about a beauty therapy treatment. A quiet, relaxing facial should be as pleasurable to give as it is to receive. A good therapist will gain satisfaction from a tranquil hour and you will find that giving a facial massage is very soothing to both of you.

As a quality check after a treatment, a good therapist should ask herself:

○ Would I like to be treated as I have just treated that client?

○ Would I pay for the treatment I have just given to that client?

○ Could I have improved upon the quality of my service?

○ Was it as restful and as peaceful as it could have been?

○ Has the client rebooked?

Effective communication

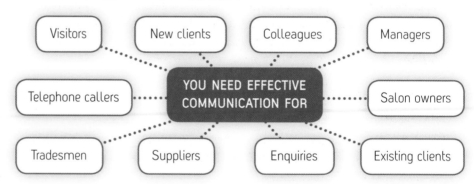

Communication at work will be with many different people

Whatever your position at work, you will need to communicate with others. If your business is to be successful, you will need to communicate effectively with a variety of different people, as can be seen in the diagram. This communication can be verbal, non-verbal or written.

Verbal communication

This refers to what you say and so it must be:

○ clear and to the point

○ easily understood, using everyday language – avoid jargon; technical terms should be put into simpler terms, wherever possible

○ spoken in a friendly manner, with a relaxed facial expression and a smile where appropriate

○ carefully enunciated, that is spoken clearly and with good projection

○ spoken while facing the client – try to direct your conversation only at the person to whom you are speaking; the whole salon does not need to hear

○ considerate of those who may be hearing-impaired – eye contact can reinforce your message.

Try to avoid:

- using slang
- talking down to the client or treating her as if she is stupid — this is patronising and is a bad habit to get into
- using endearing terms such as 'dear', 'love' or 'darling' — such terms are inappropriate in the workplace, and some clients may find them patronising.

Non-verbal communication

This is another term for body language. Your body conveys messages through your:

- general demeanour
- posture
- facial expressions
- gestures.

These unconscious gestures tell you a lot more about the client than verbal communication can. The therapist should be aware of the client's body language and learn how to interpret it.

Watch for signs that understanding is not clear, or the client is not satisfied or following what you are saying. If the client is new to the salon, she may be nervous, and this can be picked up through body language — look for continuous facial touching, hair stroking or nervous gestures with the hands. New clients may need reassurance and a calm manner to make them feel comfortable.

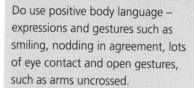

Think about it

Do use positive body language — expressions and gestures such as smiling, nodding in agreement, lots of eye contact and open gestures, such as arms uncrossed.

Avoid negative body language — frowning, tension, no eye contact and closed gestures such as arms crossed.

Body language – what this means

For the therapist:

- Use open hand gestures and ensure you look approachable — crossed arms and legs, and/or a closed facial expression or a scowl on your face will discourage the client from coming over to you.
- Smile and make eye contact — body language that avoids eye contact with the other person gives the impression of being shifty or dishonest.
- Give the client her own personal space — avoid getting too close, which may make her feel uncomfortable.
- Read the signs from your client — she may be saying one thing with her voice, but her body language will give away her true feelings. Is the client nervous? Look for hair twiddling and agitation with the hands. Is the client looking confused? Watch for frowning and puzzled facial expressions. Adjust your body language to suit the client's and you will reassure her. Be calm and smooth in your actions — this shows confidence.

For the client:

- If the client sees you as open and friendly, she will feel able to approach you and will be less nervous or intimidated.
- The client will be more confident about you and your abilities if look like you are an honest person.
- The client will be more likely to rebook and spend more money if you are a welcoming, responsive therapist — and she will probably ask for you again!

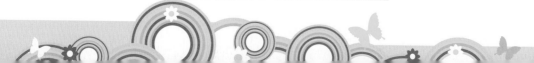

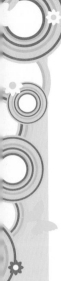

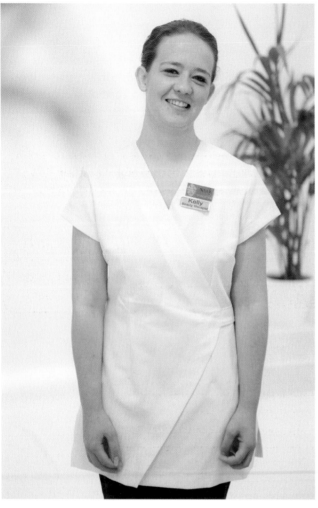

Positive body language

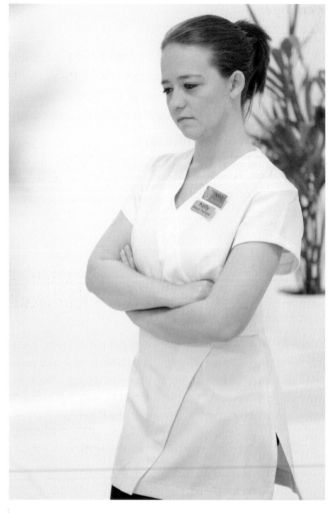

Negative body language

For your portfolio

Observe those around you and take time to study their communication skills – both in your learning environment and outside, especially if you have a part-time job.

Look at someone you admire and consider to have good communication skills – what do they do that makes it easy for you to get on with them and relate to them in a positive way?

Write a 150–200-word summary of how your boss communicates with you. How could you improve your own communication skills?

Whether your body language is good or bad, it will create a lasting impression on the client – so make sure it is good!

Communicating and working together

When you work in a salon you will have a manager or a senior staff member, who supervises what you do, or you may have junior staff who you guide through the working day. Good communication means being understood: the message sent out is the message received.

Working under supervision
This means that you:

○ accept that someone is in charge

○ should take instructions and act upon them

○ communicate effectively

○ take responsibility for your job role and do it to the very best of your ability.

Working together

Good teamwork means:

○ supporting each other, not being in conflict with one another

○ giving the salon a good atmosphere, which the client senses

○ providing a reliable service

○ giving effective results.

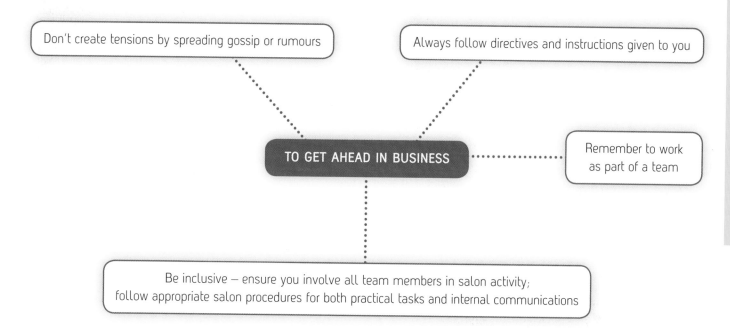

Don't create tensions by spreading gossip or rumours

Always follow directives and instructions given to you

TO GET AHEAD IN BUSINESS

Remember to work as part of a team

Be inclusive — ensure you involve all team members in salon activity; follow appropriate salon procedures for both practical tasks and internal communications

The ability to listen

The ability to listen is a dying art! In our fast-paced world we often only half listen when someone is speaking, forming our reply even before the other person has finished talking. A good listener will be attentive, look interested in what is being said and be still, so that the information can be absorbed.

If you try to clear your work area or prepare for the treatment while doing your consultation, the client will know that you are not listening thoroughly and are distracted by the job you are doing. This does not show a caring or supportive manner.

To be a good listener you should:

○ be attentive — it is very off-putting if, when talking to someone, they look uninterested, so avoid yawning or looking bored

○ avoid assuming you know what the client is going to say — whenever you take something for granted and presume knowledge, you are more likely to make a mistake

○ try not to be distracted by others or by external noise

○ try not to form your reply before the speaker has finished — you may miss an important piece of information

○ be genuine.

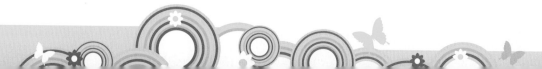

Professional basics

To have effective listening skills means:

○ knowing when to stop talking and listen to what is being communicated

○ listening with interest and understanding

○ having the right body language to show you are interested – be still, face the client and make eye contact

○ providing encouragement and confirming you have understood what has been said, e.g. nodding or agreeing with the point being discussed

○ confirming the statements the client is saying to show you have been listening and you understand, e.g. 'So, you have never had a full facial before, Mrs Chapman?'.

Written communication

Communication that is written down must be:

○ clear and easy to understand

○ concise – only information that is required should be given

○ legible and easy to read

○ well presented – handwritten or word processed

○ correct – all the information should be included.

Avoid using texting language – not everyone understands this shorthand, and it is a bad habit to get into. Write the words in full to avoid any confusion.

Written communication must be clear and concise

> INTERNAL MEMO
>
> | **Date:** 24th Feb 2010 **Time:** 10.30am | **Taken by:** Rasheda | **For:** Saskia – senior therapist |
> |---|---|---|
> | **Message:** Can Mrs Kaminski change her appointment from tomorrow to next week as she has just been signed off by her doctor with a nasty virus and is not going to work for the rest of the week. She doesn't want the girls in the salon to catch it and is too poorly to come in. | | |
> | **Action:** If you agree can you just confirm by phone and leave a message on the answer machine. tel: 01234 56789012 | | |

Clear written communication is important for many aspects of work within the busy salon environment, including health and safety, accident reports and record cards. For example, the client could be placed in danger if an allergic reaction warning on her record card is not readable. Messages for staff can also cause misunderstanding if appointments are cancelled or changed but not fully understood by the person receiving the memo.

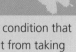

Benefits of good communication skills

For the therapist:

- It gives you the chance to develop a relationship, or a rapport with the client. The client is likely to make up her mind on your professionalism during her first treatment, so good communication is essential to build up her trust and will help to ensure that the treatment is successful.

- It means there can be no misunderstanding about treatments, **contra-indications** and health and safety issues. Misunderstanding can lead to problems and potentially be very serious: for example, if the client had a nut allergy and you mumbled through the consultation, and she did not hear the questions about allergies, there could be serious medical consequences.

- Relationships with other staff members are clear and will enable you to enjoy a good working relationship.

For the client:

- The client feels valued — she is listened to and appreciated.

- The client feels safe and secure, knowing that all personal knowledge is received and understood.

- The client is happy with how she is treated — it makes her feel special and she will want to return for more treatments.

Salon services

A good therapist is pleasant, patient, and helpful to everyone who comes into the salon. The needs of each person will vary and you must be able to give correct information. If you do not know, you must be professional enough to admit your knowledge is not sufficient, and get a salon manager to help — rather than making something up.

Treatments offered

Even if you personally cannot perform the entire treatment list, it is important to be aware of all the treatments and sell them. A professional therapist will have a thorough knowledge of the treatment process, the advantages or disadvantages of each, and each of the topics mentioned below. The salon will lose business if you just shrug and say you do not know.

Think about it

Knowledge about your salon and the treatments and products it offers is key! Read through all new literature for the salon or new treatments when they are launched. Take responsibility to be up to date with all aspects of your salon, even if you cannot perform the treatments yet. For example, you could sit in on a training exercise or volunteer to be the model so that you can talk about what the treatment feels like and how it had a great effect on your skin. The same applies with products. Take home samples and try them so that you can talk with confidence about the feel, consistency or benefits of the product.

Key terms

Contra-indication – a condition that will prevent a treatment from taking place or that will require a treatment to be adapted.

Salon services – range of professional treatments and activities available in a beauty salon or spa.

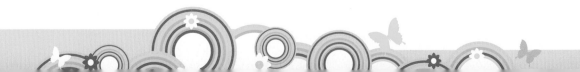

My story

Personal experience

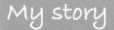

Hi, my name is Marie. I am a mature Beauty Therapy student and have returned to college after working as a receptionist in a GPs' surgery. I always wanted to do a beauty course. I am really enjoying the course. Being a receptionist, I already had good communication skills and customer services qualifications, so I was quite confident about doing a rota on our college reception.

However, what I was very conscious of was my skin. I have always had some acne, with a greasy skin, and breakouts. I covered my skin up quite well, but I was always very aware of it and would not let anyone see me without make-up.

When we started the facial unit I decided to share my worries about my skin with my tutor — she was really helpful. My tutor also takes a Level 3 group who are learning the electrical facials for deep cleansing and healing. She asked me if I would be a model for one of the students in the group and have a course of treatments. I was a bit scared at first, as I didn't know anyone in the group and they all seemed so professional, but I have learned so much about Level 3 treatments. Not only can I talk them through when I am on reception, I can say how well my skin is doing!

My confidence has grown because my skin is clearing up nicely, and because I have had a galvanic facial, I can tell clients what it feels like, and what the results are. The Level 3 student also recommended some new products for me to try at home, so I felt really supported and encouraged. I would recommend that all Level 2 students go into another, more advanced class and model for them. That way, you'll get to see the salon from the client's point of view and experience some really good treatments.

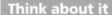

Think about it

Remember also to check for product suitability. Not all clients are suitable for every treatment or service. Clients may have allergies or food intolerances. Some aromatherapy-based products may irritate an existing eczema condition. (Refer to the lists of ingredients in Unit B4 Provide facial skincare treatment, pages 280–88.)

Think about it

Do not guess the time it takes for a treatment: if you underestimate, it will disrupt the day's running order, and the therapist will be stressed trying to catch up; if you over estimate, the treatments will finish early and there will be gaps when the therapist is doing nothing, which is not cost-effective.

Suitability of treatment

Not all treatments are suitable for every client. Some treatments require a sensitivity test, prior to the appointment, in order to assess the sensitivity of the skin or eyes. If a client has a treatment that was not entirely suitable for her, she will not be pleased. A customer who is not completely satisfied will not return to the salon and may spread bad publicity about the salon instead.

Treatment timings

The timings of treatments should be accurately given. Do not mislead the client or underestimate how long a treatment may take, or your credibility will be undermined. In addition to this, the smooth running of the salon will be disturbed if timings are not given correctly. Learn the price list and treatment menu thoroughly so you can accurately book in a client, and not disrupt the running order for the whole day.

Time is money and in order to be cost-effective the timing of treatments must be accurate. Standard timings also help maintain the quality in the salon, so that all therapists offer the same time for each treatment. Clients are then all treated equally and get the same value for money.

The frequency of treatments given should also be negotiated with the client and will be dependent upon the time available, financial considerations of the client, the condition or suitability of the area of the body to be treated, and any **contra-actions** to the treatment.

If a deluxe manicure treatment with paraffin wax takes 45 minutes, and the receptionist has booked the client in for only 30 minutes, there is very little time to offer a relaxing treatment. So, either the treatment is modified (losing money for the salon), the treatment is rushed and the client is left dissatisfied, or the therapist overruns and keeps the next client waiting. All of this could so easily have been avoided, if the treatment time had been correct in the first place.

Key terms

Contra-action – an adverse physical reaction, as a result of treatment or products. This should be recorded on the record card.

Prices

Prices will vary from salon to salon, and area to area. Price lists should always be on display. This allows the client to view the costs for herself and is also additional advertising.

Costings given should be truthful, with no hidden extras – no one likes to be conned.

Special offers

If the salon has any offers to pass on to the client, then the therapist needs to be aware of them. This helps to promote the offer and provides a chance to sell additional treatments that your client may not be aware of.

Most people like a bargain, or offer, and if they get to hear about it after the offer closes they may not be pleased.

Remember that there is legislation in place regarding sale prices (refer to the Sale of Goods Act, page 62, in the legislation section) so be careful when advertising a sale in your window.

Retail sales

Retail sales form an important part of any busy salon, and can help boost a therapist's pay at the end of the week.

Many salons offer a full retail sales service to complement the products used in the treatment. The therapist needs to be aware of what the salon sells, whether it is in stock, and what the benefits and features of each product are.

The Beauty Salon

Face and eyes

Express facial (30 minutes)	£25
Radiance boost facial (30 minutes)	£32
Anti-ageing facial (60 minutes)	£45
Deep-cleansing facial (75 minutes) £60	
Eyebrow shape	£10
*Eyelash tint	£12
*Eyebrow tint	£10
*Eyelash and brow tint	£20

Patch test required 24hrs before treatment

Clients need to know what the different treatments and services involve and how much they cost

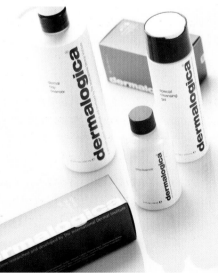

Retail sales can be an important part of a salon's business

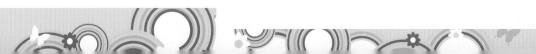

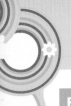
For your portfolio

Carry out a comparison between two local salons in your area – are the prices and treatments offered the same or very different? Do they have a similar client base or do they cater for different tastes?

Money will be lost if you ignore the customer who wants to buy the product that has just been used within the treatment. Most suppliers provide large sizes of product for use in the treatment room, with a smaller retail size for the client. During the consultation, the therapist will ask the client about her homecare routine and which products she uses. Continuous care at home with the right products boosts the benefits of a salon treatment and good results can be seen.

Think about it

Learners are sometimes hesitant about what they regard as 'hard selling', but it should be viewed as part of the aftercare given to a client, which involves recommending products that will enable the client to support the treatments carried out in the salon. It's a difficult skill to get right, and there is a fine balance between putting off a client with a hard-selling approach and not actually recommending anything! The skill comes with experience, confidence and belief in your products.

For your portfolio

When you sell retail-size salon products, keep a copy of the till receipt or daily taking sheet. This will be excellent evidence for your portfolio for Units G18 Promote additional services or products to clients and G8 Develop and maintain your effectiveness at work, and shows you have communicated and listened to your client's needs.

If you are employed in a salon, also keep a copy of the salon price list and all the advertising materials the salon may have. You need to be aware of what your salon offers, regardless of whether you can perform the treatment or service, and you should understand what each involves.

Complaints

Realistically, a busy salon will encounter complaints. It is therefore important for the salon to have a complaints procedure, which staff are aware of and have been trained to follow. This will mean that when a complaint does arise, however minor, the correct salon policy can be followed. Here is an example of a complaints procedure.

- Deal with any complaints pleasantly in a professional manner.
- Calm the client and remove her from the reception desk to a more private area.
- Listen to her. Be objective and not defensive – the complaint may be valid.
- Be prepared to apologise if you are in the wrong and offer some form of compensation – a free treatment perhaps.
- Try to reach a mutually satisfactory outcome. This will minimise the damage that a complaint may have on other customers, and prevent further legal action being taken.
- Should the complaint be about another person, speak to the staff member later in a calm manner. Do not blame others in front of the customer.
- Record the complaint in the customer comments book.
- Be aware of the legal implications of further action (refer to the section on insurance on page 65).

Treatment planning and preparation

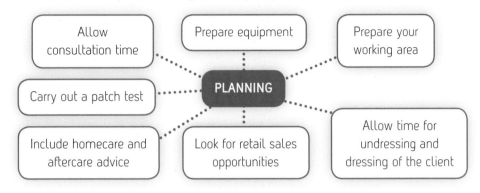

Allow consultation time	Prepare equipment	Prepare your working area
Carry out a patch test	**PLANNING**	
Include homecare and aftercare advice	Look for retail sales opportunities	Allow time for undressing and dressing of the client

Treatment and planning should include these tasks

Treatment planning is essential for the smooth organisation of a salon where there is more than one therapist working. Through good organisation, the relaxed, calm atmosphere that a salon should have will be in place, and that will be reflected in the mood of both customers and staff. Even if there is only one therapist employed, treatment planning will help with time management in order to ensure that money is not lost.

Remember the old saying:

Time = money

Treatment planning should be viewed as an investment. The more planning carried out 'behind the scenes', the more professional the treatment becomes. The key is to be organised.

Good working relationships between staff should also be part of the planning for the salon manager or owner. Teamwork is very important and regular training and team building is essential.

The receptionist

A good receptionist is worth their weight in gold. They are the first person the client comes into contact with – often called 'front of house' as in a theatre. They represent everyone else within the business and should create a welcoming and excellent first impression. Their planning also needs to be first rate.

All the planning for the treatment starts with the receptionist and the initial booking of treatments. The receptionist needs to be aware of:

○ what treatments are being offered through the day and therefore which preparations can begin early, e.g. turning on the wax heaters

○ what any treatment involves and therefore how much time should be booked out

○ if this is a first treatment for the client or the middle of a course

○ if a full consultation is needed, therefore requiring more time

○ the 'before' and 'after' time required for the treatment, that is undressing/ dressing/shoes, etc.

Extra time should be included so that a client relationship can be built up.

Last-minute alterations

An organised therapist will make the receptionist aware of any alterations to the day, any time out of the salon, and any change of plans, well in advance.

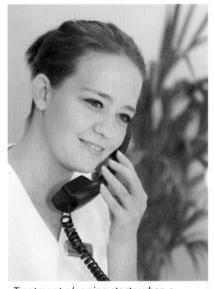

Treatment planning starts when a client is booked in

Think about it

Treatment planning and being on reception should be done in a calm and organised manner – if you are hurried and anxious, you will pass those feelings on to the client, who may be agitated and consequently not enjoy her treatment. Business may be lost.

Obviously, the uncontrollable factor is sickness. If you have a full column of clients booked in and are unable to attend work because of illness, there is very little that can be done. Therefore, the earlier you notify the salon, the better.

The receptionist should be able to rearrange some clients for another day, or at least notify them, as they may wish to cancel. The other therapists in the salon then have the task of covering all the clients who cannot be contacted. This is dependent upon the goodwill of the other staff members, and a good relationship is vital for the health, growth and atmosphere of the salon.

You should discuss at the initial job interview what the establishment policy is regarding illness and sick cover, as well as sick pay.

Good working relationships between staff should also be part of the planning for the salon manager or owner. Teamwork is very important and regular training and team building is essential.

Reliability is a valuable quality and helps to build goodwill among team members. If you are constantly relying on others to counter the effects of your bad planning or time management, then tensions may increase in the workplace.

Sickness in the salon – what it may mean

For the therapist:

- spreading of germs or disease in the salon to both clients and staff members, especially something that is highly contagious such as sickness or diarrhoea
- unhygienic practice – even if it is a minor complaint such as a running nose, you cannot afford to 'drip' all over the client!
- lost wages – especially if you have a high sickness rate for odd days off
- lost business.

For the client:

- a cancelled appointment, which can be very disappointing
- exposure to additional germs and illness if a therapist with a contagious condition comes into work
- delays and rescheduling into another therapist's column
- may decide to take her business elsewhere.

Think about it

To obtain evidence for Unit G18 Promote additional services or products and G8 Develop and maintain your effectiveness at work, you will need to spend time acting as the salon manager as part of your duties. This puts you in charge of allotting treatments and managing the bookings for the day. If you are trying to fit in a full page of treatments and half of your team is off sick, it will involve a lot of swapping about and possible cancellation of clients. You will certainly see the other side of the coin and how disappointed clients are when their treatments are cancelled.

Develop and improve personal effectiveness within the job role

You must prepare for the working day ahead and contribute to the planning of the salon. Remember, however, that treatment planning is not just about appearance and personal presentation as discussed on pages 12—13. Just as important is your approach or mind-set. Most organisational skills develop from having the right attitude.

Being organised and planning ahead can become second nature and almost part of your personality at work. Being prepared, tidy and forward thinking are very good habits to cultivate!

Benefits of personal effectiveness and organisation

For the therapist:

- At home:
  Is my appearance professional and as good as it could be?
  Do I have everything I need for the day: money, lunch, keys, handbag, loose change for parking or the bus?
  Have I allowed enough time for my journey, public transport, or time to walk?

- At work:
  What treatments do I have booked in?
  Am I prepared for them? Have I got enough of the right equipment, stock and tissues, sponges and cotton wool?
  What time is my first appointment?
  Do I need to organise a float, till roll or fill up tea/coffee?
  Is my working area clean, tidy and welcoming for the client?

- Mind-set/mental approach:
  Am I calm and relaxed to greet my client?
  Am I focused on the client and not on my own problems?
  Am I confident in what I am doing?
  Am I fully prepared?

For the client:

- They will feel calmed by the tranquil atmosphere in the salon.

- Their pace will match the therapist's relaxed approach and they can begin to unwind.

- They will feel cosseted and pampered by the therapist's undivided attention.

- Their tension will drain away as they realise their treatment is hassle-free.

- They will want to repeat the experience — and will book another appointment!

Think about it

In Unit G8 Develop and maintain your effectiveness at work, you will be expected to review your own performance at work. Ask yourself the following as you go through the day:

- What went right today and why?

- Did anything go wrong and why?

- Did I keep my clients waiting for their treatment or service to begin?

- Have I allowed enough time to give full attention to each client?

- Are my clients totally satisfied with my service?

- Is all my equipment to hand?

- Have I left my client unattended to go and get equipment?

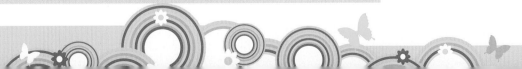

- Can I help colleagues with their set up, or do I need help with mine?
- Would I pay for the treatments I have carried out today?
- How could I improve upon my performance tomorrow at work?

By continually evaluating your answers to the above questions you will be able to recognise and improve upon your working pattern. If being disorganised is a habit that you have fallen into, with the attitude that 'it really doesn't matter, because someone else will do it', then bad habits need breaking.

Effective teamwork and relationships

During your practical sessions for Units G4 and G18, so that assessments can take place, you will be asked to run a realistic working environment (RWE), with fee-paying customers booked in, just as in the industry. These sessions will involve you acting as salon manager for a day. It needs good teamwork and an excellent relationship with your peers to be able to plan and run an RWE session effectively. How you organise the session affects everyone, and you need to be aware of what is expected of a salon manager.

The salon manager plays a vital role and it is important that you understand how what he or she does affects how the salon operates.

The manager

The role of the salon manager is vital to the treatment planning and preparation of the working day. A good manager will organise the salon, the staff and take responsibility for the well-being and safety of the clients.

For the salon, the manager will:

- have a set system in place for morning and evening preparation and jobs to be done (these should be on a rota basis for all to do)
- have procedures and rules for everyone to follow – this will provide a consistent standard of service
- have clear guidelines on treatment times and expected preparation time
- provide realistic times for specific treatments.

For the staff, the manager will:

- hold regular training sessions for everyone so that all members of staff know what is expected of them
- praise and reward those who perform well
- hold regular **appraisals** and direct those who are not organised
- instruct clearly and without favour
- instruct clearly with regard to being cost-effective, not wasting products and being uneconomical
- lead by example and be professional at all times.

For the client, the manager will:

- ensure that systems and procedures are in place for the health and well-being of all clients and visitors, including risk assessments on the salon and equipment,

Key terms

Appraisal – a one-to-one meeting between an employee and their line manager to discuss how the job role is going and identify further training required. It may involve a considered opinion, estimation or judgement of an individual or an estimate of value.

upholding the law on health and safety and holding regular fire evacuation practices (see pages 49–61 for more health and safety information)

○ hold a first aid certificate that is up to date and valid

○ protect the client with regular sensitivity testing for potential allergy-related products and ensure all staff are trained in these procedures

○ take responsibility for complaints and refunds.

Record keeping

Good record keeping is absolutely essential to any beauty salon. You should create and use good systems in order to keep track of your work and the clients.

Record cards

The functions of a record card are:

○ to record relevant contact details so as to be able to contact the client if necessary

○ to provide full and accurate information about the client to ensure client safety

○ to ensure consistency of treatment – regardless of who performs the treatment

○ to record the number of treatments in a course and the date of each – this is so that if the client changes therapists for any reason, there is a complete record of what they have had and when

○ to note changes to the treatment programme or contra-actions if they occur

○ to record the progress of the condition or treatment success

○ to safeguard the salon and the therapists – to prevent clients taking legal action for damages or negligence.

The record card should be filled out in full for every treatment or service the client has. It should be written accurately, neatly and legibly.

For your portfolio

Some Awarding Bodies will require a parent/guardian's signature on a consent form for clients less than 16 years of age, and this should be attached to the record card. You will need to make sure a copy is in your portfolio if you are treating a young person.

Think about it

A record card can also be used to record information that will enable you to develop a better relationship with your client and perhaps to avoid saying something embarrassing! For example, a note that says 'recently widowed' or 'newly married' will not only be a good jog for your memory, but if you are off sick, and another therapist treats your regular clients, they will know whether to handle the client with extra sensitivity or enquire about her honeymoon – it doesn't take much to add a personal touch to a client's day!

Think about it

The personal information on record cards should always be kept private and confidential. Under the Data Protection Act you are not permitted to pass on names and addresses and other information about your client. If the salon or therapist does so, they may be liable to prosecution.

Record systems

Most salons have a number system in place (see below), or keep records on computer. This is both for safekeeping and for easy retrieval. Most software packages for computers have a database system for easy recovery of names and storage. A computer system is a large cost to start with, but can be very easy to use, with the correct training. It is ideal for use in a larger salon, with a wide client base. However, the Data Protection Act 1998 needs to be upheld (see You, the client and the law, page 63).

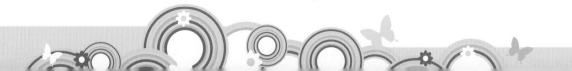

Think about it

The record card should be signed and dated, every time, to show the client gives written consent to the treatment. If the client is under 16 you must also obtain parental or guardian written consent. Some Awarding Bodies do not allow assessments to take place on minors, so do always check the age of the client when booking the treatment. The more detailed your record card, the safer and easier the treatment for all concerned.

If the data is set up in a database or spreadsheet, it is easy to print labels with client names and addresses so that you can post them details of promotions and special offers.

The storage of record cards should be given consideration. They need to be accessible to the receptionist or therapist, but not so open that others can view them. A locked filing cabinet or drawer is most common, with limited access to the keys.

The two most common ways of filing names are:

○ a number system – client 1, client 2, etc.

○ an alphabetical system – A, B, C, etc.

Alphabetical systems tend to use the first letter of the surname and if two names begin with the same letter, then the second letter is used, and so on.

Benefits of record cards

For the therapist:

- It provides a complete picture of the client. This will include: personal details, lifestyle, occupation, any medical conditions and minor health issues that may impact upon treatment.

- It gives an immediate view of potential problems: allergies to products, adverse reactions to products or treatments (known as contra-actions) and medical considerations which may affect the treatment, such as pregnancy.

- It tracks the treatments the client has and if she has had a course of specific treatments, providing a record of what the client has paid to date and how many treatments she has had – so avoiding any possible disputes.

- It provides a chart of the progress made and provides an opportunity to boost the client's morale and state how well she is doing.

- It protects the therapist against any accusation of misconduct, malpractice or negligence if filled out correctly and signed by the client – the client will have given her consent to the treatment being carried out.

For the client:

- It ensures the client's protection by providing a record of her medical history, so regardless of which therapist treats the client, all are aware of any medical problems.

- It provides a record of the client's improvement and allows her to see progress being made.

- It makes the client feel special, and it personalises the treatment – the client isn't just a number, she matters to the salon.

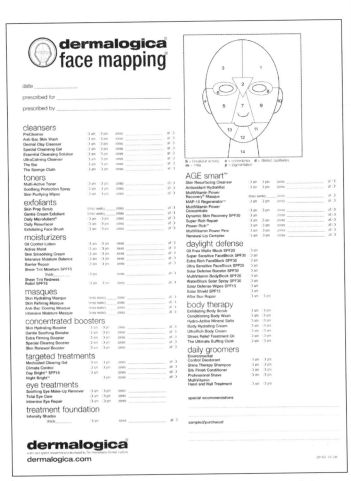

Dermalogica include a detailed skin mapping diagram on their facial treatment record card (Source: Dermalogica)

Subject specific record cards

Obviously, each client record card will be different and be personal to the clients: recording their treatment plan, skin problems, and personal history. Most product houses supply their own record cards which can be purchased in bulk. These offer a thorough checklist of contra-indications, the client's health, skin type, previous products used, retail sales history and so on. They also include a detailed line drawing of the face and body so that you can accurately highlight the problem areas – you must be as detailed as possible for both the continuity of the treatments and so that other therapists are aware of the treatment programme.

> **Think about it**
>
> Whichever treatment you are performing, the client will need a subject specific record card, so if she has a manicure, facial and eye treatments, she will need to have all three in her record file. You will need to fill out all of them as evidence for your assessments and as a written record to show her consent to having these treatments performed.

Skin mapping diagram
(Source: Dermalogica)

You and your client

> **In this outcome you will learn about:**
>
> - assessment techniques and questioning the client
> - contra-indications
> - contra-actions
> - hygiene and avoiding cross-infection
> - treatment and client expectations

Assessment techniques and questioning the client

This is a vital part of your role as a successful therapist. All treatments and services are based upon what you discover within the initial consultation. The only way to make a correct diagnosis of the client's needs is through questioning and then tailoring your plan to the information you receive. All practical assessments are based upon successful client consultations and recognising the client's needs.

All thriving salons earn their reputation by providing an excellent personal service. Care and attention to the client is the key to good business. The consultation should be carried out in privacy, and the service should be free. It is standard practice to link a consultation with a treatment plan.

The consultation also provides the initial bonding process between client and therapist. You can get to know the client a little better as well as gaining a clear picture of her for the treatment, including: contra-indications, her current skincare regime and how effective it is, and what she hopes to gain from the treatment or service. Managing a client's expectation is often a hard part of the consultation – a facial will make the skin look better and clearer, but it will not change the shape of the face, or turn the client into her favourite celebrity!

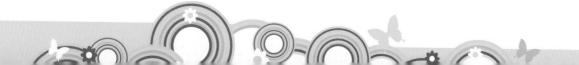

A good therapist will use all the skills mentioned and follow the client's body language to help obtain the information required for a good effective treatment plan. It must be agreed mutually that the time and money involved and the results suit both your client and yourself. If the plan is unrealistic, the client will not stay with the salon; she will go elsewhere.

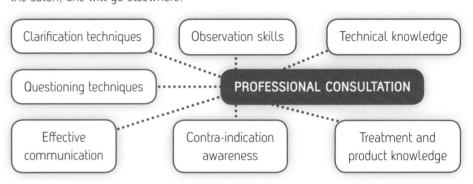

Your professional consultation should include all this

Questioning techniques

Asking questions is a skilled task. If you really want to find out what the client thinks and needs from you, you need to ask her. How you ask, what you ask and the type of question will dictate the reply you get. So, it is important that you give some care to your questioning technique.

If you ask the right questions and listen carefully to the answer, the treatment almost plans itself! All information should be included on the record card, which you will be filling out as you discuss details during the consultation. Use the record card as your guide. As already stated, verbal questioning will determine all the personal details — refresh your memory by looking at record cards above. There are two types of questions: closed and open.

Closed questions

Closed questions usually need only one-word answers. They do not allow conversation to flow, but they are good for confirming information, so they have their place. For example, 'Have you ever had high blood pressure?' will enable you to confirm or eliminate information when the client responds with 'Yes, I have' or 'No, I have not'. Sometimes you have to use a closed question if you just require facts, but try to keep them to a minimum.

Open questions

Open questions provide a hook for the other person to respond to in more detail than a simple 'yes' or 'no' answer. For example, 'How did you get to the salon today?' requires the client to give a more detailed answer, so such questions are good to break the ice. They help build a rapport with the client and put them at their ease.

A professional therapist will use open or leading questions to help put her new client at ease and draw them out ahead of the consultation. For example, the following open questions could be asked as she greets the client at the door.

A successful consultation leads to a good treatment or service

- What's the weather doing out there now?
- How far have you come?
- Where did you manage to park the car?
- How did you hear about us?

It is better to use open questions than closed questions, such as the following.

- Is it still raining?
- Have you been here before?
- Did you get the bus?
- Is this your lunch hour?

Open questions are also a good means of recommending products, as you can start a dialogue about which products they have used, how they found them, how long they lasted, and so on.

A mixture of both open and closed questions will need to be used in the consultation process, but try to use them in the appropriate context — and then they will become a great tool towards a thorough and professional consultation.

Observation skills

Diagnosis of the client's well-being is not only discovered by the consultation questions but also through observation. It can reveal as much as, and sometimes more than, questioning alone. You will be carrying out detailed observations on the specific areas of the client to be treated — these are covered in the individual practical units. However, it is not just about looking at the skin, or the area to be treated, it is about seeing the client as she first walks into the salon. The unconscious body language of the client can speak volumes about her general attitude and state of mind.

A dropped pair of shoulders and dragging feet will indicate that she is nervous, a bit low in self-esteem or worried or anxious about something. A confident client will have more direct body language, more eye contact, with a spring in the step and an upright posture. So, when your client arrives it is important to observe:

- how they walk in — what does the body language say: confident or hesitant?
- the client's general appearance — ungroomed or groomed?
- how they stand
- how they sit
- if there is a mobility issue or disability to be aware of, or any other special consideration.

In addition to this, you may be able to look at some of the area to be treated (if on the face or hands), the condition of the client's skin, the amount of care and attention previously given to the area and how well the client is groomed — her hair, nail varnish, make-up.

If the client doesn't wear nail varnish or make-up, it may mean that she does not know how to use them, or perhaps considers them too expensive or time-consuming to bother with. She might also prefer a more natural look. All this will give you an indication of which treatments are likely to best suit the client's needs.

The other important factor to look at is, of course, your client's reactions to you.

Think about it

We are all different. One client may be quite open and talk freely about herself and what she hopes to get from the treatment or service; others may be shy, and it may be some time before you fully gain the clients' trust and confidence. As in life in general, relationships take time to build.

Never assume something about the client and listen carefully to the answers given.

It's a good idea to have a practice run – ask a close family member, or someone you know really well, whether you can carry out a full consultation on them. Although you know the person, try to view them as a client. Ask about lifestyle, skincare regime, diet, and so on, to build up a good picture of them.

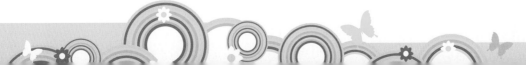

Clarification techniques

Clarification means checking the details given by the client to ensure the information that she gives you is recorded correctly. You need to do this whenever information is being passed on to you. It will happen at all stages of client contact. The following are examples.

1 When the client makes a telephone booking, all information regarding date, time, the nature of treatment or service, and the client's name and number should be repeated back as confirmation. Avoid saying what the treatment is too loudly, as it could be of a sensitive nature, e.g. if the client is booked in to have a bikini wax, she may not appreciate everyone in reception knowing about it!

2 When the client arrives at reception for the appointment, the time of the booking and the name of the therapist can be repeated to the client.

3 When the client is having the consultation.

Repetition of details will enable the correct treatment plan to be prescribed and reinforces what the therapist may already know. For instance: 'So, Mrs Lakhani, your skin has been dry for most of the winter months. What products are you using?' This also gives the client lots of opportunities to respond to your open questioning techniques and therefore rapport builds up between you.

Technical knowledge

It is very important that you fully understand the treatments you are talking about. Do not make anything up — this is very unprofessional. Always refer to the manufacturer's instructions and product information if you are unsure.

You should always have a copy of your salon's price list at hand to refer to. You could give it to the client to take home to look at later, as she may not take in everything you say during the consultation and might like to book a further treatment.

A good price list should have the treatment description, time of the treatment and the cost, along with a brief description of what happens and how it feels: for example, waxing should be highlighted as being slightly uncomfortable, like a plaster being ripped off the skin, and a deep facial massage could be described as 'total relaxing bliss'!

Product knowledge

Think about it

Try to use straightforward language when talking to your client. Use words that she will recognise and avoid jargon: for example, refer to blackheads not comedones! The client will want to know what the treatment or service can do for her and the results. Resist the temptation to show off your knowledge of technical terms – they will only confuse her.

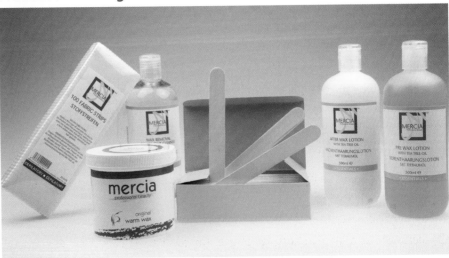

Get to know your products to talk about them with confidence

Professional basics

Products, like treatments, require some time and effort so that you fully understand what they can do and how to use them properly. Be sure the information, benefits and effects you are claiming are true. It is also professional to ensure that the product you wish to sell to your client is appropriate and in stock. Selling an unsuitable product just to close the sale is very bad practice. You will lose the client as they can no longer trust you — you may have gained a sale in the short term but lost a client in the long term.

Regular training and visits from manufacturers will ensure that your information is up to date and accurate. Many companies are happy to visit training establishments to introduce their product. It is a good idea to volunteer to model for product training so that you can talk about what the treatment/product feels like and keep experimenting with the products. It is common for therapists to have their favourite products and just stick to those, as they feel confident with them. Because they use the same products all the time, they keep on recommending them, never extending their knowledge to other products. Often it is only when a product is discontinued that the therapist is forced into trying something new — so try to keep an open mind.

Treatment and product advice

The client has come to you (and is paying) for your skill and expertise. Some of her issues may be of a personal or sensitive nature. Be gentle with her and treat her kindly. Treat her as you would wish to be treated.

When giving advice remember never to patronise or talk down to your client. All clients should be treated with the same respect and courtesy, regardless of how trivial their problems or questions may seem. Be both honest and realistic with aims and objectives in the treatment plan, especially with courses of treatment.

Make sure the client realises that results may take some time and are often not instant. Perhaps some small treatments that do have instantly visible results could be used as a morale booster, such as a nail varnish with a manicure or an eyebrow tidy.

Contra-indications

A contra-indication is the presence of a condition which makes the client unsuitable for treatment. A contra-indication means that treatment should not take place at all because it will be harmful to the client or make the condition worse, or it is a risk to others in the salon. A treatment is normally unsuitable because the client has a medical condition which may be external and/or visible, or it may be 'hidden' and discovered during the consultation.

Refer to individual practical units for full details of relevant contra-indications specific to the treatment or service. You should refer to them prior to commencing any treatment.

It is important that you do not treat the client because:

- the disease could be contagious and there is a risk of cross-infection to both therapist and other clients
- the condition may be made worse by a treatment
- there may be a reaction later, which puts the client's health at risk.

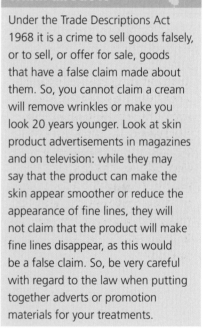

Think about it

Under the Trade Descriptions Act 1968 it is a crime to sell goods falsely, or to sell, or offer for sale, goods that have a false claim made about them. So, you cannot claim a cream will remove wrinkles or make you look 20 years younger. Look at skin product advertisements in magazines and on television: while they may say that the product can make the skin appear smoother or reduce the appearance of fine lines, they will not claim that the product will make fine lines disappear, as this would be a false claim. So, be very careful with regard to the law when putting together adverts or promotion materials for your treatments.

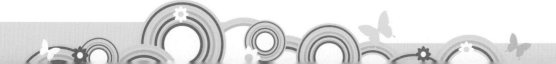

This is why it is essential to complete a thorough consultation, prior to any treatment being given.

If the contra-indication is small and localised in one area, treatment may take place with some adaptation. For example, a minor cut would be covered with a plaster. But a larger problem, such as a leg with open, weeping eczema, would be a definite contra-indication and further advice should be sought from the client's GP.

Be aware that some GP's surgeries request a small fee to cover administration costs which must be paid by the client. The salon provides a short letter outlining the treatments to be undertaken and the GP can just sign this. Most doctors are very open to their patients having beauty treatments and massage, as they recognise the health benefits — and some doctors refer clients to salons, for treatments such as electrolysis and massage.

The cost of a permission slip is preferable to risking a reaction to drugs taken, and a possible court case for negligence. The GP's permission slip could then be placed in the client's record card so that all therapists are aware of medical problems for that client and therefore all therapists are protected.

Anyone receiving chemotherapy or radiotherapy would be unsuitable for treatment as would anyone with a history of deep vein thrombosis. Always check with your Awarding Body with regard to its contra-indications policy.

General contra-indications

To help you remember different contra-indications, try to visualise looking from the outside of the body and work inwards, as shown in the table opposite. What you may see on the skin comes first, then muscles, bone, blood, and so on.

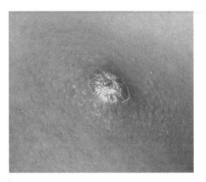

Boil

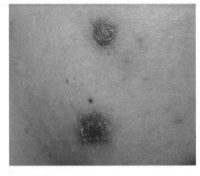

Impetigo

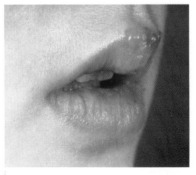

Cold sore

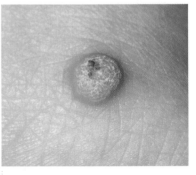

Wart

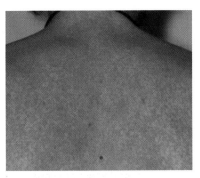

Measles

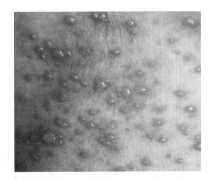

Chickenpox

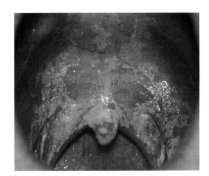

Oral thrush

Skin	Muscles	Bones	Body systems
• Skin infections, disease or disorders	• Dysfunctional muscular conditions, such as Parkinson's disease or multiple sclerosis	• Broken bones	• High or low blood pressure
• Open wounds or weeping sores		• Recent dental work, implants in the jawbone or cosmetic surgery such as rhinoplasty	• Heart conditions
• Cuts, bruising or abrasions	• Loss of sensation to the area		• Diabetes
• Raised or hairy moles or moles with uneven edges which have bled or weep	• Spastic muscle conditions		• Epilepsy
	• Dysfunction of the nervous system which affects the muscles, such as motor neurone disease		• Severe asthma
• Unknown swellings			• High fever, colds and flu
• Recent scar tissue – do not treat until GP approval is agreed			• Hormone imbalances
• Varicose veins or phlebitis	• Dropped muscular tone, such as Bell's palsy (recognised as one side of the face being lower than the other)		• Any systemic disease such as chronic liver conditions
• Medicines which impair the skin's healing properties or increase its fragility: e.g. Accutane given for acne may cause severe dryness and further treatments may exacerbate the condition; or antibiotics which can result in oversensitivity to sunlight and cause rashes or pigmentation. (Refer to You and the skin, pages 179–80, for a full list of medications and vitamins which affect the skin.)	• Recent procedures, such as Botox® injections which freeze the facial muscles and may impair sensation		• Disorders of the endocrine system affecting any of the glands, such as thyroid
	• Collagen infill injections around the eyes or mouth		• All types of cancer

It is very important you follow these guidelines when dealing with contra-indications:

○ As a therapist, it is not your place to mention specific conditions to the client, because you are not medically trained. You can recommend that the client see her GP, but do not name the condition, nor offer any diagnosis or cure.

○ It is important that the contra-indication is discovered prior to the treatment or service starting, rather than half way through. This stops the client being disappointed in not getting the full treatment and keeps your professionalism in place. It will also stop the condition from spreading to others, or putting them at risk.

○ Some contra-indications if they are minor will not prevent the treatment from taking place, either because they can be covered over, or are not in the area to be treated. A client with a bruised big toe having a facial can obviously continue with the treatment.

○ Clients may be forgetful and omit to mention they have a condition, such as high blood pressure, but may list the medication they are taking, often not remembering what it is for. Stop the treatment until you do know what conditions they have and ensure you get a GP's approval for treatment in writing and the client signs the consent form.

Contra-actions

A contra-action is the unfavourable reaction of a client to a treatment. Some treatments do cause some slight reaction, which is normal and to be expected: for example, a waxing treatment will cause the skin to go red, and there may be some blood spotting. It is a normal reaction to the slight trauma that the skin has undergone. However, an abnormal reaction to a treatment would be a severe response, as shown in the diagram below.

It is up to the therapist to respond quickly to any adverse reaction that happens within the salon, in order to minimise the problem and not make it worse. The client must also be informed of what to look for after the treatment has finished and what action to take at home.

Contra-actions can occur with the application of any product – even one your client has used for years can suddenly produce a reaction not seen before.

An abnormal reaction to a treatment can lead to unpleasant contra-actions

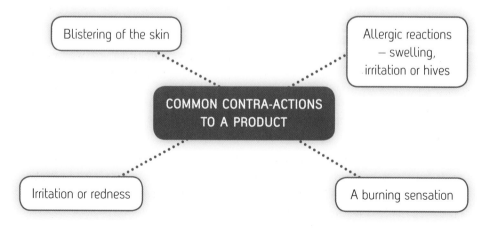

Blistering of the skin

Allergic reactions – swelling, irritation or hives

COMMON CONTRA-ACTIONS TO A PRODUCT

Irritation or redness

A burning sensation

Refer to individual practical units for specific contra-actions.

Professional basics

Allergies

One common reaction to a product used within the treatment may be an allergic reaction. Clients can develop an allergy to a product they have been using for years. It can literally occur overnight. It may be a reaction to a food, a cleaning substance or an airborne droplet such as someone's perfume. Refer to You and the skin, page 205, for a full explanation of how an allergy occurs and how it affects the body.

Some allergies can be life-threatening and the client may go into anaphylactic shock, a condition of extreme hypersensitivity, which is an emergency condition requiring urgent medical attention. Symptoms include breathlessness, fever and, in extreme cases, the person falls unconscious and the heart stops.

Clients with a severe allergy will carry an EpiPen® which administers a dose of adrenalin to counter the effects of the allergy. Allergies to shellfish, bee stings and nuts are very common, but it can be a reaction to any substance such as house dust, pet hairs, and so on.

Be very careful about using creams or oils with a nut base.

Hygiene and avoiding cross-infection

Hygiene may be defined as: 'The science concerned with the maintenance of health; clean or healthy practices or thinking.' So for you, as a professional therapist, hygiene could be described as good practice to maintain your own health, your clients' health and your colleagues' health.

However, there is no such thing as a completely sterile environment; perhaps the closest to it would be an operating theatre within a hospital. Germs are all around us and, while some are beneficial to humans, many of them are not. Beauty therapy treatments demand close human contact, so care must be taken to provide the maximum protection against cross-infection.

Expert advice on hygiene can be confusing. There have been conflicting reports in the media regarding AIDS and hepatitis, and the resistance of some bacteria, such as MRSA, commonly found in hospitals, to antibiotic treatment. (MRSA is a drug-resistant strain of a very common bacterium called Staphylococcus aureus.) The most valuable up-to-date information can be gained from your Awarding Body's code of ethics or practice (refer to it for more details). These guidelines have been established after a great deal of research on behalf of the beauty industry, and are most likely to be current.

It is important to understand the responsibilities we each have under the Health and Safety at Work Act 1974, and under the COSHH (Control of Substances Hazardous to Health) regulations. Refer to the legislation section on pages 48–64 for extra guidelines.

Micro-organisms

In order to understand how to maintain the highest hygiene standards it is important to know how infection can occur. Micro-organisms are organisms that are too small to be seen by the naked eye. These micro-organisms are ever-present in the environment and can cause different types of infection.

Think about it

During the consultation remember to ask your client whether she has any allergies.

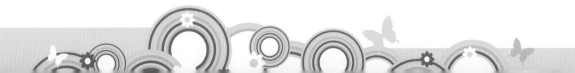

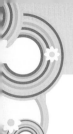

Micro-organism	Diseases
Bacteria	Boils, impetigo, sore throats, meningitis, pneumonia, diphtheria, tuberculosis, typhoid fever, tetanus (lock jaw), whooping cough
Viruses	Common cold, flu, cold sores (Herpes simplex) warts, measles, rubella, mumps, chicken pox, Hepatitis A, B and C, HIV
Fungal/yeast infections	Ringworm of the foot, body, head and nails, thrush, infection to the heart and lungs, which may prove fatal
Protozoa	Diarrhoea, malaria, amoebic dysentery

Types of micro-organism and the diseases they can cause

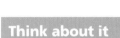

Think about it

Disposable gloves

There are a wide variety of disposable gloves on the market and therapists must ensure that health and safety legislation is adhered to, to protect themselves and their clients from cross contamination. Most Awarding Bodies also specify that gloves should be worn for treatments in which there is a possibility of contact with bodily fluids and/or if the skin is being pierced, for example epilation, intimate waxing and microdermabrasion.

- Always buy medical-standard, single-use only disposable gloves from a reputable manufacturer and use within the expiry dates.
- Gloves should be chosen to fit snuggly on the hands.
- Do not apply talc to the hands prior to use as this may cause an allergic reaction.
- Always wash and dry hands thoroughly before and after using gloves.
- Do not use the gloves if they are damaged, smell or have holes in them.
- Latex gloves should be avoided as they may cause an allergic reaction.

Micro-organisms enter the body using any route they can:

- through damaged, broken skin
- through the ears, nose, mouth and genitals
- into hair follicles
- into the blood stream via a bite from blood-sucking insects (e.g. malaria).

So, disease is spread by:

- direct contact with a person who has a disease or infection
- infection from droplets in the air, as when someone sneezes near you
- indirectly – when you touch an infected item such as a towel or cotton wool.

The symptoms and severity of the infection or disease will depend on the type of invasion, the strength of the person's immune system, whether it is able to defend the body, and their general health. If a person is run-down, then the micro-organisms have more chance of multiplying rapidly. They also thrive in poor hygiene. The best ways of avoiding these are prevention – through good hygiene practices.

Some of these diseases are life threatening, but many are not and can be prevented by good hygiene. For example, protozoa can be transmitted from contaminated food and water, which grow and infect the bowel causing ill health with diarrhoea.

Many of these diseases are also radically reduced by vaccination. Precautions can be taken against both Hepatitis B and tetanus – recommended for beauty therapists. Most school children are given immunisation against measles, mumps and rubella, unless there are medical reasons not to have the injections. Whooping cough has been dramatically reduced by the same method of immunisation.

Refer to Contra-indications, pages 35–38, for recognition of the common diseases that may prevent the treatment from taking place.

Good hygiene practices

How do you maintain good hygiene practices in a beauty salon?

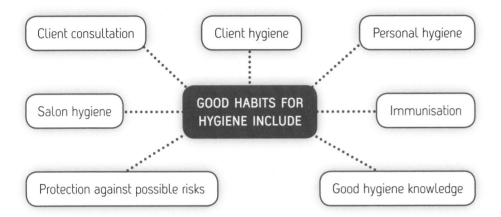

Client consultation

Client hygiene

Personal hygiene

Salon hygiene

GOOD HABITS FOR HYGIENE INCLUDE

Immunisation

Protection against possible risks

Good hygiene knowledge

Good hygiene practices must include these aspects

A guide to controlling micro-organisms

Alcohol

Alcohol-based disinfectants are very good for soaking metal instruments such as small manicure equipment. The usual dilution is 70 per cent isopropyl alcohol – or a surgical spirit base. Once it has been used, the disinfectant should be thrown away and a fresh solution made up for every client.

Isopropyl alcohol is an antibacterial solvent used in many different products, from aftershave to hand lotions and cleaners. It is made from propylene, which is obtained during the cracking of petroleum. It is a good cleaner, but the fumes can be an irritant, so surgical spirit, commonly bought over the counter at the chemist or local wholesale supplier, can be used instead.

Ammonia

Ammonia is commonly used as a base for trade liquids used to kill bacteria, e.g. barbicide that is used to soak suitable instruments in salons. The drawback with using ammonia is its strong smell!

Antibiotics

An antibiotic is a chemical substance that destroys or inhibits the growth of micro-organisms. Antibiotics are usually used to treat infections that will respond well to them, such as fungal or bacterial infections, and are given to humans and some animals for treatment. They can be taken as tablets, or as a cream applied to the area, or in an injection, or, if in hospital, they can be administered in a drip form straight into the blood stream. They are not available over the counter to buy. They are only issued on prescription from a doctor.

Think about it

All good hygiene practices should be continuously carried out to ensure that no cross-infection takes place – starting with preparation of the work area, throughout the treatment itself, through to leaving the work area and equipment clean and tidy ready for the next treatment. The client will then have total confidence in the salon and it ensures you are following all the required health and safety regulations.

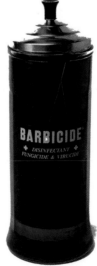

A barbicide disinfecting jar

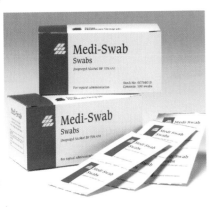

Medi-wipes

Antiseptic

An antiseptic is a chemical agent which destroys or inhibits the growth of micro-organisms on living tissues, thus helping to prevent infection when placed on to open cuts and wounds.

Autoclave

An autoclave is a piece of equipment rather like a pressure cooker, used to sterilise small metal equipment, such as eyebrow tweezers and manicure items. It works by heating distilled water under pressure to a higher temperature than 100°C, so creating an environment where germs cannot survive.

Ideally, the autoclave should heat up to 121°C for 15 minutes. There is a stacking system of baskets in the base so that lots of small tools can be put in together, but they should be washed and clean prior to sterilisation. If several therapists use the autoclave at one time, be sure that the equipment is easily identifiable — perhaps with a blob of nail varnish, otherwise you will not know which tools belong to whom! The autoclave is most suitable for small metal tools. Refer to individual manufacturer's instructions for use.

My story

Cleaning your tools

Hi, my name is Anya. We were learning pedicures and had to swap partners with someone we had never worked with before. Unfortunately, although the tutor told everyone to make sure they followed the correct sterilisation procedures, the student didn't sterilise her equipment properly, and I'm fairly certain I got athlete's foot from her tools — I didn't see her put them in the autoclave, but I couldn't prove anything. I told my tutor about it, and she reminded everyone in the group how important it is to clean and sterilise tools properly. Too late for me though!

Bactericide

This is a chemical that kills bacteria but not necessarily the spores, so reproduction may still take place. It can also be called biocide, fungicide, virucide or sporicide.

Chlorhexidine

Trade names for chlorhexidine include Savlon and Hibitane. Chlorhexidine is widely used for skin and surface cleaning and some sunbed canopies. Check individual manufacturer's instructions for cleaning.

Detergent

A detergent is a synthetic cleaning agent that removes all impurities from a surface by reacting with grease and suspended particles, including bacteria and other micro-organisms. Detergents need to be used with water but are ideal for cleansing large surface areas.

Disinfectant

This is a chemical that kills micro-organisms but not spores — most commonly used to wash surfaces and to clean drains. Disinfectants can only work against bacteria and fungi. They reduce the number of organisms, minimising the risk of infection. In medicine, disinfectants (e.g. Triclosan) are used to clean unbroken skin.

Hypochlorous acid is a weak unstable acid, occurring only in solution, which can be used as a bleach and disinfectant. Products containing sodium or calcium hypochlorite can be used on large surfaces, such as floors and walls, as they are relatively inexpensive to buy. They can however be corrosive and are not suitable for soaking metal instruments or applying directly on to the skin.

Phenol compounds

Phenol compounds are ideal for large areas that need cleaning, but phenol does have a chlorine base and should not be used on the skin. It is used in industrial cleaning preparations and the old-fashioned carbolic soap.

Sanitation

Sanitation is a generic term relating to health and the measures for the protection of health, that is to be free of dirt and germs, and to be hygienic. The word comes from the Latin *sanitas*, meaning health.

Sterilisation

Sterilisation is the complete destruction of all living micro-organisms and their spores.

Surgical spirit

Surgical spirit is widely used and easily available from chemists. It can be used for skin cleansing, and to remove grease on the skin. Surgical spirit comes in varying strengths of dilution. A 70 per cent alcohol base concentration is acceptable for cleansing.

Ultraviolet boxes

Some salons use an ultraviolet (UV) light box to destroy bacteria. UV rays are generated from a quartz mercury vapour lamp (similar to a mini sunbed) with a low rate of penetration. The tools have to be thoroughly clean and dry before they go into the box, otherwise germs will cling to the dirt or dead skin cells on the surface and form a barrier preventing sterilisation from fully taking place. The tools also need to be turned around after 15 minutes because the rays only clean the surfaces of the tools. Only metal tools such as cuticle nippers are suitable for UV sterilisation and, of course, once you touch them taking them out of the box, they are no longer sterile.

UV rays are harmful to the eyes, so the box should be switched off before you open it. UV bulbs have a limited life, so a log of usage should be kept and the bulbs replaced when recommended by the manufacturer. Always follow manufacturers' instructions.

There are a great many commercial products on the market for cleaning and sterilisation — with lots of different trade names. This is merely a general guide. Please consult the manufacturer's instructions for each individual piece of equipment. Most companies have their own particular favourites that they recommend.

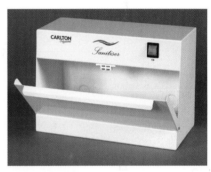

An ultraviolet box can be used to sterilse small tools

Professional basics

For your portfolio

Investigate the recommendations of beauty wholesalers and suppliers for cleaning and sterilisation products. Look at the advantages/disadvantages of each. Which is the most effective? Which has the most pleasant smell? Which is the best value for money? Which is the most versatile and can be used on lots of surfaces? Which ones would you use if you had your own salon?

Use the internet to research advice on cleaning and sterilisation, e.g. the Health and Safety Executive, your Awarding Body and Habia websites.

Think about it

Germs and disease can be found in all sorts of unlikely places. Even a cracked cup will contain germs, so if you give the client coffee in a chipped mug, or water in a cracked glass, you are not upholding good hygiene practices. Always dispose of chipped or cracked cups/mugs/glassware.

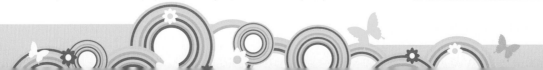

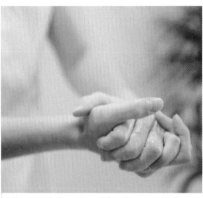

Thorough handwashing is essential to good hygiene

Your personal hygiene

- Always wash your hands – ideally with bactericidal gel – before and after every treatment.
- Wear disposable gloves for treatments if there is a possibility of an exchange of body fluids, e.g. waxing.
- Wear protective clothing for protection and to ensure a professional appearance, e.g. an apron for waxing.
- Cover cuts or broken skin with a waterproof plaster.
- Keep nails short and scrub under them with a nail brush.
- Do not come into work if you know you have an infection or disease likely to put anyone else at risk, e.g. impetigo.
- Wash hands thoroughly after every visit to the toilet.
- Follow the guidelines given in the section on professional presentation (pages 12–15) for clean uniform, etc.
- Attend training programmes about hygiene and the use of sterilising equipment.
- Do not use equipment that is cracked or broken, as germs will be present. This includes chipped cups, plates or glasses.

Salon hygiene

- Sanitise used equipment as fully as possible. This means following the manufacturer's instructions for individual equipment, such as using the recommended cleaner for make-up brushes so that the bristles do not fall out. Some cleaners will dissolve the glue that holds them in place.
- Tools should always be washed in hot, soapy water, rinsed well and dried thoroughly, before using a sterilising fluid or a UV box.
- Invest time and correct training in the use of sterilisation equipment, such as an autoclave or sanitising unit.
- Clean the treatment area or room thoroughly. Clean it daily and also wipe generally after each treatment has taken place. There are many preparations on the market for use on walls, floors and work surfaces, trolleys and couch and stool.
- All work surfaces should be cleaned regularly with hot water and detergent.
- Couch roll and towels can be used as a barrier between blankets and the clients – they can then be disposed of, and fresh ones put on for each client.
- Tissues tucked into the headband or turban can be disposed of after use, so keeping the headband/turban looking fresh.
- Towels should be washed after use – so your salon needs to invest in plenty of towels to ensure you do not run out.

An autoclave can be used to sterilse metal instruments by using a high temperature to kill bacteria

Professional basics

○ The same applies to towelling robes for clients. Big fluffy robes are very luxurious, but the image would soon be spoilt if dirty ones were given to clients. Soft cotton robes are easier to wash and keep clean.

○ When carrying out a facial and wrapping the client up in blankets, for hygiene purposes use a cotton sheet as a barrier between the blanket and the client. The sheet can be washed on a boil wash, therefore washing and drying times and costs are saved as you do not have to keep drying heavy blankets. Some salons use duvets to cover clients and the covers can be easily replaced.

○ Disposable brushes for applying make-up will prevent cross-infection from lips and eyes.

○ Make-up pencils should be wiped clean with spirit and re-sharpened to get rid of any contamination.

○ Powder eye shadows and blushers need to be scraped on to a palette and then applied to the client, to avoid contamination.

○ Creams and oils need to be decanted into a smaller bowl, using a spatula, and any excess should be thrown away. Never pour back into the original container any product that has been in contact with your hands or the client. In order to be cost-effective, be careful not to pour out too much, as it may be wasted.

○ Disposable spatulas should be used for waxing, that is one use from pot to client, to avoid contamination.

Client hygiene

○ It is a good idea to have some form of notice in the reception area asking clients to inform staff if they are suffering from any contagious diseases.

○ Always carry out a full consultation to discover any contra-indications.

○ Always perform a physical check of the area to be treated for infection, etc.

○ Do not treat if any unrecognised problems are present.

○ Ask the client to sign the declaration on the record card stating that all medical and other information is correct to date, to avoid possible repercussions later.

○ Before you start, always wipe the area to be treated with the appropriate lotion, e.g. surgical spirit, Hibitane or the recommended choice of your establishment.

○ Provide all possible protection for the client and insist that clients use the recommended procedure, e.g. treading on the couch roll with bare feet to avoid touching the floor surface.

○ Discourage the client from having a treatment if she has the beginnings of an illness – she may really want the treatment but spreading a cold or flu to you and to other clients and therapists is not sensible.

Think about it

Most commercial washing powder manufacturers now make a washing powder which is antiseptic/bacterial at a 40-degree wash – use it for all linens and you will be safeguarding the clients' hygiene.

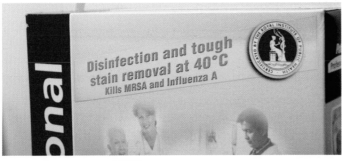

Disinfection and tough stain removal at 40°C
Kills MRSA and Influenza A

A good washing powder keeps laundry disinfected and is eco-friendly in that it works at low temperature

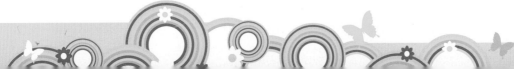

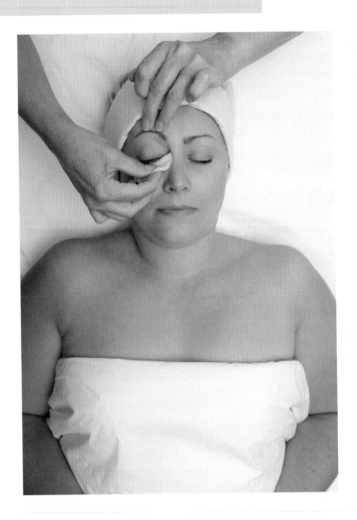

Make sure the client feels secure and relaxed before you start

Client modesty

Whatever treatment your client is having, remember to preserve her modesty and dignity. This is especially important on the first treatment, as the client may be very unsure of the procedures.

○ Explain fully to clients how they will be positioned and how much clothing they will need to take off – a facial would not require the removal of the lower garments, but a wax treatment would. Make sure clients understand this.

○ Always allow clients to get undressed and into a robe in privacy behind the curtains.

○ Cocoon the client in a blanket and towels, with couch roll if required for treatment, and only expose the area of the body being treated. This will not only ensure the client is cosy and secure, but will also preserve modesty and provide warmth.

○ Provide full instructions and a modesty towel if carrying out a more intimate treatment, such as a bikini wax. Ask the client to place protective couch roll in the panty line rather than just assuming she won't mind you doing it.

○ Ensure your working area or cubicle is private and that others are not able to see in. No one having a bikini or leg wax wants to feel that they can be seen by the general public. Even a facial is not a very relaxing treatment if the client feels exposed.

- Respect clients' modesty by keeping personal details, information and record cards confidential and private. It is a privilege to be a party to certain information – do not abuse the clients' trust by sharing information with others unless it is necessary for a professional referral.

- Allow the client time and personal space to dress and prepare to meet the outside world after the treatment. Do not pull back the curtains and tell her to get up as your next client is waiting – this is very bad practice.

- Finally, treat your client as you yourself would wish to be treated – with dignity, respect and as a valued customer.

Treatment and client expectations

It is important to explain the treatment thoroughly to the client. It is equally important that the client understands what the treatment involves. This will help to ensure client satisfaction, avoid misunderstandings, dispel any unrealistic expectations and give the client confidence in the salon and the therapist.

Honesty between therapist and client is part of the ethical conduct that is expected of all beauty therapists in order to maintain high professional standards. The table below gives some examples of unrealistic and realistic expectations.

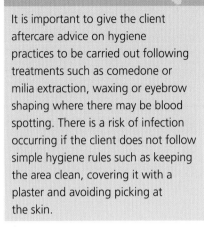

Think about it

It is important to give the client aftercare advice on hygiene practices to be carried out following treatments such as comedone or milia extraction, waxing or eyebrow shaping where there may be blood spotting. There is a risk of infection occurring if the client does not follow simple hygiene rules such as keeping the area clean, covering it with a plaster and avoiding picking at the skin.

Treatment aim	True	False
Waxing is a permanent method of hair removal		✓
Regular waxing makes the hair grow weaker		✓
All the hairs grow back at the same time.		✓
The hairs grow back feeling stubbly and spiky.		✓
Waxing does not hurt.		✓
Waxing lasts for 4–6 weeks depending upon your hair growth.	✓	
As the blood supply to the hairs is stimulated when waxing, it is possible the hair will grow back slightly thicker.	✓	
Waxing does not change the hair colour.	✓	
Shaving causes a blunt end to the hair shaft and it feels spiky, but waxing allows the hair shaft to grow back with a tapered end so it still feels smooth.	✓	
Tinting makes the eyelashes thicker and looks like mascara has been applied.		✓
Tinting the eyelashes is permanent – you never have to do it again.		✓
Regular facials makes the skin grow older faster.		✓

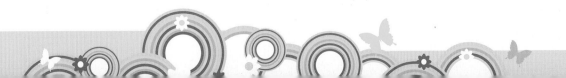

Professional basics

Think about it

A satisfied customer will return and will also tell everyone else about how good their salon experience was – word-of-mouth advertising is invaluable and free! A good reputation starts with positive feedback and grows from there.

Be truthful with your clients and they will always respect and trust you.

Key terms

Legislation – laws passed by parliament.

Think about it

None of us can get away with claiming ignorance about the law. We should each take responsibility for our deeds and actions and must face the consequences if we act recklessly or endanger others. Insurance cover may be null and void if you are proven to be negligent or if legislation or establishment rules have been broken or ignored. An accident or injury to others could be the result with serious implications to you personally and your employers.

The client must also be aware of:

○ the time involved in a treatment
○ the total cost of the treatment or course of treatments
○ the position she will be in – on the couch, seated, etc.
○ the expected outcomes
○ the length of time the treatment should last
○ the possible contra-actions to the treatment
○ the aftercare and home care for the treatment
○ the cost of items that may be purchased
○ the cost of maintenance, e.g. for artificial nail structures
○ how often the treatment should be given for maximum effect
○ the reasons for a sensitivity test, consultation and record cards.

The entire list above has a part to play in creating the complete picture for the client, so that the therapist gains the client's full trust and confidence.

You, your client and the law

In this outcome you will learn about:

- legislation
- local by-laws
- insurance
- independent regulators
- industry codes of practice
- salon guidelines.

There are many regulations and lots of **legislation** covering you and your work in the salon. Any person dealing with members of the public and working with other people has to be aware of the law, and how to use it to be safe. You do not need to know all the regulations in detail, but you do need to know what your responsibilities are.

Legislation

All businesses are covered by laws as set down by the government in Acts of Parliament. These Acts of Parliament are continually being updated to fit into modern society, so you will find that Acts have dates after their title stating when they were updated, such as Trade Descriptions Act 1968 (amended 1987).

These Acts are the law of the land. Breaking or ignoring them is therefore an offence, and can lead to punishment. You could be fined, your business could be closed or you could go to prison.

As well as UK law, there is European Union law to follow, too. The European Union (EU) is made up of 27 countries, including the UK, which joined the EU in 1993. EU laws are decided in Brussels, where the European courts are based, and all EU member states follow the same legislation.

In order to be fully competent in employment it is essential that you have a sound knowledge of the basis of consumer protection and health and safety legislation. You need to understand how these laws protect you, your colleagues and your clients. The specific legislation that you need to know is given on the following pages.

Health and Safety at Work Act 1974

This requires all employers to provide systems of work that are, as far as is reasonably practicable, safe and without risk to health.

The employer's duty is to provide safe:

- premises – a safe place to work
- systems and equipment
- storage and transport of substances and material
- access to the workplace exits
- practices in the workplace.

The employer's duty to other persons not in employment includes not exposing them to health and safety risks – this includes contractors, employees, and self-employed people.

The employee has a responsibility to:

- take care during time at work to avoid personal injury
- assist the employer in meeting requirements under the Health and Safety at Work Act
- not misuse or change anything that has been provided for safety.

The employee has a duty to herself/himself, to other employees, and to the public.

The Act allows various regulations to be made, which control the workplace. It also covers self-employed persons who work alone, away from the employer's premises.

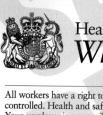

Health and Safety Law
What you need to know

All workers have a right to work in places where risks to their health and safety are properly controlled. Health and safety is about stopping you getting hurt at work or ill through work. Your employer is responsible for health and safety, but you must help.

What employers must do for you

1 Decide what could harm you in your job and the precautions to stop it. This is part of risk assessment.

2 In a way you can understand, explain how risks will be controlled and tell you who is responsible for this.

3 Consult and work with you and your health and safety representatives in protecting everyone from harm in the workplace.

4 Free of charge, give you the health and safety training you need to do your job.

5 Free of charge, provide you with any equipment and protective clothing you need, and ensure it is properly looked after.

6 Provide toilets, washing facilities and drinking water.

7 Provide adequate first-aid facilities.

8 Report injuries, diseases and dangerous incidents at work to our Incident Contact Centre: **0845 300 9923**

9 Have insurance that covers you in case you get hurt at work or ill through work. Display a hard copy or electronic copy of the current insurance certificate where you can easily read it.

10 Work with any other employers or contractors sharing the workplace or providing employees (such as agency workers), so that everyone's health and safety is protected.

Your health and safety representatives:

Other health and safety contacts:

What you must do

1 Follow the training you have received when using any work items your employer has given you.

2 Take reasonable care of your own and other people's health and safety.

3 Co-operate with your employer on health and safety.

4 Tell someone (your employer, supervisor, or health and safety representative) if you think the work or inadequate precautions are putting anyone's health and safety at serious risk.

If there's a problem

1 If you are worried about health and safety in your workplace, talk to your employer, supervisor, or health and safety representative.

2 You can also look at our website for general information about health and safety at work.

3 If, after talking with your employer, you are still worried, phone our Infoline. We can put you in touch with the local enforcing authority for health and safety and the Employment Medical Advisory Service. You don't have to give your name.

HSE Infoline: **0845 345 0055**

HSE website: **www.hse.gov.uk**

Fire safety
You can get advice on fire safety from the Fire and Rescue Services or your workplace fire officer.

Employment rights
Find out more about your employment rights at: **www.direct.gov.uk**

HSE

Health and Safety Executive

(Source: Health and Safety Executive)

Employers' responsibilities	Shared responsibilities	Employees' responsibilities
Planning safety and security	Safety of all individuals in the workplace	Correct use of systems and procedures
Providing information about safety and security	Safety of the working environment	Reporting flaws or gaps in the system or establishment procedures
Updating systems and procedures with five or more employees	Never knowingly endangering anyone	Taking reasonable care of themselves and others
Regular training and information for all staff	Following all Health and Safety at Work Act directives	Cooperating with employers in the discharge of their obligations

Health and safety responsibilities

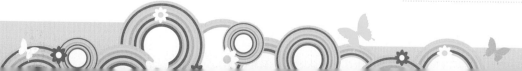

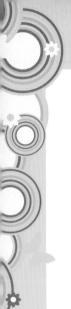

In 1992 EU directives updated legislation on health and safety management and widened the existing acts. These came into force in 1993. There are six main areas:

○ provision and use of work equipment

○ manual handling operations

○ workplace health, safety and welfare

○ personal protective equipment at work

○ health and safety (display screen equipment)

○ management of health and safety at work.

Some provisions of the EU directives are:

○ the protection of non-smokers from tobacco smoke

○ the provision of rest facilities for pregnant and nursing mothers

○ safe cleaning of windows.

The Management of Health and Safety at Work Regulations 1999

These regulations place responsibility firmly on the employer to make significant risk assessments for the health and safety of employees and others working in the salon, record any significant findings, and instruct and train employees in the correct way to ensure all are protected. Codes of practice and systems need to be monitored, reviewed and adjusted to suit. All employees should be informed of these, and a statutory poster for health and safety displayed in the workplace.

The regulations cover a great deal of information for employers including:

○ risk assessment

○ principles of prevention to be applied

○ health and safety arrangements

○ health surveillance

○ health and safety assistance

○ procedures for serious and imminent danger and dangerous areas

○ contact with external services

○ information for employees

○ cooperation and coordination

○ persons working in host employers or self-employed person undertaking work

○ capability and training

○ employer's duties

○ temporary workers

○ risk assessments for new or expectant mothers

○ protection of young persons

○ exception certificates

○ provisions of liability

○ exclusion of civil liberties

○ extension out of Great Britain

○ amendments to the Health and Safety (First Aid) Regulations 1981.

Employment Rights Act 1996

This Act covers all aspects of an employee's terms and conditions after they have been employed for a month or more. After two months' employment, an employee should have a written contract with their conditions of work including:

- details of payment, along with commission and incentives
- hours of work and expected holiday entitlement
- the amount of notice an employee is expected to give
- the amount of notice the employer expects the employee to give
- the date the employment started
- a full job description
- the employee's workplace location.

If an employee does not receive a contract of employment in writing, they can apply to an industrial tribunal and the employer is obliged by law to provide one.

The Workplace (Health, Safety and Welfare) Regulations 1992

The employer should ensure the workplace complies with the requirements of these regulations by:

- maintaining the workplace and all equipment and systems used there
- ensuring adequate ventilation
- keeping the workplace at a reasonable temperature (minimum 16°C)
- making sure employees have sufficient light to work comfortably
- keeping the workplace clean and tidy
- ensuring employees have enough space to work comfortably
- keeping floor and 'traffic routes' in a reasonable condition (no holes, slopes or uneven surfaces)
- ensuring workstations and seating are suitable
- providing suitable washing and toilet facilities (with soap and a means of drying hands)
- making sure employees have accommodation for clothing (worn at work) and changing facilities
- providing employees with facilities for resting and eating (if meals are to be eaten on the premises)
- providing clean drinking water and cups
- regularly removing waste materials
- keeping employees safe from falling objects
- making sure all doors and gates are suitably constructed and fitted with any necessary safety devices
- making sure windows are protected against breakage and signs (or similar) are incorporated where there is a danger of someone walking into them
- making sure escalators and moving walkways have safety devices fitted so they can be stopped in an emergency.

Think about it

In most settings separate toilet facilities must be available for men and women. However, in small, mostly female salons, men and women can use the same facilities as long as the toilet is a separate cubicle and it can be locked. In larger health clubs and spas the toilet and locker facilities would be separate.

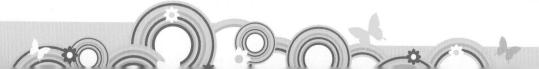

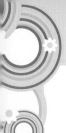

(For further information on the safe disposal of waste products, refer to Unit G20 Make sure your actions reduce risks to health and safety, pages 87–104.)

Heat stress

The Health and Safety Executive draws attention to heat stress at work. The best working temperature in beauty therapy is between 15.5 and 20°C.

Humidity (the amount of moisture in the air) should be within the range of 30 to 70 per cent, although this will vary if your salon has a sauna and steam area. These should be in a well-ventilated area away from the main workrooms, while still being accessible to clients. There should also be sufficient air exchange and air movement, which must be increased in special circumstances, such as chemical usage. Treatment rooms used for nail art, aromatherapy, bleaching or eyelash perming will need specialist ventilation methods.

Physical effects	Psychological effects
Headaches	Irritability
Sweating	Aggressive behaviour
Palpitations	Fatigue – resulting in mistakes being made
Dizziness	Lethargy
Nausea, vomiting	Lack of concentration
Feeling faint	

The effects of heat stress

○ Mechanical ventilation – extractor fans, which can be adjusted at various speeds.

○ Natural ventilation – open windows are fine, but be careful of a draught on the client.

○ Air-conditioned ventilation – passing air over filters and coolers brings about the desired condition, but of course this is the most expensive method!

A build-up of fumes, or of strong smells (for example from manicure preparations), will cause both physical and psychological problems, which affect not only clients but staff, too!

The Manual Handling Operations Regulations 1992

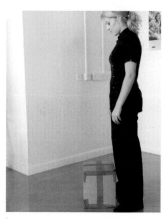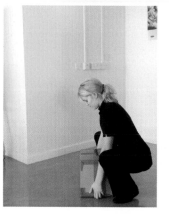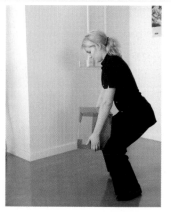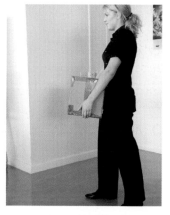

Safe lifting procedures must be followed

The Health and Safety Executive (HSE) has drawn attention to skeletal and muscular disorders caused by manual handling and lifting, repetitive strain disorders and unsuitable posture causing low back pain. The regulations require certain measures to be taken to avoid these types of injuries occurring.

Think of all the situations that may apply in the salon:

○ stock unpacking and storage – lifting heavy objects

○ couch height adjustable for individual therapists

○ chairs or stools used in the treatment rooms

○ trolley height

○ reception desk and chair

○ rotation of job roles so that the therapist is not in the same position for every treatment

○ height and size of nail art desk.

The Personal Protective Equipment at Work Regulations 1992

Every employer and self-employed person must ensure that suitable personal protective equipment is provided both for themselves and for their employees in situations where they may be exposed to a risk to their health or safety while at work. This is particularly relevant to waxing (refer to Unit B6 Carry out waxing services, page 407) and where there is a risk of contamination by body fluids (see also Environmental Protection Act 1990, The Controlled Waste Regulations 1992 and The Special Waste Regulations 1996 below).

Protective clothing

This covers both equipment and protective clothing provisions to ensure safety for all those in the workplace. The regulations also provide that workplace personnel must have appropriate training in equipment use. Protective clothing, such as white overalls for work wear, ensures cleanliness, freshness, and professionalism. For certain treatments it may be advisable to wear extra disposable coverings. The client's clothing must also be protected.

> **Think about it**
>
> Research what your Awarding Body states about protective clothing. It may invalidate your insurance if you do not follow the rules – and it may ruin your own clothing if tint or wax were to be spilt on your uniform or trousers, for example.

Protection against infectious diseases

It is essential to protect against all diseases that are carried in the blood or tissue fluids. Protective gloves should be worn whenever there is a possibility of blood or tissue fluid being passed from one person to another, that is through an open cut or broken skin. Two specific infectious diseases to mention are:

○ **AIDS (Acquired Immune Deficiency Syndrome)** – this disease is caused by HIV (Human Immunodeficiency Virus). The virus is transmitted through body tissue. Most people are aware of AIDS because of media coverage. The virus attacks the body's immune system, and therefore carries a strong risk of secondary infection, such as pneumonia, which could be life threatening. As there is no known cure, prevention through protection is vital.

○ **Hepatitis variants (A, B and C)** – hepatitis is an inflammation of the liver. It is caused by a very strong virus transmitted through blood and tissue fluids. This can survive outside the body, and can make a person very ill indeed; it can even be fatal. The most serious form is Hepatitis B and you can be immunised against this disease by a GP. For those who can prove they need this protection for their employment there is no cost involved. Most training establishments will recommend this.

> **Think about it**
>
> It is worth considering all of these factors when purchasing equipment, as you then have to work with the consequences!
>
> When purchasing a couch for home or mobile use, it is worth pretending to carry out a facial, complete with client lying on the couch, to find the right height. Working at a couch at the wrong height is very bad for the back in the long term, and may cause considerable discomfort.

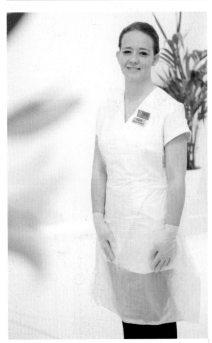

Always use protective clothing for hygiene and good client care

> **Think about it**
>
> Always cover cuts with a plaster to prevent cross-infection.

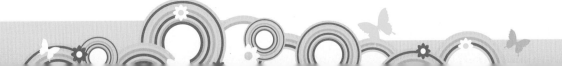

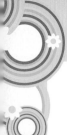
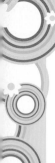
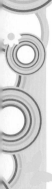

Professional basics

The Control of Substances Hazardous to Health (COSHH) Regulations 2002

The COSHH Regulations require employers to control exposure to substances that are hazardous to health in the workplace. Exposure can be prevented or reduced by:

○ finding out what the health hazards are

○ deciding how to prevent harm to health by carrying out a risk assessment

○ providing control measures to reduce harm to health

○ making sure they are used

○ keeping all control measures in good working order

○ providing information, instruction and training for employees and others

○ providing monitoring and health surveillance in appropriate cases

○ control exposure to hazardous substances in the workplace

○ planning for emergencies.

Most products used in the salon are perfectly safe, but some products could become hazardous under certain conditions or if used inappropriately. All salons should be aware of how to use and store these products.

Employers are responsible for assessing the risks from hazardous substances and must decide upon an action to reduce those risks. Proper training should be given and employees should always follow safety guidelines and take the precautions identified by the employer.

The COSHH regulations require that the containers of hazardous substances are labelled with warning symbols. These symbols are shown opposite.

Here are some examples of potential hazards.

○ Highly flammable substances, such as solvents, nail varnish remover or alcohol steriliser, are hazardous because their fumes will ignite if exposed to a naked flame.

○ Explosive materials, such as hairspray, air freshener or other pressurised cans, are also highly flammable and will explode with force if placed in heat, such as an open fire, or even on top of a hot radiator.

○ Chemicals can cause severe reactions and skin damage – if chemicals are misused, vomiting, respiratory problems, and burning could be the result.

For your portfolio

Take a look at 'Working with substances hazardous to health: What you need to know about COSHH' available on the HSE website. Look also at the HSE's COSHH essentials web tool.

Dust

Toxic

Flammable

Irritant

Corrosive

Oxidising agent

Symbols showing types of hazardous substances

COSHH precautions

Employers must, by law, identify, list and assess in writing any substance in the workplace. This applies not only to products used for treatments in the salon but also to products that are used in cleaning such as bleach or polish. Potentially hazardous substances must be given a hazard rating, or risk assessment, even if it is zero.

It is essential that you read all of the COSHH sheets used in the salon, and be safe: follow what they say, never abuse manufacturers' instructions and attend regular staff training for product use. You never know when you might need it!

Health Act 2006

This law has been introduced to protect employees and the public from the harmful effects of 'second-hand' smoke inhalation (passive smoking). Below is a summary of its key points.

○ From 1 July 2007 it has been against the law to smoke in virtually all enclosed and substantially enclosed public places and workplaces.

○ Public transport and work vehicles used by more than one person should be smoke-free.

○ Non-smoking signs should be displayed in all smoke-free premises and vehicles.

○ Staff smoking rooms and indoor smoking areas are no longer allowed, so anyone wanting to smoke will have to go outside.

○ Managers of smoke-free premises and vehicles have legal responsibility to prevent people from smoking.

○ Anyone not complying with the smoke-free law is committing an offence and can be issued with a fixed penalty notice – up to a maximum of £200 if prosecuted and convicted by a court.

○ Failure to display non-smoking signs carries a fixed penalty of £200, or a maximum fine of £1000 if prosecuted and convicted by a court.

○ Failing to prevent smoking in a smoke-free place has a maximum fine of £2500.

The Gas Safety (Installation and Use) Regulations 1998

These relate to the use and maintenance of gas appliances. You may think that this does not apply to you as a therapist, but read on! The Gas Safety (Rights of Entry Regulations) 1996 & 2004 give gas and Health and Safety Executive (HSE) inspectors the right to enter premises and order the disconnection of any dangerous appliances. The inspectors themselves are not usually trained gas fitters, so they will instruct you to contact your local service engineer. Gas fumes are silent, with no smell, and deadly.

The Fire Precautions (Workplace) Regulations 1997 (as amended 1999)

The Fire Precautions (Workplace) Regulations bring together existing health and safety and fire legislation to form a set of dedicated fire regulations which aim to achieve a risk appropriate standard of fire safety for persons in the workplace.

The regulations were amended in 1999 in order to confirm the concept of employers having unconditional responsibility for the safety of employees. As a result, most workplaces are now subject to the legal requirements of the above regulations. They require small business owners to adequately assess the fire risks associated with their work activities and to decide what needs to be done to control these risks. The steps to be taken for a fire risk assessment are similar to those taken for general risk assessments, although the business also has a general duty to the public (refer to Unit G20 Make sure your actions reduce risks to health and safety, page 71).

Staff need to be aware of the procedures involved in the event of a fire, preferably through the displaying of a notice. It is recommended that you have some form of fire-fighting equipment – even if it is just a fire blanket. Contact the fire authority in your area, who will be happy to assist you.

Think about it

- Manufacturers have to supply a COSHH sheet containing product data for each product. The COSHH sheets should be kept together in a central folder in the salon so that everyone can refer to them.

- A reaction can happen if a client has recently used a chemical at home and it reacts with the products used in the salon, e.g. home hair colours.

- Clients on long-term medication are more likely to have a reaction. Triggers include hormone replacement therapy, the contraceptive pill, heart and blood pressure medication – this should be recorded on the client's record card.

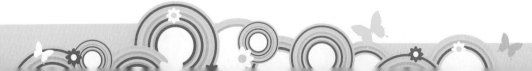

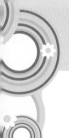

The Provision and Use of Work Equipment Regulations 1998

The key points here are to ensure that all equipment at work is properly maintained, fit for purpose and in a good state of repair, as explained below.

Suitability of equipment

Employers must ensure that equipment is suitable for the purpose for which it is used or provided. When selecting equipment, they need to be aware of the working conditions and the risks to health and safety in the premises in which the work equipment is to be used and any additional risk posed by the use of the equipment.

Maintenance

Equipment must be maintained in efficient working order and good repair. Wherever possible, maintenance should take place when equipment is switched off to avoid risks to the person's health and safety; if maintenance can only take place when the equipment is switched on, precautions should be taken to protect the person carrying out the work. Where equipment has a maintenance log, this must be kept up to date.

Inspection

Where the safety of equipment depends on the installation conditions, it must be inspected after installation and before being put into service for the first time; or after assembly at a new site or in a new location, to ensure that it has been installed correctly and is safe to operate. This is also to ensure that health and safety conditions are maintained and that any wear and tear is detected and remedied in good time. Inspections that take place under this regulation should be recorded and kept until the next inspection takes place and is recorded.

Equipment should be used only for the purposes of the employer's business, and if equipment is obtained from another business, it should be accompanied by an inspection certificate.

Specific risks

Where the use of equipment is likely to involve a specific risk to health or safety, the equipment must only be used by staff trained to operate it. Where appropriate, employers need to provide training.

Any repairs, modifications, maintenance or servicing should only be carried out by a competent person.

Information and instructions

Staff operating equipment must be provided with adequate health and safety information and, where appropriate, written instructions on how to use it. This also applies to employees who supervise or manage the use of equipment.

Training

For health and safety reasons, staff should be given adequate training to operate equipment, including training in the methods which may be adopted when using the equipment, any risks involved and precautions to be taken. This also applies to employees who supervise or manage the use of equipment.

Protection against specified hazards

Employers are responsible for taking measures to ensure that staff using equipment should be protected from hazards that might endanger their health and safety. If it is not possible to prevent the risk, then it needs to be adequately controlled.

High or very low temperature

Where equipment, or any article or substance produced, used or stored in work equipment, is at a high or very low temperature, it needs to be protected so as to prevent injury to any person by burn, scald or sear.

Controls for starting equipment

Where appropriate, equipment should be provided with one or more controls for the purposes of starting it (including restarting after a stoppage for any reason).

Stability

Equipment should be stabilised by clamping, or another method, where necessary for health or safety purposes.

Lighting

The work area where equipment is to be used should have suitable and sufficient lighting.

The Electricity at Work Regulations 1989

These regulations affect the use of electrical equipment in every salon, clinic or health club. Regulation 4 of the Act states: 'All electrical equipment must be regularly checked for electrical safety.' In a busy salon this may be every six months. The check must be carried out by a 'competent person', preferably a qualified electrician. All checks must be recorded in a book kept for this purpose only.

Types of equipment to be checked include:

- wax heaters
- autoclaves
- thermal boots
- infrared lamps
- foot spas that plug in
- paraffin wax heaters
- fast nail UV dryer boxes.

A 'competent person' need not be a qualified electrician, but must be capable of attending to basic safety checks. Manufacturers often supply their own technical staff to attend to safety checks.

PAT Testing (Portable Appliance Testing)

All companies and organisations should comply with the Electricity at Work Regulations. Each electrical appliance should be comprehensively tested to meet the exacting requirements of the IEE code of practice for In-Service Inspection and Testing of Electrical Equipment.

Ideally, the electrician or competent person should be a member of both NICEIC and NAPIT (National Association of Professional Inspectors and Testers). All engineers should undertake a NAPIT technical assessment and be subject to regular inspection and monitoring of their work and records.

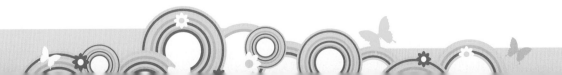

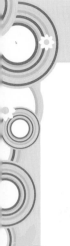

Professional basics

All electrical equipment to be tested has to be disconnected from the mains supply. This may be inconvenient so ideally it should be carried out of normal salon hours.

If electrical apparatus is found to be faulty, the equipment must be withdrawn from service and repaired. An electrical safety record book should be used to record dates, the nature of the repair and by whom it was done. It should also contain a list of tests carried out on the equipment under inspection, the results of those tests, and be signed by the competent person who carried them out.

This is essential for public liability insurance purposes and in case of legal action being taken for accidents due to negligence.

The Pressure Systems and Transportable Gas Containers Regulations 1989

Steam sterilising autoclaves fall under this Act. You are required to have a written scheme of examination carried out or certified by a competent person.

Environmental Protection Act 1990

The Controlled Waste Regulations 1992 (as amended in 1993)

The Special Waste Regulations 1996 (as amended)

These Acts require all clinical waste to be kept apart from general waste and to be disposed of to a licensed incinerator or landfill site, by a licensed company. This includes:

- waste which consists wholly or partly of animal or human tissue
- blood or other body fluids
- swabs or dressings
- syringes or needles.

The Reporting of Injuries, Diseases and Dangerous Occurrences Regulations (RIDDOR) 1995

These regulations cover the recording and reporting of any serious accidents and conditions to the local environmental health officer, whose remit covers beauty therapy and hairdressing salons. This officer will investigate the accident and make sure that the salon prevents the accident from happening again in the future. The officer can also assess the risk factors in each instance.

An accident or death at work must be reported within ten days. If the accident does not require a hospital visit, but the person is absent from work for more than three days, a report still needs to be made.

If an employee reports a work-related disease, a report must be sent: a work-related disease could include occupational dermatitis, asthma caused through work or even hepatitis. Accidents as a result of violence or an attack by another person must be reported. A car accident when on company business is reportable in the same way as an accident at work.

A dangerous occurrence in which no one was actually injured must also be reported: for example, if the ceiling of the salon collapses overnight.

If you are a mobile therapist working in someone's home and you have an accident yourself or you injure the client you must report it.

The Health and Safety (Display Screen Equipment) Regulations 1992 (amended 2002)

These regulations implement an EU Directive and were amended in 2002. They require employers to minimise the risks in visual display unit (VDU) work by ensuring that workplaces and jobs are well designed with specific thought given to position of the monitor and height of chair in relation to how the workplace station is set up.

There is no the difference between a VDU, a VDT, a monitor and display screen equipment (DSE). All these terms mean the same thing: a display screen, usually forming part of a computer and showing text, numbers or graphics. Some users may get aches and pains in their hands, wrists, arms, neck, shoulders or back, especially after long periods of uninterrupted VDU work. Repetitive strain injury (RSI) is the term used to refer to these aches, pains and disorders, but can be misleading as it means different things to different people. A better medical name for this group of conditions is 'upper limb disorders'. Usually these disorders do not last, but in a few cases they may become persistent or even disabling.

Problems can often be avoided by good workplace design, so that you can work comfortably, and by good working practices (like taking frequent short breaks from the VDU). Prevention is easiest if action is taken early, before the problem has become serious.

Extensive research has found no evidence that VDUs can cause disease or permanent damage to eyes. But long spells of VDU work can lead to tired eyes and discomfort.

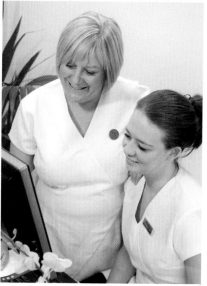

Many salons now use computers for bookings and stock taking – ensure it is set up correctly for good health and safety

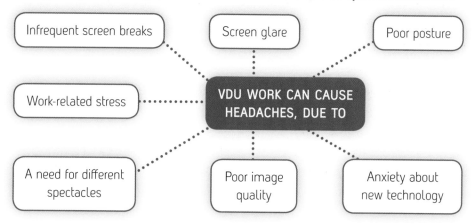

- Infrequent screen breaks
- Screen glare
- Poor posture
- Work-related stress
- A need for different spectacles
- Poor image quality
- Anxiety about new technology

VDU WORK CAN CAUSE HEADACHES, DUE TO

Once the employer recognises these considerations to the positioning of screens, any problems can be easily put right. People who suffer from photo-sensitive epilepsy and are susceptible to flickering lights and striped patterns may be affected by the use of VDUs in some circumstances.

Employers have to analyse workstations, and assess and reduce risks. They should look at:

- the whole workstation including equipment, furniture, and the work environment – workstations need to meet minimum requirements
- the job being done
- any special needs of individual staff
- planning work so there are breaks or changes of activity
- arranging eye tests, on request, and provide spectacles if special ones are needed

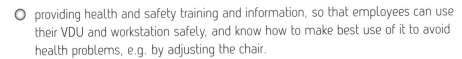

O providing health and safety training and information, so that employees can use their VDU and workstation safely, and know how to make best use of it to avoid health problems, e.g. by adjusting the chair.

Employers' Liability (Compulsory Insurance) Act 1969

Employers and self-employed persons must by law hold employer's liability insurance. This will reimburse them against any legal liability to pay compensation to employees for bodily injury, illness or disease caused during the course of their employment.

Employers must insure for at least £2 million per claim, but check with your own insurance company. Also follow the recommendations of your professional association.

It is worth remembering the following points.

O A legal claim made against your salon could result in very large financial losses and possibly the sale of the owner's business or even private home.

O Public prosecution results in a heavy fine for those not having this essential insurance cover.

O Damage to the salon could be so great that the business might never recover.

O Some cases can take up to ten years to come to court and with inflation the claim against you could be very much more than your original cover, if you only take the minimum requirements.

Consumer Protection Act 1987

This Act follows European laws to safeguard the consumer in three main areas: product liability, general safety requirements and misleading prices.

Before 1987 an injured person had to prove that a manufacturer was negligent before suing for damages. This Act removes the need to prove negligence.

An injured person can take action against:

O producers

O own brand manufacturers

O importers

O suppliers such as wholesalers or retailers.

In the salon this means that only reputable products should be used and sold. Care should be taken in handling, maintaining and storing products so that they remain in top condition.

It is important that all staff are aware of consumer protection laws when selling products and when using products in a treatment.

The Cosmetic Products (Safety) Regulations 2004

The Cosmetic Products (Safety) Regulations 1996 defined 'a cosmetic product as any substance/preparation that is used on the skin, teeth, hair, nails, lips … with the intention to cleanse, perfume, and change the appearance of, to protect, keep in good condition or to correct body odours' – which covers just about everything that is found in a salon!

A cosmetic product must be clearly labelled with the following information:

- a list of ingredients – either on the outer packaging of the product, or if there is no outer packaging, on the container itself
- name and address of the manufacturer/supplier
- minimum shelf life – on both the outer packaging and the container itself
- storage instructions – to help the consumer to maintain the product at its best
- warnings and precautions – on the outer packaging and the container
- batch number or lot code – this would allow a manufacturer to recall a batch of products if necessary
- its function
- its weight.

Medicines Act 1968

This Act deals with the supply and use of topical anaesthetics and is enforced by the police and the Medicines and Healthcare product Regulatory Agency (MHRA). Product licence conditions are for medical application only and not for cosmetic use, therefore their use by a beauty therapist can be unlawful.

Trade Descriptions Act 1968

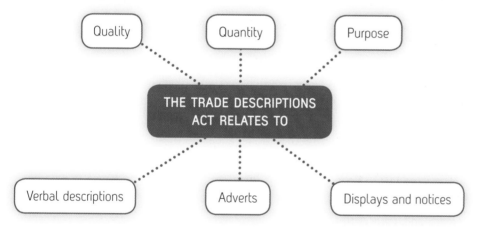

This Act is concerned with the false description of goods. It is important to realise its relevance. It is illegal to mislead the general public. This also applies to verbal descriptions given by a third party and repeated. So, if a manufacturer's false description of a product is repeated you are liable to prosecution. The law states that the retailer must not:

- supply information that is in any way misleading
- falsely describe or make false statements about either a product or a service on offer.

The Consumer Protection from Unfair Trading Regulations 2008

The European Union adopted the Unfair Commercial Practices Directive (UCPD) in May 2005 in order to strengthen laws on trade descriptions within Europe, as these varied from country to country. In the UK, the directive was implemented as The Consumer Protection from Unfair Trading Regulations, which came into force on 26 May 2008.

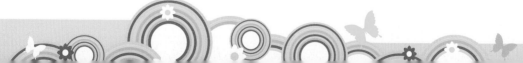

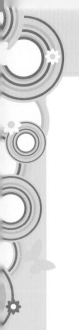

The regulations maintain good practice and are specific about what retailers may or may not do. The retailer may not:

○ make false contrasts between present and previous prices
○ claim to offer products at half price unless they have already been offered at the full price for at least 28 days prior to the sale.

Be mindful of using statements saying something is 'our price'. Comparison of prices can be misleading and can be illegal – be sure that the product is identical in every way. You should also check that products are labelled with their country of origin.

Related acts: Supply of Goods and Services Act 1982 amended 2003; Sale and Supply of Goods Act 1994; The Sale and Supply of Goods to Consumers Regulations 2002.

○ Wherever goods are bought they must 'conform to contract'. This means they must be as described, fit for purpose and of satisfactory quality (that is not inherently faulty at the time of sale).

○ Goods are of satisfactory quality if they reach the standard that a reasonable person would regard as satisfactory, taking into account the price and any description.

○ Aspects of quality include fitness for purpose, freedom from minor defects, appearance and finish, durability, and safety.

○ It is the seller, not the manufacturer, who is responsible if goods do not conform to contract.

○ If goods do not conform to contract at the time of sale, purchasers can request their money back 'within a reasonable time'. (This is not defined and will depend on circumstances.)

○ For up to six years after purchase (five years from discovery in Scotland) purchasers can demand damages (which a court would equate to the cost of a repair or replacement).

○ A purchaser who is a consumer (that is they are not buying in the course of a business) can alternatively request a repair or replacement.

○ If repair and replacement are not possible or too costly, then the consumer can seek a partial refund, if they have had some benefit from the good, or a full refund if the fault(s) have meant they have enjoyed no benefit.

○ In general, the onus is on all purchasers to prove the goods did not conform to contract (e.g. was inherently faulty) and should have reasonably lasted until this point in time (that is perishable goods do not last for six years).

○ If a consumer chooses to request a repair or replacement, then for the first six months after purchase it will be for the retailer to prove the goods did conform to contract (e.g. were not inherently faulty).

○ After six months and until the end of the six years, it is for the consumer to prove the lack of conformity.

Disability Discrimination Act 1995, as amended by the Disability Discrimination Act 2005 and the Equality Act 2006

This Act makes it unlawful to discriminate against disabled people in employment, the provision of goods, facilities and services, education, and the buying or renting property or land. In 2007, the promotion of civil rights for disabled people became the responsibility of the new Equality and Human Rights Commission.

It is illegal for an employer (employing 20 or more staff) to discriminate against a disabled person or prospective employee on the grounds of their disabilities. If a person is suitable for the job, it is up the employer to make the necessary arrangements and adjustments in the workplace to ensure there is no disadvantage for the disabled person.

It is also unlawful to harass a person on the grounds of their disability. All employers must take positive steps to avoid harassment happening in the workplace.

The Working Time Regulations 1998

The Working Time Regulations (1998) merged with the European Working Time Directive into UK law. The regulations were amended with effect from 1 August 2003.

The regulations control how employers organise the average working week, minimum daily and weekly rest breaks, and paid holiday entitlement – which before the regulations were introduced, was left very much up to what the employer wanted to do. The law applies to full-time, part-time and casual workers. You should not work more than 48 hours in a week, with a rest period of 11 hours between each working day, with a minimum of one day off a week. If working for more than six hours, you are entitled to a 20-minute break.

Performing Rights – within Copyright, Designs and Patents Act 1988

This Act is designed to protect the people who write music but then do not get the royalty payments they should when the music is played! Any use of music in the treatment room, reception or in exercise groups is classed as a public performance.

PPL is the body that is responsible for collecting licence payments from people wishing to use music on behalf of artists and record companies. Under the Copyright, Designs and Patents Act 1988, PPL can take legal action against anyone who does not pay a licence fee to use music – and it does! This can mean a considerable fine for those who try to avoid paying. So all salons and exercise/aerobic instructors need to purchase music that has a built-in licence. Although more expensive to purchase in the first place (a CD can price can vary from £10 up to about £30) it does save all the worry of a heavy fine, if caught!

Most good specialist music shops have a section of licensed music – just ask.

Data Protection Act 1998

The Act states that every organisation (data controller) that uses and processes personal information (personal data) must notify the Information Commissioner's office, unless they are exempt. Failure to do so is a criminal offence.

The main purpose of registration is to ensure that the eight principles of 'good information handling' are being followed – that data should be:

1 fairly and lawfully processed
2 processed for limited purposes
3 adequate, relevant and not excessive
4 acurate
5 not kept longer than necessary

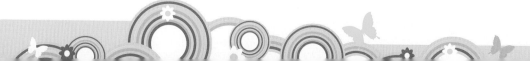

6 processed in accordance with the person's rights

7 secure

8 not transferred to countries outside the European Economic Area (EEA) without adequate and proper protection.

The fee for notification and annual renewal of a register entry had been £35 for all data controllers, but from 1 October 2009, this was replaced by a two-tier payment charge: for businesses employing fewer than 250 staff the cost remains at £35; a higher fee of £500 is payable by businesses with more than 250 employees. The fee paid also relates to turnover — businesses with a turnover of £25.9 million will go into tier two, but this does not apply to charities and public authorities.

Any person can ask to see the information held by an organisation about him or her within 40 days for a fee that is now only £2. It is possible to gain compensation through a civil court action if you feel there has been any infringement of rights, in which information that was given for a specific purpose has been abused.

Local Government (Miscellaneous Provisions) Act 1982

This relates to the local authorities in your particular area. Section 8 of the Act is concerned with the registration of any practitioners who pierce the skin. This applies to:

- ⊙ acupuncture
- ⊙ tattooing
- ⊙ ear and body piercing
- ⊙ epilation.

It applies to both salons and mobile therapists.

The concern of most local authorities is that through registration they will be able to keep some control of hygiene regulations and ensure that people have recognised qualifications. The enforcement of these regulations will depend upon the individual authority, as does the amount of inspection that takes place, and the scale of fees for registration.

This does not include people working in hospitals.

Local by-laws

Local government **by-laws** are laws decided by the local authority or borough council of an area, and they can differ from region to region. Therefore, Manchester has different local by-laws from Birmingham. However, both these authorities have a register of salons offering body massage as a treatment. This is to maintain a professional, qualified salon base and to eliminate the 'massage parlour' image.

You need to investigate the by-laws in your own area from your borough council — these by-laws relate to hygiene, and the registration of ear piercing, and epilation salons, as well as tattoo parlours.

London Local Authorities Act 1995

This Act requires all premises in London that carry out treatments to be licensed by their local authorities. This is for any skin piercing treatments, acupuncture, tattooing and ear piercing — and some local authorities also expect salons to register if they offer massage, too. So contact your local authority to check whether you need a licence when you start your new salon.

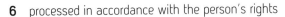

For your portfolio

To find out more about data registration visit the Information Commissioner's website, or contact the Information Commissioner's Office, Wycliffe House, Water Lane, Wilmslow, Cheshire SK9 5AF.

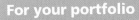

Key terms

By-laws – laws decided by the local authority for your area.

Professional basics

Insurance

Professional indemnity insurance

Every single professional beauty therapist should have this **insurance** protection, regardless of how few or how many treatments they carry out.

The best deal for these kinds of insurance policies can usually be found via your professional body – professional bodies are often able to offer the best rates because they negotiate on behalf of members and get a considerable discount.

As an employee you need to check with your employer whether you are covered on the company's business insurance, or if you need to organise your own cover. A salon owner or employer should include this in the public liability policy, so that all employees are protected against claims made by clients.

Public liability insurance

This insurance is not compulsory, but it is certainly advisable. It will protect the employer should a member of the public be injured on the premises. This could be something as unexpected as a roof tile hitting the client on her way into the salon. If this results in the client being unable to work for a long period of time, the client can sue the salon owner for compensation.

Insurance is important – so protect yourselves and your clients. Contact your professional association for guidance on all aspects of insurance.

Independent regulators

Advertising Standards Authority (ASA)

The ASA is an independent body set up to regulate the content of advertisements, sales promotions and direct marketing in the UK.

It is responsible for maintaining the quality of advertising standards through codes of practice for television, radio and other types of adverts, such as interactive adverts. The ASA can stop misleading, harmful or offensive advertising, ensure that sales promotions are run fairly, and help to reduce unwanted advertising sent through the post, by email or by text message. It also deals with mail order problems. Part of its role is to investigate complaints made about advertising, sales promotions or direct marketing.

The advertising standards codes especially apply to beauty products. Advertisements must be careful not to mislead or misdirect the consumer into believing that wrinkles will disappear, that skin will look ten years younger or that lines can be permanently removed. Adverts may refer to temporary prevention of the skin drying out, but any long-term or permanent correction of the lines or wrinkles is not possible and therefore not allowed in advertising.

ACAS (Advisory, Conciliation and Arbitration Service)

ACAS is an independent organisation that offers impartial advice to individuals and organisations to help resolve disputes or disagreements at work. It aims to encourage better and more direct workplace communication and to help businesses improve their employment practices. From April 2009, ACAS will concentrate less on how

Key terms

Insurance – whereby the beauty therapist (or salon) pays an annual fee to an insurer (insurance company) to compensate them in case of loss incurred during the course of their work.

Think about it

Never assume anything when it comes to insurance cover.

Always check whether you have cover as a therapist working in a salon. Would you be personally liable if things go wrong?

Check you are covered if you are a mobile therapist entering clients' homes. What if you were to spill wax on their new bedroom carpet? Are you covered?

If you are running a business from home, do not automatically think your household insurance will cover your work and clients coming to your home. What if a client were to fall in the driveway, and hurt herself? Would you be covered?

Accidents can and do happen – and many clients have heard of these 'no win, no fee' solicitor firms willing to take legal action against you. Better safe than sorry! Be covered and you have security and peace of mind. One of the advantages of joining a professional association is that they negotiate better and reasonably priced insurance cover.

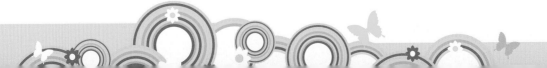

to manage disciplinary issues, grievances and dismissals and more on resolving problems in the workplace at an early stage, so saving businesses time and money.

BSI British Standards

BSI British Standards is the UK's national standards body, which brings together representatives from a range of organisations to develop formal standards for the benefit of UK business and consumers. Standards are there to help industry, and society at large. So even if you are not involved in developing or manufacturing products, you are bound to come into contact with BSI Standards every day. The aim of the Standards is to:

○ promote and share best practice, so designers can focus on developing better products

○ set benchmarks for performance, quality and safety

○ ensure similar products work together (e.g. making sure all CDs are the same dimensions)

○ make technical requirements

○ reduce risks

○ reduce costs.

Industry codes of practice

Key terms

Industry code of practice – a guide to correct procedures and etiquette within a particular industry.

Industry codes of practice or ethics are a guide to correct procedures and etiquette as dictated by professional therapists' associations, of which there are several. Which professional body you join is a matter of personal choice, and may depend upon the one favoured by your training establishment.

The cost involved in joining depends on your level of entry – a student membership is normally available and with your joining pack you will be given a code of ethics or a code of practice.

This code is a book of rules that the therapist agrees to abide by, as part of the contract of membership. If these rules are broken or ignored, membership can be withdrawn.

Being a member of a professional body brings benefits, which can include:

○ a good insurance deal negotiated on the members' behalf

○ support and advice upon leaving college

○ a monthly magazine, with useful articles and adverts for jobs and equipment

○ regular legal updates

○ free legal helplines, for all aspects of your business

○ discount cards for suppliers

○ a business guide for setting up on your own.

The following is a typical set of rules and regulations for a professional therapist organisation.

Federation of Holistic Therapists Code of Ethics and Professional Practice

The Federation of Holistic Therapists (FHT) is the UK and Ireland's largest and leading professional association for beauty, complementary and sports therapists. Professional therapist members of the FHT agree to abide by the FHT Code of Ethics and Professional Practice and any amendments or additions that may be made in the future.

Duties as a professional therapist

The definition of a professional therapist concerns the welfare of clients and the protection of the public from improper practice. This includes;

- making the care of your client your first concern
- providing a high standard of care at all times
- clients being treated with respect, as individuals
- professional knowledge being kept up-to-date
- acting lawfully in your professional and personal practice
- personal accountability for your professional activity

Failure to abide by this Code will result in disciplinary procedures being applied by the FHT Professional Conduct Panel ranging from a warning with sanctions according to conditions of practice, suspension until further training is completed, or termination of membership, depending on the nature of the breach. When an allegation is made against a professional therapist, the FHT will always take account of the standards set out in this Code when considering that allegation.

Guidelines to advertising your services

All advertising undertaken in relation to professional practice must be accurate, must not be misleading, false, unfair or exaggerated. Personal skills, equipment or facilities cannot be promoted as being better than anyone else's. Advertising any product or service requires promoting knowledge, skills, qualifications and experience in an accurate and professionally responsible way without making or supporting unjustifiable statements. Any potential financial rewards should be made explicit and play no part at all in the advice or recommendations of products and services that clients and users receive.

Limits of competence

A professional therapist must only carry out treatments and give advice within their area of training and competence. Clients' consent should be obtained before introducing new treatments into their existing treatment programme. A professional therapist has the right to refuse to treat a client if the treatment is outside of their competency level. In such circumstances they should refer to an appropriately qualified professional therapist or suggest that they contact their GP.

Regulation

Holistic therapies are not currently regulated by statute that provides protection of title. Protection of title prevents anyone calling themselves a 'doctor', physiotherapist, chiropodist, chiropractor etc, without being registered with the relevant statutory regulator under the provisions of an act of parliament. Membership of a professional association for a therapy that is not regulated enables the therapist to demonstrate to clients that they are suitably qualified, insured and participating in Continuing Professional Development (CPD).

(Source: Federation of Holistic Therapists; www.fht.org.uk, January 2010)

Salon guidelines

All the legislation mentioned above should be considered within the normal working life of the beauty therapist. Working safely and following the correct legal procedure is very important.

It is also very important to follow the **salon guidelines** for the particular establishment you are in – be it a training establishment, salon or spa, ocean liner or renting a room in a health suite.

It is vital that you are aware of the policies on health and safety, safety training and what exactly is expected within the job role. Normally salon rules are very similar, regardless of where the salon is located, but the safety procedures to follow if your salon happens to be floating in the Caribbean Sea will be very different.

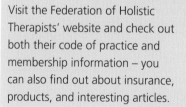

For your portfolio

Visit the Federation of Holistic Therapists' website and check out both their code of practice and membership information – you can also find out about insurance, products, and interesting articles.

Key terms

Salon guidelines – policies and procedures followed within the salon.

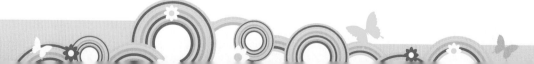

It is very important that the salon expectations and the required behaviour for therapists are set out at the beginning. This could be at your induction training, or even at the initial interview.

Regular reviews of policies and regular training for updates is essential, as is your attendance. If a member of staff continually ignores safety requirements, whether through negligence or through ignorance (if they have not attended training), this could form the basis for dismissal. Worse still, should an accident happen through negligence, injury may occur, and the person responsible may be found liable.

Health and safety rules

These will encompass all aspects of the Health and Safety at Work Act, plus COSHH guidelines and the Electricity at Work Act.

You should be in no doubt about:

- therapists' responsibilities
- salon procedures
- treatment safety
- equipment safety
- protection against cross-infection.

Client safety	Storage procedures	Stock regulations
Positioning of client	Electrical equipment	COSHH regulations followed
Minimum risk of hazard for bed height – getting on and off	Chemicals	First aid procedures in place
Correct use of equipment and products	Valuables	Stock rotation
Correct diagnosis for treatments	Stock	Spillage management
Correct evacuation procedures	Money	Correct storage and containers

Salon procedures for health and safety

Your employer or head of the training establishment should have all these standard procedures in place. If you are not instructed within your first few weeks of beginning your new post – then ask.

Check your knowledge

1 Which of the following statements is correct?
   a) All products should have a list of ingredients on them if they contain nuts.
   b) Products do not need any ingredients listed on the outside.
   c) Products only need a list of ingredients on them if they are bought at a chemist or through a salon.
   d) All products must have all ingredients listed on them.

2 The Data Protection Act states:
   a) all information on the record card must be accurate and correct
   b) clients must be kept safe at all times
   c) all personal information must be kept private and confidential
   d) all consultation forms must be the same.

3 What does the Consumer Protection Act state?
   a) The consumer must be kept safe while on the premises.
   b) The consumer must be protected from unsafe products.
   c) The consumer must be protected against unfair prices.
   d) The consumer must be protected against disease.

4 What does the Health and Safety at Work Act state about responsibility?
   a) Both the employer and employees are responsible for health and safety in the workplace.
   b) It is the responsibility of the employer to be responsible for health and safety.
   c) It is the client who is responsible for their own health and safety.
   d) It is the salon owner who is responsible for health and safety.

5 The Trade Descriptions Act states:
   a) It is illegal to make false claims about a product or service.
   b) It is illegal to put an advert on television.
   c) It is illegal to employ a foreign person without a work permit.
   d) It is illegal to offer unsafe treatments.

6 An example of a viral infection is:
   a) athlete's foot
   b) a cold sore
   c) scabies
   d) impetigo.

7 A bacterial infection is the cause of:
   a) ringworm
   b) diarrhoea
   c) warts
   d) boils.

8 A contra-action is:
   a) a condition which is present and means the treatment cannot go ahead
   b) a condition that the client is born with
   c) a reaction which appears during or just after treatment
   d) a condition which means the treatment has to be adapted.

9 An autoclave is:
   a) a waxing pot
   b) an effective sterilisation method
   c) a hot towel heater
   d) a chemical sterilising agent.

10 Sterilisation is:
   a) the removal of dirt and being ultra clean
   b) the removal of bacteria
   c) the removal of viruses
   d) the removal of bacteria, spores and viruses.

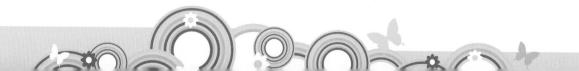

Section

2

The workplace environment

Unit G20

Make sure your own actions reduce risks to health and safety

What you will learn

G20.1 Identify the hazards and evaluate the risks in your workplace

G20.2 Reduce the risks to health and safety in your workplace

HSE

Health and Safety Executive

Five steps to risk assessment

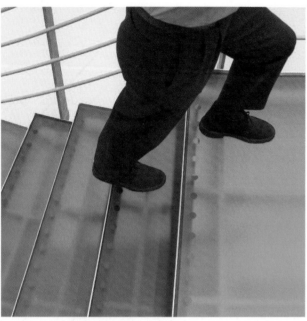

Advice is available from the Health and Safety Executive (Source: Health and Safety Executive)

Key terms

Health and Safety Executive (HSE) – an enforcing authority responsible for health and safety regulations in Great Britain. It ensures that risks to people's health and safety from work activities are properly controlled.

Introduction

A beauty salon should be a haven of tranquillity where the client can relax, unwind and enjoy her treatment, secure in the knowledge that she is in good hands and her professional therapist is in total control. Part of setting the scene is ensuring not only that the treatment is of the highest quality but also that the client is safe and not at risk.

Unfortunately, because of the very nature of its business a busy beauty therapy salon has the potential to be a dangerous place. Any business whose livelihood involves dealing with the general public, that is, the customer, could be viewed as an accident waiting to happen! The types of treatments involved in a salon are also a potential hazard: most equipment relies on electricity to work, we use chemicals when eyelash tinting and perming, we work with hot wax, and so on – each of the units carries its own potential hazards and risks.

It may not be obvious to the client that lying on a couch having a relaxing facial is potentially dangerous. In fact, it should not even cross the client's mind, but the therapist should view all treatments as a possible risk, and then minimise that risk. Your motto should be: 'Prevention is better than cure.'

This unit is for everyone at work, regardless of whether they are a paid worker, a volunteer, part-time or full-time employee or a self-employed therapist in a mobile business. Everyone within the workplace has an obligation by law to secure their own and others' health, safety and welfare. This unit is about identifying the factors that contribute to you becoming a responsible employee.

The Health and Safety at Work Act 1974 covers the legal requirements of an employer. **The Health and Safety Executive (HSE)** gives lots of advice for those considering going into business and employing others.

But what about you? Who are you responsible for? As a professional therapist, you are as liable as your employer, perhaps more so as you have regular direct contact with the customer. You are just as accountable to legal action should a client be able to prove you were negligent.

Individual salons usually have their own 'house rules' and favourite methods of doing things that are largely governed by the owners' preferences. The uniform, the décor and the daily running of the salon are personal and the working pattern will differ from salon to salon. The health and safety policies should not.

This unit is not a guide to completing a full risk assessment – that should be done by a trained professional who specialises in that field. The aim of this unit is to make you aware of the significant risks in the beauty salon, and to show you how to identify the risks and deal with them appropriately.

Identify the hazards and evaluate the risks in your workplace

Unit G20

In this outcome you will learn about:

- identifying which workplace instructions are relevant to your job
- identifying those working practices in your job which could harm you or others
- identifying those aspects of your workplace which could harm you or others
- checking which of the potentially harmful working practices and aspects of your workplace present the highest risks to you or to others
- dealing with hazards in accordance with workplace instructions and legal requirements
- correctly naming and locating the people responsible for health and safety in your workplace
- reporting to the people responsible for health and safety in your workplace those hazards which present the highest risks.

The three key areas to consider are:

- ○ a **hazard** in the salon
- ○ the **risk** that the hazard will be harmful
- ○ the **control** by which you reduce the risk where possible.

A firework is an example of a hazard — it has to be lit using a naked flame. It ignites to create patterns in the sky because it has explosives within it that create the noise and colour. So, the potential to cause harm is high — it can, and unfortunately often does, cause burns to the skin, loss of sight and even death. However, if the firework display is professionally organised, then the potential for harm is lessened. The spectators are behind barriers, the fireworks are set off in proper containers of sand using long tapered ignition sticks, and fire extinguishers are near — the risk is controlled to minimise damage.

Should the fireworks be set off in the street by people with no experience and no supervision using a domestic lighter, then the risk becomes greater — there is a real possibility of someone getting hurt. This is the fundamental difference between a hazard and a risk.

So, the skill is not only to recognise the potential of the hazard to cause injury or harm but also to know how to act in the most sensible manner to neutralise the risk, or to make it as low as possible.

Looking for a risk, and acting upon a risk assessment, is not necessarily a complicated matter, but it does need to be thought through thoroughly. Be logical. Start with the most obvious risks. Visualise making a cup of tea. What is the most hazardous part? Boiling the water and pouring the boiling water is the most obvious answer, as the boiling water has the potential to burn the skin quite seriously. You may get a tummy upset if the milk has gone off, or the handle on the teacup may break, or the spout on the teapot may leak, but these are secondary probabilities. Go for the main hazard, even if you think it is probably too obvious, and you cannot go far wrong.

Key terms

Hazard – anything that can cause harm or that has the potential to cause harm.

Risk – the chance, however great or small, that the hazard will cause harm to someone.

Control – the means by which risks identified are eliminated or reduced to acceptable levels.

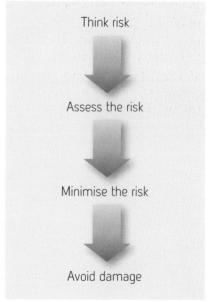

Think risk

Assess the risk

Minimise the risk

Avoid damage

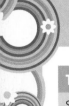

Unit G20 Make sure your own actions reduce risks to health and safety

Think about it

Simple precautions can often be the most effective, and common sense will always help to prevent accidents. Ignorance is not an acceptable excuse, nor is it accepted as a defence against misconduct or a damage claim within a court of law. There is no justification for not being fully aware of your responsibilities and duty to yourself, your clients and your colleagues.

Promoting a safe working environment

A sensible and intelligent question to ask when attending a job interview for any salon position is what staff training is available, not just for advancement of skill areas but also for health and safety training.

Regular guidance for all levels of staff will help to identify and minimise the hazards. All salons should have a workplace policy to include:

- the workplace/environmental factors
- safe working methods and equipment use
- the safe use of all hazardous substances in the workplace (not just for your particular job role)
- general policies for eating, smoking, drinking and drugs
- expected personal presentation
- what to do in the event of an accident, breakage or spillage
- all emergency procedures
- behaviour policies for all personnel
- corrective action where required.

If you are told at interview not to worry about any of the above and that it really doesn't matter, then you need to consider whether you want to work in a place that has so little regard for the safety of staff and clients, as well as health and safety legislation.

Identifying workplace instructions relevant to your job

'Employers have a general duty under section 2 of the Health and Safety at Work etc Act 1974 to ensure the health, safety and welfare of their employees at work so far as is reasonably practicable. People in control of non-domestic premises [e.g. beauty salons] have a duty (under Section 4 of the Act) towards people who are not their employees but use their premises [e.g. clients]. The Regulations expand on these duties and.are intended to protect the health and safety of everyone in the workplace, and ensure that adequate welfare facilities are provided for people at work.

These Regulations aim to ensure that workplaces meet the health, safety and welfare needs of all members of a workforce, including people with disabilities. Several of the Regulations require things to be 'suitable'. Regulation 2(3) makes it clear that facilities/the workplace should be suitable for anyone. This includes people with disabilities. Where necessary, parts of the workplace, including in particular doors, passageways, stairs, showers, washbasins, lavatories and workstations, should be made accessible for people with disabilities.'

(Source: Health and Safety Executive (2007), *'Workplace health, safety and welfare: A short guide for managers'*)

A salon only has a legal requirement to have written risk assessments and documentation if it employs five or more people. However, the sensible salon owner will have that in place regardless of how many staff are employed. Many insurance companies insist on written risk policies before they will agree to insure the business.

The other health and safety requirements for a small business are:

○ to inform the HSE area office or the local authority's environmental health department of the business's name and address

○ to inform the HSE area office or the local authority's environmental health department of any new employees

○ to display the health and safety law poster (available at your local Trading Standards Office) or hand out leaflets containing the equivalent information

○ to make an assessment of the risks at the workplace – which must be acted upon and kept as a written record if the business has five or more employees (this includes fire risks)

○ to bring the business's written statement of its health and safety policy to the attention of employees, and keep it up to date

○ to register with the local health authority if appropriate – this will apply in particular to therapists who carry out skin piercing.

Workplace health, safety and welfare

In each of the practical units you must take into account the lighting, ventilation, heating and general comfort of the client – refer to Organisational and legal requirements in the section 'What you must know' of the National Occupational Standards. This is not only for client safety but also for yours. The client may be in the sauna for a ten-minute treatment and you will be looking after her. Not only is her body temperature rising, yours is too, but she will be able to relax and rehydrate while you will be working!

Although you may think that salon ventilation and lighting is not part of your job role, these environmental factors affect you, your colleagues and the clients, so you need to be aware of them. You will therefore need to consider all aspects of the salon, both for client comfort and safety and for all workers in the salon. These include:

○ ventilation

○ temperatures in indoor workplaces

○ environmental factors, e.g. humidity and sources of heat in the workplace

○ personal factors, e.g. the type and quantity of clothing a worker is wearing and how physically demanding their work is

○ thermal comfort in the workplace – this applies to both workers and clients

○ supervision – to ensure the implementation of precautions put in place to safeguard workers' health in the workplace environment

○ lighting

○ automatic emergency lighting, powered by an independent source, should be provided where sudden loss of light would create a risk

○ cleanliness and waste materials

○ room dimensions and space

> **Think about it**
>
> All aspects of the workplace are pertinent to you, and should be researched.

> **Think about it**
>
> Therapists who work in large salons within department stores are expected to unpack their own deliveries in loading bays, so health and safety for this area should also be researched – it is all part of your job role in a salon.

Unit G20 Make sure your own actions reduce risks to health and safety

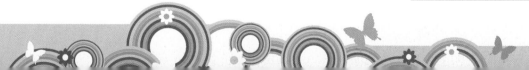

Unit G20 Make sure your own actions reduce risks to health and safety

- ○ workstations and seating
- ○ safety and training in the precautions to be taken
- ○ maintenance
- ○ floors and traffic routes
- ○ loading bays
- ○ open sides of staircases — these should be fenced with an upper rail at 900 mm or higher, and a lower rail
- ○ transparent or translucent doors, gates or walls and windows
- ○ windows and skylights — these should be designed so that they may be cleaned safely
- ○ doors and gates — internal and external
- ○ escalators and moving walkways
- ○ sanitary conveniences and washing facilities
- ○ drinking water
- ○ accommodation for clothing and facilities for changing
- ○ facilities for rest and to eat meals — canteens or restaurants may be used as rest facilities provided there is no obligation to purchase food
- ○ suitable rest facilities for pregnant women and nursing mothers. (Source: Health and Safety Executive (2007), 'Workplace health, safety and welfare: A short guide for managers'.)

For your portfolio

The questions below are from students who have just started work in a salon. Research each question to find out how the law can help them.

Maria: My salon is very stuffy. I often feel light-headed and sometimes think I'm going to faint. Can I complain to my employer, or will I get into trouble? What are my rights, if any?

Nicky: There is nowhere for me to eat lunch, and my boss says I am lucky to get a lunch break at all. I thought the salon should have a rest room for staff, am I right? How would I find this out?

Shreena: My work station is right next to a store cupboard. Staff are always going in and out, and the cupboard door keeps crashing into the back of my seat. It disrupts my treatments all the time, and I'm usually feeling a bit sore by the end of the day. What do the rules say about working areas? Surely we have to be safe?

Sam: In my salon we just put all the waxing strips (even the ones with blood spots on them) into the normal bin. I don't think that is hygienic or allowed by law. What do we have to do and how can I find out about this?

Jasmine: The lighting in the passageway to the stock cupboard is very dull and I think it is a bit of a hazard. Someone could easily fall over the step leading into the cupboard. What does the law state?

Think about it

When you inform your local Health and Safety Executive office that you are going into business, they will check out your business premises. This will depend on the authority within your own area, whose requirements would affect you whether you work from home or in a salon. The level of inspection may vary from area to area, and will also depend upon the types of treatment your salon is going to offer; for example, face and body massage will require registration in large cities such as London, Birmingham and Manchester to show you are a legitimate massage business, but may not if you are in a small village. The same is true of treatments which involve skin piercing and the disposal of contaminated needles, ear piercing and electrolysis and milia removal.

My story

Taking a risk

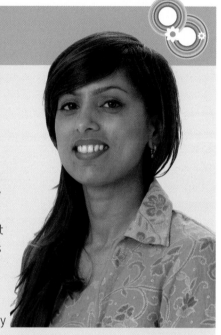

Hi, my name is Ruminda. I have witnessed a horrible accident that shows why risk assessment is so important in the workplace.

To help my finances while at college studying beauty therapy, I work part time in the local newsagent's. Last summer, a boy came in and bought his usual comic. He started to read it and was so engrossed that he wasn't paying attention to where he was walking. Unfortunately, he walked straight into the glass front of the shop instead of the open door. His shoes and head hit the glass and it shattered – the noise was really loud and frightening. He fell through the glass, and ended up lying face down on the pavement. There was a stunned silence and then the owner rushed out to see if the boy was all right. I was too scared to look as there was quite a lot of blood on him. He was lucky in one way, as the shards of glass hanging down could have done some real damage. We called an ambulance and he was taken to hospital.

The police and fire-fighters made the glass safe by knocking it all into the shop, and we had to close for repairs. The boy only had some cuts and bruising – he made a full recovery.

I had to give a witness statement to the insurance company and the police. Because the owner had not installed safety glass and did not have enough stickers on the glass front to show it was a glass window, he is to be prosecuted for negligence. That young boy could have died – I see him sometimes and often think how differently that day could have turned out.

Make sure your own actions reduce risks to health and safety **Unit G20**

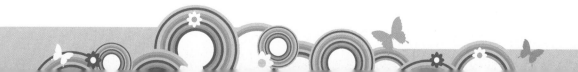

Identifying aspects of the workplace which could be harmful

Here are a few of the many hazards in a beauty salon:

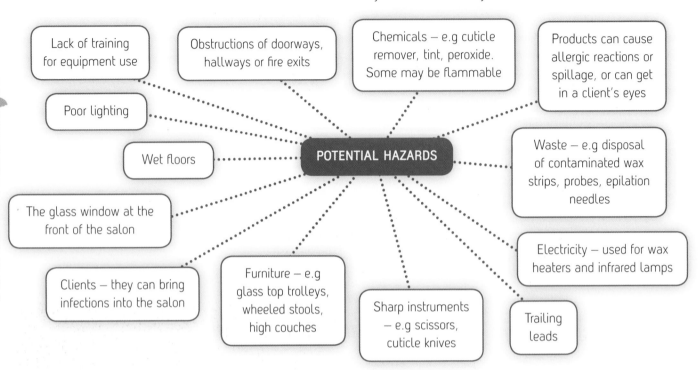

POTENTIAL HAZARDS

- Lack of training for equipment use
- Obstructions of doorways, hallways or fire exits
- Chemicals — e.g cuticle remover, tint, peroxide. Some may be flammable
- Products can cause allergic reactions or spillage, or can get in a client's eyes
- Poor lighting
- Wet floors
- Waste — e.g disposal of contaminated wax strips, probes, epilation needles
- The glass window at the front of the salon
- Electricity — used for wax heaters and infrared lamps
- Clients — they can bring infections into the salon
- Furniture — e.g glass top trolleys, wheeled stools, high couches
- Sharp instruments — e.g scissors, cuticle knives
- Trailing leads

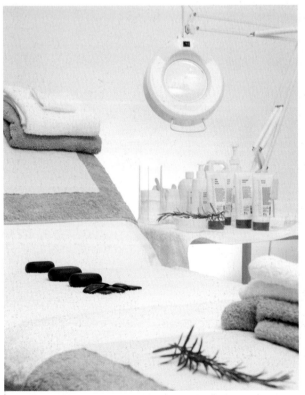

A safe work station

Although these are identified as possible hazards, not all of them will become actual hazards, and certainly not all at the same time! For example, in all the years an experienced therapist works in a salon, there may not be a fire caused by faulty equipment overheating and bursting into flames. But the important thing is that the therapist will have recognised the possibility and will have her equipment regularly checked by a competent person. She will also keep a safety logbook with all equipment checks dated and signed, as recommended in the Electricity at Work Regulations 1989. The risk has been minimised, and should a fire start, the logbook will show that responsibility has been taken and the therapist or salon owner has not been neglecting her duty.

In this unit the Health and Safety at Work Act 1974 is the only piece of legislation specifically referred to, as it is the main piece of legislation under which nearly all of the other regulations fall. However, you should also refer to 'You, your client and the law' (see Professional basics, pages 48–68) for other health and safety legislation. This includes the Electricity at Work Regulations 1989 and Environmental Protection Act 1990 for safe disposal of contaminated clinical waste.

Each practical unit has its own particular hazards which will be addressed in the unit itself. These risk factors are often out of the control of the therapist and should be the responsibility of the salon owner, for example ventilation required for nail varnish and artificial nail chemicals, or adequate ventilation in the sauna and steam suites.

However, if the sign to the salon was hanging off and about to drop onto a client or unsuspecting passerby, you would be neglectful if you did not report it. Structural damage does happen to older buildings. If the salon is in, say, a Tudor building, which may be protected and listed, then the amenities will not be as modern as in later buildings. Oak beams and lead windows may be very attractive, but if water is dripping down a wall into an electricity socket, the building is not safe! Older buildings may be very expensive to maintain and can present many more hazards.

Identifying aspects of the workplace which present the highest risk

Some areas of the salon will be more high risk than others. For your own personal safety and that of others, it is up to you to know, understand and carry out workplace instructions particular to your job role, to identify those areas which are potentially harmful and control the risks, to be responsible and to be safe.

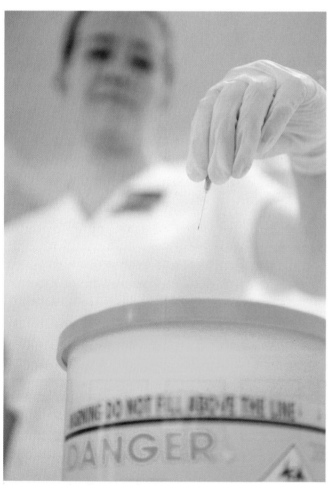
Waste must be disposed of safely

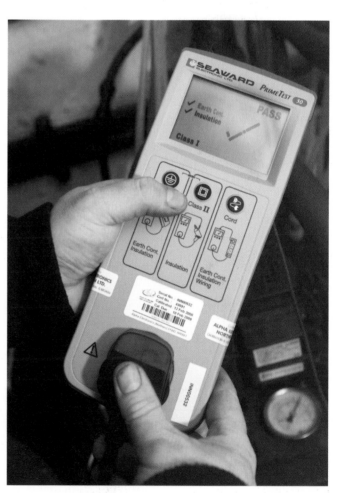
Electrical equipment must be installed by a competent person and regularly checked

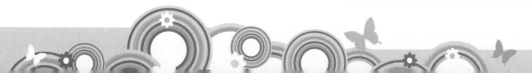

Unit G20
Make sure your own actions reduce risks to health and safety

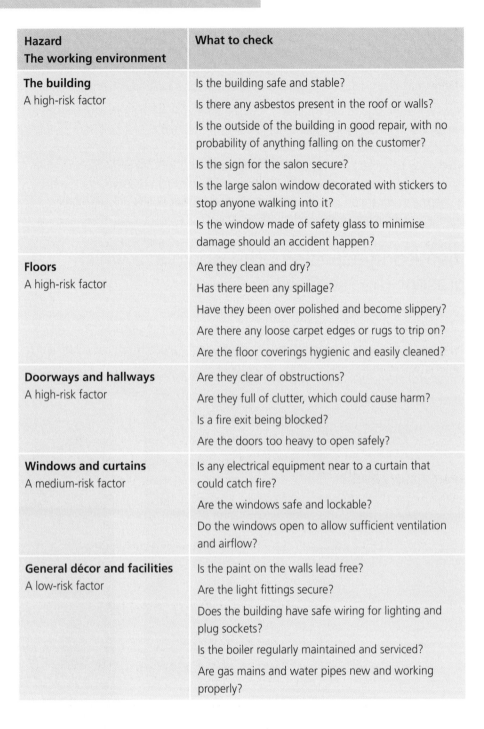

Hazard The working environment	What to check
The building A high-risk factor	Is the building safe and stable? Is there any asbestos present in the roof or walls? Is the outside of the building in good repair, with no probability of anything falling on the customer? Is the sign for the salon secure? Is the large salon window decorated with stickers to stop anyone walking into it? Is the window made of safety glass to minimise damage should an accident happen?
Floors A high-risk factor	Are they clean and dry? Has there been any spillage? Have they been over polished and become slippery? Are there any loose carpet edges or rugs to trip on? Are the floor coverings hygienic and easily cleaned?
Doorways and hallways A high-risk factor	Are they clear of obstructions? Are they full of clutter, which could cause harm? Is a fire exit being blocked? Are the doors too heavy to open safely?
Windows and curtains A medium-risk factor	Is any electrical equipment near to a curtain that could catch fire? Are the windows safe and lockable? Do the windows open to allow sufficient ventilation and airflow?
General décor and facilities A low-risk factor	Is the paint on the walls lead free? Are the light fittings secure? Does the building have safe wiring for lighting and plug sockets? Is the boiler regularly maintained and serviced? Are gas mains and water pipes new and working properly?

Dust

Toxic

Flammable

Irritant

Corrosive

Oxidising agent

COSHH symbols showing the different types of hazardous substances

Hazard Equipment	What to check
Beds A high-risk factor	Are the brakes on? Is it at the right height for the therapist to work comfortably, and not too high for the client to get on to easily? Is the bedding a danger by being too long and trailing on the floor, ready to trip someone up? Is the bedding easily cleaned, protected during the treatment and hygienic?
Chairs A high-risk factor	Are chairs secured and at a suitable height? Are hydraulic chairs regularly maintained? Are all chairs stable? Are they on castors? Are they hygienic and easy to keep clean?
Trolleys A low-risk factor	Are they glass topped and liable to shatter? Are they secure on their castors? Are they regularly maintained? Are they hygienic and easy to keep clean? Are they up to the job given to them, or is the equipment too heavy?
Electrical appliances A high-risk factor	Are they regularly maintained by a competent person? Are they used by qualified personnel only? Are they safely stored? Are they used with the correct products only? Are they bought from a reputable manufacturer to ensure safety? Are they used at the correct socket with the right plugs and fuses? Are there any trailing leads? Are they placed on a safe surface, rather than balanced on a windowsill?
Bins for disposal of waste products A high-risk factor	Are the correct bins available for different waste products? Is contaminated waste separated from other waste (e.g. body fluids, blood, etc. from waxing or eyebrow shaping)? Who is responsible for emptying the bins and how regularly will they empty them? Is infection control in place to minimise risk?

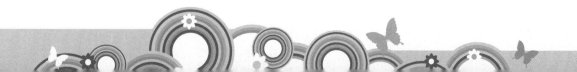

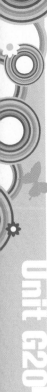

Hazard	What to check
Products A very high-risk factor	Are they clearly labelled?
	Are they stored safely and correctly?
	Has a COSHH (Control of Substances Hazardous to Health) sheet been completed for each product?
	Do therapists know how to use them correctly?
	Are they stored in the proper containers, not in other bottles?
	Is the shelf life taken into account?
	Are lids secured properly?
	Is a designated first-aider available in case of accidents?
	Do staff know what to do in cases of personal injury caused by poor product use?
	Are correct patch tests being carried out to prevent allergic reactions?
	Is regular product training being offered?
	Are toxic products stored correctly?
People A very high-risk factor	Should they be there?
	Are they going to create a hazard (e.g. workmen doing repairs and leaving tools out where clients are walking by)?
	Do they know where they are going?
	Are they aware of steps and the salon layout?
	Is their behaviour suitable for the salon, or are they using threatening behaviour?
	Are they intruders?
	Is there a risk they may be able to steal something?
You – the therapist	Do you lead others by giving a good example in health and safety matters?
	Does your behaviour endanger others?
	Are you fully trained to use equipment/products?
	Are you as hygienic as possible to avoid cross-infection?
	Do you follow the correct procedures for the workplace?
	Do you actively take part in regular training sessions for health and safety?
	Do you report possible hazards to the correct person?
	Is your uniform a health or safety hazard?
	Do you wear safe shoes?
	Do you wear a lot of jewellery?
	Do you walk around with sharp scissors in your pocket?
	Do you look out for the safety of others?
	Do you keep up-to-date client record cards?
	Do you use the correct lifting posture, i.e. keeping your back straight and bending your knees?

Who is responsible for health and safety in your workplace?

Health and safety regulations apply to all businesses all the time. They should not merely be referred to when there has been a near accident at work — they should be a full-time concern.

The Health and Safety at Work Act 1974 is largely about employers — but since you may be an employer yourself one day, the following extracts from the Act will be very important to you.

The general duties of employers to their employees are set down in section 2(1) of the Act:

'It shall be the duty of every employer to ensure, so far as is reasonably practical, the health, safety and welfare at work of all his employees.'

In addition to responsibilities to employees, an employer has a duty to protect other persons, for example members of the public. These are stated in section 3(1) of the Act:

'It shall be the duty of every employer to conduct his undertaking in such a way as to ensure, so far as is reasonably practical, that persons not in his employment who may be affected thereby are not thereby exposed to risks to their health or safety.'

All persons who are self-employed also have responsibilities under the Act. These are dealt with under section 3(2):

'It shall be the duty of every self-employed person to conduct his undertaking in such a way as to ensure, so far as is reasonably practical, that he and other persons (not being his employees) who may be affected thereby are not thereby exposed to risks to their health or safety.'

Even if you have no intention of owning a salon, employing anyone, or becoming self-employed, you still have responsibilities as an employee. These include:

○ correct use of systems and procedures
○ reporting flaws or gaps within the system or procedure when in use.

Employers and employees have a shared responsibility for:

○ the safety of individuals being cared for
○ the safety of the working environment.

Employees also have responsibilities to take reasonable care of themselves and other people affected by their work and to cooperate with their employers in the discharge of their obligations.

The employee has a responsibility to:

○ her/himself   ○ other employees   ○ the public.

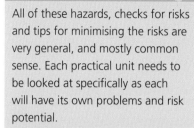

Think about it

All of these hazards, checks for risks and tips for minimising the risks are very general, and mostly common sense. Each practical unit needs to be looked at specifically as each will have its own problems and risk potential.

By asking yourself the questions given here, you will soon start to identify and then rectify any risks.

Make sure your own actions reduce risks to health and safety Unit G20

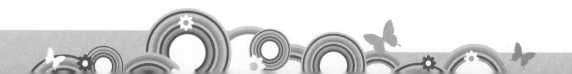

Dealing with hazards in accordance with workplace instructions and legal requirements

All professional salons should have a set of rules and procedures for everyone to follow. Employees should be familiar with these rules and regulations for the safety and protection of all within the salon.

By law, the salon has to:

○ display the health and safety rules and regulations on the wall in a prominent position (see Professional basics, page 49, for an example of this poster)

○ display fire evacuation procedures.

Professionally, the salon will also have:

○ codes of practice to follow from its professional body with regard to set procedures

○ certain standards to maintain for insurance cover to be valid, which are usually linked to the codes of practice.

Legally, the employer is responsible for putting into place the rules covering the health and safety of all employees and clients and ensuring that safe practice is followed by all staff. These responsibilities may be carried out by:

○ providing regular training, with staff meetings to update on safety issues

○ giving a clear outline at the initial interview as to what is expected

○ maintaining records of injuries or first aid treatment given

○ monitoring and evaluating health and safety arrangements regularly

○ providing a written health and safety booklet

○ consulting the experts and being knowledgeable — ignorance is not an excuse.

Refer to 'You, your client and the law' (see Professional basics, pages 48–64) for a full breakdown of legal obligations of the employer and employee.

Reporting hazards of high risk

Hazards can and do happen and everyone should be aware of the safety implications.

As part of their personal responsibility, the therapist needs to be able to recognise when the hazard can be dealt with immediately and when help may be needed. It is very important to know who to go to when a salon problem arises that is a potential health and safety issue and there is any risk of harm. Salons will have different staff members with different areas of responsibility. One or two staff members will be trained in first aid, one person will assume responsibility for filling out the accident and report book and keeping health and safety records up to date, another will be responsible for building maintenance and the replacement of light bulbs, and so on.

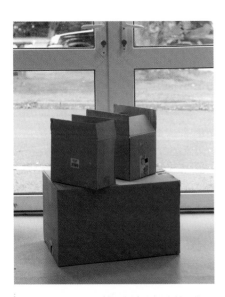

If something obstructing access is too heavy to be moved, it should be reported

ACCIDENT / ILLNESS REPORT FORM

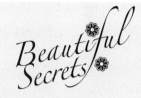
Beautiful Secrets

This form is to be completed by the injured party. If this is not possible, the form should be completed by the person making the report. If more than one person was injured, please complete a **separate form for each person**.

Completing and signing this form does not constitute an admission of liability of any kind, either by the person making the report or any other person.

This form should be completed immediately and forwarded to the Health and Safety Officer and Salon Manager.

If it is possible that an accident has been caused by a defect in machinery, equipment or a process, isolate / fence off the area and contact the Health and Safety Officer or Manager immediately.

SECTION 1 PERSONAL DETAILS

Surname: __Lung__ (Mr/**Mrs**/Ms/Miss) Forename(s): __Jenny__

Date of birth: __29/01/57__ Address: __89, New Street, Glasgow__

STAFF ☐   CONTRACTOR ☐   VISITOR ☐   GENERAL PUBLIC ✔

SECTION 2 ACCIDENT / INCIDENT / ILLNESS DETAILS

Accident (Injury) ✔   Illness ☐   Date: __19/04/10__   Time: __13:07__   (24-hour clock)

Location: __Salon room 3__

Nature of injury or condition and the part of the body affected:

__Slipped on floor, twisted ankle__

Account

Describe what happened and how. In the case of an accident state clearly what the injured person was doing.

__Small patch of water on the floor – client got off couch and__
__slipped on it.__

Name and address of adult witness(es): __Jo Benfield, Beautiful Secrets__

Details of action taken

Ambulance summoned ☐   Taken to hospital ☐   Sent to hospital ✔

First aid given ☐   Taken home ☐   Sent home ☐   Returned to work ☐

SECTION 3 PREVENTATIVE ACTION

Recommended: __to ensure that all spillages are mopped up straight away__

Implemented: **Yes**/ No   Date: __19/04/10__

Report raised by

Name: __Catrina Waldron__

Position: __Therapist__

Signature: __C Waldron__   Date: __19/04/10__

FOR OFFICE USE ONLY	
Copy sent to: Salon Manager	☐
Health and Safety Officer	☐

An accident report form

Make sure your own actions reduce risks to health and safety

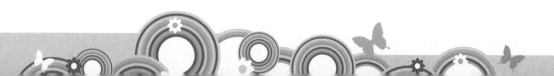

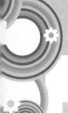

Examples of hazards which need reporting:

Hazard	Way to avoid hazard	When referral may be necessary
Breach of security	Shut windows, lock cupboards and doors	When something is found open or something is believed to be missing
Faulty or damaged products, tools, equipment, fixtures or fittings	Handle correctly, store correctly, treat with care Follow manufacturer's instructions	When something is found to be broken
Spillage	Take care when mixing, pouring and filling	When spilled material is corrosive or irritant
Slippery floors	Make others aware by blocking the area with a chair to prevent an accident Sweep up powder spills, mop up spills of liquid; refer to COSHH sheets for correct method	When acid, grease or polish is spilt
Obstruction to access and exit	Move large equipment away from doorways if able to do so Put bags and coats on a rack or shelving	When object is too heavy to be moved, it should be reported

These hazards should be reported to a manager or the health and safety officer within your workplace. There are also hazards that need to be reported to the local health officer or the Health and Safety Executive – refer to 'You, your client and the law', Professional basics (see pages 48–68) for more information.

Dealing with hazards of low risk

This is largely common sense. If the risk is low and you can deal with it straight away, then do so to prevent an incident occurring. This could be something very straightforward, such as a client's handbag on the floor which could trip someone up. Pick it up off the floor, put it under the trolley out of the way and carry on with what you were doing.

This low-risk hazard does not need reporting, but it still requires prompt action to prevent it becoming a bigger problem.

Always act within the policy of your workplace. For example, if there is a policy on where clients' handbags and coats are stored to prevent congestion in the salon, then use the correct place.

For your portfolio

Any low-risk hazard has potential to become a high risk – if action is not taken. What would you consider to be a low-risk hazard in your salon? Look around your place of work and have a detailed review of possibilities. What would be a high-risk hazard? Keep a risk assessment form handy and write down what you see – in many companies bonuses are paid to workers who prevent accidents from happening.

Reduce the risks to health and safety in your workplace

In this outcome you will learn about:

- carrying out your work in accordance with your level of competence, workplace instructions, suppliers' or manufacturers' instructions and legal requirements
- controlling those health and safety risks within your capability and job responsibilities
- passing on suggestions for reducing risks to health and safety to the responsible people
- making sure your behaviour does not endanger the health and safety of you or others in your workplace
- following the workplace instructions and suppliers' or manufacturers' instructions for the safe use of equipment, materials and products
- reporting any differences between workplace instructions and suppliers' or manufacturers' instructions
- making sure that your personal presentation and behaviour at work protects the health and safety of you and others, meets any legal responsibilities and is in accordance with workplace instructions
- making sure you follow environmentally friendly working practices.

This section looks at how to reduce or minimise the risks relating to the hazards you identified within the first part of this unit. You need to know how to carry out risky tasks safely, following both suppliers' or manufacturers' instructions and your workplace requirements.

Think about it

Your legal responsibilities form the first part of every practical unit – refer to Organisational and legal requirements in the section 'What you must know' of the National Occupational Standards. Reducing the risks to health and safety in the workplace is part of your legal responsibilities, so it is important to link this to your treatments.

You must also have a thorough understanding of the health and safety policies within your salon that affect your working day. This includes your conduct and personal presentation, which will ensure the health and safety of yourself, your clients and your working colleagues.

You should always carry out your work in relation to your level of competence, your workplace instructions and manufacturers' instructions, as well as the legal requirements. You should be capable and know your job responsibilities; this will allow you to control health and safety risks where you can. Never knowingly endanger the health of others and do pass on to your supervisor or manager any suggestions that you think might help to reduce risks to yourself or others.

Reducing risk by taking appropriate action

In the first part of the unit we looked at the various hazards and what to check for. We will now look again at those hazards and see how to minimise the risks by taking the appropriate action.

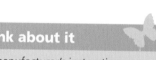

Think about it

If a manufacturer's instructions do not comply with the practice in your salon, then always ask for clarification from your supervisor or manager, rather than endanger a client.

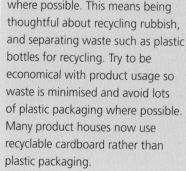

Think about it

You should always follow environmentally friendly practices where possible. This means being thoughtful about recycling rubbish, and separating waste such as plastic bottles for recycling. Try to be economical with product usage so waste is minimised and avoid lots of plastic packaging where possible. Many product houses now use recyclable cardboard rather than plastic packaging.

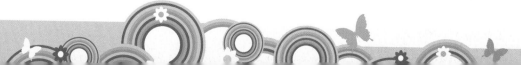

Unit G20 Make sure your own actions reduce risks to health and safety

Hazard The working environment	Actions to minimise risk
The building A high-risk factor	Take out property owner's liability insurance, often known as buildings insurance. This covers damage to the outside of the salon building such as roof repairs, wall repairs, etc. Internal major fittings such as toilet facilities and kitchens are also often covered. Maintain and check the outside of the property regularly and repair small damage before it becomes a major hazard.
Floors A high-risk factor	Only use the correct products for floor cleaning and allow plenty of drying time. Major stripping and recovering of the floor surface can be done outside normal salon times. Repair or avoid carpets and rugs with frayed edges and those not easily kept clean. Pay for professional cleaning companies to chemically clean carpets outside normal salon hours.
Doorways and hallways A high-risk factor	Have a regular inspection from your local fire safety officer who will advise the salon on the correct walkway exit route in case of fire. Keep corridors tidy and clutter free. Ensure stairs and corridors are well lit, and replace blown light bulbs immediately.
Windows and curtains A medium-risk factor	Keep all electrical equipment away from the window area. Employ a handyman to ensure the windows open, are hinged properly and are safe and secure. Invest in double-glazing if possible, or make sure older style windows are properly maintained. Loose windows are the ideal entry for a potential thief. If your salon has a large window front and glass doors, remember to put lots of display stickers on them. Magnification mirrors without covers placed near to a window can become a fire risk if the sun's rays pass through the window, through the middle of the lamp and then on to a couch or curtains – the material may smoulder, then catch fire. Always cover the magnification lamp and do not leave by unshielded windows.
General décor and facilities A low-risk factor	Invest in safe decorating products bought from a reputable DIY store, not from the boot of someone's car. Lead-based paint is hazardous to health and should not be used. Avoid positioning product displays, ornaments and plant pots where they are likely to be in the way of heavy traffic flow of people through the salon – they could be tripped over or knocked. Regularly check and maintain the utility services – many companies provide a regular service agreement for a yearly overhaul of gas and electricity parts including boilers and central heating, etc.

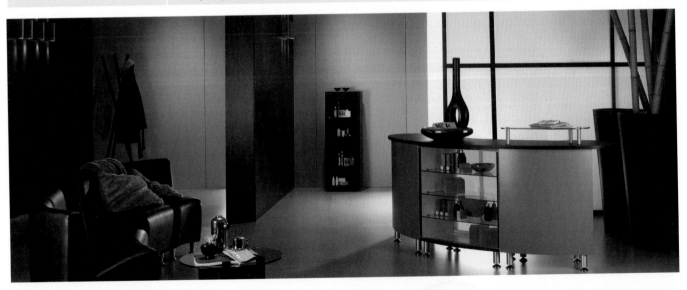

Hazard Equipment	Actions to minimise risk
Beds A high-risk factor	Buy from professional suppliers only, with guarantees, and maintenance and repair agreements. Ensure the bed is the correct height to avoid back problems and buy an adjustable bed where possible. Use protective coverings that are washable, and minimise the risk of cross-infection by regularly disinfecting the bed and covering.
Chairs A high-risk factor	As above. The recommended chair for use by professionals is the five-castor movable chair with adjustable height and backrest, often called the 'super secretarial chair'. Make sure the height of the chair is suitable for you – you should be able to sit squarely with your bottom at the back of the chair and your feet firmly flat on the floor. Regularly maintain the chair and lubricate the castors.
Electrical appliances A high-risk factor	As above. Always buy from a reputable manufacturer who provides training, suitable products and an after-sales service, and offers repairs and servicing. Comply with the Electricity at Work Act 1989 and have the equipment tested by a competent person. Keep a logbook of testing, dated and signed, with a system of labelling and removing faulty equipment from use. Ensure regular training to update all staff as well as training in fire fighting and the use of an extinguisher. Make sure staff know who to report to in case of electrical fires.
Disposal of waste products A high-risk factor	Environmental Protection Act 1990 The Controlled Waste Regulations 1992 The Special Waste Regulations 1996 This legislation requires all clinical waste (waste which consists wholly or partly of animal or human tissue, blood or other body fluids, swabs, dressings, syringes and needles) to be kept apart from general waste and to be disposed of to a licensed incineration or landfill site by a licensed company. A contract can be arranged with a local firm who will take away yellow bins with contaminated waste and replace them on a daily or weekly basis.
Products A very high-risk factor	The Control of Substances Hazardous to Health Regulations 2002 require you to assess the risk of all hazardous substances used in the workplace as well as those that you may become exposed to during your work activities or which are produced at the end of any work or process. Keep manufacturers' data sheets and ensure that products are used in accordance with the manufacturers' recommendations. COSHH sheets also have a space for the recommended first aid requirements if the product is in contact with the skin, is ingested (swallowed) or enters the eye. Learn these and be prepared for any eventuality. Proper labelling and clearly identifiable bottles or tubs for caustic ingredients will help to prevent accidents. Keep thorough and up-to-date record cards for clients' treatments and products, especially if there has already been a reaction or allergy to a particular product, or if the client has a severe allergy to a specific substance, such as nuts. Go on regular commercial training to keep abreast of new products, and never guess a product use or equipment usage.

Unit G20

Make sure your own actions reduce risks to health and safety

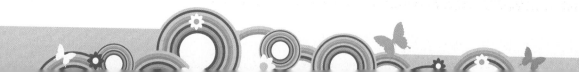

People	There are many risks involving people – operator error with equipment, visitors to the salon, untrained people using equipment they shouldn't and even opening windows they shouldn't.
A very high-risk factor	With visitors, be informed about who is coming and going in the salon. Many salons employ a badge or name labelling system to identify visitors, sales reps, trades people, delivery drivers and so on. They may be expected to sign in using a visitor book and have suitable identification with them.
	Minimise the risk of client harm by asking workers to carry out repairs in the quieter part of the day, or when the salon is closed. Major repairs would necessitate the salon being closed, as the clients' safety cannot be compromised.
	Do not be intimidated by a person shouting or by abusive behaviour. Firmly ask the person to leave, or consult with the manager or salon owner, and if necessary call the police.

Risk assessments in the workplace

A risk assessment is simply a careful examination of what, in your workplace, could cause harm to people, so that you can weigh up whether you have taken enough precautions or should do more to prevent harm. You are legally required to assess the risks in your workplace so that you put in place a plan to control those risks. According to the Health and Safety Executive's leaflet 'Five steps to risk assessment', 'The law does not expect you to eliminate all risk, but you are required to protect people as far as "reasonably practicable".'

Think about it

You cannot blame anyone else for your own actions – you need to take responsibility for everything that you do. Suing for damages if there is an accident is becoming common practice, so do not allow yourself to be vulnerable or open to a negligence claim. The law is very clear on what amounts to negligence, so be well informed and knowledgeable to minimise risk in all you do.

How to assess the risks in your workplace

'When thinking about your risk assessment, remember:

- a **hazard** is anything that may cause harm, such as chemicals, electricity, working from ladders, an open drawer etc

- the **risk** is the chance, high or low, that someone could be harmed by these and other hazards, together with an indication of how serious the harm could be.

Follow the five steps:
Step 1 Identify the hazards
Step 2 Decide who might be harmed and how
Step 3 Evaluate the risks and decide on precautions
Step 4 Record your findings and implement them
Step 5 Review your assessment and update if necessary'

(Source: Health and Safety Executive (2006) 'Five steps to risk assessment'.)
(This leaflet is available to download from the HSE's website.)

Using the scale of probability, severity and danger ratings, you can clearly identify the potentially harmful working practices and aspects of your workplace which present the highest risks to you or to others.

The risk rating is:	The probability rating is:	The severity rating is:
Low = 1–7 Medium = 8–16 High = 17–25	1 – Highly unlikely 2 – Possible 3 – Probable 4 – Likely 5 – Inevitable	1 – trivial injury (no first aid required) 2 – minor injury (first aid required) 3 – major injury (hospitalisation) 4 – major injury to many persons 5 – death (of one or more persons)

Scale of probability, severity and danger ratings

Using the ratings, a risk assessment would look like this:

RISK ASSESSMENT FORM:

NAME OF EQUIPMENT:

A magnifying lamp

STEP 1 WHAT ARE THE HAZARDS?

Accident:

- placing the lamp too close to the client's face during the consultation
- the hinges not supporting the lamp head so risk of dropping / not staying in position
- trailing wires from lamp to wall socket

Fire: if placed by window with no cover on the lens, there is a risk of the sun's rays being magnified, heat being produced and a risk of smouldering /fire

STEP 2 WHO MIGHT BE HARMED?

Client

Therapist

All in the salon if fire occurs

WHAT IS ALREADY IN PLACE?

Lamps are covered when not in use

Lamps are not stored near windows

Equipment is regularly maintained

Extension leads used where necessary if workstation is far away from wall socket

WHAT FURTHER ACTION COULD BE TAKEN?

Training in use of equipment

Health and safety notice put up

Fire precaution and evacuation procedures put in place

| The **risk rating** is: 10 | The **probability rating** is: 2 | The **severity rating** is: 2-5 |

You should now begin to see how you can reduce the risk of harm by following some basic steps, being responsible and thinking about your actions.

Make sure your own actions reduce risks to health and safety **Unit G20**

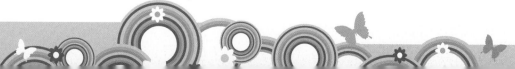

Key terms

Level of competence – the limits of a person's authority; usually the extent of a person's responsibility as set out in their job description and workplace policies.

Reducing risk through your personal presentation and behaviour at work

It is your responsibility to carry out your work in accordance with your **level of competence**, workplace instructions, suppliers' and manufacturers' instructions and legal requirements.

Refer to Professional basics (see pages 12–15) for full information about professional presentation. In this section you will be looking at the safety aspect of your presentation and how it contributes to safety in the salon.

Hazard	Actions to reduce risk
You – the therapist	Be professional at all times.
	Have short nails, minimal jewellery, safe shoes and clean, hygienic uniform.
	Follow the Health and Safety Act and be responsible in actions and consequences for both yourself and others.
	Go on regular training courses to be safe and competent.
	Be knowledgeable and use your knowledge: know the correct person to inform in case of an accident, who to contact for first aid and the salon policies on health and safety.
	Be as hygienic and as thorough as possible when protecting the client.
	Fill out a full consultation card and carry out a contra-indication check prior to every treatment.
	Never knowingly endanger others.

Think about it

Never exceed your own level of competency as it may make any insurance claims invalid. It might also jeopardise your own or someone else's health or become a risk to safety in the salon.

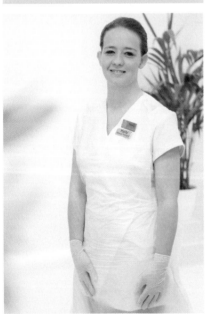

Personal appearance should be a combination of safety and professionalism

It is not only the employer's responsibility to provide health and safety management, it is also the responsibility of each employee to follow the rules.

All beauty therapists work very long hours and are often on the go all day. They are in a busy salon environment with other people present all the time – their own clients, other therapists' clients, other staff, outside representatives, management, receptionists, cleaners and so on. If the therapist does not have a sense of personal safety and respect for the safety of others, accidents will occur.

To be safe the therapist should consider the following:

○ Make sure personal appearance combines safety with professionalism.

○ Wear shoes that are smart but comfortable. High heels are not only uncomfortable but also not particularly stable to walk on. Open-toe sandals will not protect the toes from damage from either spillage or impact injury.

○ Avoid stooping and slouching. This will prevent back problems occurring.

○ Have good posture and distribute body weight evenly by standing correctly with feet slightly apart. This will prevent accidents and injury.

○ Always wear the correct protective clothing to shield a uniform.

○ Always wear gloves when using chemicals or if there is a possibility of coming into contact with body fluids.

○ Always follow the correct disposal regulations for gloves and waste materials.

○ If an establishment provides a uniform as part of a corporate image, wear it!

○ Keep hair tidy and wear it short or tied back. Loose long hair may fall in the eyes and cause eye problems.

A high standard of cleanliness will ensure no cross-infection can occur. This should include the following:

- Wash hands between clients.
- Keep nails short.
- Cover cuts or open wounds.
- Do not attend work with an infectious disease.
- Do not spread cold or flu germs.
- Do not wear dangling jewellery that may be a hazard.

Good conduct cuts down any risks:

- Do not run in the salon or rush.
- Use equipment properly.
- Follow manufacturers' instructions at all times.
- Do not take short cuts when cleaning the salon and equipment.
- Always leave the equipment ready to be used by the next person.
- Do not block fire exits for any reason.
- Do not deliberately endanger anyone – even as a joke.
- Do not behave negligently – such as playing with fire!
- Use proper lifting procedures.
- Do take responsibility for yourself, machinery and problems such as spillage that may occur – do not expect someone else to clean up after you!

Salon security and reducing workplace risks

There are many areas to keep secure in a business.

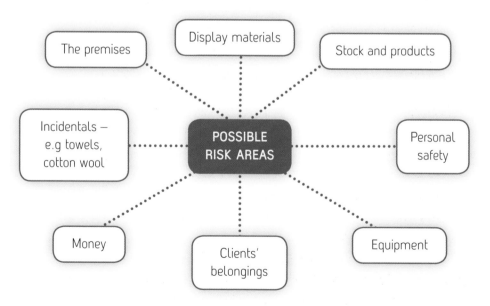

POSSIBLE RISK AREAS

- The premises
- Display materials
- Stock and products
- Incidentals – e.g towels, cotton wool
- Personal safety
- Money
- Clients' belongings
- Equipment

> **Think about it**
>
> According to the government's Labour Force Survey, between July 2007 and June 2008, around 5.8 million working days were lost to sickness or injury. This amounts to 1.5 per cent of all working days.

Make sure your own actions reduce risks to health and safety **Unit G20**

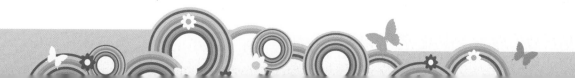

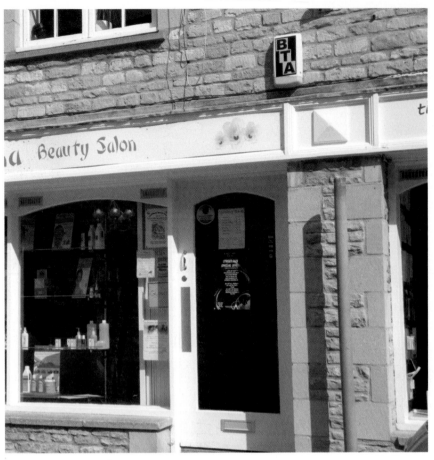
Fit a burglar alarm if possible

The premises

For insurance and mortgage applications the salon owner must have adequate security measures in place for the salon. It is worth consulting the local police station for guidance. The crime prevention officer will survey the premises and give advice regarding the most vulnerable areas and the most common forms of entry by a burglar.

Externally

○ Deadlock all doors and windows. Double-glazing is expensive but is more difficult to break into — the older the window and frame, the easier the entry.

○ Fit a burglar alarm if possible, or even a dummy box on the wall, which will deter a burglar.

○ Closed circuit television (CCTV) may be available if the premises are in a shopping area with other stores.

○ Metal shop front shutters are probably the most effective deterrent. If the premises have a shutter system, use it.

Internally

○ Internal doors can be locked to prevent an intruder moving from room to room.

○ Fire doors and emergency exits should be locked at night, and reopened by the first person to arrive in the morning.

○ A light left on in reception may deter would-be burglars, who may feel that well-lit premises will make them more easily seen.

○ Stock and money should be locked away or should be in the bank so that nothing is visible to entice a burglar in the first place.

○ Lock expensive equipment away in treatment rooms or in the stock cupboard.

○ Very large businesses employ night security guards to patrol their premises, but as with alarmed infrared beams, these are not affordable for the average small salon owner. If, however, the salon is situated within a shopping centre or business park, night patrols may be included in the lease or purchase agreement or offered at a set fee per year. Costs would need to be considered, but it may be a worthwhile investment and save money in the long term.

○ The local police station can be contacted and the police patrol vans will regularly check the building as part of their normal evening beat.

Stock and products on display and in use in treatment rooms

Of all the temptations to the thief, these smaller items may prove irresistible. They are small enough for a pocket and are very accessible. Unfortunately, this form of shoplifting costs many businesses a great deal of money, as stock can be expensive to replace and can be a big chunk of the capital outlay of a salon.

A sad fact is that the average thief may be rather closer to home than is comfortable. Staff may 'borrow' an item of stock for home use and think that their behaviour is acceptable. Also clients may like the look of a lipstick and 'forget' to pay for it!

Stealing small items is referred to as 'pilfering'; a polite word for stealing, and stealing larger items is referred to as 'shoplifting'. Either way, it means the salon has bought an item of stock from the wholesaler that has not been paid for by a customer, so it has to absorb that financial loss. If unchecked, it could eventually bankrupt the business, so tight precautions such as the following are called for:

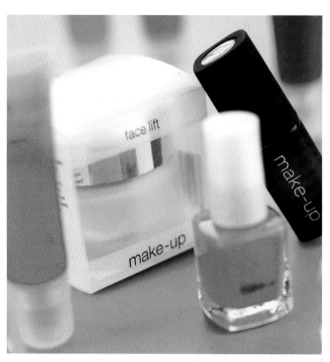

Small, attractive items may prove tempting to a thief

- Have one person, usually the senior therapist or senior receptionist, in control of stock and limit keys and access to stock.

- Do a regular stock check, daily for loss of stock and weekly for stock ordering and rotation.

- Use empty containers for displays, or ask the suppliers if they provide dummy stock – this will also save the product deteriorating while on display.

- Keep displays in locked glass cabinets that can be seen but not touched.

- Encourage staff and customers to keep handbags away from the stock area, usually at reception, to stop products 'dropping' into open bags or supply lockers so they bags can be safely locked away.

- Have one member of staff responsible for topping up the treatment products from the wholesale tubs.

- Hold regular staff training on security and let staff know what the losses are and how it may affect them – some companies offer bonus schemes for reaching targets of both sales and minimising pilfering. Heavy losses may affect potential salary increases.

- Bank money from the till at different times of the day and do not keep too much money in the till at any one time.

- Do not leave the till key in the till if the reception is to be unmanned for any length of time – it is too easy to get into.

Reducing risks for staff

The salon should provide lockable storage cabinets or similar so that personal belongings can be locked away. Handbags and purses are always vulnerable to the opportunist thief, who may look like an ordinary member of the public, come in off the street and be gone in no time with someone's valuables. Large amounts of cash should not be brought into work.

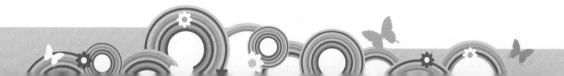

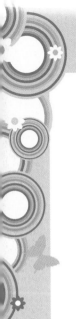

Staff should be discouraged from wearing expensive jewellery to work. This will have to be removed during treatments and is therefore vulnerable to loss or theft.

Large amounts of takings should be removed from the salon daily and put into a bank or night deposit. Avoid taking the same route to the bank at the same time of day. Someone may be watching!

Be very aware of clients' jewellery – let them see that their items of jewellery are placed in a bowl on the trolley and make sure you return them after finishing the treatment. Do not risk being called a thief by slipping them into your overall pocket!

Be aware of suspicious packages left unattended – inform a supervisor and if necessary call the emergency services. The salon should have a list of telephone numbers by the phone in case of emergency, such as the local police station or security guard room. This will save time in an emergency situation.

Make sure you are protected – do not leave outside doors open when working in a treatment room, do not leave the till drawer open and do not be naive enough to think that it could not happen to you! If unsure, seek professional advice from the local crime prevention officer who will be able to advise you on both building security and personal safety hints for staff and clients.

As a professional therapist do not allow yourself to become a victim – follow your professional guidelines:

- Do not treat a male client alone in the salon late at night.
- Always work in pairs, at least on winter evenings.
- Always lock up the premises together.
- Be aware of where you have parked your car. In daylight that alley may look fine, but it may not be in the dark after work.
- Do not walk home alone in the dark – phone a taxi or friend.
- Do not put yourself at risk in any way.

My story

Security conscious

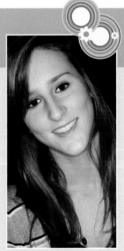

Hi, my name is Amelia and I work in a small salon in the high street, which is quite busy. We get a lot of walk-in customers off the street for treatments. I was just on my way out to do some shopping in my lunch hour when I realised I needed the toilet. I left my handbag and shopping bag on a chair in reception. I was only gone two minutes. During that time the receptionist went into the salon to see a client – and my purse was stolen from my handbag! I just couldn't believe it – it all happened so quickly. I was devastated. I lost my cash, my bank cards and receipts for work, which I needed to claim back, my loyalty cards, which had quite a bit on them, and a lovely photo of my Mum, who died last year. I was as upset about that as much as anything. You can always replace bank cards and I immediately stopped them with my bank so no one could use them – but you never get back the personal things that are irreplaceable, do you?

Health and safety procedures

Fire procedures

The Fire Precaution (Workplace) Regulations 1997 require all premises to undertake a fire risk assessment. If five or more people work together as employees, this risk assessment must be in writing. Employers must also take into account all other persons on the premises, not just employees.

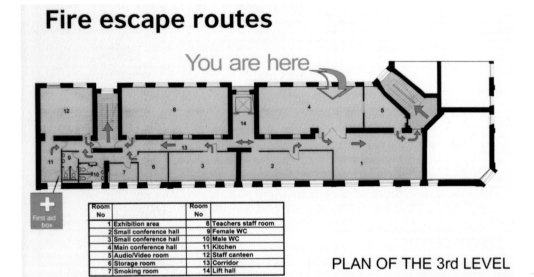

Fire escape routes

You are here

Room No		Room No	
1	Exhibition area	8	Teachers staff room
2	Small conference hall	9	Female WC
3	Small conference hall	10	Male WC
4	Main conference hall	11	Kitchen
5	Audio/Video room	12	Staff canteen
6	Storage room	13	Corridor
7	Smoking room	14	Lift hall

PLAN OF THE 3rd LEVEL

In premises of any kind, staff must be aware of evacuation procedures

There must also be a fire and evacuation procedure. In every period of one year there must be at least one fire drill, which involves everyone. Everyone must be fully informed, instructed and trained in what is expected of them and some people have special duties to perform.

All employees, trainees, temporary workers and others who work in any business must, by law, agree to cooperate with the employer so far as is necessary to enable them to fulfil the duties placed upon them. This means cooperating fully in training courses and fire drills, even when you know it is only a practice.

Most large training establishments will have their own policy on fire evacuation procedures and may carry out a fire drill once a term, that is three times per year. This is especially important with large groups of people or students, and any people with disabilities who will need special consideration.

Many fire-training exercises are organised with a fire safety officer from the local fire station. Often the fire engines will take part in the exercise to test their own attendance time from the station to the premises. Everyone should be made aware of their own particular roles in the evacuation.

When joining any business or establishment the new person should be briefed on all health and safety issues, especially fire evacuation procedures. It is standard practice to include the information in a handbook containing all the establishment's policies.

Unit G20 — Make sure your own actions reduce risks to health and safety

Think about it

Take precautions with all electrical equipment:

- Make sure there are no trailing leads to trip over.
- Carry out regular maintenance checks to ensure machines are working efficiently and safely.
- Follow manufacturers' instructions.
- Follow health and safety guidelines.

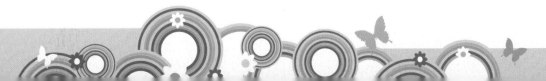

Below is an example of an evacuation procedure.

Building evacuation procedures in the event of fire or bomb alert

The following procedure has been agreed and must be followed. Any staff member who does not comply is committing an infringement of the college disciplinary code. Whenever a fire occurs, the main consideration is to get everybody out of the building safely. Protection of personal or college property is incidental.

Raising the alarm

Anyone discovering a fire must immediately raise the alarm by operating the nearest fire alarm and report to the controller the fire location.

On hearing the alarm the receptionist will immediately contact the emergency services and then evacuate the building.

In the event of a fire being discovered when the reception is unmanned – the premises officer on duty will contact the emergency services and assume control.

On hearing the alarm

All those in senior positions proceed to the control point, normally at a main entrance to the building – where one person must take control of the proceedings.

All other staff: close windows; switch off machinery and lights, and close doors on leaving the room.

Assist less able colleagues, leave the building by the nearest marked route and proceed quickly to the appropriate assembly point. Staff must supervise their class.

Staff evacuating the building must check their locality is clear.

Assembly points

Everyone must remain at assembly points well away from buildings and clear of access roads.

Report to control in person or via two-way radios where allocated.

Everyone must remain at assembly points until further instructions.

DO NOT re-enter the building until you are told it is safe to do so.

An evacuation procedure

Emergency procedures

Fire drill relevant to the working area:

- Switch off all electrical equipment.
- Close all windows.
- Lead clients to a safe area and wrap them up warmly if necessary using blankets and towels. This is especially important when the client has been having a body treatment.
- If possible, take the client's valuable possessions with her, such as her handbag and jewellery, but not if they are safely locked away, or if it puts the client or therapist in any danger (usually clients' belongings are kept under the trolley and therefore are within easy reach).

○ Be aware of the treatment being performed during the evacuation – if the client has chemicals on the skin, it may be easier to remove them immediately. This would need to be at the judgement of the person in charge of the workshop – certainly a client having an eyelash tint will need to have it removed before being able to proceed to the assembly point. Take appropriate remover and damp cotton wool or tissues to remove products on the skin such as facemasks. While it is not dangerous to the skin if left on, the client will probably be more comfortable and the skin less dry if it can be removed.

○ Be aware of the client's footwear, and if possible encourage the wearing of shoes to prevent an accident occurring during the evacuation.

Bomb alert:

○ Follow the procedures for a fire drill.

○ Do not look inside a suspect package but do act quickly if an abandoned parcel or bag arouses suspicions.

Gas leak:

○ Open all windows.

○ Evacuate the building following the fire drill instructions.

○ Do not turn off or on any electrical equipment as it may cause a spark which may ignite the gas.

Sensible fire precautions:

○ Be informed – know what to do and where to go when the evacuation begins.

○ Be sensible and do not panic – this will only make the client feel panicky too.

○ Make sure that the location of the fire bell, fire extinguishers and fire exit are familiar.

○ Never ignore smoke or the smell of burning – it is far better to have a false alarm.

○ Do not misuse or mistreat electrical appliances that are a potential hazard – a healthy respect is needed.

○ Do not ignore manufacturers' instructions for the storage and use of highly flammable products that are very common within the salon.

○ Do be sensible with naked flames and matches or the disposal of cigarette ends – a smouldering tip can burst into flames that will destroy the salon in minutes.

○ Be able to account for clients – the appointment book can be taken outside to check which clients should be present. A college lecturer or trainer should do the same with the class register to check the correct numbers of students are present.

○ Do not use a lift for the evacuation – the fire may affect the electric mechanism which then becomes another emergency.

○ If you are not at the correct location for the fire evacuation, please return to the correct assembly post or you may not be accounted for. This may mean a fire-fighter taking risks to go back into a burning building to check – and all the time you are around the corner!

Unit G20 Make sure your own actions reduce risks to health and safety

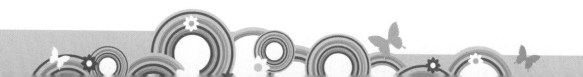

Level 2 Beauty Therapy

Fire-fighting equipment

Not every fire extinguisher is suitable to fight every fire – using the wrong one can make the situation worse.

Only a person specially trained in the use of a fire extinguisher should attempt to use one. Never put yourself at risk. Personal safety is more important than saving material items that can be replaced – a human life cannot be replaced. It is better to evacuate the building and call the fire service than it is to use the wrong extinguisher. Fire service safety leaflets recommend you never endanger life or stay in an area with a fire in an attempt to put it out – it is safer to leave it to the professionals.

In small premises, having one or two portable hand-held extinguishers of the appropriate type readily available may be all that is necessary. In larger, more complex premises larger equipment will be needed, training should be given and the location should be indicated. This is usually in a conspicuous position on an escape route, near the exit doors.

Fires are classified by the type of material that has caught alight. The class of fire determines which fire extinguisher to use.

Class of fire	Fire extinguisher
Class A: Fires involving solid materials, e.g. wood, paper or textiles	Extinguishers with an 'A' rating, e.g. 13A Water extinguisher, foam extinguisher, dry powder extinguisher (size according to risk) Water extinguishers are the cheapest and most widely used, but are not suitable for Class B fires or fires involving electricity
Class B: Fires involving flammable liquids, e.g. petrol, diesel or oils	Extinguishers with a 'B' rating, e.g. 34B Foam extinguisher, CO_2 extinguisher, dry powder extinguisher (size according to risk) Foam extinguishers are more expensive than water, but can be used on both Class A and Class B fires
Class C: Fires involving flammable gases, e.g. propane, butane	Foam extinguisher (according to risk). Seek specialist advice Dry powder extinguishers are multi-purpose and can be used on Classes A, B and C fires. However, they can obscure vision
Class D: Fires involving metals	Special powder extinguishers (size and type according to risk), dry sand (quantity according to risk). Seek specialist advice
Class E: Fires involving electrical apparatus	CO_2 extinguisher
Class F: Fires in cooking appliances, e.g. oil	Extinguishers with an 'F' rating, e.g. 15F Wet chemical extinguisher

Water with additive
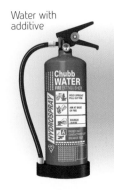

Foam
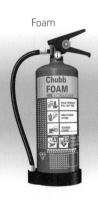

Powder
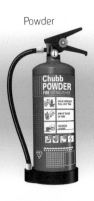

CO² gas
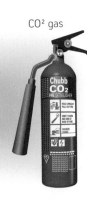

Different types of fire extinguisher

A quick guide to selecting an extinguisher:

Type of fire	Type of extinguisher	Colour	Uses	NOT to be used
Electrical fires	Dry powder	Blue marking	For burning liquid, electrical fires and flammable liquids	On flammable metal fires
	Carbon dioxide	Black marking	Safe on all voltages, used on burning liquid and electrical fires and flammable liquids	On flammable metal fires
Non-electrical fires	Water	Red marking	For wood, paper, textiles, fabric and similar materials	On burning liquid, electrical or flammable metal fires
	Foam	Cream/yellow markings	On burning liquid fires	On electrical or flammable metal fires

Fire blankets are made of fire resistant material and are intended to extinguish cooking oil fires or to wrap around a person whose clothing is on fire. A fire blanket must be used calmly and with a firm grip. If the blanket is flapped about, it may fan the fire and make it flare up, rather than put it out. The hands should be protected by the edge of the cloth and the blanket should be placed, rather than thrown, into the desired position.

Never lean over the fire. Remember – if you cannot control the fire, leave the room, close the door and phone the emergency services.

Fire blankets conforming to British Standard BS 6575 are suitable for use in the home. These will be marked to show whether they should be thrown away after use or used again after cleaning in accordance with the manufacturer's instructions. Fire blankets are best kept in the kitchen or in the salon rest room, where there are likely to be domestic appliances such as kettles, microwaves and cookers, and where small fires can occur.

A bucket of sand can be used to soak up liquids that are the source of a minor fire. However, it is impractical to have large quantities of sand available to try to stop a major fire, so the instructions would be the same as for fire blankets – if in doubt never risk injury.

First aid

The Health and Safety (First Aid) Regulations 1981 set out the essential aspects of first aid that employers must address, because people at work can suffer injuries or fall ill. It does not matter whether the injury or illness is caused by the work they do. It is important that they receive immediate attention and that an ambulance is called in serious cases.

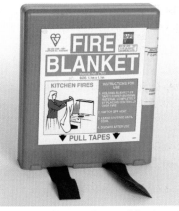

A fire blanket can be used for smothering a fire

First aid can save lives and prevent minor injuries becoming major ones. First aid in the workplace is the initial management of any injury or illness suffered at work. It does not include giving tablets or medicines to treat illness. This means that sufficient first aid personnel and facilities should be available to:

- give immediate assistance to casualties with both common injuries and illnesses and those likely to arise from specific hazards at work
- summon an ambulance or other professional help.

This will depend upon the size of the workforce, the type of workplace hazards and risks, and the history of accidents in the workplace.

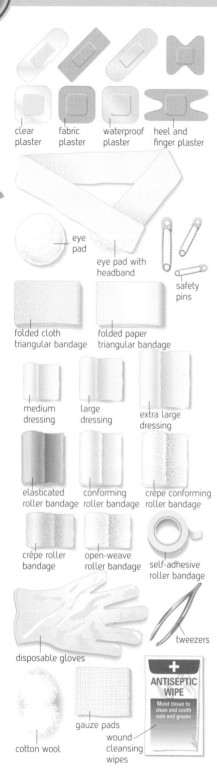

clear plaster · **fabric plaster** · **waterproof plaster** · **heel and finger plaster**

eye pad

eye pad with headband

safety pins

folded cloth triangular bandage · **folded paper triangular bandage**

medium dressing · **large dressing** · **extra large dressing**

elasticated roller bandage · **conforming roller bandage** · **crêpe conforming roller bandage**

crêpe roller bandage · **open-weave roller bandage** · **self-adhesive roller bandage**

disposable gloves

tweezers

cotton wool · **gauze pads** · **wound cleansing wipes**

ANTISEPTIC WIPE
Moist tissue to clean and sooth cuts and grazes

Items that your first aid box should contain

Two aspects of first aid need further consideration:

○ Trainees – students undertaking work experience on certain training schemes are given the same status as employees and therefore are the responsibility of the employer.

○ The public – when dealing with the public these regulations do not oblige employers to provide first aid for anyone other than their own employees. This means the compulsory element of public liability insurance does not cover litigation resulting from first aid to non-employees. Employers should make extra provision for this themselves. Education establishments must also include the general public in their assessment of first aid requirements.

First aid kits

The minimum level of first aid equipment is a suitably stocked and properly identified first aid container.

First aid containers should be easily accessible and placed, where possible, near to hand-washing facilities. The number of containers will depend upon the size of the establishment, and the total number of employees in that area. The container should protect the items inside from dust and damp and must only be stocked with useful items. Tablets and medications should not be kept in there.

There is no compulsory list of what a first aid kit should contain, but the following would be useful:

○ a leaflet giving general guidance on first aid (such as the HSE leaflet 'Basic advice on first aid at work')

○ 20 individually wrapped sterile adhesive dressings (assorted sizes) appropriate to the type of work

○ two sterile eye pads

○ four individually wrapped triangular bandages (preferably sterile)

○ six safety pins

○ six medium-sized individually wrapped wound dressings

○ two large sterile individually wrapped unmedicated wound dressings

○ one pair of disposable gloves

○ antiseptic cream or liquid

○ eye bath

○ gauze

○ medical wipes

○ a pair of tweezers

○ cotton wool.

Do not forget that if in doubt, do not treat – phone for an ambulance immediately.

First aid training

First aid certificates are only valid for a certain period of time, which is currently three years. Employers need to arrange refresher training with retesting of competence before certificates expire. If a certificate expires, the individual will have to undertake a full course of training to be re-established as a first aider. Specialist training can also be undertaken if necessary.

Records

It is good practice for employers to provide first aiders with a book in which to record incidents which require their attendance. If there are several first aiders in one establishment, then a central book will be used. The information should include:

○ date, time and place of incident

○ name and job of the injured or ill person

○ details of the injury or illness and what first aid was given

○ what action was taken immediately afterward (e.g. did the person go home, go to hospital, get sent in an ambulance)

○ name and signature of the first aider or person dealing with the incident.

> **Think about it**
>
> A first aid kit should be kept in a proper first aid container – an old biscuit tin will not do. It needs to be regularly checked to keep it fully stocked. You shouldn't be finding out that your kit is not fully stocked during an emergency!

Check your knowledge

1 Who is responsible for ensuring gloves and an apron are worn during waxing treatments?
 a) Salon manager
 b) Client
 c) Therapist
 d) Salon owner

2 A hazard is defined as:
 a) something that will harm you
 b) something that will kill you
 c) something which has the potential to cause harm
 d) the risk you take at work.

3 The two fire extinguishers suitable for use on any electrical fire are colour coded:
 a) blue or black
 b) red and cream
 c) blue and red
 d) black and cream.

4 Which of these is just the employer's responsibility?
 a) Report faulty goods or equipment.
 b) Wear protective clothing or work wear.
 c) Provide information about health and safety and security.
 d) Take care to ensure the health and safety of others.

5 The definition of a risk is:
 a) the likelihood of a hazard's potential being realised
 b) the risk of an accident occurring
 c) the elimination of an accident occurring
 d) the potential to cause harm.

6 Your job description should have within it:
 a) your national insurance number
 b) your driving licence
 c) your health and safety responsibilities
 d) your qualifications listed.

7 The symbol for a toxic substance is:
 a) a big red cross
 b) a big black cross
 c) a skull and cross bones
 d) a flame.

8 If there are blood spots on a wax strip, you must:
 a) wrap it in newspaper and put it in the bin
 b) put it in a bin liner and put it in the dustbin
 c) put it in the contaminated yellow waste bin
 d) take it to the hospital for disposal.

9 How many steps are there in a risk assessment?
 a) Ten
 b) Six
 c) Five
 d) Eleven

10 HSE stands for:
 a) Housing Standard Economy
 b) Health and Safety Executive
 c) Health and Safety Election
 d) Human Safety Executive.

Unit G20

Make sure your own actions reduce risks to health and safety

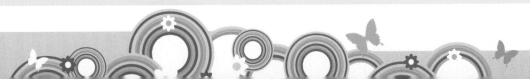

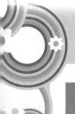

Getting ready for assessment

The first part of Unit G20 requires that you identify the hazards and evaluate the risks in your workplace and gather evidence to support your work such as:

- Take part in an evacuation procedure following all the guidelines safely. This will have to be a simulation as hopefully the building will not actually be on fire! Keep a log or diary of the date, time and exactly what happened, and the assessor will accept this as evidence.

- Attend a health and safety training day as part of your job role outside college. A formal letter from your part-time employer confirming that you attended the training day, dated and signed, will also provide evidence. It may be an accident procedure demonstration, a risk assessment training day or a training day covering maintenance of equipment. This will ensure your performance criteria — what you must do — will be covered.

- You should be able to show you can identify the possible risks of your own working practices. This means you should immediately report a spillage in the salon, a frayed wire, a faulty piece of equipment or a blocked fire exit. You could be in the middle of a facial assessment when you notice the wire to the steamer, which you are about to use, is a potential risk. Follow the set procedures for reporting it, and you will have an assessment for both Units G20 and B4.

In the second part of Unit G20 you must show you have taken steps to reduce any possible health and safety risks within your own job role/responsibilities. Any of the following duties will count towards an assessment:

- If, during the course of your reception duties, your job is to decant products from large wholesale tubs into smaller ones for use by other therapists, then make sure all labelling is correct, the storage is suitable for the product and that the COSHH sheets are up to date. By volunteering to check these details you will collect evidence for both Units G20 and G4.

- If you are designated salon manager for a day, volunteer to carry out a risk assessment on the working salon. As well as organising equipment and matching clients to therapists, look at equipment, working stations and staff with a critical eye. Are there any improvements that could be made to minimise risk? Are staff as vigilant as they could be?

- Look at the bigger picture outside the working stations. Even a light bulb blowing out could be a risk if it illuminates a stairway. Report it, minimise the risk, identify the solution. This will ensure your performance criteria will be covered.

- Be inventive. Are there risk assessment solutions that you use in your place of work that would help you at college? For example, a better design of record cards with allergy or medical conditions highlighted, better storage facilities or a particular training programme that you would recommend? Write up a proposal — the assessor can then investigate it and if it minimises risk, this will ensure your performance criteria will be covered.

Think about it

Advice is available from the Health and Safety Executive.

Unit G18

Promote additional services or products to clients

What you will learn

G18.1 Identify additional services or products that are available

G18.2 Inform clients about additional services or products

G18.3 Gain client commitment to using additional services or products

Introduction

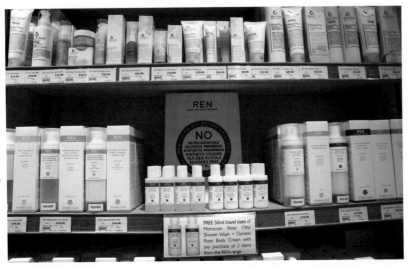

You can help the client benefit from a range of services or products

This unit looks at the backbone of any successful beauty therapy business — customer service and meeting clients' needs and expectations in terms of both product use and beauty therapy services. Keeping the client informed about all the possible treatments and products available within your salon is vitally important. Not only is it enlightening for the client, allowing her to make informed choices, but it is also essential if your business is to survive in a very competitive market.

Nowadays, supermarkets, local chemists and high street shops sell both skin care and make-up products, so people can purchase without a therapist on hand to guide them through their needs. This is a very competitive market and when you start work in the beauty industry your employer will set you targets for sales and for increasing your client base. No business can afford the luxury of standing still — to do so would mean losing out to the competition.

Clients are more informed about what is available on the market and because of extensive media coverage of treatments, beauty editors are more aware of salon treatments: this combined with celebrity endorsements of brands, makes beauty therapy a very competitive arena. Why should your client stay with you for treatments and buy products from the salon? The answer is: Because you are knowledgeable, caring and offer a more personal service with prescriptive skin care than an over-the-counter store can!

For your portfolio

Celebrity endorsements for products are big business for both skincare and haircare products. Some are genuine and the celebrities are paid to promote the products; others are linked to products in a more subtle way: the celebrity photo is placed on the page with a product, diet or lifestyle, which encourages the reader to believe that the celebrity is using the product. Have a look at both a genuine advertising campaign and one of association, and write up a critique: would the celebrity sell the product to you? Ask family and friends. Does the power of fame link the subject of the advert to the person so strongly that the client feels that if they use the product, they will actually have the same super stardom? Name two examples of such products. What makes the advert so attractive?

One of the few negative comments that salon owners make about employing newly trained therapists is that the therapists do not feel confident enough to 'sell' themselves and the products or services available to the clients. Students feel embarrassed or frightened of what they perceive as pushing themselves upon the client.

This unit will help you feel differently about the promotional side of the beauty therapy business. Don't think of it as selling in the formal sense of the word – it is more to do with helping the client gain as much as she can from her range of treatments. It really is mutually beneficial for the salon and the client if the client can make fully informed decisions on the basis of what exactly is available. The client will then be able to maximise the treatment potential with the use of complementary products.

As consumers, we all want the very best deal we can find. We not only want value for money, we also want to make sure our purchases are the most suitable for our needs and budget. We also want to know that we have been given the best advice, rather than feeling that we have been sold to and that we really don't matter as long as the sale is made. The old saying 'Buy cheap – buy twice' is certainly true with lots of items, and no one wants to buy something that falls to pieces the moment you start to use it. There is a balance to be struck between price, quality and suitability of any purchase. The client will feel so much better about their purchases if they feel supported by expert advice and guidance of how to use the products correctly, and that they have bought exactly what they need for their skin.

Benefits for the client:

- ⭘ informs the client of what is best for her
- ⭘ offers a personal service and makes the client feel valued as a customer
- ⭘ empowers the client to make informed decisions about her products and treatments
- ⭘ brings out the best of her salon treatments by continuing good skin care at home.

Benefits for the therapist:

- ⭘ helps her to focus on the needs of the client and identify what is best for her
- ⭘ increases her interest in the client and builds up a rapport
- ⭘ develops knowledge and additional training
- ⭘ promotes and increases experience and personal development
- ⭘ boosts salon income through **sales**.

Identify additional services or products that are available

> **In this outcome you will learn about:**
>
> - updating and developing your knowledge of your salon's services or products
> - checking with others when you are unsure of new service or product details
> - identifying appropriate services or products that may interest your client
> - spotting opportunities for offering your client additional services or products that will improve their client experience

> **Think about it**
>
> Promoting products and services isn't purely about selling – it involves recommending the best for your client and doing this will become second nature to you. Not only will the client gain more from her salon treatments if she is using the right homecare, but it will help maintain her skin between visits. You will be cutting the benefit of her treatments in half if she is not using good skin care at home.

> **Key terms**
>
> **Sales** – revenue from the sale of goods and services.

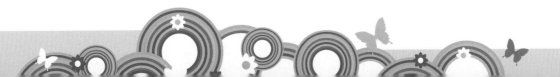

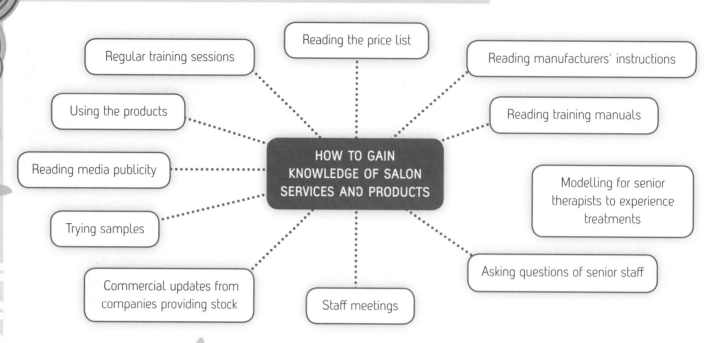

Regular training sessions

Using the products

Reading media publicity

Trying samples

Commercial updates from companies providing stock

Reading the price list

Staff meetings

HOW TO GAIN KNOWLEDGE OF SALON SERVICES AND PRODUCTS

Reading manufacturers' instructions

Reading training manuals

Modelling for senior therapists to experience treatments

Asking questions of senior staff

Key terms

Salon services – range of professional treatments and activities available in a beauty salon or spa.

Updating and developing your knowledge of your salon's services or products

There are many ways to ensure that as a new therapist in your salon you are able to identify additional **salon services** and products:

Knowledge is the key to being able to offer advice and guidance to clients; you must know what you are talking about, and you should never make up what you don't know! Insincerity can be spotted a mile away. Should you guess, make something up about a treatment or lie about it, your advice may be unsafe. You will lose the respect of the client and your credibility will be in tatters. Professionalism should be the theme running throughout your training, and integrity plays a big part in this. Integrity means being honest, acting with honour, and being reliable and truthful in all that you do.

Knowledge allows you to fulfil your entire professional obligation to your client. Ignorance is not an excuse for losing a client or her interest in other treatments. Just because you personally do not do the treatment, or have not yet trained in a certain skill area, does not mean you cannot discuss it with your client. Don't guess or recommend a treatment you are not yet qualified to carry out – realise the limits of your own authority, and be sensible. Find the right person to advise the client, even if it means making a separate consultation with the senior therapist or specialist within the salon. This will be seen as an investment in time rather than a waste of time.

Working with others to ensure your information is up to date

Be proactive in your learning about the services and products that your salon offers.

You need to be aware of your salon's procedures and systems for the use of additional services and products. Speak to your line manager about the expectations for sales and marketing and how you can 'learn and earn' by recommending to clients further services and, even if you cannot yet use them, products.

Learning opportunities within the job include:

- attending training sessions – in house and with external companies
- promotional work – designing a course of treatments suitable for a wedding, summer holiday, etc.
- making a presentation and giving it to the other staff in your salon
- acting as a spokesperson for the salon
- writing a report on the benefits of a treatment for the local paper for additional publicity
- learning the price list or designing a new one
- visiting a supplier to keep up to date with new launches
- spending the day with the salesperson
- showing people around the salon
- stocktaking.

Learning opportunities to be gained by extending your job role include:

- standing in for a receptionist/senior therapist
- shadowing/work experience
- job sharing
- job rotation
- modelling for treatments at demonstrations
- taking part in open evenings at your salon
- attending open evenings at other salons
- watching the experts in action
- applying for extra training courses.

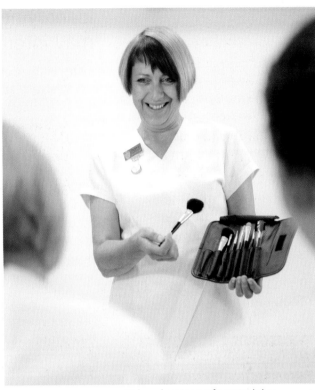

Take advantage of any training opportunities

Think about it

Recommending products is all about timing and when within the treatment plan to start. Always have eye contact, so you know the client is listening and understanding what you are saying. During a relaxing facial massage is not the time to do it – you will just spoil the treatment and irritate the client!

Think about it

If you have difficulties in remembering what the benefits are of a treatment or product, then make up some flash cards, about the size of a postcard, and list the key points of the service or product. Not only will writing these down help your memory, it will be a good way of doing some revision – if you have a quiet time on reception, you can look through your notes, so that you are fully informed when you take the client through it.

Checking with others when you are unsure of new service or product details

Seeking help and asking questions of others with more experience than you should never be seen as a weakness – quite the opposite. Within the salon there is a wealth of experience and knowledge. Checking with others will ensure your information is correct and give you wisdom, which you, in turn, can pass on. (Refer to Unit G8 Develop and maintain your effectiveness at work, pages 123–48 for other ideas on how to increase your knowledge base and how to learn from others.)

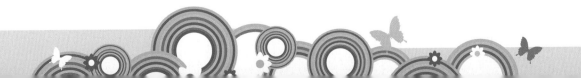

Think about it

Try grouping similar products together for the client's benefit so they are aware the products match, for example cleanser, toner, moisturiser, or day and night cream. This is known as link selling.

Identifying appropriate services or products that may interest your client

With a little experience and knowledge of the products and salon treatments, you will be able to advise your client about services and products that will suit her needs, budget and lifestyle. For example, if your client comes regularly for a facial but just cleanses her skin using soap and water and no moisturiser, she would definitely benefit from using homecare products – she will soon see and feel the difference these make to the skin's condition.

It is important that you match up client needs to the correct product, so that the products work and the client will benefit. We have all had impulse buys and then not used or worn them: the therapist must be sufficiently well informed to be able to advise and instruct the client that she does *need* and will *use* the products. You should always have the client's best interests at heart and should be genuinely interested in improving her skincare – it is not about making a quick sale and your personal gain.

Use your intuition when discussing additional services or products, just as if you were talking to an old friend. Develop an insight into what to mention to different clients and which treatment or product would be most beneficial. Tread carefully – going through the whole price list and reciting every single treatment the client could have can be overwhelming and put her off. If the choice is too large, she may become confused or deterred by the costs or time involved. Being aware of her constraints, such as time and budget, will help you make an informed choice about what to recommend. The client may not have the time to come in every week for a manicure, or she may only be able to afford a monthly manicure. However, her contribution to keeping her nails in good condition may be as simple as wearing gloves to do the housework and using a basecoat and a hand cream nightly.

My story

Getting enthusiastic about products

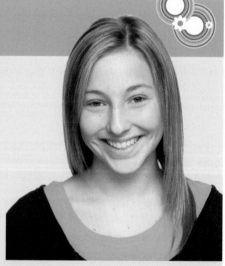

Hi, my name is Vanya and I am a Level 2 Beauty Therapist. I have just completed a commercial certificate in facial products with my group, as we use and sell them in our client workshops. I feel so much more confident now about what I am telling customers, and I really think the system of face mapping for the skin analysis is good. We were all given the "book" which is their training manual and because I knew we were going to have a test at the end of the training, I really swotted up and read it every chance I got. Having a good knowledge base now of all the creams and their benefits and features was very good for my selling skills: I never let a client leave the salon now without giving a sample of something, and it works – they do come back and buy it! Really, it is so good and I believe in it, that all I am doing is recommending what I know is right – it sort of sells itself!

We were given samples to try and I have passed some of mine on to my sister, who is suffering with a few spots at the moment. She wants to buy the products and so does my mum. It's amazing what a bit of training and knowledge can do – I am top of the chart for retail sales at the moment. Every month we have a prize for the best-selling therapist and I want to win it, so that I can give the products to my mum.

For your portfolio

Look at the additional products or services your training establishment offers. Do you use them in your salon workshop session with clients? Pick one additional product or extra treatment (e.g. thermal booties, a hand mask, a foot scrub) and introduce it to three clients in the next session. Don't view it as trying to make a sale; treat it more as an information exercise. Talk to the clients about the benefits, and what a difference they will see to their feet/hands/face. Be informed and enthusiastic! Check if any of the clients books in for the treatment and make a note of it on your treatment sheet for the client or record card. If the clients aren't aware of lovely pampering treatments, they cannot book them!

Spotting opportunities for offering your client additional services or products

Spotting opportunities for offering clients additional products or services is easy if you are receptive and have your ears and eyes open. Very often they will ask. Either they have heard about a treatment from another client, or they see something going on that they want to know more about. A special day or occasion will trigger extra interest, such as a wedding, a party, a holiday or a Christmas function. (Refer to Professional basics, pages 31–35, for further questioning techniques to use during your consultation.)

In the salon, there are many opportunities to discuss the range of services and products on offer. In particular, treatments such as manicures, pedicures and waxing, where there is time to talk and lots of eye contact between therapist and client, are ideal and can lead so well into other treatments. Here are a few possible links:

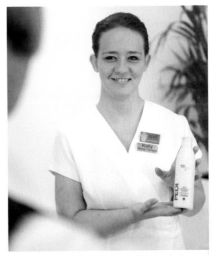

Use your product knowledge to help the client buy appropriate products

Treatment	Possible links to suggest
Manicure	Deluxe manicure, hot oil cuticle treatment, matching pedicure, nail varnish or treatment purchases, e.g. nail strengtheners, base coat, top coat Arm wax, paraffin wax
Pedicure	As above. Leg waxing, massage
Leg waxing	Full leg waxing, bikini and intimate waxing, pedicures, massage
Facials	Eyelash tinting, perming, eyebrow shaping or waxing Makeover or make-up lesson Steam treatment or hot oil mask with infrared lamp Electrical facials, Level 3 treatments: microdermabrasion, galvanic facials or non-surgical face lifting (although you are not yet trained in these areas, that should not stop you recommending them, or being knowledgeable about them!)

Other opportunities may arise from:

- the client looking at the product display at reception
- the client asking about a particular product that she has heard about or seen in the media
- the client observing another treatment as she is walking through the salon, e.g. nail extensions

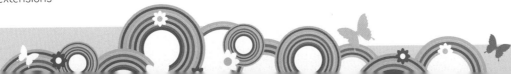

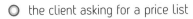

- the client asking for a price list
- a friend recommending a particular treatment
- an open evening or promotional demonstration creating interest
- a commercial company holding a training day for which you request your favourite clients to model.

Use all of these openings as a chance to inform, educate and offer your clients the best products and services for their needs.

> ### Think about it
>
> A very easy and effective way to gain additional clients is through word-of-mouth advertising. Once you have a good recommendation from a satisfied client, her friends are going to want to know all about it, and will want to come in for themselves!

Key terms

Seasonal promotions – special offers that change throughout the year and are based on a season, an occasion or specific time such as Mother's Day, Valentine's Day, Christmas presents, summer pampering.

Seasonal promotions

Promotions are an excellent way for the salon to create interest in products and services. It is important to look at the whole year and to plan ahead so that no opportunity is missed. The calendar offers a number of sales opportunities.

Season	Promotional activity or discount to offer
Spring	Mother's Day – gift vouchers for treatments and pampering sessions Get ready for summer – leg waxing, fake-tan application and pedicures Slimming programmes and treatments for the summer
Summer	Bikini bodies – waxing, tanning and pedicures Matching manicure and pedicure in the new season's colours French manicures on tanned toes Hen parties – pamper sessions, a day out for everyone with lovely treatments Wedding packages – bride and mother-of-bride pamper days
Autumn	Get ready for the Christmas party season with a make-up lesson Birthday treats – gift vouchers Repair the signs of the sun with a course of soothing facials Bonfire night party – come and learn how to look glamorous Halloween – face painting available for children: become a witch or a warlock for the night!
Winter	Christmas parties – make-up and manicure treatments Christmas gift vouchers Avoid winter problems that cold does to the skin with a warming and relaxing facial

For your portfolio

Put together a proposal for a promotion in your training establishment. Have a look at the time of year and what is coming up, or is there a special charity you would like to contribute to by setting up a pamper day and advertising it? Think about what you would need. How would you advertise it and where? What are the health and safety/risk assessments? How could you make it a success? Be thorough and think the whole thing through: would you have enough therapists, staff and products to make the promotion a success? Put it to your tutors – if they agree, you could run it and make it a great event!

Inform clients about additional services or products

In this outcome you will learn about:

- choosing the most appropriate time to inform your client about additional services or products
- choosing the most appropriate method of communication to introduce your clients to additional services or products
- giving your client accurate and sufficient information to enable them to make a decision about the additional services or products
- giving your client time to ask questions about the additional services or products

Choosing the most appropriate time and method of communication

You will need to pick the right moment to communicate with the client. This should be when you have good eye contact with her, not when she is trying to relax with eye pads and a face mask on, or when she is running late and trying to get dressed. This will only irritate the client and she will not be interested. The consultation is always a good time to ask lots of questions, and some treatments lend themselves better to chatting than others — manicures, pedicures and waxing give a lot of opportunity as the client is your captive audience!

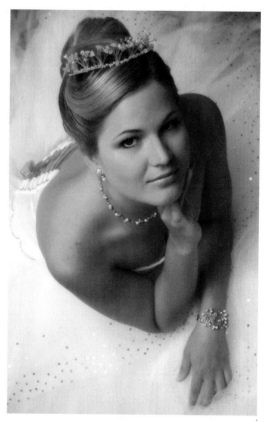

You will also need to be able to communicate easily with your clients if you are to let them know about the services and products offered by the salon. If the client does not understand you, then she will not be listening fully to your recommendations. You should have enough accurate and detailed information to help her make decisions. This will also help you to build up a good rapport so that the client feels able to ask questions about how and when to use the products you are suggesting.

Open questions will help draw out the client's needs. These could include:

- How long is it until the wedding/party/holiday? Do you feel ready? What can we do to make you feel more fully prepared?

- Have you read about our special bridal top-to-toe package? How do you want to look on your big day?

- What are your worries about your party? What are you wearing? How can we help you?

- Have you seen any pictures of how you would like to look, as a guide for make-up, eyebrow shape and nails?

- Do you have any particular concerns about your skin/nails that we can help with?

If your client is getting married soon, she may wish to find out more about bridal make-up

For a full explanation of open and closed questions, refer to Professional Basics, pages 31–33. You will need these skills to identify the needs of your clients and to communicate fully with them — you cannot guess what they want or need! Also see Professional basics, pages 16–24, for more information on communication and aftercare advice.

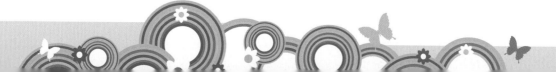

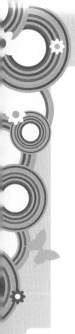

Pointing out options

If the client does not ask directly, it could be she is shy about asking, or does not know you offer a certain treatment. Tell her all about it — and use the current treatment to start the discussion. The consultation always provides a good opening to talk through alternative options to the client's normal treatments. Below are some examples:

'Did you know that an eyebrow wax is great for giving a clean finish to the shape and lasts a long time? I know you have booked in for an eyebrow tidy with tweezers next week.'

'I notice your skin is very dry on your feet. How about a pedicure and warm paraffin treatment to soften and moisturise the skin? We have a special offer on at the moment.'

'For your honeymoon, why not have a French manicure finish on your toes to match your manicure. It looks lovely with tanned feet and open-toed sandals.'

By providing the link to additional treatments, you are not introducing lots of different options all at once. The client will be pleased to receive any suggestions related to her big event or particular concern. She will be pleased you are taking such an interest (which you are) and will not view it as an intrusion or a hard-selling technique (which it is not).

Remember to pick the best form of communication, too. The client may not have time for a long chat about aftercare and sales; instead, a brochure or a handwritten list of suggested products and how and when to use them gives her something to refer to later on, when she has more time. If the client is in a hurry to get back to work, she may feel rushed and not show much interest. However, a sample used may make her think about how good the results are and encourage her to return to you for more advice and purchasing. Verbal communication may be forgotten, but a brochure/leaflet/pamphlet or sample won't.

Giving your client accurate and sufficient information

Do try to be as accurate as you can when giving information. Not only is your professional reputation at stake but you also have a legal obligation not to give any false or misleading information to the client. As a consumer, your client has legal rights to protect her, and you, or your salon, will be liable for prosecution if found to be in breach of the law.

Not only that, you will lose your clients very quickly if they have no faith in the information you are giving them, and if the products you recommend are unsuitable for their needs. If you give clients the right information, you will help them to make an informed decision and ensure they trust your ability and the salon.

Salon and legal requirements

Underpinning all the product knowledge and treatment skills you have to pass on to your clients are the legal aspects of promotion, selling and client and consumer rights. (Refer to 'You, your client and the law' in Professional basics, pages 48–68.)

Think about it

It is essential that you do not give misleading information, directly or by implication. In all your promotional activities you must always protect your client, yourself and the salon's reputation.

The specific laws relevant to this unit are:

- ○ Health and Safety at Work Act 1974
- ○ Consumer Protection Act 1987
- ○ The Cosmetic Products (Safety) Regulations 2003
- ○ Trade Descriptions Act 1968
- ○ Sale of Goods Act 1979
- ○ Sale and Supply of Goods Act 1994
- ○ Supply of Goods and Services Act 1982.

Refer to Unit G4 Fulfil salon reception duties (pages 157–58) for information on dealing with clients with special needs.

As a professional, you need to work within the guidelines of your industry and code of practice. (Refer to Professional basics, pages 66–68, for further information.)

Giving your client time to ask questions

It is important to give the client the time to ask questions, so choose an appropriate moment to discuss her queries. During a treatment is fine if it is one where you can maintain a conversation and have lots of eye contact. A manicure, pedicure or waxing is ideal for this, as the client is awake, upright and alert. Talking during a facial will detract from the quality of the treatment and all relaxation properties will be lost. Do not pick moments when the client is distracted, that is when she is trying to get dressed or pay for her treatment. Where possible, keep the question and answer session quiet and confidential – not everyone in the salon should hear about her future bikini wax! It is important to hold the client's attention and focus entirely on her questions. This will give her the confidence of knowing that your suggestions really are in her best interests.

Gain client commitment to using additional services or products

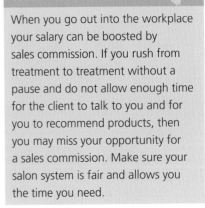

Think about it

When you go out into the workplace your salary can be boosted by sales commission. If you rush from treatment to treatment without a pause and do not allow enough time for the client to talk to you and for you to recommend products, then you may miss your opportunity for a sales commission. Make sure your salon system is fair and allows you the time you need.

In this outcome you will learn about:

- closing the discussion appropriately if your client shows no interest
- giving relevant information to move the situation forward when your client shows interest
- securing client agreement and checking client understanding of the delivery of the service or product
- taking action to ensure prompt delivery of the additional services or products to your client
- refer your client to others or to alternative sources of information if the additional services or products are not your responsibility.

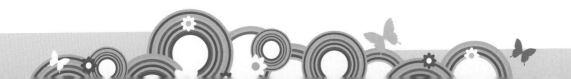

When promoting additional services or products you will need to be able to judge client commitment, how much time she has, even if she is interested in purchasing or not. You cannot force the client into something she does not want. With experience you will be able to close the discussion informally if she shows no interest or is in a hurry to leave — you cannot chase after her with products that she doesn't want to buy!

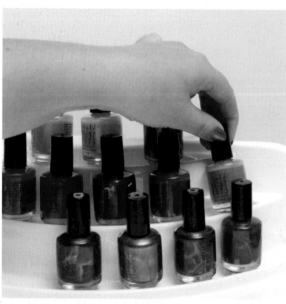

When you recommend a product, be clear whether it is in stock

Closing the discussion if the client shows no interest

While it's important to give time and enthusiasm to the client's enquiries, it's also just as important to know when to stop if she shows no interest. If the feedback from the client is minimal, or she says 'No thanks, not just at this moment', then take your cue and stop. Nothing is more irritating to the client than a hard sales pitch; you will lose her altogether if you come across as pushy.

As a double check, ask yourself the following questions:

- Am I giving the relevant information for my client's particular needs?
- Am I explaining myself clearly, or am I confusing the client?
- Am I being too technical in my explanation?
- Have I chosen a good time to give advice?

My story

A snap judgement

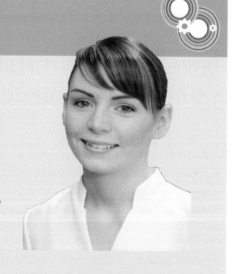

Hi, my name is Sophie and I have a story that I am rather ashamed of, but it is a valuable learning curve for us all, so I feel it needs to be told!

I was at the reception desk when a scruffily dressed lady walked in. She was wearing old clothes and had bad hands — torn cuticles, cuts and very dry skin. The lady wanted some products to help her hands. She told me, 'I want to look a little more decent, as I have a lunch in London to attend and I have been doing a lot of gardening.' I was rather offhand as she wasn't one of my regular clients and didn't look well groomed. Without much enthusiasm, I offered her hand cream and cuticle oil but did not suggest a manicure later in the week when the cuts had healed over. I am ashamed to say I didn't pay her much attention as I was sure she couldn't afford very much.

The client agreed to pay for the recommended items and handed over her credit card. She turned out to be the owner of a large estate and had been getting her huge garden ready to receive the summer crowds who visit the estate. She also dropped into the conversation that her lunch was at Buckingham Palace! Needless to say, I soon realised my mistake and tried to rectify my not-so-kind attitude. The lady was very gracious and did become a regular client in the salon. I felt like a complete fool — not because she would have spent a lot of money but because I had made a really snap judgement and was not very professional. Who am I to judge a client, just because her hands were in bad condition through lots of gardening?

Review your techniques to answer the above questions satisfactorily.

○ Try to make the information relevant to the client's needs.

○ Make your explanation of the treatment or product crystal clear.

○ Avoid being too technical — explain the benefits of the product, not the way it works.

○ Stop the conversation if necessary and choose a better time to discuss the client's needs — this will show her that you are aware of her time constraints.

If a client is not interested in a treatment, it may be because she does not have the time to discuss it, because she cannot afford it or because the treatment just does not appeal to her. Knowing when to back off and stop giving information is essential to maintaining good communication.

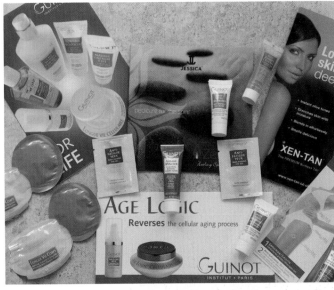

Be ready to show clients a range of products and/or leaflets

Not judging your client

Do not prejudge what your client may want or what she can afford. Until you open up clear lines of communication and discuss this with her, you do not know how best to help her, whether she can afford a course of treatment or how much she already knows. While we all tend to judge one another within a few seconds of meeting, it is certainly not up to you to judge a client's financial state and decide what she can or cannot afford. Do not underestimate a client's commitment to the treatments — it is not up to you to decide that your client does or does not have the time, money or inclination to attend her appointments.

Moving the situation forward when the client shows interest

A client will indicate that she agrees with your recommendations in several ways. She may:

○ book an appointment for the recommended treatments

○ purchase the suggested products

○ book a consultation

○ order a product if not in stock

○ put a deposit on a course of treatments

○ buy a gift voucher.

Be guided by the client. Once she has made up her mind, the client will clearly indicate the route you should take: escort her to the till or to the receptionist who will book her follow-up appointment, or fill out the purchase order for whatever product she is having. If the item is not in stock, make it quite clear at the beginning — this will avoid disappointment and she will keep her faith in you. Try not to recommend a product and then backtrack and suggest an alternative once you realise that you do not have the item in stock. That is not fair to the client and it will put you in a bad light — it looks as though you are only after her money, rather than providing the best possible product or service for her.

> **Think about it**
>
> The way to close the discussion is to offer some literature, such as a price list or a leaflet. Always make sure your client has samples and promotional materials if you are about to offer a special price or discount.

Promoting existing treatments and products

New treatments and products are always easy to recommend to the client. You may have had training in their use, had the treatment yourself, seen the excellent results and be brimming over with excitement and enthusiasm. This becomes infectious and soon the cash registers are ringing and stock is moving very quickly.

But what about existing services and products? They may be seen as old hat, or just boring and regular, and your excitement for all the new products only reinforces that. There is a danger that the standard treatments, which are still very trustworthy and beneficial, get overlooked.

It is worth revisiting the price list to see what treatments or products have not been recommended very often recently. A paraffin wax incorporated into a manicure and pedicure has lots of pamper appeal to someone who has never had one before but can easily be overlooked if you consider it to be bordering on the mundane.

Key terms

Feature – the attractive aspects of a product, e.g. its anti-ageing properties, designed for dry or oily skins

Benefit – the advantages of a product or what the product is doing for the skin, e.g. exfoliator, deep cleanser

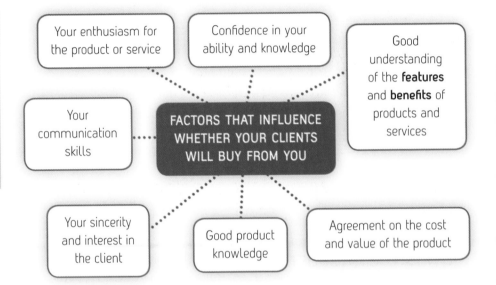

- Your enthusiasm for the product or service
- Confidence in your ability and knowledge
- Good understanding of the **features** and **benefits** of products and services
- Your communication skills
- **FACTORS THAT INFLUENCE WHETHER YOUR CLIENTS WILL BUY FROM YOU**
- Your sincerity and interest in the client
- Good product knowledge
- Agreement on the cost and value of the product

Least-used treatments and products

A very useful exercise is to do a 'favourites' chart of treatments carried out in the last month. Often a pattern emerges – a therapist may have a favourite treatment or product and always recommend that, rather than other options. Does the top therapist's pattern on the chart match her passion for waxing or facials and show her least favourite treatments less frequently?

A chart will clearly show the most common and the least-used treatments and products. A promotional period of a month could be used to generate interest in those trailing behind. Remember, stock sitting in the cupboard is dead money, generating neither income nor interest if the client does not know it exists.

The same applies to machines and equipment. A client will not ask what a brush cleanse machine does if it is sitting on the top shelf of the storeroom, with all its related creams and washes, so she can't see it. Dust it off, do a demonstration of its use, revisit the manufacturer's instructions and offer it to clients to enhance their facial. Or think laterally and offer alternatives – have a back treatment promotion at the beginning of the summer when clients are coming out of winter woollies and showing off their backs in swimming costumes.

This is how many salons improve their business: through analysis of turnover and ensuring movement of static items. Most salons set targets, either within sales or treatments. It is important, through regular meetings and agreed personal goals, that you understand what is expected of you. It should be agreed at the time of your interview what your personal goals are, what incentives there are for achieving those goals, and what happens if you do not achieve them. (Please refer to G8 'Develop and maintain your effectiveness at work', page 123, for information on personal goal setting, how to work with your manager and how to develop your job role for personal satisfaction.)

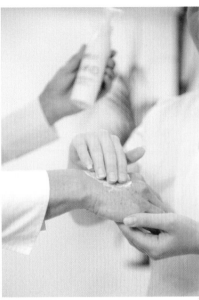

Always demonstrate the use of machines and equipment on the hand

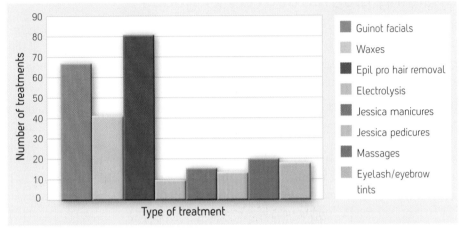

Legend:
- Guinot facials
- Waxes
- Epil pro hair removal
- Electrolysis
- Jessica manicures
- Jessica pedicures
- Massages
- Eyelash/eyebrow tints

Produce a monthly chart of salon treatments to find out which are the most popular

Securing client agreement and checking their understanding of the service or product

To get the best from the product, the client should fully understand how to use it, when to apply it, and its benefits and advantages. For example, a rich eye cream needs a delicate application using the ring fingers of both hands. A tiny amount of product should be warmed between the fingers before it is patted on, starting from the outer eye and working inwards. If too much product is applied, the eye area absorbs it and becomes puffy. Using heavy strokes to apply it will pull the fragile skin around the eyes causing damage. Little is definitely more in this case!

When talking through the method of application with the client, and possibly demonstrating, look for lots of eye contact and nodding, which the client will do if she has understood. If the client looks confused, bored or distant, you have lost her interest. She will not use the product and may even return it.

To ensure the client has understood your instructions, remember to ask if she has any questions or whether what you said was clear. Use the famous five questions to help you: How? When? What? Why? Who?

Ask your client:

How do you apply this cream?

When will you need to use it?

What will it achieve for your skin?

Why do you need to use it?

Who is it most suitable for?

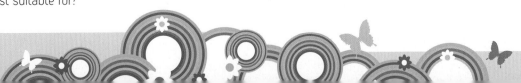

If you have provided this information properly, and the client can demonstrate that she has understood, then she will understand all there is to know about using the product. This will affirm her information and show you she fully understands. Write in her record card that she has purchased the product. The next time you treat her, ask her how she found it and if she is pleased with the results. Be interested in her efforts and comment on the effects of her product use. This will confirm your recommendations were correct.

Ensuring prompt delivery of goods

If, following your advice, the client wishes to purchase either a product or treatments, you need to ensure she understands the time restraints or delivery expectations. If the client has to wait, perhaps because it needs to be ordered, you should keep her fully informed to avoid misunderstandings.

Delivery dates vary considerably. They are dependent upon the company, its resources and stock levels, and how local they are to you. It may be a next-day delivery if the supplier is in your area, or there may be a wait of several weeks if the suppliers are awaiting a shipment themselves. Problems arise when the client is not kept fully in the picture and is kept waiting. She will not be happy if she thinks she is being 'fobbed off' with poor excuses. Honesty is the best policy – if the client is told she has to wait two weeks, then at least she knows and is not irritated by what she would see as a late delivery.

Key terms

Epilation – hair removal

If the client has booked an additional or new treatment, ensure she understands the time restraints there too. The nail technician may be fully booked for a week in advance, so the treatment is not instant. Match up the appointment booking to suit both your client's needs and the therapist's column. Squeezing a client in late on a Friday evening because you promised her that week will not make you popular with the therapist, and there is no guarantee of a quality treatment.

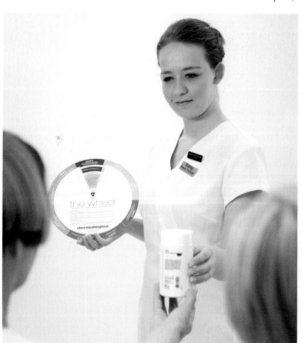

In both instances, take responsibility for your actions. Ensure you know how to order the correct goods, or give the task to someone who does, and take a little effort to juggle the appointment system to suit everyone. A little consideration and kindness goes a long way and is always appreciated.

Referring clients to alternative sources

There are times when you cannot recommend or offer the client what she needs. This may be because you are not yet trained in the particular treatment or because your salon does not offer that treatment. If you think another member of staff may be able to help, do ask their advice. Should the client require a sunbed session and you do not have one, or want a specialist **epilation** treatment and you do not offer it, then recommend somewhere else, but only if you know of a reputable therapist.

You could offer to give a short presentation to colleagues on new products or services

There is always the possibility that you will lose the client altogether of course, but she may approve of your professionalism and remain loyal to you for all other treatments. That should be viewed as the best of compliments to your customer relationship.

If there is sufficient demand and the salon is losing clientele by not offering the required treatment, this is also the time to recommend to the salon manager or owner that the salon should investigate the possibility of introducing it to expand business opportunities.

Do some research yourself on the cost of equipment and training, profit margins and expected returns, and then do a short presentation to the staff. You will learn a lot and so will they — as well as being impressed with your initiative.

Check your knowledge

1 The most important reason for offering aftercare advice is to ensure:
    a) you get good sales commission
    b) the client gets value for money
    c) the effects of the treatment last longer
    d) the client spends more time with you.

2 Additional training in the workplace will give you:
    a) more confidence through knowledge
    b) more holiday allowance
    c) more weekends off
    d) promotion.

3 If you make up information because you do not know something, you are likely to:
    a) increase the risk assessment on products
    b) increase the damage costs to the salon
    c) put the client at risk through poor information
    d) increase the advertising revenue for the salon.

4 It is important to gain full information about the client's needs so you can:
    a) sell her lots of products
    b) take lots of money through the till
    c) make lots of sales commission
    d) give her the best products for her skin type.

5 You should make sure your client knows how to use a product by:
    a) asking her to buy a magazine in which it appears
    b) telling her to watch the adverts
    c) asking her questions about it before she leaves
    d) making her sit a test.

6 A bar chart of top-selling lines will allow you to:
    a) keep stock levels high to meet sales
    b) buy lots of other stock to the same level
    c) get rid of old stock on the shelf
    d) spend more money on other stock.

7 A calendar of promotions will allow you to:
    a) plan staff holidays
    b) organise activities to promote seasonal sales
    c) organise a work rota
    d) plan ahead for expansion.

8 Link selling means:
    a) putting all the products in one bag
    b) linking the products up to the computer
    c) linking the products up to the till
    d) linking sales to each similar category.

9 The best time to talk to your client about offers is when:
    a) they have a face mask on
    b) when they get dressed
    c) when you can make eye contact
    d) on the phone.

10 A feature of a product is:
    a) what it does to the skin
    b) its good qualities
    c) its price
    d) its value.

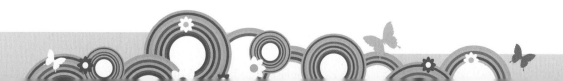

Unit G18 Promote additional services or products to clients

Getting ready for assessment

Sources of evidence could be the following:

- On the client's record card, make a note of any products purchased, any recommendations you make for the future, and other services that would be suitable for your client's needs.

- During your consultation, or during the course of a treatment (where suitable), let the assessor hear you recommending suitable products and treatments. The client does not necessarily have to have them; rather it is your verbal recommendations that form the evidence as well as the correct knowledge that you are imparting.

- Design a questionnaire to show client knowledge of treatments. This will indicate how little or how much the client knows about her options. You could then highlight staff weaknesses in knowledge of products or services and recommend a training day. For example, of the 17 clients having a manicure this week, only five of them realised they could have a warm oil treatment to help dry cuticles.

- Design a poster to promote a particular product or service, perhaps with a seasonal theme – a free nail polish application with every Christmas makeover, or a pedicure polish carried out with every Spring waxing treatment. Make the poster as informative as you can to attract new business.

- Design an aftercare and homecare leaflet for a treatment, suggesting suitable products for home use that will carry on the good work of the salon treatment.

- Organise a training seminar for other staff or students where you promote a particular treatment or product that you feel confident in, which perhaps is not selling as well as it could. Make it very 'hands on' – get others involved in using the product and demonstrate how to promote it.

- Copy and enclose in your portfolio the order form or delivery note that you may have had to complete if a product was out of stock or it was a special order.

- Include any evidence of outside selling seminars or lectures you have attended while in employment. Enclose any training certificates from commercial training you may have received.

These suggestions will show you understand the requirements and mechanics of selling and linking your treatments with retail sales. It is not only important you learn how to do it but that you record it, too.

Unit G8

Develop and maintain your effectiveness at work

Introduction

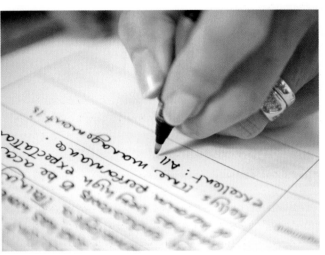

Your appraisals will contribute to your personal development

This unit is all about you and your professional growth, which will, in turn, lead to your personal growth too. As your skills develop, so will your confidence. This gives you courage to tackle new training and experiences, which provide certain self-assurance. Before you get to that stage, you have to go through a professional growing period during which you start as a student and end as an employee.

As part of the transition from student to potential employee, you have to step outside your own sphere to realise that you are joining a business and that it is vital to contribute to the effectiveness of that business if you want to stay employed.

This is not always an easy change to make: as a student the only responsibility you have is for your own learning, and the framework for this is already put into place by your tutors. This unit will help you take more responsibility for your own development in the workplace — your employer will expect this, and you will no longer have the safety cushion of asking your tutor all the time! However, just like all skills, the more you take responsibility for your own development, the better you will become at it, and the more training you have, the more confidence you will gain.

Improve your personal performance at work

In this outcome you will learn about:

- identifying your own strengths and weaknesses and discussing them with the relevant person
- finding out more information from relevant people to perform a task when the instructions you have are unclear
- seeking feedback from relevant people about how you can improve your performance
- asking your colleagues for help and taking opportunities to learn when they are available
- seeking help from relevant people when you are unable to obtain learning opportunities relating to your work
- regularly reviewing developments in beauty therapy and related areas
- agreeing realistic work targets with the relevant person
- regularly reviewing your progress towards achieving your agreed targets
- using the results of your reviews to develop your future personal development plan.

How to become employable at work

To learn how to become a good employee and develop a business focus, we will look at the differences between your life at the moment – as a student – and the working life of a therapist in a busy salon.

A student – your life at college	An employee – your life at work
In the safe college environment you are the main focus of attention: quite rightly, college is all about you working towards your portfolio collection.	In the world of work, you are not working with your best friends (in fact, you cannot choose your work colleagues and there is no guarantee that you will like all of them or that they will like you). There is a shift away from you personally towards what is expected of you.
You are developing your skills through practice and receiving lots of positive feedback from your tutor. You also become used to working with your friends, you know your lecturers or trainers very well. There is little business pressure as you are concentrating on gaining your qualification, rather than building up a company.	Instead of working towards a qualification, you are working to increase a client base and helping to grow the profit of a salon. This is an ongoing process – no one in business can afford to stand still. A business quickly dies if it is not nurtured and developed by enthusiastic, motivated staff giving a professional service, which separates your salon from its competitors.
This might seem like pressure, as you may be concerned about completing all your practical ranges, but you are well supported and if you are non-competent in a treatment, you will have the opportunity to practise and then repeat it at a later date.	It is not your business yet, but by being the very best employee you can, *you* can gain invaluable experience for when you do own your own salon or go into a mobile business. You can then become a good employer to others.
Tutors are well trained in supporting learners and will take into consideration if you are having an 'off day'. Learners bring many problems into college: for example, child care problems, lateness to class because of transport delays, and so on. This is allowed for, to an extent, and your assessments may be altered to reflect your needs. It is not that easy in the workplace!	As an employee, there is an unwritten expectation that you will be punctual, highly motivated and leave all your domestic problems at home in order to concentrate on the business. You cannot let your first client down because you didn't get up early enough.
	So, you can see there is a real shift away from your personal needs to those of the business you are joining. However, becoming a good employee does involve your growth: of skills, confidence and ability. Certain tools are needed to nurture and cultivate this growth. A good manager will guide you and help you develop your new skills as long as you play your part too.

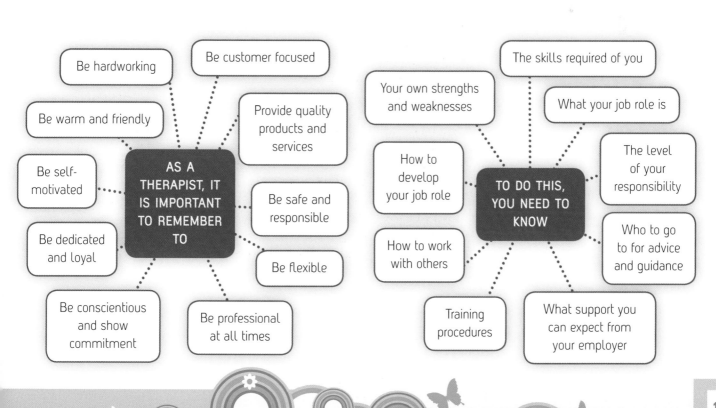

Think about it

It is a fact of life that no one gets to choose who they work with unless they own the salon! It isn't like a college/training environment where you are very close to your best friends and tend to stick in little groups. You may enter an established salon that has a variety of employees with different backgrounds, skill areas and ages, who may have more experience than you and may have been in the job role for many years. Be open and receptive to what they have to teach you – learning doesn't stop when you leave college. You should never stop learning, whether it is a new skill or the skill of getting on with people – even if you would not choose to socialise with them, you do have to work with them. Working with others is a hard lesson to learn, and is something that you will be expected to do.

Carrying out your job role to salon and National Occupational Standards

When you first start work in a salon, it is very important that you have a full understanding of what exactly is expected of you; only then can you carry out your duties well, and to the best of your abilities.

What are National Occupational Standards?

National Occupational Standards (NOS) are the beauty therapy standards that all students taking a Level 2 qualification work to. They cover all the practical ranges within each unit, or areas you must cover. This gives you a good practical grounding in each area of work, in turn making you very employable. In fact, employers have a great deal of influence over what topics are included within the standards. They consult with Habia (Hairdressing and Beauty Industry Authority), and all training establishments nationally teach to those same standards, giving equality and uniformity of learning. Carrying out practical skills using the correct procedures is not only professional, it is also essential for health and safety. Deciding to take short cuts or ignoring the safe methods will invalidate insurance cover and leave the therapist open to negligence charges.

So, the training is the same wherever you are in the country, and employers have told the trainers what they expect from a new employee. Because your training has been so thorough, you have the confidence to apply for jobs.

For your portfolio

Every time you use your assessment book, you are automatically working with the National Occupational Standards. Every time you take an assessment and are given verbal and written feedback on your progress, you are making your own developmental plans. Your tutor may also give you action plans on what you need to do to complete your unit.

Keep all your feedback sheets together – they are an important part of your evidence. You may not always be competent in every treatment, but your feedback charts your development and you will be instructed on what to do to improve your performance. It may be that you give a very good treatment but are not yet within the commercial time for that treatment. Next time, you could concentrate on timing and become competent. That shows excellent progression and development, and you will have the evidence to prove competency.

Additional knowledge

Visit Habia's website at www.habia.org and look up the guidelines for the beauty therapy industry. Habia also offers information on career advice, the latest business developments, salon safety and guidelines for hygiene and waxing, and all the latest legislation. It also provides revision and learning materials and holds forums for students' comments.

Salon standards

Your salon standards of behaviour and work philosophy will be the same as the NOS and you will be expected to carry out every treatment to the highest standard. However, as you develop a commercial understanding of products, the manufacturer's recommendations for certain products may differ from the NOS, or the method in which you were trained. Be flexible and follow the manufacturer's instructions when using products – providing you have received a certificate of training from the company, your professional association or federation insurance will still cover you. (Refer to Professional basics, pages 65–68.)

The Government Minister for Education sets out the policies for further and higher education.

The Quality and Curriculum Authority (QCA). This is the government body that regulates all the qualifications, which are reviewed for authenticity and equality. Awarding Bodies must submit their qualifications to QCA for approval.

The Hairdressing and Beauty Industry Authority (HABIA) work with Awarding Bodies to set the standards. These are drawn up via consultation with employers who know what the market trends are.

Awarding Bodies can then plan and print assessment books and written papers for students.

Your college or training provider can then decide which Awarding Body to go with. The college will be inspected and approved, and will then receive the support it requires to offer beauty qualifications.

The people involved in setting and interpreting the National Occupational Standards

For example, many companies offer very good manicure/pedicure training using their products. It will differ from your basic manicure training at college, as you are following the company's recommended procedures. Do not be frightened of learning new techniques – there is more than one way to do things. As long as the company fully trains you to its standards and provides a certificate of competence to allow you to use its techniques, you are covered by your professional indemnity insurance. In most commercial training there is a practical skills test and a short written paper to prove you have understood the theory of the techniques: even on a short one-day course, expect both tests.

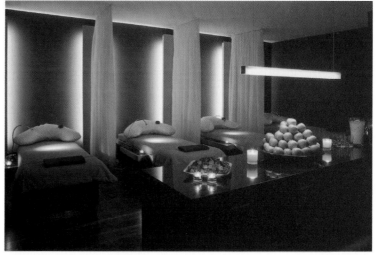

> **Think about it**
>
> Do not think that if you have seen another therapist using the product, it is acceptable for you to attempt a treatment in the same way. You will not be covered by your professional indemnity insurance if you are not commercially fully qualified. This could be expensive should damage occur and the client decides to sue you or the salon. It is not worth the risk.

Performing your task – salon job roles and procedures

A good salon, and certainly the larger health farms or salon chains, will provide a **job specification** as part of your contract. You then sign the contract, which not only lays down the working terms and conditions, such as annual holidays, but also gives a framework of duties that you are expected to carry out.

Smaller salons may do this orally at your interview. However, there is a danger that you won't take it all in at once – a written list of duties is much easier to refer to.

Speak to your salon manager and gain clarification on what you are expected to do on a daily basis and how this fits in with the rest of the team. If you don't do something because you are not aware it is part of your job, at best you will be perceived as lazy or not a team player, at worst you could endanger clients, especially if your job role involves sterilisation and hygiene procedures.

Taking opportunities to learn

(Refer also to Unit G18 Promote additional products or services to clients, pages 108–09, for more tips on how to take opportunities to learn your expected tasks.)

> **Key terms**
>
> **Job specification** – a list of tasks or roles that the job holder will be expected to do as part of their employment.

> **Think about it**
>
> When you first start in a salon, it is usual to be in a junior position – you may have the correct qualification, but you do not yet have the same experience as a more senior therapist. It is likely that you will spend at least some part of the day assisting with treatments and 'shadowing' a more senior person. You will also be given the more menial tasks in the salon, or certainly take part in the rota for toilet cleaning, setting up for treatments and general tidying up. This can be used as a valuable method of learning.
>
> Whatever your task, if you tackle it with enthusiasm and energy it will be done well, and your endeavours will be noticed by your manager.

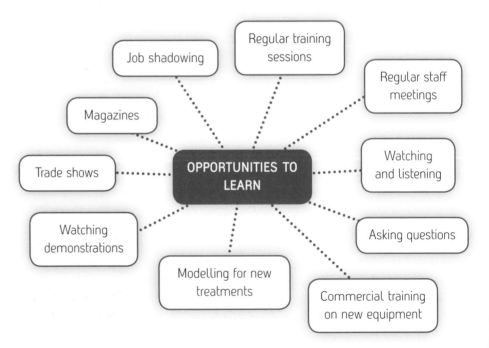

You can find many opportunities to learn the tasks you will be expected to do

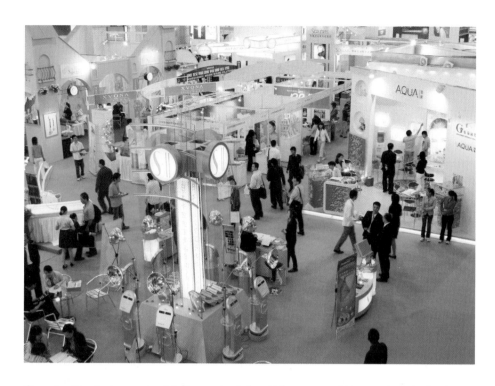

Attending beauty trade shows or exhibitions will keep you up to date

Opportunities to learn should always be taken if they present themselves in the form of a formal demonstration or watching an experienced member of staff work — we are never too old to enhance our skills and learn something new. Enthusiasm and passion for learning will soon be picked up on by your manager and this will help you to develop. The more you learn, the more confident you will become, and the positive cycle will continue. Being interested in all aspects of the business means you have more knowledge and information to offer clients; even if you are not trained in that area you will know who to refer them to. Ask the famous five questions (Who? What? When? Why? How?) and you will soon develop a confidence in salon life.

Organisation

Most successful salons — the ones that take the most money and are the busiest — are normally very well organised. The salon will run like a well-oiled machine, with everyone knowing what they have to do, tackling the jobs with enthusiasm and care, and working together as a team to make the working day run as smoothly as possible. Therefore, the most organised managers are often the most productive. A salon with a rota of jobs with names beside them, and ticks when they are completed, is giving clear instructions to the staff about expectations and essential jobs, without which the salon would cease to function.

Imagine the salon running out of towels because a junior did not turn the laundry around, or running out of couch roll, products or tissues because the manager did not make the order last week.

If you understand the importance of your specific jobs, you very soon feel that you are performing a vital function within the wheels of your industry. For example, you may be asked to count stock because a stock check is needed for stock levels. If you run out of a good selling line simply because you couldn't be bothered to do the paperwork, you are costing the salon money in lost revenue.

Think about it

I look – I see.
I listen – I hear.
I do – I understand.

Develop and maintain your effectiveness at work **Unit G8**

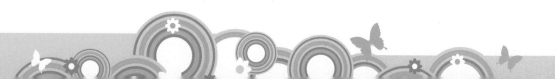

Agreeing your job role and being comfortable with it

Do make sure you know what you are going to be doing, where the equipment is to carry out your tasks, and how your responsibilities relate to the team. If your job role is not explained properly, or you do not really understand it, your only option is to ask! Do not keep quiet – it could lead to real misunderstandings. Do not make the mistake of nodding and agreeing to what is being said, and then going home thinking 'I didn't understand a word of that!'

Do not sign an agreement to your job role and duties if you are unsure of the implications.

Knowledge is very comforting and prevents worry. If given an area of responsibility, make sure you know what is asked of you. A clear understanding of issues and requirements makes for an unruffled operation and prevents confusion.

Be competent. Do the job as well as you have been trained to. Do not attempt to bluff through a job that could put a client or colleague at risk. This comes back to knowledge – do not attempt a job you have not been taught to do.

Skills and knowledge can be kept up to date through regular training, reading trade journals, attending beauty trade shows or exhibitions and through the media. Be enthusiastic to learn new skills and regard it as a challenge rather than a chore. The more skills therapists have to offer, the more employable they are.

My story

Beauty therapy at sea

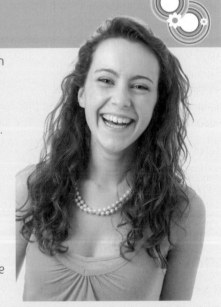

Hi, my name is Victoria and I trained in Level 2 and then Level 3. After a year's salon experience I joined a company that provided staff for cruise ships. My beauty therapy job has taken me all over the world!

When I first left college and went to work in the salon, I was just so tired every night. College was great; we finished most days by 4 o'clock and we got a morning off and one late start – so it was quite a cushy time. When I went into the salon and had clients booked from nine in the morning until six or seven in the evening, it was non-stop and I was lucky if I got a lunch break. However, I did learn a lot from my colleagues and made some great friends, too. I did lots of commercial training with different companies, which gave me lots of confidence as I gained more experience. Then, when I did my sea training and had to take a seaman's safety course (everyone on board has to), I thought being in the salon was easy!

Working on cruise ships taught me so much: I had to do presentations to large groups of people about what the salon had to offer – I was really nervous the first time as I had never used a microphone before. However, after doing a few presentations, my colleagues would grumble I was hogging the limelight and never wanted to get off the mike! It was certainly very long days, but on days off in the Caribbean we would swim with dolphins and go to beach barbeques. Well worth the hard work – I would recommend it to anyone. College gave me a really good career.

Flexibility is a skill worth cultivating. Try to accommodate the client who arrives without an appointment with help from colleagues. Do not make her feel it is just too inconvenient or that she is stupid to even ask. Reschedule the appointment if you cannot help at that particular time. If a client is late for her appointment or there is an overbooking, then do the same. Rescheduling of appointments can work both ways – clients may have to be juggled into other time slots due to staff sickness. If this is done in an open, genuinely apologetic manner, most clients will be just as flexible. If a client changes her treatment booking, again be flexible. If time permits, and the client's needs can be accommodated, then do so. The receptionist may need to be made aware of the change so she doesn't double book the time slot, but flexibility is the way to keep encouraging new business.

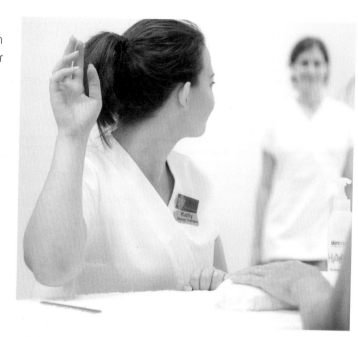

Knowing when to ask colleagues for help

It is just as important to know what you cannot do, as it is to know what you can do! To maintain a hierarchy within the salon, there has to be a person in charge who takes responsibility for the larger problems in the salon. Dealing with complaints, banking the takings and ordering stock may be some of the duties you are not expected to take part in. There is a good reason for this – you may not have the knowledge or people skills to handle a serious complaint, or not enough stock knowledge to predict what the salon is going to need in the next month.

Some things are best left to those who have the experience and get paid for taking on that extra duty. Always refer to those in a higher authority and involve management in decisions or judgements that you are not experienced in. For example, giving away complimentary treatments may only be done by the manager. If no one was coordinating gift vouchers, the business could suffer a severe financial loss.

Accept that you are not able to perform certain tasks or duties, and be aware of the limits of your own responsibilities – the only exception to this is health and safety, which is everyone's responsibility. (For information on Identifying your own strengths and weaknesses and discussing them with the relevant person, see page 136.)

Contracts of employment

All responsible employers have a contract of employment, which has a section on discipline, the possible consequences of breaking your contract of employment and the route to a better performance at work. Most salons expect a certain amount of commercial professional development, and their contracts of employment allow time away from salon duties for additional training (see page 135). The salon will often agree to help fund the training, provided the therapist agrees to stay in the salon employment for a fixed period of time – say a year. It is a good way of gaining commercial training without the personal expense.

It is always good to know the basis of your employment. There is usually a scale of disciplinary action, which can vary from a verbal warning for, say, continual lateness, to instant dismissal if caught stealing or physically assaulting a client. Rather like in a college, a good salon has to have discipline and rules and regulations to function.

Minor indiscretions are usually discussed and may result in a good telling-off, and provided it does not happen again, there are no major consequences. A poor standard of work, or a regular occurrence such as absenteeism, may result in pay being stopped or bonus incentives being withdrawn.

Your rights as an employee, and salon grievance and appeals procedures

Major problems need to be sorted out using the salon grievance and appeals procedure. It is important you are aware of how to use it, should the need arise. Equal opportunities laws are designed to give everyone the same rights, whether they are defending or justifying their actions, or appealing against unfair or biased judgements. This is much the same as when you are a candidate taking assessments. If, as a candidate, you do not agree with the decision your assessor has made, there is a format for appeal, just as there is in employment.

The bigger cases of employees suing their employer are reported in the national media, as judgement against employers for unfair dismissal or other charges often results in large amounts of money being awarded, and is seen as newsworthy.

Employee rights

Employment law is very specific in many areas. Regardless of whether you are employed full or part time, or are on a fixed-term contract, you have the right to:

○ a written statement of employment
○ pay and itemised pay statements
○ payment on medical suspension (when you are unable to work through illness)
○ reasonable time off for antenatal care
○ statutory maternity leave and statutory maternity pay
○ return to work after a full period of maternity leave
○ parental/paternity leave
○ paid adoption leave
○ four weeks' paid holiday, and daily and weekly rest breaks
○ request flexible working hours
○ time off for public duties
○ time off for trade union duties and activities
○ statutory redundancy payment after two years' continuous employment
○ time off to look for work or arrange training during a redundancy notice period
○ time off for family emergencies
○ statutory notice of termination of the contract of employment
○ complain of unfair dismissal
○ be treated fairly and in accordance with proper procedures.

You also have the right not to:

○ suffer unlawful deductions from pay

○ be dismissed for asserting a statutory right

○ be unfairly discriminated against on the grounds of sex, age, race or disability

○ be dismissed for trade union involvement or taking action on health and safety grounds.

Qualifying periods of employment are needed as follows:

○ minimum period of notice – one month

○ not to be unfairly dismissed – one year (there is no qualifying period where a breach of contract or discrimination occurs)

○ written statement of reasons for dismissal – one year

○ redundancy payments – two years

○ statutory maternity pay – 26 weeks (at the 15th week before the expected date of birth).

These are the basic legal guidelines for employment. They are designed to protect you as an employee. However, employment law is complex and subject to change, so always seek professional advice before deciding on action if you are considering a court case.

> ### Additional knowledge
>
> Does your salon have an equal opportunities policy? Most small businesses do not have a written one. However, all the salon's written policies and procedures should have equal opportunities running through them. Review these and see if there is any discrimination that you feel should be eliminated. Advice on discrimination is available from the Equality and Human Rights Commission – have a look at its website.

Agreeing realistic work targets

Being commercially aware

The old saying 'Time equals money' applies to treatment times as well as your preparation time (refer to Professional basics, 'Treatment planning and preparation', page 25).

Most therapists are perfectionists in their approach to any treatment: a leg wax has to be the best the client has ever had, the make-up application a work of art. This is highly commendable – except that if it takes several hours to achieve, the treatment time is not commercially viable.

Commercially viable treatment times are part of the criteria of student assessment. You have to try to reach a happy medium between an excellent treatment and a time factor that is realistic in the world of work.

Not only does it cost the salon money if you take too long (you could have squeezed another treatment into the extra half hour that you ran over time) but you are also infringing upon the client's rights as a consumer. The Supply of Goods and Services

> #### Think about it
>
> Each of us must take responsibility for our actions, and we are liable for any damages that occur if we do not. Insurance cover will be void if it is proven that legislation or salon rules have been broken, so you must be aware of the limits of your own role.

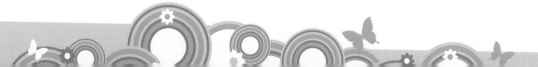

Act 1982 (refer to Professional basics, page 62) states that the person providing a service (such as a beauty therapist) must:

○ charge a reasonable price

○ give the service within a reasonable time

○ give the service with reasonable care and skill.

The aspect we are concerned with here is the time it takes to carry out a treatment, so this means no two-hour manicures.

Salon targets and treatment times

Most price lists contain a description of the treatment, the product used and the length of time each treatment will take. This is the guide for the customer, who can then allow enough time to relax and enjoy the treatment. It is reasonable, within the law and the commercial viability of the salon, to expect that the service will actually be carried out in that stated time.

Of course, there is a little give and take – the client is running late, she falls asleep during her facial and needs waking up time, or your appointments are overrunning slightly. However, if the client is in her lunch hour and has to dash back to work, having had a rushed treatment which she really didn't enjoy, you may have lost your customer altogether. It is also well within her rights to complain. Experience will speed up your technique – the more you use your practical skills, the more automatic they become. It is easy to spot students who have a Saturday job in a salon, because they are quicker at treatments, have good customer awareness and good communication skills! Remember that practice makes perfect: more senior therapists are able to carry out the treatment while chatting to the client, clearing up as they go and producing excellent results. It will come to you, the more experience you gain.

Productivity targets and timescales

We all react well to incentives and praise – for most domestic animals (and small children!) training is based around rewarding good behaviour and ignoring, or punishing, bad behaviour.

We want, and should have, goals to work towards. We then feel we have achieved something knowing that all our efforts will be recognised, and we benefit from all that hard work. This applies in all types of work.

Beauty therapy is no different. A keen therapist will want to increase her client base and product turnover, if she knows that not only will her work be rewarded with praise, but there is an extra incentive to do so.

Targets should be realistic and achievable if they are to work. They should be mutually agreed between you and your manager, with a set target over a defined period of time. This could be a month, every two months or every quarter of the year, depending upon how you both feel it works best. Short-term goals are often the favourite: they feel more achievable and reinforce the work ethic when reached. This target setting will be both personal, for your own growth and development, and commercial for the salon – sales targets, number of treatments per day and so on.

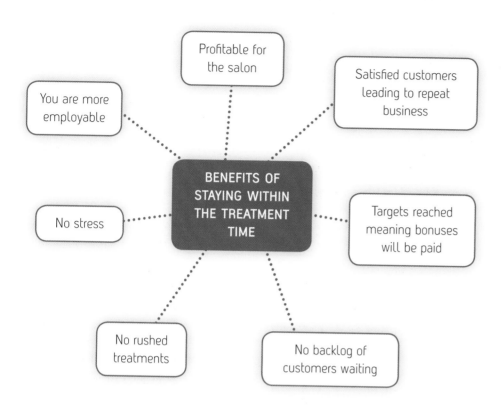

There are many benefits to staying within the treatment time

The diagram shows **BENEFITS OF STAYING WITHIN THE TREATMENT TIME** connected to:
- Profitable for the salon
- Satisfied customers leading to repeat business
- You are more employable
- No stress
- Targets reached meaning bonuses will be paid
- No rushed treatments
- No backlog of customers waiting

Rather than view this as a negative aspect of work, most therapists look forward to the challenge, knowing that they can only benefit by trying their hardest to achieve their target. Most salons have an incentive for achieving targets, which can be anything from free products or a free treatment to a weekend break, shopping vouchers or even a trip abroad. If you read the trade magazines, you will find some fabulous prizes given by commercial companies, rewarding a therapist who has become therapist of the year or salesperson of the year.

It is important that you try to achieve your targets: it not only keeps you employed, but it makes you very commercial and gives you invaluable experience should you decide to run your own salon or develop a mobile business. Only doing two treatments a day on a mobile beauty round is soon going to put you out of business.

Improving your performance and identifying training needs

Improving yourself requires self-awareness and analysis. It's not easy to look outside yourself and see yourself as others do.

As you gain experience in a salon, your performance improves. You should also specifically target your improvement, which is rather like setting a training programme for an athlete before the Olympic Games. If the athlete does not push the boundaries a little more every time, the performance will stay static so will not be good enough to beat the competition.

Think about it

It is important to know your **productivity** targets and the timescale for achieving them so you can plan ahead and become comfortable in your job role. If you were to leave a large sales target until the last week of the month, you will be putting additional pressure on yourself and may not perform as well as you could. If you pace yourself and plan your targets in an achievable manner, you will be less pressurised and are therefore less likely to put pressure on your clients.

Key terms

Productivity – the amount of work achieved or a measure of a worker's efficiency.

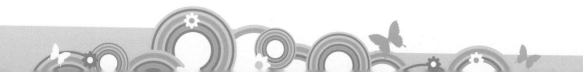

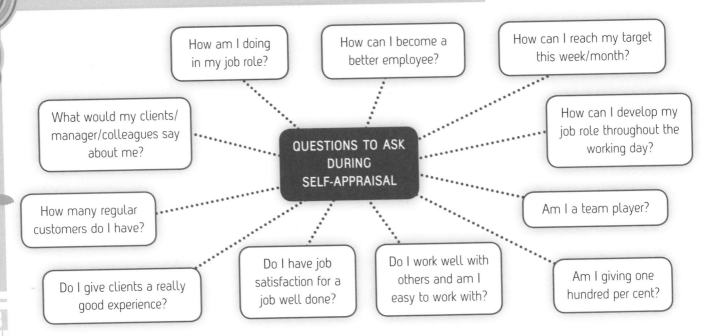

QUESTIONS TO ASK DURING SELF-APPRAISAL

- How am I doing in my job role?
- How can I become a better employee?
- How can I reach my target this week/month?
- What would my clients/manager/colleagues say about me?
- How can I develop my job role throughout the working day?
- How many regular customers do I have?
- Am I a team player?
- Do I give clients a really good experience?
- Do I have job satisfaction for a job well done?
- Do I work well with others and am I easy to work with?
- Am I giving one hundred per cent?

Self-analysis is essential for your development as a therapist

Unit G8

Develop and maintain your effectiveness at work

Think about it

Training and assessment should be viewed in a positive light – they provide opportunities to learn and progress in personal growth and the maintenance of good working relationships.

It is important to react in an optimistic way to any feedback or review.

Nobody likes criticism, but it is important to listen carefully to what is said.

Key terms

Appraisal – a performance review of a job role, usually carried out yearly.

Self-analysis and self-development are essential for your growth and maturity as a therapist within a salon environment. This is often referred to as professional development. Some companies provide a commercial professional development folder – rather like a record of achievement. All the training certificates and qualifications can be kept in the folder, and it helps you spot where your gaps in training may be.

Identifying your own strengths and weaknesses

If a therapist keeps making the same mistakes again and again, and clients complain or stop coming into the salon altogether, this is a strong indication that something is wrong. Often, with experience, it is easier to be reflective and spot our own mistakes and then change the action, or reaction, to break the cycle of behaviour. Sometimes it is not so easy to be inward-looking, and this is where a good manager will help by giving regular work-related reviews. This is called an **appraisal**.

As your practical skills grow and your confidence develops, you may find some treatments harder to master than others. This can become a training cycle: the treatments you enjoy and do well you want to do more of, but the ones you find difficult to get to grips with you stop practising because you do not feel comfortable with them. This forms a good basis for your strengths and weaknesses analysis. Is there a topic or treatment that you are sailing through? That will be one of your strengths. You may also count being good with people, enjoying the client sessions and earning lots of tips!

Now look at any topics or treatments you are not doing a lot of, and may be falling behind on. These would be considered your weaker areas: the ones that need some work. You may not know how to operate the till, so you avoid volunteering to cash up at the end of the session. However, your weaknesses will not go away by themselves. Look at them in a non-emotional manner. Why is this happening and how can you correct it? It may mean shadowing someone who is good at that particular skill, but sometimes you may just have to tackle the problem head on with supervision. You may need more demonstrations, more practice or more instruction.

The appraisal

Appraisal or team reviews should take place regularly, perhaps once a month or every three months.

The appraisal should be:

- ○ at a mutually agreeable time, not an inconvenience to either party
- ○ constructive and open, not conducted in fear or terror of job loss
- ○ objective and as non-personal as possible
- ○ a review for both parties, not just a performance judgement
- ○ constructive and positive.

The appraisal process should leave the employee feeling enthusiastic and not depressed.

Many large companies provide both self-assessment sheets for the employee to fill in throughout a set period, and a joint review sheet to be completed with the manager, to help improve performance. A self-assessment form can contain whatever the employer or manager feels is relevant to the job role. Here is an example of a common format:

> **For your portfolio**
>
> Copy out this self-assessment form (or ask your tutor for one) and use it to analyse your own performance.

Salon name: Beauty Within, The High Street, Sale, Cheshire LA13 7PQ

Date: July 2010

Position held: Junior Beauty Therapist

Therapist: Jasmine Abrams

Self-appraisal

Please add comments on how you feel you are progressing in each area listed. Thank you.

Appearance   Good. I do try to look professional every day. I like the new uniform and it is comfortable and easy to wash.

Absences   Could be better, as I have had a week off with flu this month. I haven't had any more time off.

Time keeping   Could be better. I have been late 5 times this month.

Job performance   Good. I feel my regular clients always ask for me, and I have worked hard this month. Since I did my training I have really enjoyed doing more facials and selling products.

Sales   Good, as above. My sales are from my regulars. We all love the new product range.

Strengths   I am confident with my treatments and I especially enjoy facials. I am outgoing and get on well with others and I feel I am progressing as I should.

Weaknesses   Time keeping. I have missed my bus quite often in the mornings. They aren't that regular and I can't drive to work every day as it would cost me a fortune in parking.

Any areas of change   I have been in the wet area putting clients in the sauna this month, as Jane seems to have the flu bug that I had and is still off sick.

Staff development request   I would like to go on an eyelash perming training day if possible, as we have been asked for the treatment by our regular clients.

Action plan for the next review   To improve on time keeping and do my course.

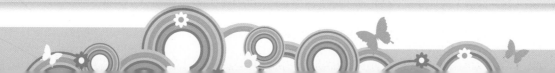

Here is an example of the salon manager's appraisal of Jasmine:

Salon name: Beauty Within, The High Street, Sale, Cheshire LA13 7PQ

Date: July 2010

Position held: Salon Manager

Therapist: Jasmine Abrams

Professional / technical knowledge and understanding

Excellent – your skills are current and you show a great understanding of the work in the salon. Your technical abilities are commercial, delivered with enthusiasm and a thorough understanding of your subject area.

Quality / accuracy of work and performance   Again, excellent. I appreciate how much care and attention goes into all areas of your work and how much effort you put into ensuring accuracy.

Time / task management   This could be better, Jasmine – your time keeping is not good. I know you have transport problems, but we cannot afford to let down the first client of the day and then it makes you late because you are playing catch-up all day.

Team working skills   Jasmine, your team working skills are very good and you are a valued colleague to all who work with you.

Problem solving / decision making   You are not yet able to make decisions on your own as a junior staff member. However, when you have had a bit more experience, it will come. It is good that you understand your level of responsibility and you do always ask and clarify, which is very good.

Communication skills   Excellent. Your communication with everyone is outstanding. You are outgoing and social and have a lovely client manner. Your client base for regulars is growing nicely and people are beginning to ask for you.

Leadership and management skils   N/A at this time

General performance
eg
– self motivation
– initiative
– commitment

Your general performance is very good and I am pleased with your progress in this six months. The training has been good. I will pay for you to do the eyelash perming course and we will run a promotion on it for the rest of the summer.

Think about it

A self-assessment appraisal is not just about achievement within the job role and the number of sales that have been completed – that is really only a part of being a therapist (even though an important aspect of remaining profitable). It is also about short-term plans and development of the individual and it opens up many areas for discussion of future plans between a manager and an employee.

It should highlight how well the individual is coping within her job role and whether the salon is asking too much of an employee. It also provides an opportunity for the therapist to offer her opinions on improvement. It should be viewed very much as a two-way discussion, not a telling-off for a bad performance at work.

Linked into the appraisal system is the setting of targets for the action plan to improve performance at work.

The SMART rule

Follow this simple SMART rule. Targets should be:

S = Specific

Have particular aims in mind rather than too grand an idea. Set a goal specific to you. For example, I want to complete two assessments each week.

M = Measurable

Make sure they are aims you are able to measure with a start and a finish. Assessments can be measured against NVQ performance criteria and ranges. You must know where you are now, and where you want to be. For example, product sales might be on average £50 per day now, and a 10 per cent increase would take that up to £55 per day.

A = Achievable

Do not set an aim that cannot be realised. A short-term target may be to complete an NVQ unit by a certain date.

R = Realistic

Doing ten treatments per hour is not realistic – be sensible with your aims. For example, how long will it take you to cover all the performance criteria and ranges in one unit?

T = Timed

For the target to be achieved there should be a timescale for you to aim towards. For example, by next month I will improve my timekeeping by 50 per cent; by Christmas I am going to have my portfolio for G8 ready to be signed off by my assessor.

A joint review

The self-assessment form provides you with the opportunity to identify your own strengths and weaknesses and to set your own personal targets.

A joint review with a relevant person, that is a manager, assessor or tutor, can then identify whether your personal targets are realistic and achievable using the SMART formula. These targets can be either short term or long term.

Short-term goals are easier to measure and judge. They can bring a very positive glow to the therapist who achieves them and that will encourage her to go on and improve further. A short-term goal for our therapist Jasmine, from the self-assessment form on page 137, is to complete an eyelash-perming course and gain her certificate, and so offer her clients another service. This is rewarding and achievable.

Long-term goals are not so easy to measure and may be harder to keep in view. They require much more dedication to achieve. A long-term goal for Jasmine may be to gain two years' salon experience and then apply for a job as a therapist on a cruise ship. This is still achievable but will take two years.

Think about it

Some companies ask for anonymous peer reviews where you are asked to write an appraisal on a colleague or a manager. Always be professional and objective. This is not the time to air personal grievances like 'she always makes Jo a coffee but not me!'. A peer appraisal also reflects on you and how you think, so don't be rushed or attack the person you are writing about.

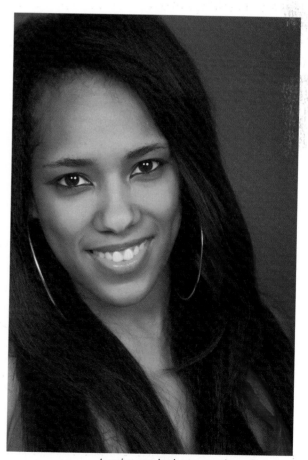

Jasmine can look at a number of different things to achieve her goals

Develop and maintain your effectiveness at work **Unit G8**

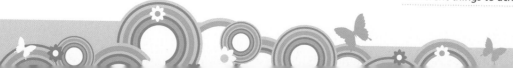

Unit G8 Develop and maintain your effectiveness at work

For your portfolio

Companies also use peer appraisals for teamwork and to check how everyone gets along. In pairs, using these headings – professional and technical knowledge, communication skills, team working skills, problem solving and decision making, self-motivation and quality of work – conduct a peer appraisal on each other. Write a short paragraph, be constructive and fair, and keep a copy of your peer appraisal. Put a copy of the appraisal of you in your portfolio of evidence.

Remember, this is not reflective practice: that means it isn't how you think you are doing, it is someone who works with you reflecting upon your performance, but it is a very valid form of appraisal.

Short-term goals are like a carrot dangling on a stick! They provide incentive and reward. Lots of short-term goals can also help achieve a long-term goal, which is also very satisfying, and can help you get where you want to go!

For example, Jasmine could apply any of the following to help her get to work on time:

○ Buy an alarm clock and set it at an earlier time.

○ Ask if any other member of staff could share a ride with her, perhaps sharing petrol costs.

○ Put an advert in the local shop for someone from her village who works in town and would be able to offer her a car share on a permanent basis.

○ Change the appointment-booking system at the salon so that Jasmine starts at 9.30 am when she can realistically get to work, and then either finishes half an hour later or has only a short break for lunch.

○ Try cycling to work and get fit at the same time.

Any number of these possible solutions would help Jasmine achieve her goal. Now fill out your own self-assessment plan and see if you can offer your own solutions to your problems. Think clearly and try to view yourself objectively.

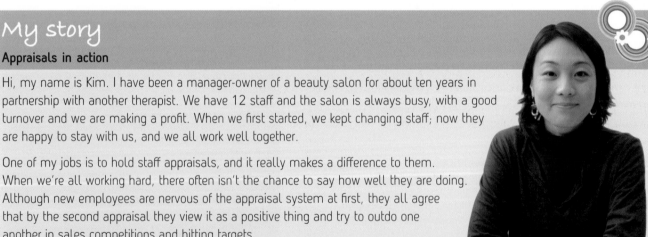

My story

Appraisals in action

Hi, my name is Kim. I have been a manager-owner of a beauty salon for about ten years in partnership with another therapist. We have 12 staff and the salon is always busy, with a good turnover and we are making a profit. When we first started, we kept changing staff; now they are happy to stay with us, and we all work well together.

One of my jobs is to hold staff appraisals, and it really makes a difference to them. When we're all working hard, there often isn't the chance to say how well they are doing. Although new employees are nervous of the appraisal system at first, they all agree that by the second appraisal they view it as a positive thing and try to outdo one another in sales competitions and hitting targets.

We came up with a target plan which was quite easy to achieve, so there are bonuses and incentives for sales and we have an 'employee of the month' reward, too. Some of the team have made some excellent suggestions on how to improve the business, and everyone is loyal and hard working. I won't have any trouble or lazy people working for us: it's too stressful without that!

The staff also get a chance to appraise my role and how we are getting along – it is a very good way to keep communication open with staff, in a non-judgemental manner.

Reviewing developments in beauty therapy

As well as doing treatments well, you must keep up to date with trends and innovations within the industry.

Clients and customers are very aware of the latest treatments, as media coverage of every aspect of beauty treatments is extensive, from **Botox**® injections to the latest in organic face creams. Beauty editors are sent hundreds of samples and given treatments to **promote** the latest fashion within beauty, so that a favourable report gives free publicity in newspapers and magazines. Advertisements in fashion magazines also keep clients aware of the latest releases, so expect your customers to ask for them in your salon.

You should ask your salon how it keeps up with the latest trends — going to trade shows in the major cities is an excellent way of seeing demonstrations of new equipment and products by commercial companies. Be warned, though — the commercial sector is always after new salons to join its sales list, and you could end up changing products or your supplier just for the sake of change. If your salon has a line of products that is popular and sells well, rather than changing brand, ask the sales representative to call. In a staff meeting they could go through the latest emerging trend and give samples or a demonstration.

Joining in national competitions is also a good way of meeting like-minded professionals and sharing good practice. You may be in opposite corners for a make-up competition, but watching someone like Bobbi Brown give a make-up master class or winning a competition will inspire those who can only stand back and watch in admiration! This can only help to raise the standard of skill levels in the industry, and to motivate and enthuse all who take part.

Key terms

Botox® – the brand name for the non-toxic botulinum toxin. When injected into the muscles, particularly of the face, it prevents movement, causing certain wrinkles to disappear completely.

Promote – to encourage sales through publicity or advertising.

Work effectively as part of a team

In this outcome you will learn about:

- agreeing ways of working together to achieve objectives
- politely asking for help and information from your colleagues, when necessary
- responding to requests for assistance from colleagues willingly and politely
- anticipating the needs of others and promptly offering assistance within your capabilities
- making effective use of your time throughout your working day
- reporting problems likely to affect salon services to the relevant person promptly and accurately
- resolving misunderstandings with your colleagues in a helpful way at the time they happen
- being friendly, helpful and respectful in the contact you have with colleagues.

Unit G8

Develop and maintain your effectiveness at work

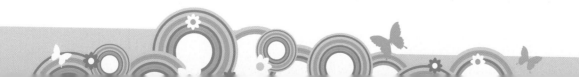

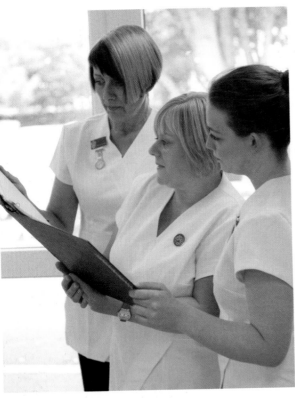

Team members need to respect and help each other

Working together to achieve objectives

(You will need to read the information in Professional basics on good communication skills, pages 16–21, and on treatment planning and preparation, pages 25–28, in conjunction with this section.)

To work well with others we must first analyse ourselves. This is a breakdown of how we see one another, and what we are judged upon:

The old saying 'Actions speak louder than words' is true!

Communication and working together

When you work in a salon, you may have a manager who supervises what you do, or you may have junior staff who you guide through the working day. Good communication means being able to get on with all your co-workers.

When working under supervision, you should:

- accept that someone is in charge
- take instructions and act upon them
- communicate effectively
- take responsibility for your job role and do it to the very best of your ability.

Working together:

- means supporting each other, not being in conflict with one another
- gives the salon a good atmosphere, which the client senses
- provides a reliable service
- gives effective results
- includes the ability to listen.

Communication is a two-way process and the ability to be an effective listener means:

- knowing when to stop talking and listen to what is being communicated
- listening with interest and understanding
- providing encouragement and confirming you have taken in the conversation
- nodding or agreeing with the point raised.

Professional staff hold the key to an effective, friendly and efficient salon. These are the skills with which they do it:

- good communication
- knowledge of client's requirements
- competence
- initiative
- responsibility
- identification of own strengths and weaknesses
- flexibility
- teamwork.

Think about it

Being a team player involves offering lots of support, getting assistance when you need it and never letting other team members down. Do you consider yourself a team player?

Think about it

Part of being a team player means working with others to achieve common goals. Attend staff meetings so you can all agree how to work together to achieve your joint aims. Be willing and polite if requested to work with someone on a project or event. It costs little to be friendly, helpful and respectful and these are the traits of a good employee.

Good communication between colleagues will build rapport, which will be reflected in the smooth running of the business.

Initiative means taking the first step or action of a task without being prompted to do so. If a job needs doing, do it without being asked. This will prove to your employer that you can be relied upon to work effectively without having to be prompted all the time.

Be responsible for all your actions. Also take responsibility for mistakes and take appropriate action to minimise damage – do not try to cover up mistakes as this will only make things worse.

Identification of your strengths and weaknesses allows for professional growth and the development of skills. This should not be seen as a personal attack, but as an opportunity for constructive guidance and evaluation of performance. A supervisor, manager and colleagues can carry this out in staff review sessions and appraisals.

Teamwork is essential for any group of people working together.

Teamwork skills – what makes a good team

To be part of a team takes patience, a willingness to help each other and respect for the others in the team. Respect cannot be bought; it has to be earned through hard work and commitment.

While a little competitiveness may be healthy in the salon (for example, the person achieving the most retail sales in a month wins a prize), a person determined to undermine her colleagues at every opportunity could not be considered a team player. The consequences may be a build-up of bad feelings between staff, resentment and ill-will – all of which are very bad for business.

As a vital part of the team you need to know:

○ who is who within the salon

○ who is responsible for what

○ who you should go to if you need information or support.

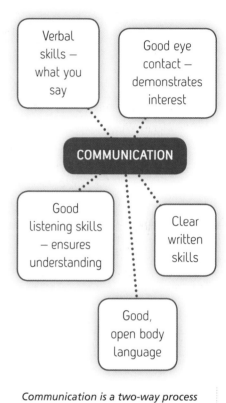

Communication is a two-way process

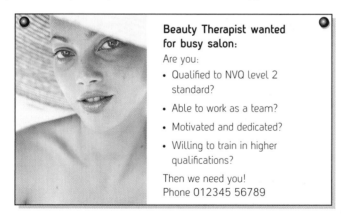

Beauty Therapist wanted for busy salon:

Are you:
- Qualified to NVQ level 2 standard?
- Able to work as a team?
- Motivated and dedicated?
- Willing to train in higher qualifications?

Then we need you!
Phone 012345 56789

Employers value the ability to work as part of a team

A good team needs:

○ an appropriate leader who is fair but decisive

○ enthusiastic, committed team members

○ good listening skills and willingness to exchange ideas

Unit G8 Develop and maintain your effectiveness at work

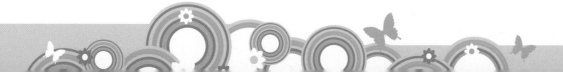

For your portfolio

Do some research into job roles and responsibility in your own salon environment. Who is responsible for stock, who for booking appointments and who for replenishing towels and blankets? Produce a flow chart to remind you of each person's job title, what the job role involves and who they are directly responsible to.

- ○ clear objectives and sense of direction
- ○ a good balance of planning and action
- ○ good communication
- ○ clear roles (you know what you are supposed to do)
- ○ flexibility and tolerance
- ○ the right number of people
- ○ the right mix of skills
- ○ a safe environment to try things, make mistakes and learn from them
- ○ a sense of humour!

Team spirit can be lost when:

- ○ group members feel that one is favoured more than others
- ○ one member of the group works on her own and refuses to join in with the team
- ○ there is a breakdown in communications
- ○ group members are unwilling to be flexible and tolerant of others' mistakes
- ○ there is too much work for too few people
- ○ job roles become blurred and people encroach upon areas they should leave to others
- ○ the team is not managed properly and resentment builds up.

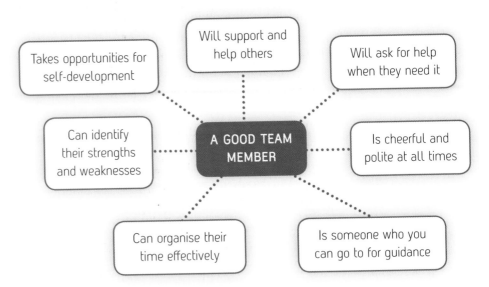

Various skills are required to make a good team member

Think about it

A bad atmosphere seeps into every corner of the salon, and the clients soon pick up on a feeling that something is not right. Any bad mood will undo the good of any treatment and spread like a poison and make the clients feel uncomfortable. Tension and ill-will between therapists will cost the salon money. Harmony and positivity are so much more relaxing for staff and clients alike. No one likes to work in an atmosphere of animosity or resentment.

Think about it

To be a fully rounded team player, you should always consider your co-workers. Think ahead! If you are organised, can you help others? If you know that your colleague has a wax treatment first thing in the morning but is running late, you could anticipate her needs and put on a wax pot to heat up for her when you do your own. Offer assistance when you can and cultivate the art of being helpful and kind without needing to be prompted. This should also make it easier to ask for help from others when you are in need.

Dealing with conflict

If you have a problem or are experiencing working relationship difficulties, what should you do?

First, tackle the problem without sulking or using angry body language and a surly tone to show your displeasure at someone. Try to keep a sense of proportion. Gossiping, spreading rumours or moaning achieves nothing; nor is it helpful to your cause.

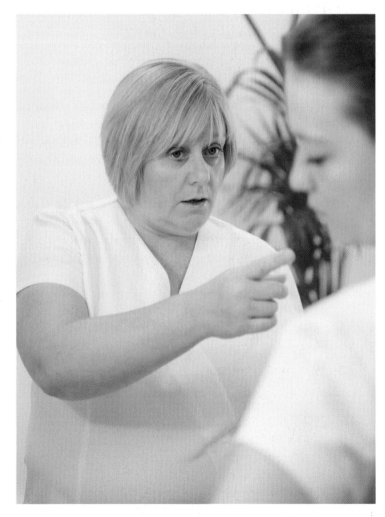

Shouting is never a good way to resolve relationship difficulties – do not tackle problems while you are still angry

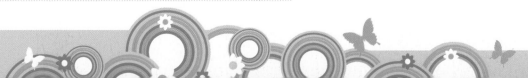

Secondly, think carefully, and do nothing while you are still angry. It may be that on reflection you realise you are in the wrong. An apology is then appropriate, and while your pride may be hurt, it will defuse the situation. It is important to learn by your mistakes and move forward, not repeating the mistakes. If you have acted thoughtlessly or caused upset without realising it, you need to make amends, and will be a bigger person for recognising that fact.

Negotiation and mediation

Often a frank, private word between the two upset parties is all that is needed to clear the air. Ask the person you are in conflict with to discuss the problem, stay calm and apologise if necessary. This will avoid prolonging the dispute. A feud that drags on for weeks is so much more difficult to resolve than one that blows over in a day or two. You can always be civil and polite and start with a 'sorry if I have upset you over this last week or so, please can we talk this through ...'

If you really feel you cannot work with the person you are in disagreement with, or feel uncomfortable or intimidated, then you must report your concerns to your manager. The manager will probably call you both in and hold a meeting where you can both air your views in a private but controlled environment. This again gives you the chance to put your case forward in a calm manner and present the facts as you see them.

The manager may wish to talk to you both individually first and then call you in together. You may find when you hear the other side of the story that you can quickly work out a solution – you may even end up laughing about the situation.

However, if the problem is of a more serious nature and you require further action, you must approach your manager in confidence and expect total privacy while you discuss your conflict. If the matter requires outside intervention, then you must be prepared to substantiate your allegations – if, for example, another member of staff assaulted you, or a staff member was stealing from the salon.

Cases of serious misconduct will, and should, be taken very seriously, and the matter should be taken to a higher authority, but such cases are few and far between. Most conflicts tend to be minor, with concerns over shirking responsibilities or not doing a job properly, or having lots of time off work, which puts others under pressure.

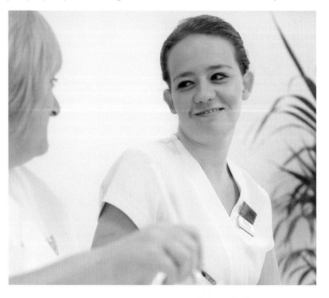

Working closely with your manager and colleagues will give you confidence

Check your knowledge

1 What does CPD stand for?
   a) Continuous professional development
   b) Constant professional development
   c) Caring personal development
   d) Constant personal development

2 When setting targets they should be:
   a) TIDY
   b) SMART
   c) ORDERLY
   d) NEAT.

3 What does NOS stand for?
   a) National Occupational System
   b) Nationwide Occupational system
   c) National Occupational Standards
   d) National Order Students

4 A contract of employment will tell you:
   a) when to get to work
   b) what your job roles will be
   c) how you should be trained
   d) which bus to catch to work.

5 A productivity target is for:
   a) helping you be productive in work
   b) incentives for sales
   c) helping you work faster
   d) helping you work harder.

6 A self-assessment appraisal is your chance to:
   a) reflect on how your colleagues are working
   b) complain about how badly everyone treats you
   c) criticise your boss and working conditions
   d) reflect on your job role and improve your performance.

7 Trends in business mean the latest:
   a) fashions
   b) magazine articles
   c) treatments and products
   d) hair styles.

8 When working with others, actions speak louder than:
   a) behaviour
   b) words
   c) body language
   d) aggression.

9 Good communication skills will build:
   a) rapport with colleagues
   b) a pay rise
   c) a licence for you to say what you like
   d) more friends.

10 When faced with a problem in the salon you should:
   a) go straight to your manager and tell her
   b) write it all down and post the letter
   c) try to sort out the problem with the person in a calm manner
   d) go straight to the salon owner and complain about the manager.

Develop and maintain your effectiveness at work   UNIT G8

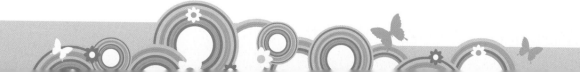

Getting ready for assessment

You cannot use any simulation within this unit, but the evidence can be gained quite easily. Remember to keep all paper evidence of any actions, showing you have actively taken part in developmental activities at work.

Your assessor will observe your contributions to effective teamwork on at least one occasion which will be recorded.

To cover the ranges you must:

- take part in opportunities to learn from colleagues and other relevant people
- actively participate in training and development activities
- actively participate in salon activities
- set targets for productivity and personal development
- offer assistance on a one-to-one basis and in a group.

Evidence could be gathered in the following ways.

- Observe a senior student carrying out a treatment that is on the salon price list that you are not yet able to do, write a report on it and then discuss it with your class, passing on the information you have learned. An assessor could observe your class discussion (very useful for key skill evidence, communication level 2).

- Attend a training day given by a commercial company and pass the trade exam at the end of the day — eyelash perming, new facial products or commercial nail training is ideal. Keep the exam paper and your certificate of competence as evidence.

- Take part in a one-to-one review in your tutorial period with either your tutor or subject lecturer. Mutually agree the target achievement date for your assessment progression, for example 'by October I will have finished all my practical waxing assessments'. Both sign and date the target date and when achieved, sign again. Include your evidence book with the assessment signed off.

- Include your treatment page from the salon, highlighting your column and indicating how many treatments you gave and how much money you took in a day. Write out a target on the page for the following weeks that includes an increase of 10% for both treatments given and money taken.

- Ask your salon lecturer to start a 'salesperson of the week' award. Have a table in the appointment book of who took the most sales in both treatments and products. A small prize could be offered to the winner, either a free eyelash tint or a nail varnish. The table would show evidence of you trying to achieve and better your previous target.

- Volunteer to become salon manager for your practical class and help your therapist colleagues set up and tidy up their treatment areas. Deal with problems as they arise. Keep a salon logbook of all activities within that salon session and your contribution.

Remember that your assessor is looking for evidence of your professional growth and ability to learn. This may be an ongoing process, and although you will be observed only once, your evidence should show progression over time and demonstrate how you have developed your skills.

Be enthusiastic, take part in any training that is offered and seek advice from people with the right experience who know more than you do. Even learning from your technician how to clean a wax pot properly can be viewed as a training experience. Soak up all you can, and this unit will present all the evidence you need.

Fulfil salon reception duties

What you will learn

G4.1 Maintain the reception area

G4.2 Attend to clients and enquiries

G4.3 Make appointments for salon services

G4.4 Handle payments from clients

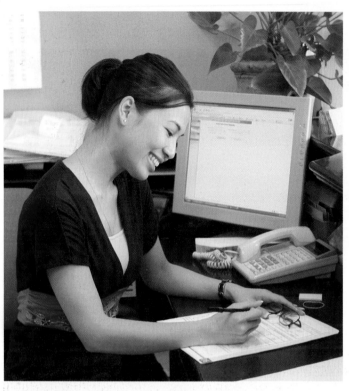

Receptionists need to be in control of paperwork and booking systems

Introduction

In this unit you will explore all the areas you need to learn about in order to become a successful beauty therapy receptionist. The reception area and receptionist are the first to be seen by the client as she enters the salon, so a warm and inviting entrance with a confident and effective receptionist is essential.

First impressions really do count – and they become lasting impressions, so it is vital that they are positive. Reception is the heart of any salon. It needs to work properly and have the right impact on clients. It should be a place of tranquillity, with order and tidiness being the key to functioning efficiently.

All visitors should be made welcome and treated with equal courtesy, so that no one feels neglected or ignored. You should acknowledge clients as they appear, even if you are unable to deal with them straight away. Every client is important to the salon, no matter what the enquiry may be – they should all be given equal attention.

You will need to learn your own salon's guidelines for dealing with general enquiries and more specific problems as they occur. You will also have to gain knowledge about each treatment, how long they take and linked services offered, as well as the system for booking appointments. All of this information will enable you to offer a professional service, guarantee client satisfaction and allow maximum cost-effectiveness to your employer.

Maintain the reception area

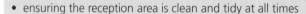

In this outcome you will learn about:

- ensuring the reception area is clean and tidy at all times
- maintaining the agreed levels of reception stationery
- ensuring that product displays have the right levels of stock at all times
- offering clients hospitality to meet your salon's client care policies.

Reception is key to the whole functioning of the salon – it will soon grind to a halt if the receptionist is poorly organised, books appointments incorrectly and is untidy.

The therapists depend upon appointments being booked correctly, with the right time allowed for each treatment. The receptionist needs to be able to produce the correct record card, the right stock request and the correct stationery to be able to order a product for the client. That means being tidy, in control of paperwork and having a thorough knowledge of the treatments as well as good **stock control**.

Refer to Professional basics, 'You, your client and the law', pages 60–62, for the relevant legislation concerned with selling retail products.

Key terms

Stock control – maintaining sufficient levels of stock, such as products, consumables and stationery, for the salon's day-to-day needs.

My story

Spa receptionist

Hi, my name is Siobhan, and I'm the receptionist in a busy spa. I run the appointments for 12 therapists, who all have different areas of expertise. It is my job to ensure their days run smoothly and the clients gain the maximum benefit from their treatments. If I were to make a mistake with the bookings, it would have a huge impact on the smooth running of the salon and the therapists would get very agitated.

My other role is to be the 'face' of the salon. I am the first point of contact for the clients, either face to face or on the phone, so I need to be calm, smiling and polite at all times. A client can even tell over the phone if you are not smiling! I also need to keep up to date with the treatments, services and products offered by the salon to ensure clients receive the treatments and products that are the most suitable. I enjoy my job as a receptionist. It is varied and I get to meet lots of interesting people.

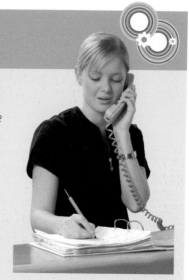

Ensuring the reception area is clean and tidy

During the course of the day a reception area can become untidy just like a living room at home: the magazines and papers soon get messy, a few coffee cups may be scattered around on the table, the odd coat is thrown over a chair, and the carpet is in need of a run over with the vacuum cleaner!

Think of the reception as part of your living area, with your clients as your guests, except that new ones are appearing more often than at home. At work, as at home, the living area takes regular upkeep to ensure it always looks clean and orderly.

Potential untidiness may be created by:

- ○ clients' coats not being put away in a cupboard
- ○ clients' umbrellas being left in a heap
- ○ magazines and papers that are not kept in a rack or in a neat pile
- ○ dirty coffee cups or water tumblers that are left on the table
- ○ tables with dirty marks or stains
- ○ delivery boxes or product trays lying around causing obstructions
- ○ a messy floor area covered with crumbs or dust
- ○ record cards being left out on the reception desk.

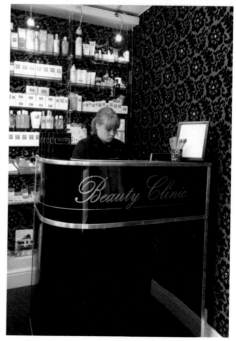

A clean and tidy reception area is inviting to clients

The key to being tidy is having the correct storage and being able to put things in their correct place. A salon should have a coat cupboard, an umbrella stand, a magazine rack, a table that is easy to clean and low-maintenance flooring. Suitable colours, which do not show the dirt, also help — all white, for example, would soon look grubby and would not be easy to keep clean.

Be careful though: there is a compromise to be found between being so house-proud that you hover over the client, waiting impatiently for the coffee to be drunk so that the cup can be washed up, and not tidying up until the end of the day when the mess has accumulated into a big job.

Tidying up should be carried out with minimum disruption to clients and at moments when the reception is at its quietest. This might be when there is a natural lull in client traffic flow, as they have gone into their treatment rooms. Do not attempt to vacuum around the clients when the reception is busy. Save the bigger jobs, such as floor cleaning, for morning preparation or evening tidying.

Morning preparation for the day ahead should include:

- switching on the lighting, both overhead and in the display cabinets
- putting out the day's newspapers
- getting the coffee pot ready, filling the kettle and filling up sugar and milk containers
- checking the appointments for the day and being ready to receive those clients
- putting the float money in the till
- emptying the dishwasher and putting cups away ready for the day
- collecting and sorting the post.

Ongoing duties throughout the day should include:

- keeping magazines tidy by putting them back in their rack
- removing used cups and glasses and washing them up or putting them in the dishwasher
- putting away record cards returned by the therapists
- topping up the kettle, filling the tea caddy, etc.
- wiping up spills on the table as they happen
- dusting around when quiet.

Evening tidying will include:

- leaving the reception area ready for the next morning
- putting on the dishwasher
- vacuuming the floor or other suitable cleaning for your type of flooring
- polishing all surfaces
- removing out-dated papers or magazines
- emptying the tea/coffee pots to avoid an unpleasant smell overnight or over the weekend
- filling any gaps in the display cabinets
- clearing the reception desk of all the day's paperwork
- tallying up the till and emptying the takings
- switching off all lighting.

Maintaining levels of stationery

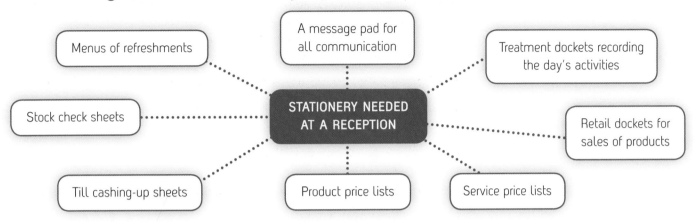

Menus of refreshments

A message pad for all communication

Treatment dockets recording the day's activities

Stock check sheets

STATIONERY NEEDED AT A RECEPTION

Retail dockets for sales of products

Till cashing-up sheets

Product price lists

Service price lists

Stationery is vital to the smooth running of reception. Running out of stationery will cause staff to use scraps of paper, or not write the information down at all, therefore forgetting vital information. Lack of the correct paperwork will affect all staff. Sales commission may be lost as the treatment and sales cannot be recorded properly. This will affect staff wages, and will not make the receptionist popular.

Vital messages may not get to the correct person, and appointments or business may be lost if there are no price lists to give out to potential clients. This is not a professional image to project. It is much better to order stationery well in advance, right down to ordering the toilet rolls! This will ensure the smooth running of all reception functions.

Ensuring product displays are stocked

Retail sales will always boost a salon's profit margin. They are a key factor in enhancing the benefits of clients' salon treatments by the use of the correct products at home. Therefore, running out of a popular line of stock or having poor displays of products neither makes good business sense nor gives the reception a professional look.

By taking regular stock checks, the receptionist can see exactly what is required. She will know which products are most popular and sell well, and which are slow moving and may require a promotion to boost sales.

Keep product displays simple but clean and neat. No one is going to be tempted to buy a dirty pot of cream, or one which looks as if it is past its sell-by date. (Refer to Unit G18 Promote additional products or services to clients, pages 105–122, for more information on this topic.)

Good product displays

Products are usually displayed in one of two ways:

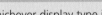

○ By product – if there are many products in the range, then use the display cabinets as storage and display the products in a logical order, by size or by type – all cleansers together, all toners together and so on. Display them by height and size so the client can easily compare the value of buying the larger, economical size (the larger the product, the better the saving – always a good selling point!).

Think about it

Whichever display type is used, the products need to be locked up to avoid potential theft. Security should be an important factor

For your portfolio

Research the display cabinets and stands that are available from various stockists. You may need to look on the internet or in salon supply magazines. Decide which would be the most suitable for your salon area and which gives you the most scope for displaying your products and displays.

○ By design – display the products for an attractive effect using 'dummy' boxes with nothing in them. Organise products in an artistic display using flowers, ribbons or even nail art gems to complement the colouring of the display cabinet. The boxes are usually clustered to form a small display within a glass case, and stock is held in a cupboard underneath for easy access.

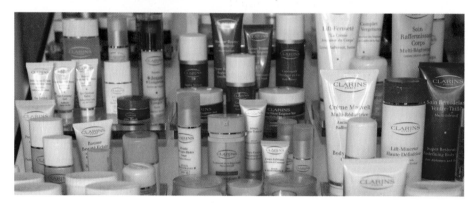

Display products for an attractive effect

Offering clients hospitality

Client care and **hospitality** are all about treating your client as you would wish to be treated yourself. No matter how good the salon treatments may be, if the client feels rushed, unwanted or is made to feel uncomfortable in any way, you will lose her business. Your salon will have a client care policy on the correct way that clients are to be greeted, both on the phone and in person. This will cover making appointments, handling payments and dealing with complaints, as well as where you store clients' coats and belongings while having a treatment and the offering of beverages in the salon.

There is a fine line between being professional, yet friendly, and being too familiar and possibly careless with your client's feelings. The old saying that 'familiarity breeds contempt' is true in business: regardless of how long you have known your clients, you must remember they are still paying for a service and deserve the best of care. The beauty therapist often learns quite personal, intimate details about her client, and there is a danger that this information could lead to a familiarity that is inappropriate.

Good client care and hospitality will ensure your clientele returns to the salon regularly, as they feel welcomed, pampered and cosseted.

Refer to Professional basics, pages 25–28, for treatment planning and preparation, which is all part of your client hospitality, pages 31–35 for other factors that contribute to client care, and page 24 for how to handle complaints.

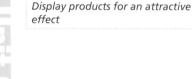

Key terms

Hospitality – being welcoming, warm and friendly, and ensuring that the clients' needs are met by offering refreshments or magazines.

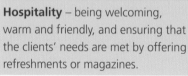

For your portfolio

Plan a summer promotion to promote waxing and pedicure treatments and a cabinet display. Design a poster promoting the special offer to enhance your display. You could link this to the research you have conducted on local salons and department store displays.

Effective product displays will pay dividends in increased sales

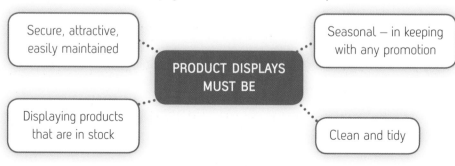

Secure, attractive, easily maintained

Seasonal – in keeping with any promotion

PRODUCT DISPLAYS MUST BE

Displaying products that are in stock

Clean and tidy

Attend to clients and enquiries

In this outcome you will learn about:

- attending to people promptly and in a polite manner
- correctly identifying the purpose of enquiries
- confirming appointments and promptly informing the relevant person
- promptly referring enquiries which cannot be dealt with to the relevant person for action
- recording messages correctly and passing them to the relevant person at the right time
- giving accurate information clearly
- giving confidential information only to authorised people
- balancing the need to give attention to individuals while ensuring others are not left without attention

The client's first impression of the salon is often formed by the way she is greeted rather than just the décor. Receiving clients into the salon is a little like greeting a guest into your home. The hospitality and friendliness should be the same. It may be the client's first or twenty-first visit; the polite and welcoming greeting should be the same. All visitors should be made welcome and treated with equal importance. This is achieved through verbal and non-verbal communication, good listening skills and questioning techniques. (These topics are fully covered in Professional basics, pages 16–21 and 31–35.)

It is important to maintain a balance between giving the correct amount of attention to individual clients and your responsibilities towards other clients during busy trading periods.

In this section you will look at good practice in handling the wide range of clients and their enquiries — a vital requirement of a successful business.

Handling enquiries

The approach to clients and visitors can be summed up in a simple word: PLEASE.

How to approach clients and visitors

Posture	This should be good, both to give a good impression (slouching gives the impression of boredom or not caring) and to protect the spine.
Listen	Listen with your whole body, not just your ears. Look as if you are listening. Eye contact encourages the talker to continue and facing the visitor shows you are giving her your full attention. You are saying to your visitor 'you are important to me and the salon and I give you my full attention'.
Expression	This should be welcoming, open and positive. You are not there to challenge the visitor or make her feel threatened. Smile and look as if you are pleased to see her.
Appearance and attitude	These should reflect total professionalism and mirror the high standard of the salon.
Speech	Speak clearly. Your speech should not be patronising in any way, and free of any technical terms a client may not understand.
Eagerness to help others	This is a positive quality and very flattering to the client. Use it wisely to give attention without appearing insincere.

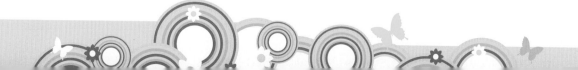

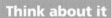
Unit G4 Fulfil salon reception duties

Think about it

Making a client angry is a sure way of losing them.

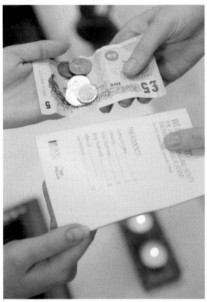

Always provide a receipt of payment

Think about it

- Always have a pen and paper handy to take messages.
- Answer the phone promptly, even if you are busy.
- If you do feel harassed, pause, take a deep breath in before lifting the receiver and put a smile in your voice. (It is very easy to sound abrupt on the telephone.)
- Identify the salon quickly, after making sure you are connected properly and the caller can hear you.
- Be cheery – no matter how pressurised you may feel, it should not show in the tone of your voice. No one wants to be greeted by a miserable-sounding receptionist.
- Redirect the call quickly when putting it through to another extension. If the call cannot be put through, ask the caller if they wish to leave a message.

The visitor should be dealt with as soon as possible and the right action taken or the appropriate staff member informed. Eye contact and a pleasant greeting are important. Introduce yourself to the visitor as you ask about the nature of the visit, for example 'Hello, welcome to Blissed Out salon. My name is Nyesha. How can I help you this morning?'

Do not:

○ ignore the client

○ act as though serving the client is the last thing you want to do

○ patronise the client by talking down to her.

The receptionist

For the receptionist to be professional and capable, she needs to know everything her job role demands. As with all life skills, knowledge leads to confidence.

A receptionist may be employed for her managerial and office skills. She may not be a beauty therapist. However, to be able to book in a client and talk knowledgeably about treatments, she must be fully aware of everything contained within the salon price list. The receptionist needs to know the limitations of her authority and when to refer to the manager or salon owner.

The receptionist should understand:

○ each treatment on the price list

○ what it involves

○ how long it takes

○ how much it costs

○ what the benefits and effects are

○ the aftercare and homecare needed

○ what products can be sold in conjunction with the treatment.

This will allow the receptionist to talk with confidence about each treatment, to book appointments correctly, to schedule the working day into a logical sequence and to advise clients appropriately.

Dealing with telephone enquiries

The telephone is now second nature to us all and mobile phones are commonplace. Not everyone can use one effectively, however. The telephone can be a very useful business tool and should be used wisely.

How to use the phone

There are key steps to a good telephone manner. These ensure that the person on the end of the phone is treated courteously, efficiently and accurately.

Identifying the purpose of the enquiry

The receptionist should ask herself these questions about her visitor in order to identify the purpose of the enquiry.

○ Why has the client come?

Do ask to use the phone if it is a quick personal call.

Do answer with a smile in your voice — just as if you can see the person's face.

Don't forget that calls may come out of office hours. Most people are comfortable leaving a message on an answer phone. Enquiries can also be made electronically via the salon's website. Remember that revenue may be lost if no one follows up the message.

Don't sigh into the phone. This gives the impression that the caller is a nuisance and you are doing them a favour by answering.

DOS

Don't use the telephone for private calls. Itemised phone bills now show who made a call, for how long and to whom. No employer would mind the odd local call or emergency message, but do not abuse an employer's goodwill.

DON'TS

Don't be curt, rude or irritated when you first pick up the phone.

Do remember that all calls are from existing or prospective clients.

Do write a message down so that anyone can read it, and make sure it is complete.

Don't make up an answer if you don't know. Honesty really is the best policy. If you make something up you will only get caught out and lose credibility.

Don't slam down the phone, cut someone off or talk about the caller in a rude manner.

The Dos and Don'ts of dealing with telephone enquiries

○ Where has the client come from?
○ Has she come for her appointment?
○ Is the client here for a price list or to purchase a product?
○ What action do I take to help the client?

Eye contact and an approachable expression will encourage the visitor to give the required information so that a decision can be made as to the proper course of action. You might say:

'Please take a seat; the manager won't keep you a moment.'
'Would you like a drink or magazine while you wait?'
'I will inform your therapist you have arrived for your appointment, Mrs Smith.'

If a client is making an enquiry by telephone, ideally the phone should be answered within four rings. All enquiries should be dealt with in a professional manner and the same courtesy should be shown to the client as if they were in the reception area.

Email enquiries should be dealt with in the same manner as soon as practical after receiving them. Ensure that full details are given to the client to ensure that they are happy with the reply. It is worth remembering that you can email at any time of day, and clients who have to cancel an appointment out of hours will often use this method, so, along with the answer phone, emails should always be checked first thing in the morning

Customers with different needs and expectations
Customers with disabilities
People with disabilities may require some help negotiating doorways and assisting into the treatment area. Always offer to help, but do not assume they cannot manage — and never patronise or talk down to the client.

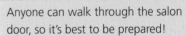

Think about it?

Anyone can walk through the salon door, so it's best to be prepared!

When dealing with clients, both face to face and on the phone, it is likely that at some time you will deal with a client who may have different needs and expectations of the service they wish to receive and will challenge the receptionist. Clients may appear confused or angry, or may have a complaint. Remember to remain polite and calm at all times.

Unit G4 Fulfil salon reception duties

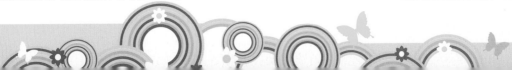

157

Wheel chair access

Deaf person

Customers with special needs may require extra assistance

Unit G4 Fulfil salon reception duties

Think about it

It can be as easy to give a bad impression over the phone as in person – perhaps more so, because the caller only judges what is heard, and may not know the background to an irritable manner.

For your portfolio

In pairs or groups, role play the following clients: angry; confused; English as a second language; complaint; hard of hearing.

The hard of hearing are usually good lip readers, so the receptionist should face the client and speak clearly so the client can see the words forming. Depending upon the severity of the disability, a pad could be provided to jot down a message. A price list could be a good visual aid to help clarify what the client wants.

People who speak English as an additional language might have difficulties communicating with you. Again, speak clearly, and use visual materials to help clarify and seek help if available.

Older clients may have problems with mobility or hearing. However, never assume this to be the case – never judge! Be on hand to offer assistance. If the client is very frail, then explain that some treatment adaptation might be needed.

Clients who appear angry

Never shout at clients. Be calm and precise when dealing with them. If they are in reception and appear angry and agitated, try to take them somewhere quiet, out of the public view, as an angry client, even if their anger is unfounded, does not do the reputation of the salon any good. Remember, if you cannot deal with the client's complaint, find someone in a more senior position to assist you.

Clients who appear confused

There may be a number of reasons for the client's confusion: for example, the client may speak English as a second language (see above) and have difficulty understanding; it may be related to an illness or a disability; or it could be something as simple as getting the date and time of the appointment wrong. It is important for the receptionist to remain calm and clarify things as many times as the client needs to ensure that they understand.

A client with a complaint

Clients with a complaint should be treated with respect and, however agitated and angry they might be, never shout or retaliate. At times, this may be difficult, but remaining calm will always give the receptionist the upper hand.

Listen carefully to the client's grievance and try to resolve the problem. If this is out of your capability, refer the complaint to someone more senior. If you are dealing with a phone complaint, you may need to say that you will ask someone more senior to phone back – if you promise this, then it's important someone does phone, as it will only annoy the client further if they do not receive the promised call.

Confirming appointments

Appointment details always need to be confirmed. Names, times and services can sound similar, and confirming the details involves double checking, which may save confusion later on.

You will need to make sure that you confirm all the details with the client: 'So, Mrs Patel, just to confirm your appointment for Wednesday the 10th, at 4 pm, for a facial with Shauna – can I give you an appointment card with that on?' Look to the client and she will usually agree with you, 'Yes, that's correct, and yes, you had better put it on a card for me, thank you.' When making appointments over the phone, as with clients in the reception area, always confirm the service and the date and time of the treatment.

Many salons now send text messages to clients the day before their appointment to remind them. The text message acts as a prompt and allows the client to reschedule the appointment if necessary, therefore saving precious salon time through missed appointments and lost revenue.

If the client has just arrived for her appointment, acknowledge her presence and inform the therapist her client has arrived. If there is a slight delay, then keep the client informed, take her coat, make her a drink and give her a magazine.

If the client's treatment is personal, then you should not repeat it too loudly. Just confirm her arrival.

Referring enquiries and recording messages correctly

Enquiries cannot always be dealt with by the receptionist, and in these cases you should refer the enquiry to someone who can help. However, if the relevant person is not available you will need to take a message and pass this on at an appropriate time. During the course of your reception duties you will be asked to take messages for other staff members, the manager, or even a client having a treatment.

This valuable service also provides evidence for your portfolio. Make sure you get your message signed and dated by the person it should go to (and include the assessor number where appropriate) and it can go into your evidence portfolio.

It is very important to write down the whole message exactly as you heard it, even if you think it sounds odd, or it is difficult to understand.

You will need to include:

- ○ the date and time of the call
- ○ how important the message is — if necessary, write 'urgent' on it
- ○ a brief description of the nature of the message
- ○ whether the caller needs a reply — a return telephone number is then essential.

It is important to listen carefully and to ask the caller to repeat any part of the message you did not understand or hear properly. Always repeat the whole message back to the caller to make sure you have all the details correctly on the pad — especially the return number.

Passing on messages manually and electronically

Many large companies have internal computer systems that allow staff to email internally. Provided each person has access to a computer, and the system is set up centrally, anyone can receive a message on their computer. An address book is set up, you type in your message and send it, and it goes to the person's inbox.

Computer technology has the advantage of saving paper and allowing several people to be given the same information at once without having to write several messages. However, the drawback is that you cannot guarantee that the person you emailed will be able to open the email that day, or that they are in the office to do so.

Many salons use a system of a personal pigeonhole with the name above or below it. Messages can be left in the pigeonhole and can be collected throughout the day.

MESSAGE

FOR	Deepak
FROM	Mrs Alessi
TEL NO.	0208 321 145

TELEPHONED ✔   PLEASE RING ✔

CALLED TO SEE YOU ☐   WILL CALL AGAIN ☐

WANTS TO SEE YOU ☐   URGENT ☐

MESSAGE: Needs to speak to you asap – you can call her on the tel. no. above up to 5.30pm

DATE: 10.05.10   TIME: 9.03am

RECEIVED BY: Amber

A message pad can be useful for recording messages

Think about it

Salons may also use email to let clients know of special offers by sending a monthly newsletter containing promotional information.

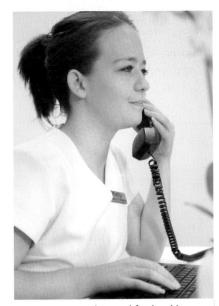

Computers can be used for booking appointments

Fulfil salon reception duties **Unit G4**

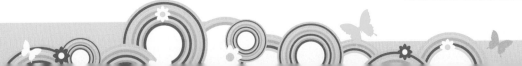

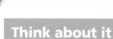
Unit G4 Fulfil salon reception duties

> **Think about it**
>
> Urgent messages, appointment cancellations and accident or emergency messages should be given in person.

> **Think about it**
>
> Professionalism should be the theme running throughout your training, and integrity is a major part of professionalism. Integrity means being honest, acting with honour and being reliable and truthful in all that you do.

> **Think about it**
>
> If a client's health status or other sensitive or personal information is not kept private, you are breaking confidentiality. You need to be aware of, and abide by, the Data Protection Act. If you break this confidentiality, you may be subject to criminal proceedings. (Refer to Professional basics, pages 63–64 for further information.)

A pin board for messages also works well – confidential messages can be sealed in an envelope and addressed as personal so that no one opens them by mistake.

Computer technology can also be used for booking appointments and taking payments. In addition, software programmes can be installed to keep stock records and client record cards, and to print off price lists and gift vouchers. Many salons also have websites advertising the treatments that they offer, with price lists and the option for clients to make enquiries and book appointments. Websites can be built fairly easily today and there are a number of companies that design websites to meet any need and fit any budget, so even a mobile therapist may consider having a website to promote her business. There are also a number of companies available that work exclusively with therapists to help promote their business. Your professional body will have details of such companies. (Refer to Professional basics, 'Data Protection Act 1998', pages 63–64.)

Regular computer training is essential so that all staff know how to access and use the information stored in a computer.

Giving accurate information

Try to make sure that information you give about products or services is as accurate as possible. If you make something up to keep the client happy, your advice may be unsafe and you will lose the confidence of the client. (Refer also to Unit G18 Promote additional products or services to clients, pages 114–15.)

Dealing with confidential information

It is essential to be sensitive to all confidential information. This includes the client's medical details and personal information as well as their treatment history held on record cards or electronically on the salon's computer.

A client's address, telephone number, health status/problems, medication and other personal details are all classed as confidential. You are allowed to give these details to authorised people only, such as your salon owner, manager or therapist colleagues. No persons outside the salon must have access to your clients' personal details.

Make appointments for salon services

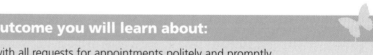

In this outcome you will learn about:

- dealing with all requests for appointments politely and promptly
- accurately identifying client requirements for the service requested
- scheduling appointments in a way that satisfies the client, the therapist and ensures the most productive use of salon time
- confirming that the appointment details are acceptable to the client
- recording appointment details accurately, clearly and to meet your salon's requirements.

It is usual for the appointments for each therapist to be recorded in a large book with either a column or a page for each. This allows the therapist to see at a glance the treatments booked in for the day and to make the appropriate preparation.

The golden rule is to have a system and make full use of it. Requests for appointments should be dealt with promptly and politely.

Filling in the appointments pages

Pages should be set out for several weeks in advance so that clients booking ahead or wanting special days (pre-wedding make-up, etc.) can book in confidence. It is useful when planning a course of treatments for a client — say twice a week for six weeks. This also allows the therapist to do some advanced planning should she need time off.

Many salons now use a computer booking system to record the appointments of their clientele. This method is used in the same way as an appointment book. There are a number of advantages over a manual system: the computer can be used to generate a mailing list and keep a record of treatments and has numerous other facilities that an appointment book alone cannot offer, such as stock levels, sales figures, recent orders and delivery times and dates.

When booking the appointment the receptionist needs the following details:

○ client's name

○ client's contact details

○ service or treatment required

○ date and time of appointment

○ therapist booked for service or treatment.

It would be advantageous to the client to know the estimated price of the treatment/ service when booking.

The receptionist also needs to know the length of the appointment she should book in order to ensure the most effective use of the therapist's time, thereby maximising the salon's productivity. She should also check with the client that she has enough time for the treatment/service to be carried out: for example, not booking an hour and a half treatment if the client only has an hour available. Time must also be allowed for:

○ greeting the client and the consultation

○ client undressing

○ client preparation during the treatment

○ client getting dressed, and being given homecare and aftercare advice.

The appointments page may look like the one on page 162.

Remember that if the salon has a system of coding, it should be used — it will make life easier. For example: C = cancellation, L = late arrival, A = client has arrived, and so on.

Some salons do not have columns for each therapist; instead they allot a workstation number or couch position and then fit the staff around the treatments that need to be completed. The advantage of this system is that the workload can easily be

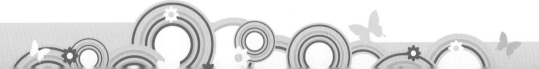

Date: Tuesday 12th October 2010

	Lucy	Hellena	Anetta	Siobhan	
AM **9.00**	Mrs Khan	Mrs Hughes			**9.00** AM
9.15	full	full			9.15
9.30	Bodywax	B/Massage			9.30
9.45	0123445678	223335			9.45
10.00					**10.00**
10.15					10.15
10.30		Mrs Inder			10.30
10.45	Miss Jones	Pedicure			10.45
11.00	Aroma	+ ½ leg wax	Miss Westerby		**11.00**
11.15	Backmassage	01235 771540	French		11.15
11.30	357928		Manicure		11.30
11.45			+ facial		11.45
12.00			01329 815242	Mr. Vallete	**12.00**
	LUNCH	Mrs Green Eyetint 444321		Backmassage + pedicure 02271881570	
13.00	Mr. Walsh Manicure + backwax 02392815815	LUNCH	Miss Rudman Miss Allen X 2 eyebrows	Miss Binder waxing	
14.00	Mrs Suline Eyebrow tidy 413927	Miss Murphy Arm wax + u/arm wax	335215 LUNCH	e/b + lip & chin 07807577211	
15.00		223792	Miss Nair Bridal	Mrs Pattel Sugaring	
		Miss Woolford Basic facial +	Top to toe 447812	to X 2 leg 221335	
16.00	Mrs Wang Non-surg. facial lift 08729815111	eyelash tint 445877			
17.00		Mrs Townsend M/up lesson 315579 ext. 222			

A page from an appointment book

distributed between staff, and the manager can allot the jobs as fairly as possible. The disadvantage is that regular customers do not always get the same therapist.

When booking an appointment, it is important to do the following.

- ◯ Fill out the details in pencil. This allows alterations or cancellations without making the page illegible.
- ◯ Have an easy code to identify any potential problems (see above).
- ◯ Make sure that everyone can easily understand start and finish times.
- ◯ Make sure that all names and numbers are clear and legible.
- ◯ Allow the hard-working therapist a break for lunch.
- ◯ Do not be pressurised by a persistent client into giving a lunchtime appointment to a therapist who has had no other break during the day. Good practice is to stagger the lunch breaks, so that there is always a therapist covering a busy lunchtime session.
- ◯ Do give an appointment card to the client with all the details recorded on it so she has a record of when she has to come in. This cuts down the possibility of a missed appointment.

Date	Time	Treatment booked	Therapist
14.2.10	11:00am	Warm oil facial + manicure	Saskia

An appointment card

Missed appointments

Have a clear salon policy on missed appointments. Some salons make a small cancellation charge if the appointment is missed – rather like dentists or physiotherapists. This is usually in the region of £30. There is usually no cancellation fee if the appointment is cancelled with 24 hours' notice. Both staff and clients need to be clear on this policy and it could be displayed in the reception area. This is when text messages or email reminders to clients are helpful: they are less likely to forget their appointment or can rearrange if necessary.

Be flexible and be prepared to fit in the client who arrives without an appointment. The receptionist should always check first and then fit the client into a suitable slot. She should then inform the therapist, who may not be aware that another client is waiting for her.

Think about it

If time is not allowed for all aspects, the first treatment of the day will overrun, making the next appointment late. This can continue all day and the knock-on effect may be that the last client is kept waiting far too long. The therapist is put under pressure, the client may feel rushed and the benefits of the treatment will be lost.

Think about it

Be aware of the new client and have a code to alert the therapist. This allows patch testing (if required) to be carried out as well as a full consultation if needed.

Unit G4 Fulfil salon reception duties

Handle payments from clients

In this outcome you will learn about:

- accurately totalling charges to the client
- informing clients of charges clearly and in a courteous manner
- visually inspecting purchases for condition and quality as they are processed for payment
- establishing the client's method of payment and acknowledging receipt of payments
- ensuring accepted payments are correct
- recording information about the sale accurately, clearly and to meet your salon's requirements
- gaining authorisation for accepting non-cash payments when the value exceeds the limit you are able to accept
- tactfully informing clients when authorisation cannot be obtained for non-cash payments
- identifying and resolving, where possible, any discrepancies in payments within the limits of your authority
- promptly referring payment discrepancies which you cannot resolve to the relevant person for action
- giving the correct change and issuing receipts when required by clients
- following cash point security procedures at all times
- identifying and reporting low levels of change in time to avoid shortages.

How the financial side of any business is approached is as vital as the treatment side. The client should be treated as courteously at the end of her treatment as at the beginning. Politeness is of prime importance when she is paying for her treatment.

Methods of payment

Several methods of payment are available. How the client pays is very much her choice and the receptionist must be prepared and able to cope with any payment method. The client should always be told the amount politely and asked which payment method is going to be offered.

All payment methods are equally acceptable and should be handled with care. However, it will be up to the individual salon to state which payment methods it wishes to accept. Salons often have a sign in the reception area and on their price lists stating the payment methods that are accepted. Clients who phone with an enquiry or to make an appointment should be told of the methods of payment that are available to them.

Cash

When a customer is paying cash (a rarity these days), there are several aspects to be aware of. A large denomination bank note, that is £20 or £50, should be checked to ensure it is genuine and not counterfeit.

○ Look for the watermark – every note has a watermark that can be seen when the note is held up to the light.

○ Look for the metallic strip which is woven into the paper – it should be unbroken.

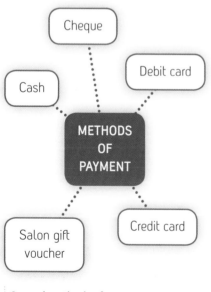

Several methods of payment are possible

- Compare the feel of the bank note paper – often a forged note is not printed on the same quality paper and may have a thin feel.
- Often the police circulate a list of forged note numbers to be on the lookout for. The numbers are on a stop list and this list should be kept near the till, so that numbers can be compared.

At the end of the day's business the till must be totalled and the takings matched against the recorded amount taken, either through the till roll or a docket system. If a float has been used to provide small change at the beginning of the day, then it needs to be deducted from the total takings. This can then be used for the next day's trading. The balance of the takings should be paid into the salon bank account. Most large banks offer a night safe facility, where the takings can be deposited. It is not ideal to keep large amounts of money and cheques on the premises overnight – there is always the risk of a burglary.

If there is a problem with a bank note, it will normally be because the client has accepted this money from another source, and the authorities should be notified. It is important that the note is removed from circulation and the police are informed. Ask the client quietly to step into the office away from reception to avoid embarrassment. Ask the supervisor, manager or owner to deal with the situation. The receptionist can then return to her duties at the front desk.

Even when accepting money from very regular customers, you should still check it thoroughly. Dealing with cash involves a lot of responsibility, and care must be taken to avoid errors.

Procedure for handling cash payments

Place the client's money on the till ledge to ensure you remember the amount given to you. Do not place the money straight in the till drawer as this may lead to confusion – was it a £10 or a £20 note? Count the change required from the note, and then re-count it into the client's hand. Place the client's money in the till drawer and close it. Give the client the receipt to confirm the cost of the treatment, how much was given to you, and the change you gave.

Cheques

A cheque is no more than an instruction to the bank telling it to pay a specific sum to a specified person. Most banks and building societies offer a cheque service, although a debit card service is also available (see below).

A cheque payment is acceptable to a salon, providing certain checks and precautions are carried out. Always check that:

- the date is correct (day, month and year), especially important around New Year
- the name of the salon is spelt correctly – the client could be offered a stamp with the full name pre-printed on it
- the amount of money is correct, and is in words as well as numbers
- the signature is completed correctly and matches the signature on the cheque guarantee card.

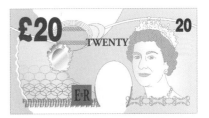
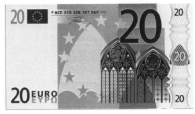

Large denomination bank notes should be checked carefully

Think about it

It is important not to feel embarrassed when checking money; it will save the salon and protect the customer.

Think about it

Payments for all treatments need to be acknowledged by a handwritten or a till receipt, regardless of the method of payment used.

Unit G4 · Fulfil salon reception duties

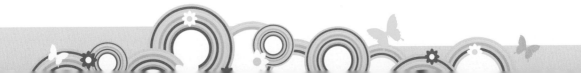

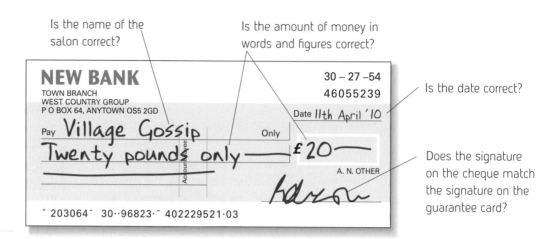

Is the name of the salon correct?

Is the amount of money in words and figures correct?

Is the date correct?

Does the signature on the cheque match the signature on the guarantee card?

Look carefully at all these items on a cheque

Unit G4
Fulfil salon reception duties

Think about it

If a cheque is faulty in any way, the bank will reject it and return it to the salon. It is up to the salon to contact the customer and inform her of the fault. The customer will then need to call into the salon and alter and initial any necessary changes. It may be wise to rewrite the cheque altogether. So it is much easier to get it right first time.

A number of business have recently stopped accepting cheques as a form of payment favouring the use of debit cards, if your salon has decided not to accept cheques as a form of payment, you should advertise the fact in the salon and on price lists. This will prevent potential embarrassment if the client does not have another method of payment.

What is a cheque guarantee card?

A cheque guarantee card should always support a cheque. It has two functions.

○ It acts as proof of identity.

○ It guarantees that the bank will honour the cheque up to the limit of the card. The limit on bank cards is either £100 or £250.

Always check the expiry date on the card, written as 03/12 for example, for the month and year the card needs to be reissued. Also check that the signatures match and the card type is the same as the cheque; that is, both are issued by the same bank. The cheque is then treated exactly like cash and put into the till. A receipt is given and the till is closed.

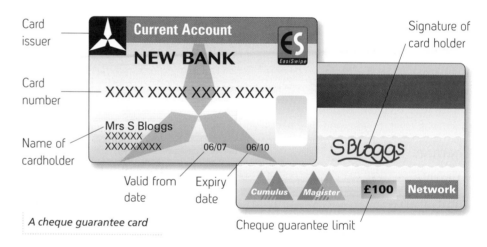

Card issuer

Card number

Name of cardholder

Signature of card holder

Valid from date

Expiry date

Cheque guarantee limit

A cheque guarantee card

Credit cards

Credit cards are often referred to as 'plastic money'. Credit card companies offer credit cards to those customers they consider creditworthy.

How credit cards work

If your salon has a contract with a credit card company, it will usually display a sign stating that credit cards are accepted. Most salons use the chip and pin linked to their computerised till for credit or debit card transactions (see below). If the amount is large, the chip and pin facility will check to see if the client has enough credit before the payment is authorised.

Debit cards

All banks now offer the convenience of a debit card. In a number of businesses these have taken the place of both cheques and cash transactions. The payment is made electronically by transferring money straight from the customer's bank account to the salon's account.

Debit cards are usually the same as the cheque guarantee card, should the customer wish to write a cheque.

The card is inserted into a chip and pin machine and the amount is entered by the receptionist taking the payment. The customer then enters their unique pin number and electronic authorisation is given by the bank. The customer is given a copy of the receipt and the business has a duplicate, which is used when calculating the takings at the end of the day.

The salon may impose a minimum spend on debit or credit cards as the business has to pay for every transaction by this method of payment either to the bank or credit card company. This is usually 1.5–2 per cent of the transaction. In some cases, this is passed on to the customer by the business, but salons do not normally charge the client for using a debit card.

Cash equivalents and pre-paid cards

Salon gift vouchers

> **Think about it**
>
> Be careful with credit and debit cards. All the information is stored in the chip and this can sometimes become damaged and the information destroyed.

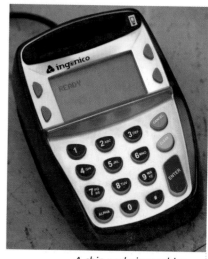

A chip and pin machine

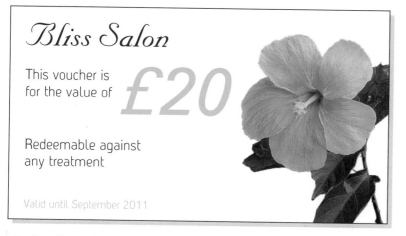

Bliss Salon

This voucher is for the value of **£20**

Redeemable against any treatment

Valid until September 2011

A salon gift voucher

A gift voucher is a good alternative to giving someone cash as a present. As the name suggests, it is a voucher to the value of a set sum of money. The voucher usually includes a card with the salon details on it. The amount of money to be exchanged will also be prominently displayed. When the lucky person who has received a gift voucher presents it to the salon, the receptionist will treat it exactly the same as a cash transaction. For security, the vouchers have serial numbers to avoid duplication or reuse. This makes them easier to track.

When the voucher goes into the till, it should be kept in a separate compartment from the notes. The receptionist or therapist should put a line through it and give her initials to state that it has been used.

Pre-paid cards

There are new advances in technology that could make plastic cards obsolete within the next few years. Manufacturers in phone technology have designed a phone that thinks it's a credit card! It works by sending bank details — which are now contained in the chip on your credit or debit card — in an infrared beam from the phone to the till. After purchases are scanned at the checkout as normal, the customer selects the 'banking' menu on his or her phone, chooses the payment function and enters a personal four-digit pin code into the keypad. Pushing the 'send' key beams the information into a receiving unit in the till. This passes the information to the account to be debited, in much the same way as completing a normal chip and pin transaction. As with the chip and pin debit/credit card, no signature is required. Some salons have now adopted this increasingly popular payment method. It is hoped that fraud and stolen cards will be a thing of the past, as the process is so easy to manage.

Invalid payments

Unfortunately, there may be times when payment discrepancies and disputes arise. They should be dealt with calmly, without causing embarrassment to the client. If you are unable to resolve the dispute refer to a senior staff member, salon manager or owner.

Possible problems may include the following.

- Invalid currency is presented — perhaps a foreign note or even a forged note.
- An invalid card is presented — it may be out of date, or not match the cheque details.
- A cheque is filled out incorrectly, or does not have a current cheque guarantee card.
- The client has entered the incorrect pin for their card.
- Fraudulent use of a payment card is suspected — perhaps it has been put on to the stop list.

Discounts and special offers

A good way of promoting a slow-moving product, or of getting the new season off to a good start, is to offer either a discount on a service or a free service to entice clients into having the full treatment. Often supermarket promotions will be 'buy one — get one free', or you get a free small conditioner when you purchase shampoo. A salon can offer the same type of discounts: for example, at the start of summer, when everyone wants leg waxing and pedicures, a salon could offer a free bikini wax with every half-leg wax. The wax is already on, the therapist can perform the service in a short time while doing the leg wax, and the client is very happy to be receiving a free treatment! A pedicure could include a free polish — very little outlay for the salon, but again a good gift to pass on to the customer.

All these variations of costs need to be carefully put through the till, so that the stock and money add up at the end of the day. If the client has been given a free nail polish by the therapist and the receptionist tries to charge it to the client, she is not going to be very happy! The receptionist needs to know what is going on, and how to work the till to show discounts and free products.

A course of treatments often includes a free one, or payment in full for a course might offer a 10 per cent discount, so the receptionist will need to know how to work out a percentage.

How to calculate a discount

Fractions, decimals and percentages are just different ways of saying the same thing: $\frac{1}{2}$ is the same as 0.5 and 50 per cent.

These three you should know straight off without any problem:

Diagram	Fraction	Decimal	Percentage
	$\frac{1}{4}$	0.25	25%
	$\frac{1}{2}$	0.50	50%
	$\frac{3}{4}$	0.75	75%

Converting fractions to decimals to percentages

For the ones you don't know, you must be able to convert them like this:

Fraction e.g. $\frac{1}{5}$ → Divide using the calculator $(1 \div 5)$ → **Decimal** $= 0.2$ → $\times 100$ (0.2×100) → **Percentage** $= 20$ per cent (%)

Fraction	Decimal	Percentage:
$\frac{1}{4}$	0.25	25%

Diagram	Fraction	Decimal	Percentage
1/4	$\frac{1}{4}$	0.25	25%
1/2	$\frac{1}{2}$	0.50	50%
3/4	$\frac{3}{4}$	0.75	75%

Fraction e.g. $\frac{1}{5}$ → Divide using the calculator (1, 5) → **Decimal** $= 0.2$ → · by 100 $(0.2 \cdot 100)$ → **Percentage** 20%

Fraction e.g. $\frac{1}{8}$ → (1, 8) → **Decimal** $= 0.125$ → $(0.125 \cdot 100)$ → **Percentage** $= 12.5\%$

Converting fractions to decimals and percentages

Salon services and available products

Refer to Unit G18 Promote additional products or services to clients, pages 108–09, for information on how to gain knowledge on which treatments your salon offers.

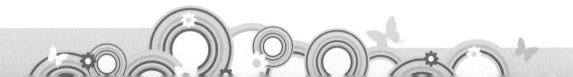

How the till works

Tills come in all shapes and sizes and vary in their functions, depending upon their age and what they are required to do. Scanning tills are automated to pick up a bar code on goods and products. The bar code includes the price and the stock levels, making reordering and analysis of sales easy. The operator has little work to do except for clearing the till when mistakes occur and loading the till roll.

Supermarket tills have a discount system built into the software. The scanner picks up the price and then automatically takes off the appropriate discount. Any till receipt will show the deductions at the end. Some larger salon chains now offer a discount or loyalty service that is often used during promotions to entice clientele.

Smaller salon tills do not often have a scanner facility. Discounts should be done manually and clearly marked on the receipt with the therapist's or receptionist's initials to verify the date and amount.

Manual tills do have an adding-on button, usually a + sign, so that items that are listed separately can be added up for a final total. The whole front button panel looks a little like a calculator and includes a percentage button and a subtotal button. Staff till training should be available for all, with regular updates as the technology changes. It is important to ensure the bill is accurately totalled, before confirming the price with the client and accepting, the payment.

Dealing with damaged goods

When finalising a transaction with a client, it is good practice to check products for faults, damage or leaks. It is both disappointing and inconvenient if a product has to be returned. (Refer also to the Sale and Supply of Goods Act in Professional basics, page 62.)

Often clients do not mind if a box is slightly damaged as long as the quality of the goods inside is still perfect. Do not try to sneak the purchase into the bag without telling the client — it looks as though you have something to hide. Point out the damage and explain to the client that it will not affect the goods. Providing it is within your authority to offer a discount, offer to reduce the item if the client is unhappy. If you cannot give deductions, you must ask the manager and obtain a signature on the till receipt.

If the goods themselves are damaged or leaking, they should be replaced. It can be frustrating if the product is the last one in stock and the client really wishes to purchase it. Again, some form of discount could be suggested, but details must be written on the till receipt to avoid the goods being brought back for a full refund.

All stock should be checked when unpacking the bulk purchase from the salon supplier, as the damage may have been caused in transit and not be the salon's fault. If you sign for a parcel and do not check it before the delivery person leaves, then it is unlikely your supplier will accept responsibility for the damage. If the stock arrives damaged and you have checked it and discovered the damage, you can send it back.

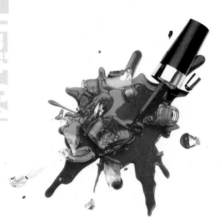

Accidents can happen and goods can be damaged or broken

If stock has been around a long time and the packaging is not as good as new, then the solution is often to have a bargain basket. Prices are reduced and the goods put in a basket on display. People will often be tempted to buy as everyone loves a bargain! Do be careful, though, that the basket is not left unattended as items are liable to be stolen. Damaged stock that is reduced in price will have to be written off against profits, so try to keep accidental damage to a minimum.

Money matters – a float

At the end of the day's business, the takings in the till must be totalled and matched up with the recorded sales and treatment dockets. A set amount of money is put into the till every morning, called a float, to provide change for clients paying in cash. It is usual to count out the float and replace it in the till for the next day's trading.

A typical float would consist of a mixture of change (for example):

- 2 × £10 notes
- 4 × £5 notes
- £30 in £1 coins
- £10 in 50p coins
- £5 in 20p coins
- £5 in 10p coins
- £1 in 5p coins
- £1 in 2p and 1p coins.

This will, of course, depend upon the size of the salon, how busy it is, and how many people pay in cash. Most transactions are carried out by debit or credit cards – very few small businesses handle a lot of cash unless the cost of goods is small, such as in a greengrocer's shop.

Security procedures

Security in the reception area is important, both for stock and for the till itself. Never leave the till drawer open when leaving the area, or leave it with the key in for easy access – unfortunately not everyone is honest. Presenting a thief with an open till will invalidate an insurance claim, as adequate measures were not in place.

Some salons have a wall or floor safe to keep the takings in and store the daily float money. The takings need to be banked frequently, but avoid taking them to the bank at the same time every day. This may make you a target for a thief, who may be watching your movements. Most banks offer a night safe facility, where takings can be deposited. Again, be safe, do not go on your own, and do not go at the same time every day.

Larger salons employ security firms to collect the moneyboxes from the salon and deliver them to the bank. Security guards have special headwear, eye goggles and often body suits to protect them against attack.

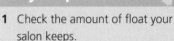

For your portfolio

1 Check the amount of float your salon keeps.
2 Count your takings at the end of the day. How much money have you taken? Remember to deduct the float.
3 How much have you taken in debit and credit card payments?
4 How many gift vouchers or pre-paid cards have you taken?
5 How many products have you sold?

Unit G4 Fulfil salon reception duties

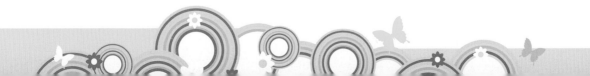

171

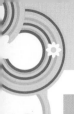

Check your knowledge

1   List five things you could do to help keep the reception area tidy.

2   Why would it be important to check emails first thing in the morning?

3   Name two benefits of text reminders for the salon?

4   List six items of stationery that are essential for the receptionist.

5   What are the two types of displays of products most commonly used?

6   What does client hospitality mean?

7   Which Act of Parliament do you need to uphold when storing client's details on a computer?

8   What would you do if you knew the client was going to be kept waiting?

9   What do you need in order to use email?

10   What will happen if you do not know how long a treatment takes and you are booking a client in?

11   List four other functions that a computer can provide to the receptionist other than storing appointments.

12   What is your salon policy on missed appointments?

13   What is the gift voucher or pre-paid card the same as?

14   How does a credit card work?

15   Your salon usually charges £17.50 for a facial. It is currently running a seasonal promotion offering a 10 per cent discount on facial treatments. How much is the discount and what is the new price of the treatment?

Getting ready for assessment

The evidence gained for this unit is quite straightforward. The best way of covering all the ranges is to spend a set time at the reception desk at your place of training. Ideally, a rota of students with no experience can be drawn up and matched with experienced students, who will pass on the skills needed to greet clients, make appointments and tend to all reception duties. An assessor can then observe your activities, and very quickly a portfolio of ranges starts to develop.

Even though a new student will have little experience of booking appointments and handling payments, a day spent observing others and being guided through the process is the only way to learn these new skills.

An assessor will expect you to be professionally presented, polite and courteous, with open body language and good interpersonal skills. Those qualities are far more important than getting the till operation correct at the first attempt. Think of it like taking a driving test – stalling the engine is not the end of the world as long as the correct procedures are followed. Seeking clarification from a more senior staff member, or asking for help if you think the problem is outside your own authority, will not mean you are considered incompetent – rather it shows you are mature enough to seek help and you have an understanding of your own personal limitations (which is actually a range you need to cover).

- Keep a reception diary of events, problems sorted, and how you dealt with situations such as an angry customer or a disabled client. Get it signed by the senior reception staff or your assessor at the end of the day.

- Be as helpful as you can and volunteer for any extra duties – they may cover a range you are unable to cover in the normal course of the day. For example, escorting a client on a conducted tour of the facilities may be classed as handling a confused client if she is unsure of prices, what the treatment consists of, or even how to find her way to the toilet!

- If you help on the reception desk in your place of work, then an employer's letter can be invaluable as evidence. It may not be in a beauty salon, but could be anywhere where you deal with members of the public, take payments and use a till, book clients in for hair appointments or doctor's appointments, or deal with telephone enquiries. The employer's letter should clearly outline your duties in as much detail as possible and be dated and signed.

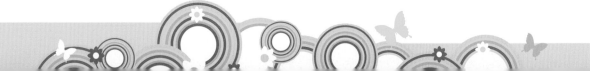

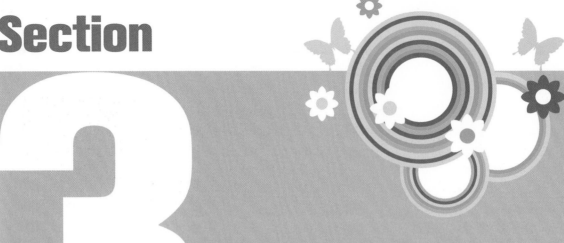

Section

3

Anatomy, physiology and the skin

You and the skin

What you will learn

- How skin type and colour is determined
- Impact of environment and lifestyle on the skin
- The pH of skin and desquamation
- How to recognise skin types and conditions
- Skin characteristics and skin types of different ethnic groups
- The photosensitivity of skin
- Tools for diagnosing skin types and conditions
- Face shapes and contours
- Contra-indications to facial treatments
- Other skin conditions – pigmentation disorders
- Allergic reactions and sensitivity testing
- Male skin
- Factors affecting the skin-ageing process
- The skin and the sun

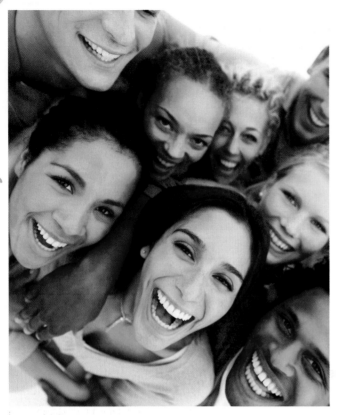

Everyone's skin is different – all clients have individual needs

Introduction

This section looks at all aspects of the skin, which is a continuing theme throughout each unit you are assessed upon. For information on the anatomy of the skin, refer to Related anatomy and physiology on pages 229–35.

The skin is a core subject for all beauty therapists to understand – not just for completing your assessments but so that you have the knowledge to offer your clients the most suitable programme for their individual needs.

Knowing how to treat the skin (and hair and nails) is essential for all the practical units, both for Level 2 and when you progress on to further treatments within Level 3. These include face and body treatments using mechanical or electrical equipment along with manual massage techniques.

A full knowledge of how the skin behaves, how it grows and what its problems or reactions may be will enable you to make sound judgements when diagnosing skin types, planning treatments and product use, and recognising potential skin problems that would prevent the treatment from taking place at all (this is called a contra-indication to treatment).

Try this quick quiz:

○ What is the largest organ of the body?

○ What is the waterproof covering for the body, stopping water getting in or out?

○ What makes vitamin D in the presence of sunlight?

○ What protects the body from harmful ultraviolet (UV) rays?

○ What makes up the majority of the contents of a vacuum cleaner?

○ What helps regulate body temperature?

○ What is dead and yet grows continuously?

○ What is found on the body that is thin, thick and has lots of layers?

○ What has a surface area of up to 6 square metres?

○ What do you lose up to 20 kilograms of in a lifetime?

○ What stops poisonous chemicals and germs from entering your body?

○ What contains sense organs that help us detect changes in our environment?

The answer to all these questions is the skin. This illustrates how amazing, hard working and versatile the skin is – and yet most of us take it for granted until it goes wrong!

How skin type and colour is determined

The type, condition and **ethnicity** of your skin are determined both genetically and environmentally. While the ethnicity of your skin is clearly inherited, your skin type

We inherit our characteristics through our parents

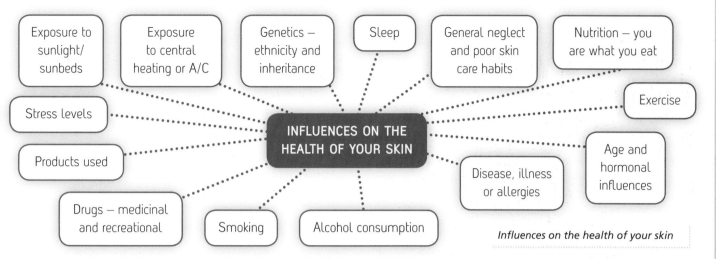

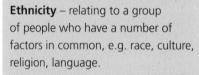

Influences on the health of your skin

may also be inherited to some extent. However, both skin type and condition can be hugely influenced by how the skin is treated, the products that are used, external conditions and lifestyle choices.

Genetics

We are all a product of our parents and we inherit all our characteristics from our families, either directly through our mother and father, or indirectly from our grandparents and sometimes further back in the family.

Every newborn baby's cells contain an inbuilt programme for its future development and growth, a set of instructions that are predetermined. In normal, healthy babies, the instructions will be the same and will make up a basic recipe for a human being. All the organs will be in the right place and working well, and, depending upon the sex of the baby, the outer appearance will be the same for us all, and reflect our family background and ethnic origins.

These instructions are found within an individual's **DNA**: an arrangement of codes that will produce an individual set of features. These are often called units of inheritance. They determine hair colour, eye colour, skin colouring and so on. It is so individual to each human being that forensic scientists are able to match DNA from tissue or hair found at a crime scene with the criminal. It is therefore a powerful tool to help fight crime. A DNA sample can be taken from the inside of the cheek lining using a sterile swab, its contents determined and the results stored on a computer.

How are the instructions in genes used? A simple way to visualise this is to think of a gene as carrying a set of instructions for the manufacture of an enzyme. This enzyme can be the difference between a characteristic being present or not: for example, if you have brown eyes, it is because you have the enzyme that helps in the production of the brown pigment. This enzyme can only be made if you have this gene.

Genes contain a mixture of influences from both parents. For example, a child may inherit the curly hair and dark colouring of its mother, and grow to be tall like its father. There may also be an inherited gene from a grandparent, perhaps if both the parents are blond but have a child with ginger or red hair. The genes of the grandparents may have influenced the colouring, as neither parent had a predominant red hair colour.

Key terms

Ethnicity – relating to a group of people who have a number of factors in common, e.g. race, culture, religion, language.

Genetics – the study of genes, the hereditary units that we receive from our parents, e.g. blood group, eye colour, height, skin colour.

DNA – deoxyribonucleic acid; a very important molecule that contains our genes. DNA is present in the nucleus of all living cells.

Think about it

Variation within humans is the result of two major influences:

the genes you inherit from your parents

the environment in which you live.

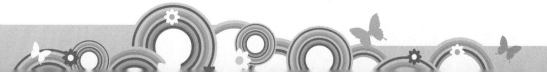

You and the skin

You can change your hair colour, or darken your skin through tanning or artificial colouring, but to begin with, like it or not, you are made up of your parents' genes! You cannot pass on something that is not natural, such as a bottled hair colour, to your children.

The environment

There are approximately 6.66 billion people on earth; we are all different, with different height, weight, shape, skin colour, eye colour and so on. To ensure survival of the human race, we have adapted as we have evolved, depending upon where on the earth we were born.

This shows within different ethnic origins. The darker the skin and eye colour, the more protection is given against the sun's rays. Those living nearest to the equator (the middle band around the earth, which is closest to the sun) have a darker skin and eye colour as the sun's rays are at their most intense.

Throughout history, nations have invaded one another. This has influenced the gene pool and therefore the skin types of people on the different continents. Immigration has also had an effect. Immigrants who settle in foreign countries and marry the people of their adopted country produce children of mixed race. If you were to look at your own family history, you may find your ancestors came from another country and your genetic inheritance comes from many different countries.

Impact of environment and lifestyle on the skin

Both the environment in which you live and your lifestyle contribute to the health of your skin.

Nutrition

Good health and therefore a healthy skin begin with good nutrition — the fuel that our bodies need to replace cells, maintain growth and repair and hydrate the skin. A variety of foods will provide the essential vitamins and minerals required to keep the body working at its optimum level. Getting vitamins in food rather than in pill form means our bodies also receive fibre, which helps the bowel to process waste products, and antioxidants, which are essential in the fight against **free radicals**. The body cannot overdose on vitamins and minerals found in food no matter how much we have, whereas too many vitamin pills can cause dangerously high levels of minerals that the liver then has to try to break down.

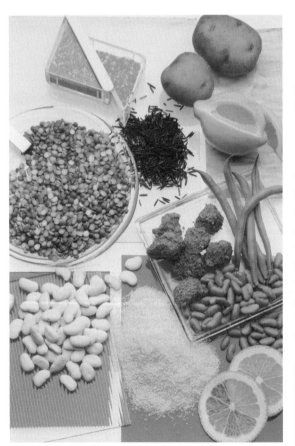

A variety of foods will ensure a healthy vitamin intake and a balanced diet

Key terms

Free radicals – highly reactive chemicals that attack molecules by capturing electrons and thereby change a cell's chemical structure. Environmental factors such as pollution, UVA rays, smoking and pesticides may cause free radical damage if production becomes excessive. Damage occurs and accumulates with age.

Nutrient	Source	Why needed
Protein	Red and white meat, dairy products, pulses and lentils, seeds and nuts	Maintains and supports body growth Essential for respiration of skin cells
Iron	Red meat, liver, egg yolk, pulses, dried fruits, e.g. apricots, raisins	With protein, forms haemoglobin to carry oxygen through the body With vitamin C taken at the same time, helps absorption Tannin and antacid medication limit absorption Deficiency causes anaemia resulting in fatigue Essential for oxygen levels in the skin
Calcium	Dairy products, whole fish (sardines), sunflower and sesame seeds	With other minerals and vitamin D, helps strengthen teeth and bones
Vitamin A (retinol)	Carrots, margarine, fortified dairy products, liver, green vegetables	Important to health of mucous membranes and resistance to infection Antioxidant essential for renewal and growth of new skin cells If applied in cream form on the skin, it can help stimulate collagen production
Vitamin B1 (thiamine)	Wheat germ, liver, whole grains, nuts, offal	Aids digestion and utilisation of energy Increases fatty acids in the skin – providing firmness to the skin and aids natural exfoliation
Vitamin B2 (riboflavin)	Milk, yoghurt, cottage cheese, liver, whole grains, green vegetables	Promotes healthy skin and eyes
Vitamin B3 (niacin)	Oily fish, whole grains, liver, fortified breakfast cereals, peanuts	Aids digestion and normal appetite needs Promotes fatty acid production
Vitamin B6 (pyridoxine)	Meat, bananas, dried vegetables, molasses, brewer's yeast, whole grains	Helps to regulate the use of fatty acids to fight infection
Vitamin B12 (cyanocobalamin)	Milk, eggs, meat, dairy products	Essential for the maintenance of red blood cells and nervous system (No vegetable source sufficient for daily needs. Vegans should see their doctor about synthetic forms)
Folic acid (folacin)	Green leafy vegetables, nuts, dried vegetables, whole grains	Essential for blood formation, therefore bringing oxygen and nutrients to the skin Vital during pregnancy to prevent possible defects in babies
Vitamin C (ascorbic acid)	Most citrus fruits (including oranges), red, green and yellow vegetables, e.g. tomatoes, peppers and broccoli	Increases resistance to infection, blood coagulation and iron absorption More required during illness Building block for collagen – the protein which provides the skin with structure, tone and elasticity
Vitamin D	Fortified milk and other dairy products, oily fish, liver, eggs, butter, salmon Sunshine on skin	Helps body to absorb calcium Calcium and phosphorus strengthen bones Essential for development of skin cells
Vitamin E	Vegetable oil, green leafy vegetables, wheat germ, egg yolk, whole grains	Protects fatty acids from being destroyed Antioxidant which helps to build and maintain good skin cells
Phosphorus	Milk products, meat, fish, whole grains, beans	Combines with calcium to strengthen bones and teeth
Iodine	Seafood, fortified salt	Regulates energy use in the body

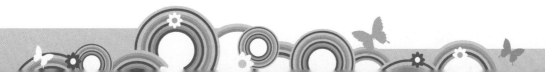

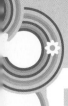

Nutrient	Source	Why needed
Zinc	Lean meat, seafood, whole grains and dried beans	Makes up some enzymes and releases vitamin A from liver
Fat – unsaturated (often classed as 'good' fats)	Unsaturated fat found in olive oil, avocadoes, fish oils with omega-3 and seeds, brazil nuts	Provides supple skin, shiny hair and softness to all the tissues

Water

Our bodies are made up of 80 per cent water, and each cell needs water to function. Water also helps blood to flow around the body. Blood should flow through the veins and arteries like skimmed milk, but with low water content it becomes thick like clotted cream, which doesn't flow well at all. Besides drinking eight to ten glasses, approximately two litres a day, water can also be found in food with high water content such as melons, fruit and soups. Drinks that include alcohol and caffeine act as a diuretic, which means they remove water and really make a big difference to the hydration levels of the skin.

Sleep

Sleep is essential to the body for repair of tissue and for growth — even though adults have stopped growing in height, cells and tissues need to repair and regenerate. Lack of sleep causes all the body functions to slow down, and both mental and physical function is impaired. You are also more likely to become run down, pick up infections and generally feel low, all of which is reflected in the skin.

Exercise

Regular exercise, which increases the heart rate and gives the lungs a good workout (cardiovascular exercise), is good for the whole body and stimulates the blood flow, which shows up in the skin. The immune system is strengthened, stress levels are reduced, and the heart functions better. General well-being is evident in a healthy, glowing skin. Walking, running and swimming are all good energy-boosting activities. Encourage your client to fit exercise into their lifestyle two or three times a week — and do some yourself and see how well you feel, with higher energy levels and the ability to cope better with your studies.

Smoking

The health risks associated with smoking are well publicised. Smoking is banned, by law, in public places, which means that the risk of passive smoking — inhaling other people's cigarette smoke — has been reduced (refer to legislation in Professional basics, page 55).

Smoking not only diminishes the lungs capacity to function well, it also affects the oxygen levels in the blood stream, showing up as a sallow, dull complexion. Smokers are depriving the skin of oxygen and their skin may be prone to line more easily and age prematurely.

Think about it

You are what you eat – how true! Nutrition is the body's fuel, so feed it well for best performance. You would not put low grade fuel into a Ferrari and expect it to work really well, and the same applies to the body.

You and the skin

Nicotine, the principal alkaloid in tobacco, impairs the circulation, slowing down the progress of nutrients and oxygen in the blood stream and the removal of waste products from the cells. Skin may look pale yellow and grey, lose its elasticity and become wrinkled, over time. Smokers also find that fingers and eyebrows become stained with a build-up of nicotine if the cigarettes are untipped and rolled without a filter. Not a good look for the skin!

Alcohol

Sustained alcohol intake can have an adverse effect on the skin as alcohol stops the absorption of essential vitamins by the body, as well as providing 'empty' calories with no nutritional goodness. This may lead to weight gain, which puts extra pressure on the skin. Alcohol can act as an appetite suppressant, and a poor diet can cause malnutrition in the long term.

There is also an allergic potential to alcohol, as it contains both salicylates and yeast, which can cause the skin to break out in hives and rashes. Yeast also feeds conditions such as thrush, irritable bowel syndrome and general irritability in the nerve endings in the skin.

Stress

We all need a little stress in our lives to function fully and get our adrenalin flowing. However, long-term and sustained stress on the body can cause ill health, mental function impairment and hormonal fluctuations, which show up in the skin. Adult acne and poor skin maintenance can be the result of long-term stress.

It is important for your client to deal with the underlying causes of anxiety and stress and manage it – and take care of the body to allow it to function properly. Exercise is a good stress buster and good nutrition is essential when the body is under stress. Regular beauty treatments are very therapeutic and regular massage will help with relaxation and improve skin function, as well as encouraging the client to maintain the skin with good product advice.

Hormones

In pregnancy, hormonal changes may affect the pigmentation of the skin and darker patches, called chloasma, may appear. These are commonly found along the hairline and on the neck or hands.

Free radicals

Free radicals or oxidants are a big factor in the ageing of the skin. They are harmful chemicals which can accumulate in the tissues. They are generated in the body as a reaction to aggressive environmental influences such as sunlight, petrol fumes, chemicals, smoking, wind and pollution, and to internal factors such as stress and tiredness. A consequence of this attack on the skin is an acceleration of the skin's ageing process, with the loss of radiance, elasticity and tone. Free radicals are controlled by enzymes, but should the production of the enzymes become poor, due to a poor lifestyle, lack of sufficient nutrition and so on, then there is a build-up of chemicals and toxins within the tissues.

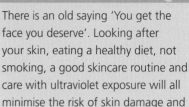

Think about it

There is an old saying 'You get the face you deserve'. Looking after your skin, eating a healthy diet, not smoking, a good skincare routine and care with ultraviolet exposure will all minimise the risk of skin damage and premature ageing.

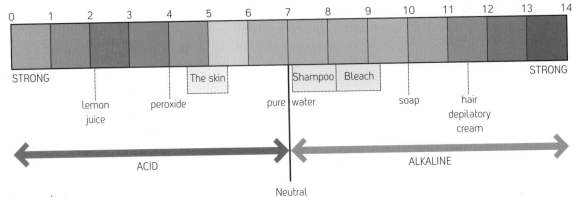

The pH of skin and some products

The pH of skin and desquamation
The pH of skin

pH stands for potential hydrogen or – if it is easier to remember – parts hydrogen, of any product. It is a number that describes whether a substance or solution is acid, neutral or alkaline. A pH of 7 is neutral, 0–7 indicates acidity and 7+ indicates alkalinity. Chemicals applied to the skin should have a pH that is neither too high nor too low to avoid skin irritation.

The acid mantle

The skin acts as a barrier against infection; this is known as the acid mantle because normal, healthy skin has an acidic pH between 4.5 and 5.5. The acid mantle is made up of a delicate mixture of sebum and moisture content on the skin – dermatologists refer to it as the hydrolipidic balance (hydro = water; lipid = fat). It helps to inhibit the growth of bacteria.

Fungi are controlled by sebum, which inhibits their growth. So it makes sense to maintain a steady pH balance in the skin to help fight off infection. Using products that are too harsh will strip the skin of its protective pH acid mantle and this will allow infections in and cause damage.

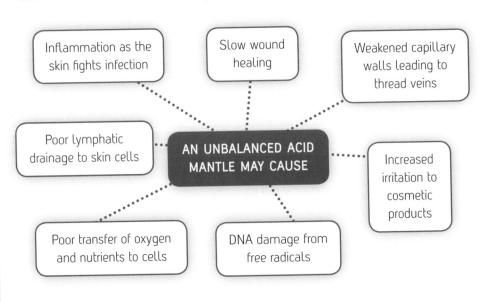

You and the skin

Desquamation

The epidermis is continually renewing itself – the lower layers are continually growing and dividing, pushing cells upward until they reach the surface, and then they are rubbed away. Friction within everyday movements, such as using a towel, getting dressed and scratching the skin will be enough to shed thousands of dead skin cells. This process is called desquamation or **exfoliation**. Getting rid of the old cells allows the new ones to come up to the surface, keeping the skin healthy and able to fight infection. This goes on daily and is not normally visible to the naked eye. Desquamation can only really be seen when a suntan is fading and the skin becomes dry and peels off in visible sheets.

The life cycle of a cell from the germinative layer to the top horny layer takes about 28 days and the cells go through a process called keratinisation. Keratin is a form of protein, and the cells get harder, flatter and eventually die. As the dead cells have no nucleus and no nerve endings, you don't feel your skin shedding itself.

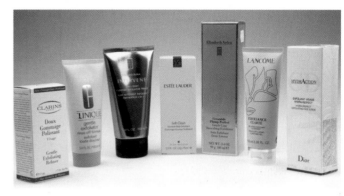

Exfoliating products

You and the skin

Key terms

Exfoliation – the manual or mechanical method of removing dead skin cells from the epidermis using techniques that may include loofah scrub, dry brushing, salt glow, enzyme masks or abrasive scrubs.

Think about it

Some skin conditions and disorders are linked to skin shedding.

Psoriasis – a common skin condition where the life cycle of the cells drops to only five days from the germinative layer to the top horny layer. This happens so fast in the cells that only the nuclei are retained. This results in itchy, red, scaly patches, most common on the elbows, knees, legs and scalp. The cause is not known, but it is thought to be stress-related. Sunlight or UV exposure from a sunbed often helps the condition and there are creams available to help, too.

Ichthyosis – a chronic condition, usually present from birth, where the skin becomes rough, dry, itchy and scaly because of the over formation of keratin and a lack of natural exfoliation. In severe forms the scales can appear all over the body.

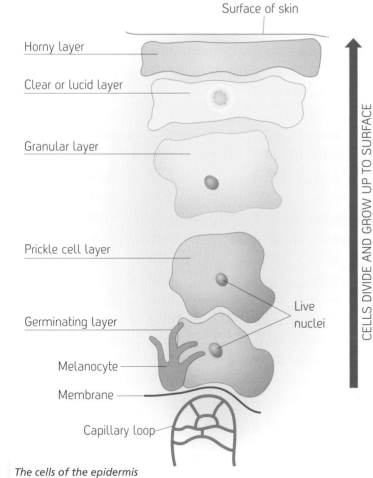

Surface of skin

Horny layer

Clear or lucid layer

Granular layer

Prickle cell layer

Germinating layer

Live nuclei

Melanocyte

Membrane

Capillary loop

CELLS DIVIDE AND GROW UP TO SURFACE

A protective layer of dead cells

Nucleus breaks down as cells die

Keratin develops in the cells: they are about to harden and die off

Cells absorb melanin in response to ultraviolet light

Cells divide by mitosis

The cells of the epidermis

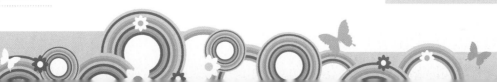

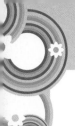

How to recognise skin types and conditions

Skin types are usually described as one of four categories:

1 Normal

2 Dry

3 Oily

4 Combination.

As well as these four basic types, skin can also be mature, sensitive, dehydrated, and may have other problems. These may include: broken capillaries, blemishes, acne, comedones, milia and other minor imperfections.

The true skin type or condition may not be very easy to diagnose at first, as all skins react to the environment, to products used, and to different lifestyles.

Skin types

Normal skin

This exists when the oil and sweat glands are working in harmony, with a working acid balance to protect the skin. This skin has a good balance of moisture content and oil to keep the skin soft, supple and flexible. It is an ideal skin type, but rare. The skin is fine textured with no visible pores and smooth to the touch.

Some experienced therapists would argue that normal skin only exists in the very young, prior to the hormonal influences brought on by puberty. However, some people are lucky enough to enjoy a balanced skin, and those who look after their skin very well and enjoy a healthy life style are more likely to experience a balanced skin type.

Normal skin can occasionally become slightly dryer or slightly greasier – it should never be assumed that it is always normal. The skin should feel warm to the touch, and it heals well if damaged.

Questions to ask your client:

1 Is your skin generally in this condition?

2 Do you feel you have any problem areas?

3 Have you had problems in the past?

4 What skincare routine and products are you currently using?

Dry skin

This type of skin is oil- and moisture-deficient, leaving the skin dry to the touch. There may be some loss of elasticity depending upon the client's age, and in extreme cases it can be rough or flaky. The texture of the skin is fine; dry skin can often be thin and small red veins (dilated capillaries) may be present on the cheek areas. Pores and follicles are often closed and inactive. The skin chaps easily and can be inclined to be sensitive. Lines and wrinkles may form early on with dry skin, especially around the eyes. The appearance of the skin is likely to be slightly dull, with a matt finish and it lacks suppleness.

Think about it

Everyone aspires to balanced skin in maximum condition and optimum health – that is the foundation of all the treatments that therapists do.

You and the skin

Dry skin can be deceiving. It may not be the client's natural state but rather the effects of internal or external influences. Factors such as ill health, poor or incorrect product use, extreme weather conditions, over exposure to UV light or a poor diet (lack of essential fatty acids) all contribute to making the skin dry. It can therefore be easy to misdiagnose this skin type.

Questions to ask your client:

1　Does your skin feel tight and drawn?

2　Does your skin sometimes flake?

3　Does exposure to cold and wind make your skin sore?

4　Do you burn easily?

5　What products are you using?

Oily skin

Oily skin is caused by overproduction of sebum from the sebaceous glands. This disturbs the acid mantle and the ratio of water to sebum on the skin. It looks shiny; it can be slightly thicker in consistency than normal skin, sallow, coarse and have problems associated with it. This skin is often referred to as **seborrhoeic**.

An oily skin often develops during puberty, when there is a surge of glandular activity under the influence of hormones. It often corrects itself when the hormone levels settle, and the use of the correct skin preparations can certainly help. Enlarged pores, congested pores, comedones and infection may occur on oily skins if the skin is not thoroughly cleansed and maintained, so care must be taken. It may also show signs of scarring, if there has been acne present.

Skin of this type is often over treated with quite harsh products, which can dry it out — it is possible to have an oily skin with dry flaky patches as a result of poor product use. This can be confusing for both client and therapist, so do check product use and previous treatments. The only advantage to having an overproduction of sebum is that in later life, as the skin sebum production slows down, the oily skin still has a good supply of sebum to moisturise and lubricate the skin — an oily skin is less prone to fine lines than a dry one.

Questions to ask your client:

1　Is your skin prone to pimples and blackheads?

2　Does the skin shine?

3　Is it difficult to keep make-up on?

4　What products are you using?

Combination skin

Some skins are a combination of two or more skin types, and the most common one is an oily T-zone along the forehead and nose, with normal or dry skin on the cheek area. This is because there are more sebaceous glands along the T-zone which may therefore show all the characteristics of greasy skin. This skin type really needs to be treated as two types.

> ### Key terms
>
> **Seborrhoea or seborrhoeic** – the name given to excessively oily skin caused by overactive sebaceous glands producing large amounts of sebum, making the skin look shiny; in some cases, may result in acne.

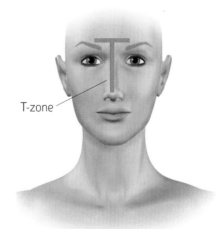

T-zone

The T-zone is commonly found in combination skin

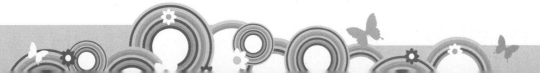

Questions to ask your client:

1 Is your nose shiny?

2 Are you prone to blackheads in the T-zone area?

3 Does the skin on your cheeks ever feel tight or dry?

Skin conditions

Sensitive skin

All skin needs to be sensitive for good health, but in beauty therapy a sensitive skin is really one that is super sensitive, that is it reacts to even mild stimulus. This condition is often associated with pale skins or a dry skin that lacks the protection of enough sebum. Sensitive skins have a highly flushed look, with a tendency to colour easily, and can react to beauty products or chemicals used within the salon.

More and more clients are developing allergies and sensitivity to chemicals and products — not just those found in cosmetic preparations but also cleaning products and perfumes — food intolerances and nickel found in jewellery.

Questions to ask your client:

1 Is your skin prone to allergic reactions?

2 Do you often have a high cheek colour?

3 Does your skin show signs of being dry but slightly red?

Dehydrated skin

Skin may have the normal sebaceous secretions and still suffer from flaking and tightness due to loss of surface moisture — a condition of dehydration. Any skin can suffer temporary dehydration, which may be caused through using products that are too harsh on the skin or through exposure to extreme temperatures, central heating or over-stringent dieting.

The most common cause of dehydrated skin is a combination of not drinking enough water and drinking too many alcoholic or caffeinated drinks (such as cola and coffee), which are also dehydrating. When the thirst mechanism kicks in and the body needs water, it very often gets a cup of coffee instead, which makes it more dehydrated.

Questions to ask your client:

1 What skincare products are you using on the skin?

2 Have you altered your diet recently?

3 How much water do you drink a day?

Mature skin

All skins will age. The general rule of thumb is that a person's cell renewal rate is relative to their age — so a 16-year-old replaces skin cells every 16 days and an 80-year-old replaces skin cells every 80 days. This is only a guide, but it gives you an idea of how an older skin behaves and why.

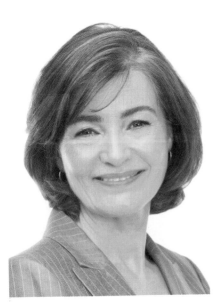

Mature skin type

There are two types of ageing.

- **Intrinsic** – this describes natural aging that occurs in the body. Your genetic programming not only dictates your colouring and height, it also dictates how fast you age. Generally, cell division stops after about 80 divisions and this cellular clock is fixed, despite our best efforts to stop or slow it down.
- **Extrinsic** – this relates to the external factors that contribute to the ageing of the skin, e.g. exposure to UV light, free radicals, extreme weather and the chemicals found in cigarette smoke.

In a fine-textured, older skin the slower rate of the sebaceous secretions, accompanied by loss of elasticity, are contributory factors in the ageing process, leading to a mature skin type. Wrinkles begin to form. The epidermis may become thinner with a lack of springiness and loss of support from underlying muscles and collagen and elastin fibres, causing the skin to sag.

However, lots of mature clients maintain their health, use the right products and have a good lifestyle, which means that you cannot always diagnose a mature skin just by looking at the client. You may find that a younger person who is a heavy smoker (thus starving the skin of vital oxygen), with a poor diet and unhealthy lifestyle, may have skin that looks and behaves considerably older than their biological age.

You can read more about the effects of ageing of the skin on pages 208–14.

Congested skin

All skin types can become congested under the right conditions. Congestion occurs because the pores become blocked and sweat and sebum cannot escape on to the skin's surface, which can be seen and felt as lumpy and coarse. Whiteheads and blackheads can build up and the epidermis may harden. Poor removal of make-up, using the wrong products and excess sweat building up all contribute to this skin condition.

Comedones

Comedones or blackheads are formed when the mouth of the hair follicle on the skin's surface becomes blocked with excess sebum and hard keratinised cells. The comedone mixes with oxygen (oxidises) and turns black, and can be quite hard and embedded, or impacted. They are not infectious and do not spread but can be numerous, especially on the forehead, nose and chin, if the client has an oily T-zone. Comedones are more common in oily skins and during puberty when hormone fluctuations affect sebum production.

Infected skin

Any bacteria, fungi or viruses can penetrate broken skin and cause infection. This is usually a sign of poor health and can occur when a person is run down or ill. The acid mantle stops offering protection and the delicate balance is disrupted. This is easily recognised as swelling or irritation, with pain and tenderness. The presence of pus is also a sign of infection.

Bacteria entering the follicle, causing pore blockage to occur, causes Acne vulgaris (see page 202).

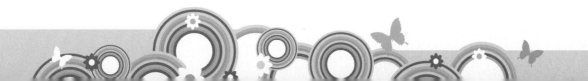

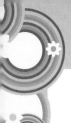

Damaged skin

Reasons for damage	Signs and symptoms to look for when assessing skin type or condition
Excessive exposure to the sun, artificial sunlight (e.g. sunbeds), alcohol intake and smoking	The skin ages prematurely, causing a breakdown in collagen and elastin which supports the skin; uneven pigmentation; excessive lines and wrinkles relative to the client's age.
Pollution from chemicals, traffic and thinning of the protective ozone layer	Contamination of the skin leads to clogged and blocked pores, irritations occur and there is a tendency to comedones and allergic reactions. This causes dehydration and overactivity of the sebaceous glands; loss of oxygen causes skin to look sallow and tired.
Heat and steam	Overstretching of the skin; pores enlarge and become congested; damage to capillaries seen as thread veins on the cheeks and chin.
Incorrect use of skincare products	Inappropriate products can cause comedones to form or lead to an oversensitive, dry or flaky skin.
Excessive heat	Chapped and dehydrated skin; damaged capillaries and vascular flushness on the skin; Spider naevus present on cheeks.
Poor diet containing insufficient nutrients or a lack of fatty acids; crash dieting	Sluggish and yellow or sallow-looking skin; lack of oxygen results in slow healing and repair of skin.
Impaired acid mantle due to poor product use or ill health	Increased inflammation and sensitisation; poor healing and infection.

The best way of caring for the skin is to:

○ avoid skin damage – picking, bruising or scratching it
○ take care of the skin internally with good nutritional habits/a balanced diet
○ drink plenty of water
○ avoid smoking
○ limit alcohol and caffeine intake
○ avoid crash diets or excluding fats from the diet
○ use the correct skincare products
○ have regular facials from an expert
○ always use sun protection on the skin when in the sun
○ maintain a good work/life balance – avoid unnecessary stress
○ take regular exercise
○ limit medication or drug use where possible
○ try to regulate hormone levels.

You and the skin

Think about it

Pigmentation is the production of colour in the body, caused by the deposit of a pigment called melanin, which protects the skin from UV radiation.

Skin characteristics and skin types of different ethnic groups

Refer to the structure of the skin in Related anatomy and physiology, pages 229–36.

The skin owes its colouring to the red **haemoglobin** found within the blood vessels, yellow **carotenoids**, subcutaneous fat and the dark brown pigment **melanin**. Various degrees of pigmentation are present in different ethnic groups. The differences are in the amount of melanin produced and are not dependent upon the number of **melanocytes** present (see below).

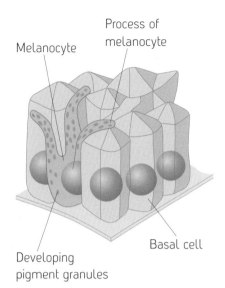

Melanocytes in skin

Pigment

Certain areas of skin are very rich in pigment, such as the genital area and the nipples, while practically no pigment is present in the palms of the hands and the soles of the feet (often referred to as 'glabrous' skin, this lacks hair follicles and sebaceous glands, and has a thicker epidermis).

Pigment is stored as fine granules within the cells of the germinative layer, although some granules may also be deposited between the cells. In white/Caucasian skin the granules occur only in the deepest cell layers and mainly in the cylinder-shaped cells of the basal row. In non-white skin pigment is found throughout the entire layer and even in the granular layer (stratum granulosum).

Melanin

All melanin is made in special cells called melanocytes and then distributed to the **epithelial cells**. The melanocytes are scattered in the basal layers of the epidermis and mature as the embryo is developing in the womb. They are influenced by the units of inheritance gene code which determines race and colouring.

Some people are born without the ability to produce melanin within their skins and with no hair pigment – a **congenital condition** called albinoism. People with this condition have pure white hair, pale skin and pink eyes.

Think about it

Not all white Caucasian skin is very light and fragile. Some skin tones are darker if the parents have brown or black hair, in which case the skin may tan more easily and be less prone to damage. Some white Caucasian skins, noticeably the Irish and Scottish, may have striking dark hair colouring with paler skin tone.

Key terms

Haemoglobin – a protein that occurs in red blood cells. It contains iron and provides the red colour. It is instrumental in transporting oxygen around the body in the blood.

Carotenoids – yellow pigment; carotene is found in yellow foods. It is also the term used to describe skin colour in relation to pigment, especially if the liver is enlarged and the body becomes jaundiced.

Melanin – pigment or colour found in skin and hair. Produced by special skin cells (melanocytes) that are sensitive to sunlight, melanin protects the body by absorbing ultraviolet radiation from the sun. The amount of melanin present determines the colour of a person's complexion: those with a large amount have darker skin, those with very little have fair skin. Melanin also determines the colour of the iris in the eyes.

Melanocytes – skin cells that produce melanin.

Key terms

Epithelial cells or epithelial tissue – specialised tissue that covers all external and internal surfaces of the body, made up of cells closely packed together in one or more layers. Epithelial tissue is separated from underlying tissue by a thin sheet of connective tissue called the basement membrane, which provides structural support and binds it to neighbouring structures. Simple epithelium is one cell thick and stratified epithelium is two or more cells thick.

Congenital condition – a condition that is recognised at birth or that is believed to have been present since birth. These include all disorders present at birth, whether they are inherited or caused by an environmental factor.

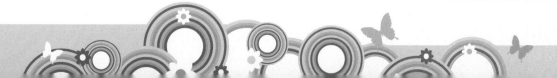

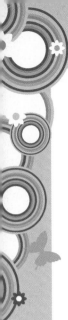

Skin ethnicity

The skin's ethnicity can be grouped into five basic categories. These are generalised only for the purposes of identification. Always remember that there are many variations within these categories.

- White/Caucasian
- Black
- Asian
- Oriental
- Mixed
- Mediterranean/Latino

White Caucasian skin

How to recognise it	Most likely origin	Features	Possible problems
White Caucasian skin is the most delicate or fragile of all the skin types, and is light in colour, often with blue or green eye colouring. It has blue and pink tones from the blood capillaries, which can be seen through the pale epidermis, and its melanin content is not as high as in other skin types.	Britain Northern and western Europe North America* New Zealand* Australia*	The skin of blonde or red-haired people tends to have a fine hair growth, and as the hair colour is light or fair, it is not usually noticeable. It tends to be fine in texture and thinner than in other skin types.	Light skins do not tan easily and are at risk of skin damage, especially if there are large amounts of freckles present. Light skins burn quickly and are less tolerant of UV light, so care should be taken in hotter climates. It is prone to early signs of ageing and wrinkles, and may bruise easily. It can be more prone to broken capillaries, especially if the skin is very light.

* People native to these countries have naturally much darker skin than those who have immigrated over the years from northern Europe. The indigenous people of Canada and Greenland are the Inuit. The indigenous people of New Zealand are the Maori and the indigenous people of Australia are the Aboriginals. They have dark skin for protection against the sunlight.

Think about it

All these basic skin categories provide only a general overview and should never be used to replace a thorough consultation with the client – and remember: there are always exceptions to the rule.

Treat each client as an individual, not just a type of skin colour. Different factors apply with each client: different lifestyles, dietary intake and use of products will determine how the skin behaves and reacts.

My story

My name is Sara-Jane.

As you can see from my picture I am a white Caucasian skin type. Being very fair, I do not tan easily. When I went to Barbados on holiday, I had to be very careful not to burn my skin. I just go a bright red and then the skin peels!

I find I am quite sensitive to some products, so I tend to stick with the products I know won't irritate me – I get a strong itchy feeling and redness over my cheeks if I use anything too highly perfumed. I am prone to patches of eczema on my body if I use anything highly perfumed or change my washing powder.

Being blonde does have some advantages. Lots of people pay their hairdresser to put highlights in their hair, but mine are natural, with no regrowth showing through!

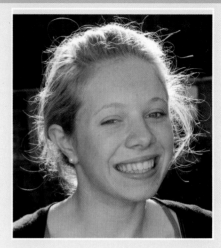

Black skin

How to recognise it	Most likely origin	Features	Possible problems
Black skins have more evenly distributed melanocytes, which are larger and more active than in a white/Caucasian skin. Black skin tends to be more robust: it has greater elasticity and strength of collagen fibres, giving support to the skin, so there is less possibility of dropped contours of the face. Black skin tends to be darker across the forehead and perimeter of the face but lighter in the middle on the cheeks.	Africa West Indies/Caribbean North America	Sebaceous glands are larger and denser, giving good lubrication and moisture, making it less prone to premature wrinkles. This also means the ageing process is usually slower in black skin, with less cell deterioration. Because black skin flakes and is shed more quickly than other skins, cell renewal also tends to be faster.	Some black skins may be quite sensitive to products and care should be taken to avoid harsh, abrasive products, or strong alcohol-based toners. These types of product are often used to treat an 'oily' skin, but black skin is not usually oily at all – the reflection of light against black skin often gives the skin a glow or sheen. As the epidermis is thicker black skin may scar more easily, which can turn into **keloid** tissue. This is seen as an overthickening of the skin, in a pink or beige colour, which is more noticeable against a darker background.

Think about it

Skin cancer is not as common in people with black skin as they are protected from the harmful UV rays of the sun. Also, the epidermis is considerably thicker than in its white Caucasian counterpart, and it is therefore less reactive and not prone to allergies or infection: warts are rarely found on a black skin.

A condition called Dermatosis papulosa nigra occurs almost exclusively in black skin, usually on the cheeks. It consists of brown or raised dark spots. Do not treat if infected – recommend that the client seeks medical advice.

Key terms

Keloid – a raised formation of scar tissue caused by excessive tissue repair in response to trauma or surgery when fibroblast cells continue to multiply and form large mounds of scar tissue. Black skins are more susceptible to keloid formation and they may appear on any part of the body.

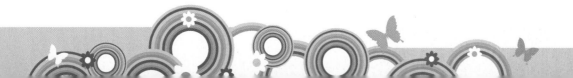

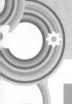

My story

My name is Ogo.

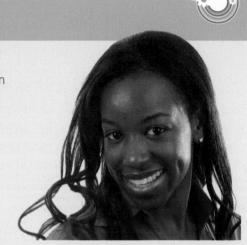

My skin is black, as my parents originally came from Nigeria in Africa.

I think I have good skin, with no real problems, although I don't wear foundation as I have trouble finding a colour that suits my skin — lots of foundations go grey on my skin tone. I can end up with darker circles under my eyes if I don't get enough sleep and my cheeks are a shade lighter than my forehead.

I use a lot of moisturiser to keep my skin from drying out — which can be a problem if I sunbathe. I do actually tan — and have a strap mark from my watch in the summer! Also if I get dehydrated I can go a grey colour because the dead skin cells build up on my skin. I need to drink water regularly and use an exfoliator to stop me looking ashen.

My only skin problem is stretch marks as I was slightly larger in my teens than I am now. They look like pink lines on my hips and tummy. I think they are fading slightly, but I am quite conscious of them, as they show up against my darker skin. I hope I have inherited my Mum's great bone structure and skin condition — her skin is great even in her fifties!

Asian skin

Asian skin can be divided into two types: dark and light or oriental.

Dark Asian skin

How to recognise it	Most likely origin	Features	Possible problems
Dark Asian skin tends to be more sallow with a darker tone than light Asian/oriental skin as there is a higher proportion of melanin present.	Pakistan India Sri Lanka Malaysia	This type of skin has more sweat glands, which are also larger, to keep the body temperature at a manageable level in the heat. It has fewer problems with oil-related conditions such as acne. The skin is often smooth and line-free, strong and adaptable, with the underlying fibres being supportive well into middle age.	Wrinkling tends to be minimal, but the skin may be prone to loss of pigmentation if care is not taken. It can have a tendency towards uneven colouring and pigmentation can cause dark circles under the eyes.

My story

My name is Poonam.

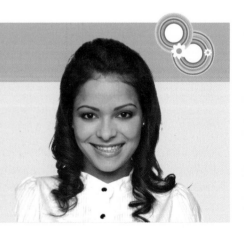

I come from a small Indian village outside New Delhi.

All of my family have very dark skin and hair. My grandmother is now greying, but both Nanna and my Mum still have a thick head of hair. My skin is quite strong and healthy. I am not very sensitive to anything and I can use most products on it with no problems, but I do have quite a lot of facial hair. I also need to have my eyebrows threaded regularly. As my Mum has grown older she has become prone to dark pigmentation patches on her face and neck.

You and the skin

Light Asian/oriental skin

How to recognise it	Most likely origin	Features	Possible problems
Light Asian/oriental skin has yellow undertones, and can develop an olive tone. The base colour is cream and this type of skin is often clear and fine in complexion.	Japan China Middle East Thailand Hong Kong	The skin is often smooth and fine, with minimal blemishes. This skin type rarely shows degeneration due to ageing. There is likely to be little or no facial and body hair. The skin has good tolerance of UV and tends not to wrinkle early.	This skin tends to scar easily and there may be irregularities in the skin's surface seen as pitting or unevenness. Hyperpigmentation may also occur; clients may be concerned about these age spots developing. As the skin can be fairly oily, especially around the T-zone, this skin type may develop a problem with open pores and comedones along the nose.

My story

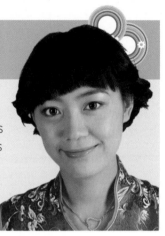

My name is Masico.

I come from Japan. Although I have an oily skin I look after it with good skincare products and I am sure my diet, which is full of fruit and vegetables, helps maintain its condition. In Japan we eat very healthily with a diet low in carbohydrates and fats/butter, so we have fewer problems with obesity or heart disease than western countries – I am sure that is also reflected in my skin's condition. I do worry about getting sun spots so I make sure I use good sun protection of SPF 30. As I have a lot of yellow surface tones if I use the wrong concealers I tend to look a bit grey – so I use a peach corrector to even my skin tone out. Still, I am lucky as I don't need to wear a lot of make-up as my skin is clear.

Mixed race (multi-ethnic) skin

How to recognise it	Most likely origin	Features	Possible problems
A client with mixed race skin will need a very thorough consultation to ensure that the skin analysis is correct, as those with this skin type are likely to have a combination of influencing factors.	Mixed parentage from any ethnic background.	These will vary considerably.	The skin will be more of a product of the mixture of parents and the environment. The correct product use will also dictate how clear the skin is, and whether the acid mantle is intact and doing its job correctly. This skin type is the easiest one to misdiagnose.

Think about it

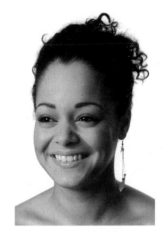

A student with one Chinese parent and one white/Caucasian parent has skin which looks quite oily, with blocked pores and comedones present. There are dry patches on the cheek area – but is this really dry skin?

The problem might be down to product use – the top layer of the epidermis is perhaps being dried out with alcohol-based toners (for an oily skin), which are too strong. They would cause the dry patches but would not address the oil production still taking place in the sebaceous glands underneath. The horny layer would not shed properly, so a build-up of cells forms the dry patches. In a case like this, good exfoliation will help, along with gentle steaming to aid extraction and then application of the correct water-based product. Avoid any oil-based products on an already oily skin.

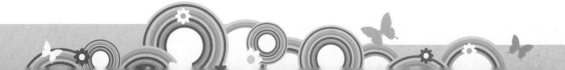

Additional knowledge

Mediterranean/Latino skin

There is one other skin type you may come across which, although it is not a range for NVQ Level 2, is still a recognisable skin type. That is Mediterranean/Latino skin.

How to recognise it	Most likely origin	Features		Possible problems
A golden skin with olive undertones.	Spain Italy Southern France Portugal Greece Southern and Central America	This skin type tends to be oilier, due to the sebaceous glands producing more sebum to keep the skin lubricated in the heat. It therefore tends not to dry out too much, and is slow to form wrinkles. As the hair colour is also darker, facial and body hair is more noticeable and often grows thicker and is coarse in texture. This skin type is robust and less prone to damage; it can withstand higher levels of UV without burning, and tends to tan more easily.		There is a tendency for excessive facial and body hair. The skin may be fairly tough and tends to thicken as it ages.

My story

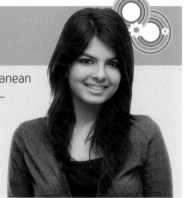

My name is Christiana.

I come from Cyprus and both my parents are originally from Greece. I have a typical Mediterranean skin – dark and tanned. I don't have to worry too much about burning and I tan really easily – we all do in my family. That is the good side about my skin – my only problem is that I tend to get blackheads around my nose and on my chin, so I am very careful to cleanse my skin thoroughly to prevent them. I have quite a lot of facial hair and have very strong hair on my head – which grows very fast, but the down side is that my leg and under-arm hair do the same. I spend a fortune on waxing!

The photosensitivity of skin

This is the term used to describe how the skin reacts to sunlight and UV rays, real or artificial. The skin may break out in a heat rash; this condition is called Photodermatosis. It may be caused by exposure to UV, or a reaction from a topical application of a product that reacts with UV, a metabolic defect within the body, a genetic disorder, which has been inherited, or a pre-existing skin disease.

The Fitzpatrick classification system for skin types

We have seen how skin can be classified by type, condition and ethnic origin. Some cosmetic houses base their product ranges – especially sun protection creams – around the Fitzpatrick classification system.

The system was developed in the US by a dermatologist, Dr Thomas Fitzpatrick of Havard University, in 1975. It is based upon melanin content in the skin and how quickly the skin burns. The system classifies the skin into six different types, ranging from extremely light-skinned people, who are highly likely to burn, to extremely dark-skinned people, who may suffer serious discoloration from laser or light treatment or other pigment-altering therapies or conditions.

For your portfolio

Of the skin types mentioned here, which colouring or skin type do you recognise as similar to your own? How does your skin react in sunlight? Look up which sun protection factor (SPF) creams would be most suitable for your skin. See pages 216–17 for more detail on SPFs. Fill out a consultation card as if you were your own client. What would you be noting as your skin particulars and needs?

You and the skin

The Fitzpatrick classification is often used by dermatologists using laser and light therapy as it can help highlight the risks of poor reactions to treatment.

A variety of questions are asked about genetic history, physical attributes such as eye colour, hair colour and freckling, and personal observations of the skin's reaction to sunlight. Depending on the answers to the questions, most people fit into one of the six skin categories, usually labelled with roman numerals I–VI.

Skin type	Typical features	Ability to tan
I Celtic, English, Northern European	Pale white, fair skin, blue/hazel eyes, blonde/red hair	Always burns, freckles, does not tan
II Nordic, North American	White, fair skin, sandy to brown hair, green, brown or blue eyes	Burns easily, tans poorly and with difficulty, freckles
III Central/Eastern European, Mediterranean, Maori (New Zealand)	Darker or olive white skin, brown hair, green or brown eyes	Tans after initial burn
IV Chinese, Korean, Japanese, Thai, South American, Indian, Filipino	Olive to light brown skin, brown hair, brown eyes	Burns minimally, tans easily
V East African, Ethiopian, Northern African, Middle-Eastern Arabic	Dark brown skin, black hair, dark brown eyes	Rarely burns, tans darkly easily
VI African type, American-African	Dark brown, black eyes, dark brown or black skin	Never burns, always tans darkly

> **Think about it**
>
> The Fitzpatrick classification system should be used as a guideline rather than a definitive analysis for determining skincare. You must always conduct a full consultation, a manual and visual examination and employ all diagnostic tools available to you as a therapist.

> **Think about it**
>
> You are not medically trained and must not recommend treatment of a medical nature. Do not pass comment on any skin irregularity you may observe; instead refer the client to her GP.

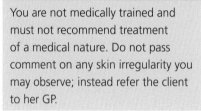

The Fitzpatrick skin-type categories

Tools for diagnosing skin types and conditions

The magi lamp

A good magnification lamp with a surrounding light is the ideal tool for examining the skin's surface; the magnification glass allows you to get a clear picture of blemishes and problems. Always check the lamp is working prior to putting it over the client's face: check the light bulb and the screws and joints so that it is safe, and not likely to drop suddenly.

> **For your portfolio**
>
> To determine your own skin type there are many websites offering complete questionnaires for the Fitzpatrick skin classification. Why not have a go to see your own skin type!

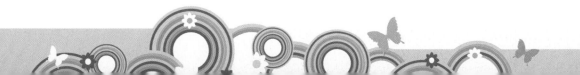

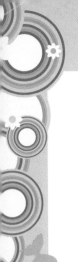

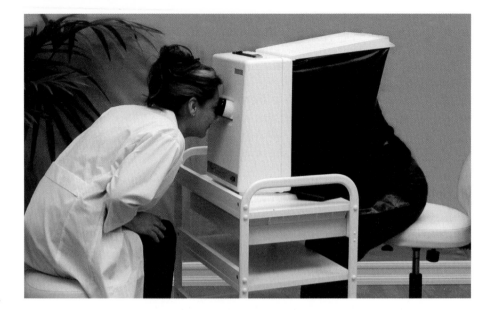

A skin scanner

You and the skin

Skin scanners and black light equipment

There are some very effective diagnostic tools for use in salons which give an in-depth analysis of black skins and for measuring the acid mantle, pH of the skin, melanin and water content, as well as density and strength of the dermis. These machines have been use by dermatologists for years and salons are finding them very useful to support the other diagnostic and consultation techniques used.

Wood's lamp or black light

The Wood's lamp (often called a black light) was invented by Robert William Wood in 1903. It was designed to produce a source of UV light and was used in hospitals to detect fungal and bacterial infections and parasites. Its clinical use in salons is to detect skin conditions.

Think about it

The colours produced by the Wood's lamp will vary depending upon the make of lamp. Always follow the manufacturer's instructions.

Colour of fluorescence	Skin type or problem
Blue	Normal balanced skin
Weak violet/light purple	Dry skin or patches of dehydration
Dark purple	Sensitive, thin, fragile areas
Coral pink	Dehydrated skin
Strong white	Thickened stratum corneum and the presence of dead skin cells
Orange	Oily skin or patches of overproductive sebaceous glands
Brown spots	Overpigmentation/sun damage
Light yellow	Acne, comedones
Green	Presence of pathogen Pseudomonas – a bacterial infection

Identifying skin conditions using a Wood's lamp

A Wood's lamp produces deep UV rays. It makes the skin glow, signifying different conditions and problems. There are both hand-held and box versions. The hand-held type is difficult to get a true reading from because the face needs to be in darkness. Ideally, the salon needs to be blacked out to operate the machine correctly, but this is rarely possible. With a box machine the client is seated, and the face is placed on a chin rest, rather like having an eye examination at the optician, and the curtain is pulled around the head so that the face is in darkness. The UV light can then be turned on to the skin. Certain colours will appear in patches which will indicate the skin's condition.

These areas can be noted down on the consultation card and the appropriate treatment and products recommended to the client.

Skin scanners

Hydration levels

The Corneometer® measures the skin's moisture content. It indicates whether the acid mantle is still intact and whether the skin's defence barrier is adequate. It also shows the enzyme action of the epidermis. The scanner looks rather like a pen, with a flat end, which is placed on the skin's surface; the reading appears on the attached machine. It is used in hospitals for patient intake of fluid.

Skin lipid levels

The Sebumeter® determines the amount of sebum being excreted by the sebaceous glands on to the skin's surface to check if the acid mantle protection is in good condition. The sebum of the skin or hair is taken by a film on the cassette's measuring head. Its transparency changes according to the sebum content on the film and is then analysed. If the skin's lipid or fat content is low, the acid mantle is unable to defend the skin properly. This could be because the client's diet is deficient in essential fatty acids. This is a good tool to use but is only one of the diagnostic procedures — your consultation will also reveal a lot about the skin's condition.

Melanin and erythema

There are also machines which measure melanin and blood flow in the skin. This can help determine which skincare and sunscreen products will be most useful to recommend to the client. This is used with the Fitzpatrick classification system of skin-burning capacity.

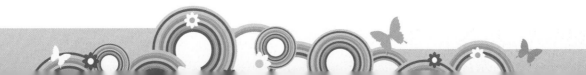

Face shapes and contours

It is not only the skin colour that characterises each ethnic identity; the shape of the skull and the bones form the contours of the face, giving the distinguishing features of different ethnic groups.

The position of the bones of the skull gives the face its shape, as the bones provide the attachment for all the muscles. The underlying bones dictate how high the cheeks are, how far apart the eyes are and so on. The jawbone dictates the shape of the face, along with the frontal bone, making the face square, round, oblong or heart-shaped. Apart from weight loss or gain, which will alter facial contours, nothing will alter your face shape unless you have corrective surgery to alter the bones themselves or have implants put under the skin or muscles to alter the contours.

For your portfolio

Identifying face shapes correctly takes some practice and may not be a skill you pick up right away. You can practise by identifying the shape of your own face.

Pull your hair back off your face. Using a biggish mirror, look at your own face shape. Try to analyse and match the shape of your face to one of the diagrams. If your forehead and jaw line are the same, you probably have a square face shape. If you have quite a pointed chin, you probably have a heart face shape. Draw your face outline on the mirror (using a pen that will rub off!) and see what shape you really are.

Face shape		How to recognise it
Oval face shape	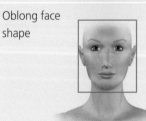	This face shape and bone structure is considered to be the ideal face shape. The chin tapers slenderly from a slightly wider forehead. The aim of make-up is to accentuate the natural shape.
Round face shape		The face is usually short and broad with full cheeks and round contours. Width at the top of the head should be provided, with height from the hair, which should be worn close at the sides. The aim of make-up is to slim the appearance.
Square face shape		The forehead is broad, corresponding with an angular jawline. This shaped face should have a little height without width and the hair should taper well towards the jawline. The aim of the make-up is to narrow the forehead and the jawline, reducing the squareness of this bone structure.
Oblong face shape		This face shape has a narrow frame. The make-up aim is to create the impression of width and to shorten the face length. A fringe with short hair would be suitable.

You and the skin

Heart face shape	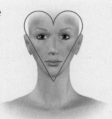	This shape usually has a wide forehead with the face tapering to a long jawline, rather like an inverted triangle. The aim of the make-up is to reduce the width across the forehead, emphasising the jawline.
Diamond face shape	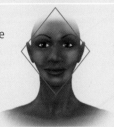	The forehead in this bone structure is narrow with the cheekbones extremely wide tapering to a narrow chin. The make-up aims to minimise the width across the cheekbones. A central fringe should be worn with hair full below the cheeks but flat at the cheekbone line.
Pear face shape	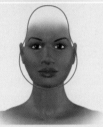	The forehead is narrow and the face gradually widens to the angle of the jaw which is broad and prominent. The make-up should aim to create the impression of width across the forehead and to narrow the jaw line. The hair should be swept off the forehead to create an illusion of width with a reverse flicking fringe.
Triangular face shape	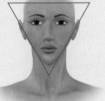	This is similar to the heart-shaped face, but not as soft. The aim of the make-up is to reduce the width of the forehead, by emphasising the jawline.

Contra-indications to facial treatments

Skin treatments must not be carried out if the client has a potential skin problem that would prevent the treatment from taking place. This is described as a contra-indication to treatment.

Contra-indications include:

○ infections — bacterial, viral and fungal infections of eyes, lips or face

○ open cuts and abrasions

○ broken bones or bruising

○ acute acne

○ severe eczema or psoriasis

○ recent invasive procedures such as chemical or medical peels (glycolic or AHA), Botox® injections, collagen or other filler injections in the face

○ recent waxing

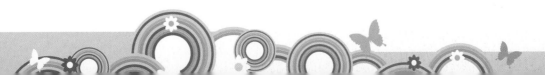

○ certain types of medication, including Retin A and Accutane used to treat topical acne

○ recent cancer treatment

○ recent dental work.

Refer to Professional basics (pages 39–40) for details of micro-organisms and the diseases they cause and also how to minimise the risk of infection.

Infections – viral

The common cold	Cold sores (Herpes simplex)	Warts
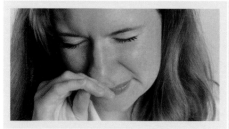	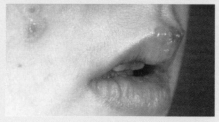	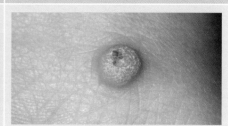
Freely recognised. Streaming eyes and nose, coughing and sneezing, easily spread.	Found on the lips, cheeks and nose. Blisters form, the skin is broken and painful; the blisters are especially likely to spread when open and weepy and then crusts form.	Small compact raised growths of skin – can be light or brown in colour, present on the face and neck.

Infections – bacterial

Impetigo	Boils	Conjunctivitis	Stye
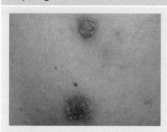	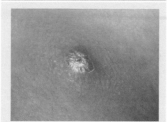	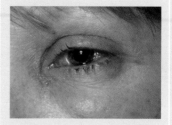	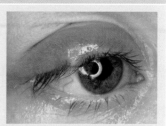
Highly infectious, this starts as small red spots, which then break open and form blisters. Most common around the corner of the mouth and, if picked, will spread. (Some strains are particularly resistant to antibiotics.) Can be spread through use of dirty equipment.	This infection forms at the base of a hair follicle. Bacteria can spread through an open scratch in the skin. The area is raised, red, and painful. Pus may be present.	This is a nasty eye condition. The eyelids are red and sore, with itching. Mainly caused by bacteria present, it can be irritated by a virus or an allergy.	This is a small boil at the base of the eyelash follicle. It is raised, sore and red; there may be considerable swelling in the area.

Infections — fungal

Ringworm (Tinea corporis)	Blepharitis
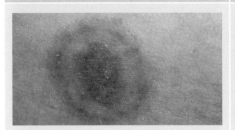	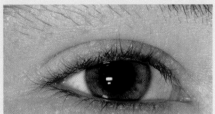
Red pimples appear and then form a circle, with clear skin in the middle. It is highly contagious and scales and pustules follow. It can be spread on to the face from any other area of the body. Can be passed on to humans by contact with domestic animals.	An infection of the lid causing inflammation, the eye will look red and sore. Depending on the severity of the condition, it may be better to avoid eye make-up application altogether, and focus attention on the mouth, with a pretty lipstick shade.

Conditions restricting the effectiveness of treatment

The following conditions are contra-indications that will not necessarily stop the treatment from taking place, but they may mean that a facial or make-up application has to be restricted and/or adapted. Most of these conditions are common sense and professional judgement can be used. If the problem is not directly on the face or neck, where the facial or make-up application takes place, then just avoid the area.

Each one will depend upon the individual case, the client granting permission, and then giving written permission on the record card. (Refer to Professional basics pages 29–31 for further information on the client record card; see also practical units on individual treatments and services.)

> **Think about it**
>
> All of the conditions mentioned would be a contra-indication to a facial treatment of make-up application to the face. The beauty therapist is responsible for protecting everyone in the salon from contamination via these micro-organisms.

Cuts/abrasions/broken skin	Bruises or swelling	Recent scar tissue
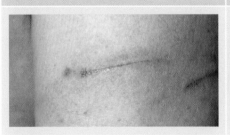	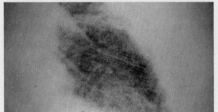	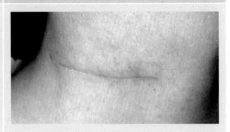
If recent, a scab will be forming, the skin may be tender and swollen in the area, and bruising may be seen. If cuts and abrasions are recent, then avoid the area altogether. If the area has healed over, and is not too recent, get the client's agreement that gentle application can take place, with careful consideration to hygiene.	Easily recognised as a swelling, with discoloration in varying shades. Avoid altogether if recent or painful to the touch. If healing has taken place, a gentle application of make-up will help to blend in the colour differences to the client's normal shade. Always ask for client's agreement.	Usually a different colour from the rest of the skin, following the line of injury. If the scar is recent, raised or angry looking, then avoid the area altogether. If the area is healing and not very large, gentle application with client's permission. Scar tissue less than six months old, or over a large area, should not be touched with make-up.

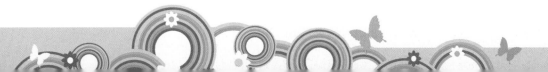

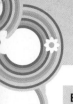

You and the skin

| Eczema | Dermatitis | Psoriasis |

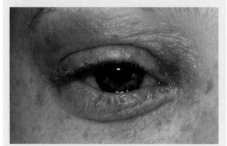 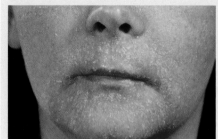 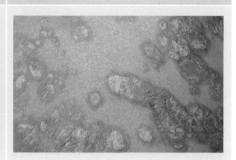

Eczema

Very dry skin, often scaly and flaky, can be red and often very itchy. If the eczema covers a large area, and is inflamed with broken skin, then leave alone, and suggest a visit to the GP. You may make it worse. If the eczema has irritated the eye area, it is unlikely the client would want make-up application. If it is only a small patch of eczema, and not angry, just exclude the area from treatment. The use of hypoallergenic products is recommended and patch test if the client is very sensitive.

Dermatitis

This is similar to eczema in appearance, but the cause is not the same. A reaction or allergy to something in contact with the skin usually causes dermatitis. See Eczema (left).

Skin allergies may result in a contra-action, so if the client's skin tends to react, do a skin patch test 24 hours prior to the make-up application. It may be advisable to use hypoallergenic make-up; ask the client to bring in her own make-up if she knows she is safe using it.

Psoriasis

Seen as scaly patches of red and/or silvery skin. This can break open and become sore. The cause is unknown but is thought to relate to the nervous system. A contra-indication would be if the psoriasis is open or bleeding. One of the common sites for psoriasis is the scalp, so the client may have a little patch visible along the hairline. If the client agrees to make-up application, and it is not directly over the area, then continue. A patch test 24 hours prior to the application of make-up is advisable to ensure that the condition is not aggravated.

| Acne vulgaris | Acne rosacea | Skin tags |

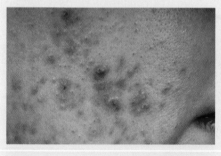 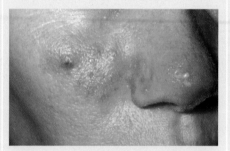 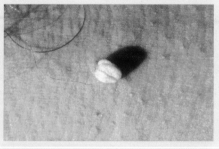

Acne vulgaris

Inflamed whiteheads, blackheads and pustules in various degrees of congestion. Mostly associated with hormones – and the presence of bacteria can make the condition infected.

Infected inflamed acne is a contra-indication. However, a client with mild acne can be treated in the salon, and a light water-based foundation applied. There may be a tendency to greasy skin, and therefore a light application of powder keeps the skin looking matt.

Acne rosacea

Seen as a flush of red over the nose and cheeks with a raised feel to the skin. Often those who have suffered Acne vulgaris in youth are prone to Acne rosacea in later life. If the skin is not tender and the client agrees, application of make-up can tone down the redness and therefore lessen the angry look of the skin.

Skin tags

Usually found on the eye area or lids and/or on the side of the neck. They resemble little 'mushrooms' of skin on a stalk which move when touched. This skin tag is under the arm.

As these are not painful or dangerous, make-up application can take place. If they become enlarged and irritating to the client they can be removed under local anaesthetic, usually at the GP's surgery.

Milia

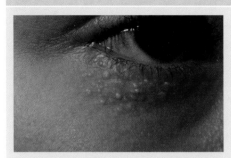

These are small white pearls under the skin, often around the eyes or on the side of the cheek, caused by a build-up of sebum. Make-up application can take place over milia, as they are not infectious.

Other skin conditions – pigmentation disorders

These disorders are caused by irregularities in the skin's melanin production. They are not infectious and are not a contra-indication to facial or make-up treatments. However, pigmentation disorders do affect the client's appearance and may make the client feel embarrassed and self-conscious; as a therapist, you therefore need to treat them sensitively. The use of remedial camouflage cosmetics may help more effectively with the matching of the pigmentation than ordinary foundations and concealers. (Refer to Unit B10 Enhance appearance using skin camouflage for more information on products available.)

Permanent make-up techniques can also help with pigmentation loss – it is a form of tattooing the skin but with the right colour of skin tone rather than coloured ink as in a tattoo. This is carried out by specially trained therapists as it is permanent and therefore there is no margin for error.

There are two main types of pigmentation disorders.

○ hypopigmentation (hypo = less than normal)

○ hyperpigmentation (hyper = more than normal).

Melanoderma

This is a general term used to describe patchy pigmentation. This is usually an increase in melanin caused by applying cosmetics or perfume which contain light-sensitive ingredients (e.g. bergamot oil used in the perfume industry) – the skin becomes extra sensitive to UV light. Some drugs have a similar effect. This can also follow inflammation and is sometimes the cause of brown patches following sunburn.

Hormones can often cause overpigmentation too. For example, there is a condition which occurs during pregnancy, called 'the mask of pregnancy', where the skin darkens in the shape of a mask or butterfly over the upper face, often into a deep brown colour, up to the hair line. It fades slightly after giving birth but will be extra sensitive to light for many years afterwards – sun creams should always be applied to the area as it will darker considerably more than the rest of the face.

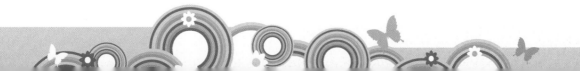

Vitiligo

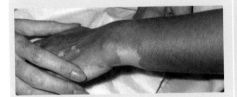

This is hypopigmentation; a condition in which small patches of skin have lost their pigmentation and appear a lighter colour than the rest of the skin. These lighter areas burn easily in the sun and need protection. They are not raised or painful to the touch. If the discoloration is in large patches a specialist camouflage make-up should be applied to conceal and match the skin tone. This may mean referral to a specialist. If the patch is small, clever choice of foundation and careful application is acceptable.

Chloasma

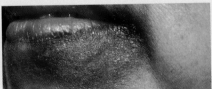

This is hyperpigmentation. It consists of irregular patches of brown pigment caused by the overproduction of melanocytes. This often appears on the face during pregnancy and is sometimes linked to the contraceptive pill. The discoloration usually disappears when the hormone balance is restored.

Freckles (Ephilidies)

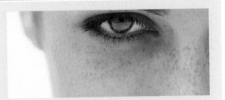

These are tiny, flat irregular patches of pigment on fair-skinned people, particularly blonde/redheads. They are due to the uneven distribution of melanin, and this becomes more noticeable on exposure to strong sunlight. The freckles often increase in size and join together. The skin between the freckles contains little or no melanin, so burns easily. As a therapist you should recommend a good sunscreen to the client.

Lentigo

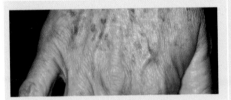

Also known as 'age spots', these are larger and more distinctive than a freckle, and may be slightly raised. This pigmentation does not increase in number or darken on exposure to UV light.

Haemangioma

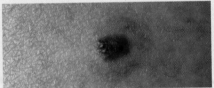

This consists of various conditions caused by the permanent dilation of superficial blood vessels. Stimulating treatments will therefore be a contra-indication to treatment, but camouflage cosmetics can be used.

Dilated capillaries

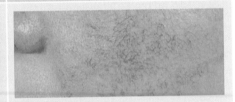

This is the result of loss of elasticity in the walls of the blood capillaries – the cheeks and the nose are often most affected. Exposure to weather, harsh handling and lack of protection, along with spicy foods and alcohol, can be contributing factors. Clients with dry/sensitive skin types are most likely to be affected.

Split capillaries

Weakening and rupturing of capillary walls – clients should avoid stimulating treatments. This condition can be treated by diathermy.

Other skin conditions – Naevus

This describes a variety of birthmarks and developmental abnormalities. It is the most common disorder involving melanocytes.

Strawberry naevus	Spider naevus	Port wine stain
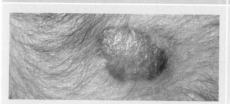	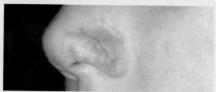	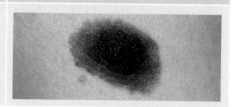
This is a raised and distorted area, often on the face, bright pink/red. It appears a few days or weeks after birth and usually clears up completely by the age of eight.	A central dilated vessel with leg-like projections of capillaries. The face and cheeks tend to be most affected and this often occurs during pregnancy due to the increase in oestrogen levels.	This is a bright purple, irregular-shaped, flat birthmark that can vary in size. It is thought to be due to damage by pressure during foetal development. These birthmarks grow with the body and can be quite disfiguring to the client. As a therapist you should always treat such marks sensitively with good cosmetic camouflage make-up.

Allergic reactions and sensitivity testing

Both in the European Union and the USA the law requires that cosmetic companies conduct very strict safety tests on materials they use to formulate products. Nevertheless, there will always be some people who are allergic to a substance that other people can tolerate without a problem.

An allergic reaction is a method of defence. The skin produces histamine – a compound derived from the amino acid histidine – found in mast cells in nearly all tissues of the body. Histamine causes dilation of blood vessels and contraction of smooth muscle: it is an important moderator of inflammation and is released in large amounts after skin damage.

A reaction could include:

- redness (erythema)
- swelling
- irritation to the area
- pain or itching in the area.

This is not a common reaction but may occur if clients have an allergy to any active ingredients within a product, or other common substances such as nickel, food or nuts. Some allergic reactions are life-threatening as the throat closes up and swells so that breathing is inhibited. Adrenalin needs to be administered in the form of an EpiPen® injection, and clients who suffer with this normally carry emergency medication to literally save their lives. This type of reaction can happen with strawberries, shellfish or even with a bee or wasp sting. It is therefore essential that you complete a sensitivity test if you are concerned that the client may react

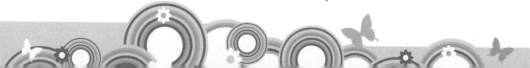

Think about it

Lots of products used within facials are nut-based – almond oil in massage, for example. Always check with the client at the consultation stage, before starting treatment, for potential allergic reactions.

to a product. This can be done by testing a small sample of the product behind the client's ear or in the crook of the elbow. If a reaction occurs within 24 hours the product should not be used.

If a client does develop a reaction, stop the treatment and treat with calamine lotion and a cold compress as necessary. Always make a note on the record card so that the product is not used again on the client. (Refer to Professional basics, page 35, for information on contra-actions.)

Choosing suitable products

Product labelling

By law, ingredients which are known to be irritants (or sensitisers) must be listed on the packaging, together with the precautions for use. Some facial and make-up products contain substances which cause allergic reactions in people who are hypersensitive. For example:

- lanolin – a fatty substance used as a softening agent in skin creams and lipsticks
- eosin – a red dye found in some lipsticks
- perfumes – particularly those containing bergamot, lavender and cedarwood
- alcohol – a grease solvent and astringent used in cosmetics and skincare products
- cobalt blue – a pigment used to produce eye make-up colours
- pearlising agents – ingredients which give products a shimmering effect
- gums – adhesives and binding agents in cosmetics.

Ingredients: Aqua (Water), Cetearyl Alcohol, Petrolatum, Caprylic/Capric Triglyceride, Ethylhexyl Palmitate, Vitis Vinifera, Stearate SE, Cera Alba (Beeswax), Stearic Acid, Ceteareth-, Carbomer, Geranium Maculatum (Geranium Extract), Lavandula Extract), Camillia Sinensis (Green Tea), Theobroma Cacao, Chinensis (Jojoba) Seed Oil, Cocos Nucifera (Coconut Oil), Gel), Parfum (Fragrance), Linalool, Alpha-isomethyl Ionone, Methylpropional, Hydroxyisohexyl 3-Cyclohexene Carboxaldehyde, Limonene, Citronellol, BHT, Tetrasodium EDTA, Lauramine Oxide, Phenoxyethanol, Methylparaben, Butylparaben, Ethylparaben, Isobutylparaben, Propylparaben, CI 19140 (FD&C Yellow No.5)

salesinfo@pbs-beauty.com

12M   code - 077334

Always check ingredients labels if you know your client is allergic to particular additives

Eye irritation

Although products used around the eye area are very strictly tested, and only safe pigments are used, some can still cause irritation to some clients.

Hypoallergenic products

If your client has sensitive or allergic skin you should use this type of product, which contains no perfume as well as fewer pigments and preservatives. Organic facial products are also freely available now, and are preferred by many clients; the only drawback may be that they lack preservatives and have a limited shelf life. Most large cosmetic and product companies recognise the need to produce quality products that are neither comedogenic nor allergy causing and so use food grade preservatives.

Products are now also more environmentally friendly, with packaging that is recyclable and biodegradable, and many companies refuse to test products on animals.

Male skin

When looking at skin types and conditions, it is important to include the male skin, as males are becoming big spenders in the skincare market. In the USA men spent approximately 10 billion dollars on personal grooming products in 2007, according to a survey picked up by the *Guardian* newspaper. Even though this includes the large number of deodorant and shaving products that most men use, it is still a lot of money. One of the fastest-growing areas within beauty is the demand for specific men's salon treatments and related care products.

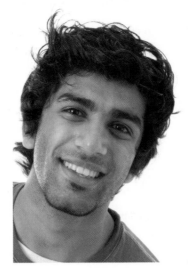

Men have become big spenders in the skincare market

Characteristics of male skin

Male skin is thicker than female skin due to the influence of the male hormones testosterone and androgen. It is therefore more resistant but can become thinner more quickly when ageing. Because of the testosterone influences, men's skin tends to be oilier than women's, so men like lighter moisturising products and products which solve their particular problems. Men also prefer less fragrance in their products or for it to have a masculine smell of cedarwood or pine.

Products for male skin

Previous generations of men would be happy to use their wife's moisturiser if their skin felt a little dry, but few would venture out into the salon or department store for a full consultation before purchasing their own products. Not any longer. The salon or company that caters for male skins is on to a winning formula — it is no longer seen as effeminate to use facial products, especially with high-profile sports personalities promoting different ranges in the media.

Products designed for men have evolved to take into account that the skin is more resistant but, conversely, may also be more fragile through neglect, misuse or total lack of protective products such as moisturisers and sun blocks.

Most men's basic product needs are for the daily routine of washing, shaving and moisturising. Calming products may also be needed for the specific treatment of blocked pores, irritation from shaving and razor burn or Folliculitis (inflammation of the hair follicle in the skin, commonly caused by an infection).

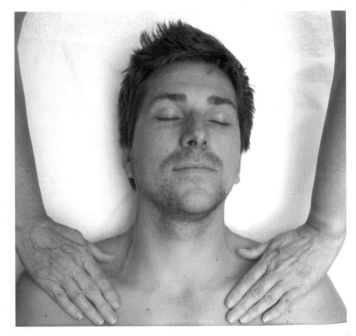

A growing number of men are visiting salons for treatments such as facials and manicures

Men who shave daily are automatically exfoliating the upper epidermal cells, so the skin stays healthy looking and clear. There are many products available for sensitive skins, both for dry and wet shaving, to avoid shaving rash, which can be very sore and unsightly.

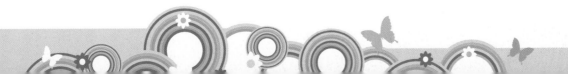

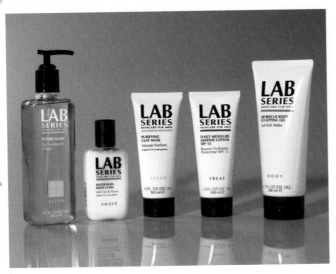

Many product ranges are designed specifically for men

Healing and soothing products, creams that reduce razor bumps, products that reduce the possibility of ingrown hairs are popular. Anti-ageing creams (although the name is misleading — nothing stops the ageing process) are also a fast-selling line. Although the signs of ageing appear later on a male face, when they do arrive the wrinkles are more intense and visible — men have fewer small lines but more deep wrinkles.

Some men use salon treatments to enhance their natural good points — eyelash tinting and the application of tinted moisturiser are very common. Manicures and pedicures are also a favourite with male clients. (Refer to Unit B4 Provide facial skincare treatment for information on how to prepare for a facial on a male client.)

Factors affecting the skin-ageing process

Along with the skin type your clients inherit, the care they take of it and their general health, age has to be the other greatest influence on the skin, not only because of the hormonal impact. Ageing is a natural part of the life cycle of a human being — it cannot yet be stopped or reversed, and is part of our evolution to keep the species going.

Unfortunately, western culture is geared up to the young and growing older is not seen as a desirable trait, unlike eastern cultures where age is equated with wisdom and knowledge. Western society tries to push back the ageing process and this has led to a marked rise in the demand for face lifts and extreme beauty treatments, such as Botox® injections and collagen infills, to delay the ageing process. However, we are genetically programmed to age, and temporary solutions are expensive, although they may provide a mental boost to the client. But we should celebrate ageing and enjoy the wisdom that age brings with it.

Ageing happens to us all and at generally the same rate, unless we have a disease that interrupts these natural processes. The inherited factor comes into play again — if your parents age well, enjoy good health and have good skin, the chances are you will too.

As well as the inheritance factor, the environment has a big impact on the ageing process. During normal metabolism, your cells make small electrically charged molecules called free radicals. These are very reactive and will react with proteins, DNA and some minerals. They can interfere with normal cell function, often causing irreversible damage that accumulates as we age. It is not yet known which chemicals within our environment stimulate free radical production: crop sprays, pesticides and household cleaning items are some of the products under investigation. Those people living in a built-up area, with exhaust fumes and lots of chemicals in their environment, are likely to have more free radicals in their body than country dwellers, who live in a less-polluted environment and on a diet of freshly grown organic fruit and vegetables.

The ageing process affects the skin in the following ways.

○ Cell renewal is always faster in youth. The older we get, the slower the renewal process becomes, until it stops altogether.

○ The genetic information in each cell gets a little diluted every time the cell reproduces, so the body cells of an 80-year-old do not have the same information as a young baby's.

○ Hormone production in both sexes varies with age and contributes to the skin's development, health and deterioration.

○ Fewer skin cells are being reproduced as a person gets older.

○ The underlying structures supporting the skin begin to offer less support – the collagen and elastin fibres in the skin degenerate, muscular tension diminishes and wrinkles appear.

○ The adipose tissue (the fat) supporting the skin diminishes and the skin starts to sag and gravity begins to win!

○ Sun damage and pigmentation disorders become more noticeable as the melanin production within the skin lessens. Age or liver spots (lentigo) may appear on the surface of the epidermis.

○ The face shape may alter if extensive dental work has been done or teeth are replaced with false ones – this causes the contours to drop and may make the face age.

Age grouping of the skin

Teenage years, 13–20 years

Just as the body is changing at puberty and getting ready for the reproduction stage of the human life cycle, so the emotional development also begins, making teenagers acutely aware of themselves and their relationships with their peers.

In females puberty is beginning earlier, often by the age of ten or twelve, which is largely due to better nutrition. Raging hormones dictate the development of the body, causing both the sexual development and the emotional highs and lows that accompany this dramatic change.

At this age the skin should be firm and compact, with a good supporting structure of collagen and elastin to give it a smooth feel. Unfortunately, the hormone levels can be unbalanced and the sebaceous glands can produce too much sebum, leading to blackheads and congested skin. Acne is common in this age group and may be directly related to high progesterone levels, so is more common in boys than girls.

Teenage boys may also cause skin problems by neglect – regular skin cleaning with the correct products can diminish skin problems but can be perceived as not a masculine pastime. However, with males taking a larger proportion of retail skin care sales than ever before, there is no reason for a male not to use a foaming facial cleanser designed for the male skin to help keep the skin clear.

A proportion of late-teen skins are not as clear as they could be for reasons that are self-inflicted. A poor diet of fast food, few vegetables and an excessive alcohol intake, combined with smoking, do nothing to enhance the skin. The only advantage is that this age group has youth on its side and the skin will recover more easily.

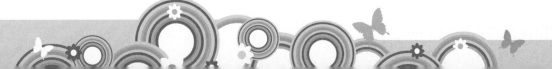

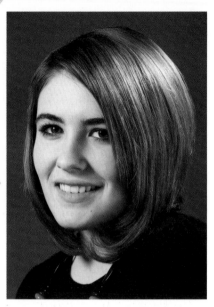

Teenagers have firm, compact skin

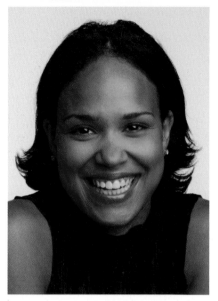

Skin is at its peak in the twenties

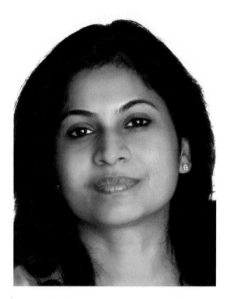

In the thirties, skin begins to dry out and fine lines appear

Adulthood, 20–30 years

This is when the chubbiness of the teenage years and the raging hormones disappear, or at least settle down, so the skin is at its peak. It looks fresh, radiant and glowing. The underlying structure is good, there are no fine lines developing yet, and providing good health is enjoyed and a healthy diet gives the body the correct nutrients, the skin is good.

Tiredness in young parents, bad lifestyle choices and simply 'burning the candle at both ends' will take its toll on this generation if care is not taken. Good choices in the appropriate skincare range and protection with a moisturiser, along with correct use of sunscreens, will be an investment for the future.

30–40 years

The skin begins to dry out and slows its reproduction down, with fine lines appearing, usually on the neck area first. The jawline is firmly defined at the beginning of the decade but can show signs of change. It may lose its definition, or if the client puts on weight, it will fill out and a double chin may form. Puffiness may be found in the cheeks — any weight gain in the face or body is instantly ageing.

The facial tissues begin to lose their fatty layer and tiredness can creep into the eye area. Creases and wrinkles remain after the depressions that form them have disappeared. Correct use of skincare products and protection against UV damage is essential in this age group as prevention is better than cure. A neck and hand cream will prevent dehydration, that is water loss. Many clients forget this — they may spend a fortune on their faces and forget that hands and neck areas are the true age reflector.

40–50 years

There is still a good clear definition of features, but 'temporary' double chins and wrinkles developed in the late thirties become a permanent feature. Elasticity and the supporting structures of collagen and elastin fibres are diminishing, especially if

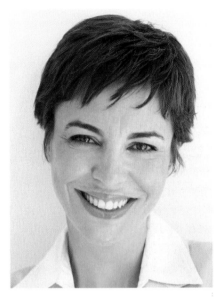

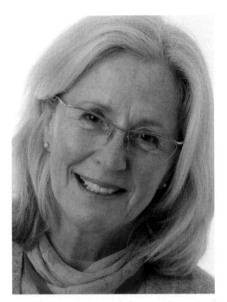

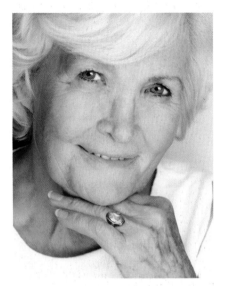

The skin's elasticity disappears in the forties

In the fifties, skin will be lined around the eyes and the mouth

When we reach sixty, care must be taken to lubricate the skin

the client is female and is undergoing the menopause, which may start towards the fifties. Oestrogen levels start to fall and this affects bone density, elasticity in the tissues and skin thickness.

The skin becomes thinner and more prone to damage from UV and the environment. Blemishes, broken capillaries and pigmentation changes begin to occur.

50–70 years

All women will have begun the menopause in this age group and the skin will be loose and thin. It may feel coarse to the touch, and the eyes are lined and puffy. The muscle tissue around the eye and mouth develop depressions, seen as wrinkles around them, and the lip line loses definition. The sebaceous glands have slowed down the production of sebum and care must be taken to keep the skin lubricated and free from infection. With ageing the skin loses some of its ability to fight infection and heal itself quickly. Facial hair growth may start to be obvious around the mouth and chin. This hair is coarse and thick because of the influence of the male hormone testosterone which is not being balanced by oestrogen.

Over 70 years

At this stage the skin has the appearance of being soft. There may be very little underlying fat to support the facial structure, and deeper furrows appear from the corner of the nose towards the lips and from the outer mouth down to the chin. Darkened patches may appear, or loss of pigment may be seen, especially on the hands and arms. The throat, neck and chest are very lined and like tissue paper, with very little sebum to lubricate the skin.

Can we slow the rate of ageing?

Evidence suggests that genes affect how long people live: long life seems to run in families. It is also known that cells have a programmed maximum number of divisions before they die off, so your life span is, to some degree, predetermined.

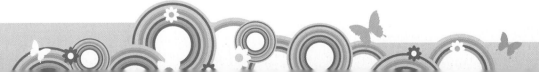

However, there are some sensible precautions you should be advising your clients to take.

- **Eat healthily** — people on lower calorie diets tend to live longer and meeting the body's additional demands as you age is important, e.g. a female who has heavy periods throughout her life will need more iron, a menopausal client will need more calcium to help keep bones healthy.

- **Keep physically active** — three half-hour aerobic sessions a week will help to keep circulation and metabolism going and will stimulate the body to repair itself (a brisk walk or swim will get the cardiovascular system working).

- **Get enough sleep or rest** — rest allows the body to repair and heal itself and the brain activity to slow and so the brain can sift through all the stimulation it has received during the day. Sleep deprivation is very harmful to the body in the long term.

- **Remain mentally active** — the more you use your brain, the better it works and the longer you remain alert. Doing a crossword, mental arithmetic, music and learning poetry is an ideal brain activity as you get older.

- **Remember good health maintenance** — this includes avoiding smoking (very ageing on the skin), moderate alcohol intake and low medication levels.

Anti-ageing treatments

The key here is 'prevention is better than cure'. In other words, encourage the client to look after their skin as early as possible, rather than waiting until the signs of ageing have begun to show. Looking after the skin in the twenties and thirties and developing good skincare habits, sun protection and work/life balance will pay dividends for a client in their sixties.

Anti-ageing treatments cannot turn back years of poor skin care and neglect, nor can they stop the ageing process. Some can significantly enhance the skin's appearance immediately. However, continuous treatments are needed for a long-term effect. The only true anti-ageing creams are sun protection creams with a high SPF factor — these prevent the skin from being harmed by the sun's rays.

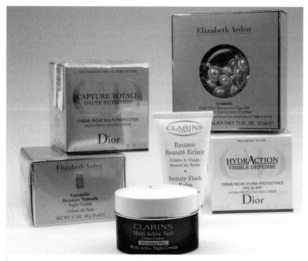

Moisturising products prevent moisture loss from the skin

Moisturisers

Contrary to popular belief, moisturisers do not add moisture to the skin, but rather they prevent moisture from being lost. This is achieved with the use of non-irritating oils and emollients such as lanolin, or vegetable-based or petroleum-based oils, which form a thin layer on top of the epidermis and stop water from literally evaporating out of the body. The result is that the outermost layers of the skin absorb the water being released by the deeper layers, so small wrinkles are filled out and the skin looks and feels a lot softer. Moisturising the skin also helps protect it from air pollution, harsh weather conditions and the drying effect of air conditioners. Most importantly, the majority of moisturisers contain ingredients that provide UV protection, which can affect the skin throughout the year, not just in the summer months.

Salon treatments

Any treatment which helps the desquamation process, that is the old cells of the epidermis being shed and new cells coming to the surface, is going to help the skin look clean and fresh. Combine a treatment that deep cleanses and then rehydrates the skin using an electrical current, such as in a galvanic facial, and the result is instant: the skin looks plump and refreshed and very, very clean. However, as we have already discovered, nothing prevents the ageing process, so all salon treatments will only last as long as the treatments are carried out on a regular basis. Scrubs, face masks and electrical treatments will work on the outer layers of the epidermis and will improve the look and feel of the skin. However, under the Trade Descriptions Act, a salon would be liable to prosecution if advertising these treatments as anti-ageing.

Alpha-hydroxy acids (AHAs) and skin peels

These treatments work by applying a chemical agent or acid (e.g. AHAs or vitamin A in the form of retionic acid) to the skin which dissolves the outermost layers, thus temporarily reducing fine lines and other superficial signs of ageing. However, the long-term effects of such skin peels are not yet known and adverse reactions are quite common, particularly if the concentration of the active ingredient is quite high, or if the product is left on the skin for too long. Peels also leave the skin far more susceptible to damage from UV rays and so sun protection is essential following treatment.

These treatments should only be carried out by trained professionals and a full aftercare programme is recommended as the skin is left vulnerable.

Dermabrasion

Dermabrasion (also referred to as 'open' dermabrasion) is a harsh skin treatment: it usually involves the use of wire brushes or diamonds to remove the epidermis down to the lowest possible cell layer. Micro-dermabrasion (or 'closed' dermabrasion) is a milder form of the same treatment, whereby minute aluminium oxide crystals are blown on to the face with the use of a vacuum unit. Again, the removal of the top cells of the epidermis will encourage new cell formation and give the skin a renewed look, but it can leave the skin vulnerable and some clients may experience soreness.

This treatment needs to be carried out by a professionally trained therapist, with a full consultation and aftercare given. Some medical treatments make this unsuitable: for example, if the client has been taking medication such as Accutane to treat acne, then the skin is already thin and dermabrasion is not suitable. If the client has recently had filler of collagen injected or Botox® injections, again do not treat. It may mean that the filler is dispersed through the tissue, and spreads!

Laser skin resurfacing

The word 'laser' is an acronym for Light Amplification by Stimulated Emission of Radiation, and laser therapy for the skin is becoming a very popular salon treatment. Laser treatment can be used for skin ageing and wrinkles, as the light stimulates the capillary level, so improving the circulation. Acne and cellulite also respond well to laser treatment, as do pigmented lesions and the removal of tattoos. The pigment is broken down into minute particles and removed through the lymphatic system.

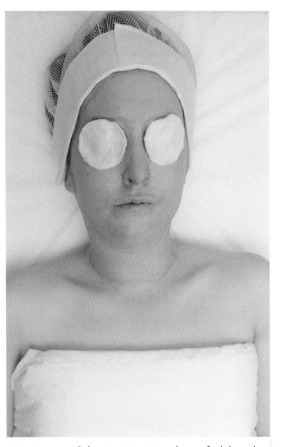

Salon treatments such as a facial mask help the skin look clean and fresh

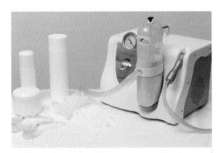

Micro-dermabrasion removes the top cells of the epidermis

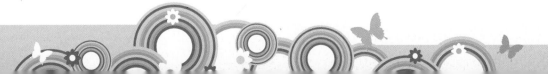

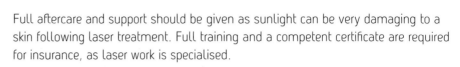

You and the skin

Full aftercare and support should be given as sunlight can be very damaging to a skin following laser treatment. Full training and a competent certificate are required for insurance, as laser work is specialised.

Collagen treatments

Collagen is a protein that is the principal ingredient of white fibrous connective tissue found within tendons, skin, bone, cartilage and ligaments. Despite any claims made by the manufacturers of collagen-containing products, it is said that the skin cannot absorb artificial collagen.

However, one collagen treatment that is temporarily effective and growing in popularity is collagen replacement therapy (CRT). This involves collagen being injected directly into the dermis to improve the appearance of fine lines and pockmarks. Collagen injections to the lips to create a 'bee sting' pout to the lip shape are common, but can go wrong if the client has an allergic reaction to the injection, leaving the lips very swollen and sore.

Avoid treating a client after a collagen treatment as there is a danger that massage movements could move the implant to another area.

Botox® treatments

Botox® works by paralysing muscles located at the site where it is injected, thus reducing lines and wrinkles in that area. It is often used to treat frown lines and crow's feet around the eyes. Once again, the effects are only temporary, and regular treatments are required.

The long-term effects of this botulinum-based treatment are not yet known. A recent report in the Journal of Cosmetic Dermatology suggests that people using Botox® to defeat the signs of ageing may simply be developing more wrinkles in nearby areas, as neighbouring muscles try to compensate for those that are paralysed.

Cosmetic surgery

Surgery is an invasive treatment and carries all the risks of any other medical operation. It is, however, considered an affordable treatment by many, and it can be very successful. Sagging contours and wrinkles can be removed by tightening the eye area or chin or having a complete face-lift, and this will reduce the signs of ageing. However, there is a danger of the skin looking too tight and not in keeping with the rest of the body — many film stars may look good in pictures of their face alone, but the neck and hands reflect their true age when a larger picture is taken. This can look most odd.

Cosmetic surgery should only be considered after a great deal of research and through a recognised medical referral. The newspapers often report that so-called 'clinics' cause a lot of pain and distress to 'patients' as they are not medically qualified to carry out procedures for cosmetic surgery, or because the post-operation care is so poor that secondary infection may occur.

In some cases, corrective surgery can be very successful and most beneficial, especially if the physical problem causes psychological distress too. The correction of a hare lip, reshaping of a broken nose or pinning back ears that protrude can give back client confidence and improve a person's self-image.

Stop the clock!

In conclusion, the ageing process is inevitable. Some treatments can suspend the process, but they cannot stop it. Take time to explain to your clients a little about the ageing process, and be honest about the limitations of any treatment they may be considering as well as its benefits. Having integrity means being honest and honouring your personal relationship with your clients. Rather than mislead or give false information about ageing and related treatments, discuss the lifestyle changes that will encourage clients to be active in preserving their quality of life: advise them to give up smoking, eat a healthy diet, drink plenty of water, take regular exercise and embark on a good skincare routine, including protection from the sun.

The skin and the sun

Coco Chanel introduced a tanned skin into high society in the 1930s when she was one of the first travellers to the south of France in the summer months. It became a sign of wealth and social standing if you could afford a tan as it meant you were rich enough to travel abroad. Going back through history the reverse is true: ladies and gentlemen of the 'upper classes' had very light faces and used powder to emphasise their whiteness. Only manual farm labourers had a tan, and this meant you had a job working outside in the sun. Unfortunately, we now think of a healthy skin as being a tanned one. This is, of course, not true. (Tanning is the name of the process used to dry out a cow's hide in the sunshine to turn it into leather!)

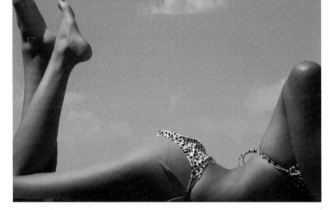

Remember – a tanned skin is a damaged skin

Except for helping to relieve certain conditions like asthma, aching joints and psoriasis, along with aiding vitamin D production, the sun's health benefits are primarily psychological. The truth is that too much sun can be positively harmful.

The immediate result of too much sun is severe sunburn, and many of us have experienced the painful blisters, fever and swelling that come from too much sun too fast. Another result of sun exposure is prematurely aged skin. The sun causes the skin to thicken and gives it a leathery, coarse appearance. With enough time, the sun weakens the skin's elasticity by cross-linking the collagen fibres in the dermis. This results in sagging and wrinkles on all sun-exposed areas.

The sun also causes dark pigmentation patches and scaly grey growths known as keratoses, which are often pre-cancerous. Sunburn and prematurely aged skin are not the worst results of constant exposure to the sun; skin cancer is. Almost all of the 300,000 cases of this disease that develop annually are considered to be sun-related. Some people are more at risk than others. Britain is fast catching up with Australia in numbers of skin cancer patients — in fact the promotion of skin cancer awareness in hotter countries is bringing down their skin cancer patient numbers as ours are growing.

People with black skins are relatively safe because the darker skin provides good protection against UV light. Those with light skin, notably redheads and blondes, are at the greatest risk due to less melanin in the skin.

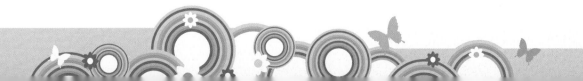

Certain drugs, such as antibiotics, medicated soaps and creams, and even barbiturates and birth control pills, can make the skin more susceptible to damage.

All clients concerned with premature ageing should be advised on the dangers of sun exposure, and a sunscreen or sun block should be recommended to them. Those clients who are avid sun worshippers should be educated to understand the relationship between the sun and skin cancer.

Once the UV light has caused cross-linking and thickening in the dermis and has predisposed the skin to premature ageing, there is no reversal of the damage. Plastic surgery techniques can help disguise the sagging by re-draping the skin, but this does not compensate for the damage that has occurred. It is, therefore, the first topic that must be discussed with the client who expresses concern about ageing. Advice on sun protection should be given verbally and in a written fact sheet. Indeed, the only cosmetic product that can legally be labelled 'anti-ageing' is a sunscreen or sun block preparation.

Concern is growing in the medical world for 'tanorexia', where young girls are becoming addicted to the use of sunbeds in tanning centres. Often, the use of these machines is not monitored and the client pays for the time on the sunbed, so they go several times a week to top up their tan. Unfortunately, this has resulted in a large increase in the incidence of skin cancers in young people, where it would not be expected under natural circumstances.

Sun preparations

While sun preparations are not included in the normal facial routine in a salon, lots of clients need the right information for homecare advice and use of the correct products, especially if going on holiday either in the UK or abroad.

Sun protection can come in the form of lotion, cream or milk, and some large manufacturers have now designed a spray-on application of sun protection.

Sunscreens filter the harmful ultraviolet rays, UVA and UVB, for a period of time. Most are water resistant and contain moisturisers to help nourish the skin. They come in various strengths, measured by a sun protection factor (SPF) ranging from 2–35. The higher the SPF number, the better the protection. The wearer can stay out in the sun for a longer time depending on the number: for example, SPF 6 permits sun exposure six times longer than with unprotected skin without burning; an SPF of 30 allows sun exposure 30 times longer. The choice of SPF depends upon the skin type and the strength of the sun. The nearer the equator, the hotter the sun, so a higher protection factor would be needed in, say, the Mediterranean than in the UK. The sun's rays are also reflected so there is a risk of getting sunburnt when sailing or skiing, even when the temperature is low.

Sun blocks are total blocks and will screen out all the sun's rays. They have become essential in some countries, for example in Australia, where there is a high incidence of skin cancer. Sun blocks are seen as coloured strips of cream that sit on the nose and forehead — very popular with cricketers.

Skin products for different types of skin

See individual products and follow individual recommendations as products do vary. As sun on the face accelerates the ageing process, clients should be advised to wear a hat or cover the face liberally with the correct SPF cream.

Most manufacturers recommend the following:

Skin type	Recommended sun preparation
Fair skin or redhead with fair skin burns easily after 30 minutes' exposure	20–35 SPF or sun block for complete protection
Sallow-skinned person who is fair will tan, but feels sore after 30 minutes	10–20 SPF
Darker skins that tan easily but tend to get sore initially	10 –15 SPF

Self-tanning creams

This is a very popular salon treatment for both face and body, and the safest way to get a tan. After exfoliation and moisturising, the tanning lotion is applied. It will develop over several hours and last for several days. Most large cosmetic houses make self-tans for the face, which are not as strong as the body self-tan. These are often in the form of an impregnated tissue, which just wipes over the facial area and leaves a residue which develops into a tan. There are also spray guns which deliver a fine mist of the product all over the body, for a speedy application.

The active ingredient is a chemical, dihydroxyacetone, which reacts with the keratin in the skin to produce a golden colour through oxidation. This has become a very popular salon treatment to offer clients. It looks very natural and lasts about a week, depending upon the depth of the application.

Think about it

Self-tanning application will only be as good as the surface it goes onto – a bit like nail varnish! If the skin is dry or rough, then the colour will come out patchy and darker in some places.

Protect children and toddlers with high SPF products and use T-shirts and hats to protect young skin

Increase exposure to the sun gradually

Sun protection is needed in the UK and abroad

Ensure all exposed skin is evenly covered with protective lotion

THE SUN

Avoid the sun between 1 pm and 3 pm in the heat of the day

Always re-apply after swimming

Apply sun protection 30 minutes before and frequently during exposure to sun

Safe sun advice

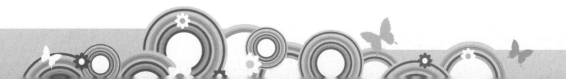

An increasingly popular treatment in the salon is to offer a complete body spray application, where the client stands in an open cubicle with three sides, and tan is literally sprayed all over the body. This application is carried out with a commercial tanning gun, which pumps the liquid tan through a nozzle turning it into a mist. The tan must be allowed to dry on the skin. A setting time is required, so the client relaxes in a reclining chair and then showers the residue off. The tan is visible immediately and develops into a deeper tan over the next 24 hours.

For your portfolio

When out shopping, pick up several samples of self-tanning preparations and try them out at home. Remember to exfoliate first and then apply moisturiser before applying the tan. Follow the manufacturer's instructions and apply the tan to your legs.

Note the different textures and smells. Which one did you prefer? Which one gave the most natural colour? (Do remember to scrub your palms if you did not wear gloves, otherwise they will be tanned too!)

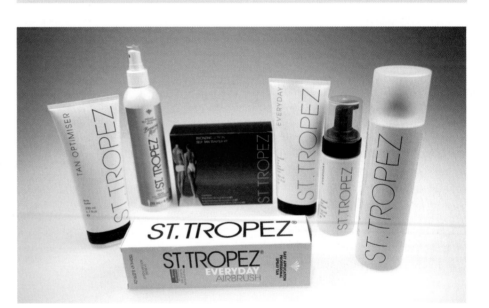

Self-tanning products

You and the skin

Check your knowledge

1 AHA stands for:
- **a)** alpha hydrogen acids
- **b)** alpha hydro acids
- **c)** alkaline help acids
- **d)** alpha hydroxy acids.

2 Chloasma is easily recognised as:
- **a)** white patches of skin
- **b)** pink patches of skin
- **c)** yellow patches of skin
- **d)** brown patches of skin.

3 Which of these is NOT a contra-indication to a treatment?
- **a)** Leucoderma
- **b)** Cancer
- **c)** Impetigo
- **d)** Dermatitis

4 Acne vulgaris is caused by:
- **a)** fungal infection
- **b)** bacterial infection
- **c)** congenital
- **d)** viral infection.

5 Eczema is a:
- **a)** fungal infection
- **b)** bacterial infection
- **c)** congenital
- **d)** viral infection.

6 A Wood's lamp gives off:
- **a)** ultraviolet light
- **b)** infrared light
- **c)** green light
- **d)** orange light.

7 The Fitzpatrick classification system measures:
- **a)** blood flow in the skin
- **b)** tanning properties of skin types
- **c)** the acid mantle of the skin
- **d)** muscle tone of the skin.

8 Intrinsic ageing of the skin means:
- **a)** the internal body clock of cells
- **b)** the external factor of pollution
- **c)** the effect of sunlight on the skin
- **d)** the importance of diet as you age.

9 Blepharitis is an infection of the:
- **a)** mouth
- **b)** ears
- **c)** eyes
- **d)** nose.

10 The function of the acid mantle is to:
- **a)** control blood flow to the skin
- **b)** produce histamine
- **c)** control bacteria on the skin
- **d)** plump up collagen levels.

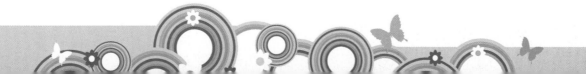

Related anatomy and physiology

What you will learn

- Bones of the head, face, neck and shoulder girdle
- Bones of the arm and leg
- The skin – structure and functions
- Structure of the nails
- Muscles of the face, neck and shoulder area
- Muscles of the arm and leg
- Hair
- Blood
- The lymphatic system

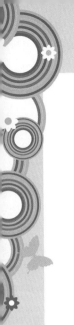

Introduction

As a beauty therapist you should have an understanding of the body and its basic functions so that you can give the most effective treatments to your client. When you can look at the body with knowledge and understanding you will be able to identify any problems and treat them with suitable products, and make recommendations to help your client.

The information in this section is compatible with the new standards for NVQ Level 2 Beauty Therapy. It can also be used in conjunction with all non-NVQ qualifications and follows the Vocational Awards International framework for anatomy and physiology.

The depth of knowledge for NVQ Level 2 is very defined; the requirements for this section have been taken directly from the standards for each unit. Therefore no other anatomy or physiology is required to complete these qualifications. The related knowledge, to support anatomy links to a specific treatment given, is contained within the book. The areas where the anatomy links into the individual units is shown in the cross mapping which follows below.

A Try it out activity is included at the end of each topic. You may like to undertake this either with your study group or independently.

Additional knowledge on the structure of a cell and the structure of the heart has been included to aid your understanding of anatomy, although this is not directly required to fulfil the Awarding Body criteria.

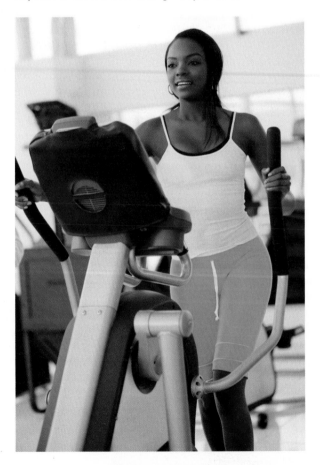

As a beauty therapist you need an understanding of basic bodily structures

Cross-mapping: anatomy and physiology

Your guide to the anatomy required in each unit.

B4 Provide facial skincare treatment	B6 Carry out waxing services	B8 Provide make-up services	B10 Enhance appearance using skin camouflage	N2 Provide manicure services	N3 Provide pedicure services
The structure and function of the skin – epidermis, dermis, subcutaneous layer, nerve endings and appendages (includes the hair follicle, the hair shaft, the sebaceous gland, arrector pili muscle, sweat gland, blood and lymph vessels)	The structure and function of the skin – epidermis, dermis, subcutaneous layer, nerve endings and appendages (includes the hair follicle, the hair shaft, the sebaceous gland, arrector pili muscle, sweat gland, blood and lymph vessels)	The structure and function of the skin – epidermis, dermis, subcutaneous layer, nerve endings and appendages (includes the hair follicle, the hair shaft, the sebaceous gland, arrector pili muscle, sweat gland, blood and lymph vessels)	The structure and function of the skin	The bones of the hand and lower arm	The bones of the foot and lower leg
The position and action of the face, neck and shoulder muscles	The structure of the hair	The skin characteristics and skin types of different ethnic client groups (Note: covered in You and the skin, pages 189–94)	The importance of recognising different skin types and characteristics (Note: covered in You and the skin, pages 184–88)	The muscles of the lower arm and hand	The muscles of the foot and lower leg
Bones of the head, neck and shoulder girdle	The basic principles of hair growth (anagen, catagen, telogen) The types of hair growth		The photosensitivity of skin and how it differs in different skin groups (i.e. the Fitzpatrick Classification System) (Note: covered in You and the skin, pages 194–95)	The blood circulation to the lower arm and hand	The blood circulation to the foot and lower leg
The position of the head, face, neck, chest and shoulder girdle bones		How to recognise the skin types listed in the range (Note: covered in You and the skin, pages 190–95)		The structure of the nail unit (i.e. nail plate, nail bed, matrix, etc.)	The structure of the nail unit (i.e. nail plate, nail bed, matrix, etc.)
The composition and function of blood and lymph and its role in improving skin and muscle condition		How to recognise the following skin conditions: sensitive, dehydrated, broken capillaries, pustules, papules, open pores, dark circles, hyperpigmentation, hypopigmentation, sun damage, scarring, erythema (Note: covered in You and the skin, pages 195–97)	The causes and appearance of skin conditions likely to need skin camouflage (Note: covered in You and the skin, pages 203–05)	The process of nail growth (i.e. nail formation, growth rate, factors affecting growth, the effects of damage on growth, nail thickness)	The process of nail growth (i.e. nail formation, growth rate, factors affecting growth, the effects of damage on growth, nail thickness)
The skin characteristics and skin types of different ethnic client groups (Note: covered in You and the skin, pages 189–94)				The structure and function of the skin (i.e. dermis, epidermis, subcutaneous layer, appendages)	The structure and function of the skin (i.e. dermis, epidermis, subcutaneous layer, appendages)
How the natural ageing process affects facial skin and muscle tone (Note: covered in You and the skin, pages 208–15)		How environmental and lifestyle factors affect the condition of the skin (Note: covered in You and the skin, pages 178–81)		The different natural nail shapes you are likely to come across during manicure services (e.g. hook, spoon, fan)	The different natural nail shapes you are likely to come across during pedicure services (e.g. hook, spoon, fan)
				The skin characteristics and skin types of different ethnic client groups (Note: covered in You and the skin, pages 189–94)	

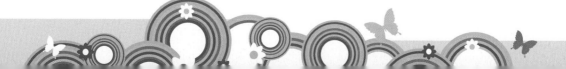

Bones of the head, face, neck and shoulder girdle

This section will teach you about the position of the bones of the head, face, neck, shoulders and bones of the forearm, hand and lower leg and foot.

The arrangement of bones that are joined together is known as a **skeleton**. The skeleton gives the body shape; it provides attachment for muscles and protects delicate organs. For good facial work the therapist needs to identify the bones of the head, neck, face and shoulders.

Bones that form the skull (cranium)

The skull, also known as the cranium, is a very hard structure that protects the brain. Although it looks like one bone it is actually made up of 22 separate bones that are fused together at ridged joints called **sutures**. The sutures are classed as fibrous joints because they only allow movement in the head of babies for ease of the head coming through the birth canal. Ten bones make up the skull and 12 form the face.

There are many openings in the skull to allow blood vessels and nerves to enter and leave. The largest of these is at the base of the skull and this is called the foramen magnum. This opening allows the spinal cord and blood vessels to pass to and from the brain. A baby's skull has soft spots called the fontanelles. Over a period of about 18 months the bones gradually join together. During this time, care should be taken to protect the baby's head.

Key terms

Skeleton – the bony framework of the body which supports and protects the tissues and organs.

Key terms

Sutures – ridged, fibrous joints of the skull.

Think about it

Skulls vary in size and shape. Your genes can dictate many features of your face shape, such as prominent cheekbones. A bigger skull does not necessarily mean a person is more intelligent.

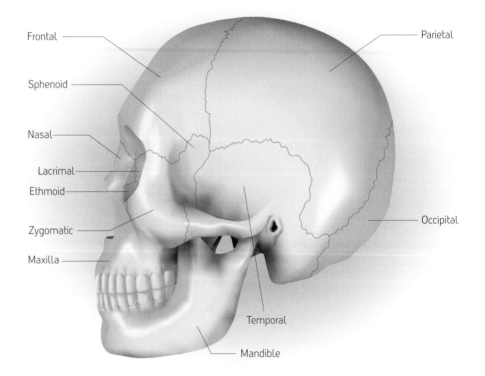

Frontal

Sphenoid

Nasal

Lacrimal

Ethmoid

Zygomatic

Maxilla

Parietal

Occipital

Temporal

Mandible

Bones of the skull

Bone	Position
Occipital bone (1)	At the back of the skull
Parietal (2)	Positioned at the back of the head and forms the roof of the skull
Frontal (1)	Forms the front of the skull, forehead, and upper eye sockets
Temporal (2)	At the side, around the ears
Sphenoid (1)	At the base of the skull, wing shaped, forms the temple
Ethmoid (1)	Positioned between the frontal and sphenoid bones and forms roof of the nasal cavities
Lacrimal (2)	One in each eye orbit These bones are fused together to form the shape of the skull, and their joins are known as sutures

The skull is attached to the body via the **vertebral column**. The vertebral column enables the head to turn and tilt. The weight of the head is supported by the neck, the shoulder girdle bones and muscles.

Key terms

Vertebral column – the spine or backbone which runs from the cranium (head) to the coccyx. It keeps the body upright and supports it, as well as protecting the spinal nerves and spinal cord.

The bones of the face

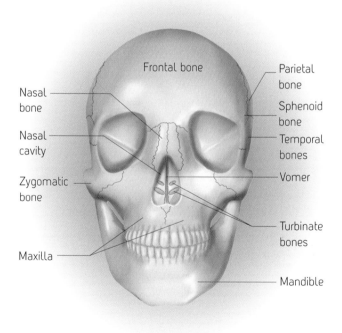

Bones of the face

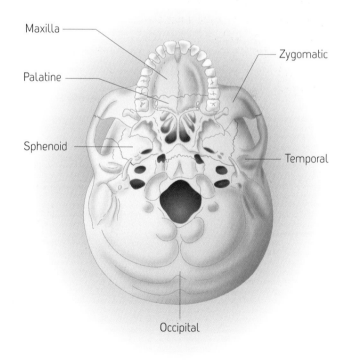

Bones of the face from below

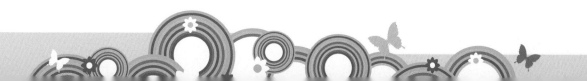

Bone	Position
1 Zygomatic bones (2)	These form the cheek bones
2 Maxillae (2)	These form the upper jaw, most of the side wall of the nose and the front part of the soft palate
3 Mandible (1)	This is the lower jaw and is the only moving bone in the face, allowing movement of the mouth for chewing and talking
4 Nasal (2)	These form the bridge of the nose
5 Turbinate (2)	The bones inside the nose
6 Vomer (1)	This forms part of the nasal septum
7 Palatine (2)	These form part of the side walls of the nose and the hard palate

The openings in the base of the skull provide spaces for the entrance and exit of many blood vessels, nerves and other structures. Projections and slightly elevated portions of the bones provide for the attachment of muscles. Some portions contain delicate structures, such as the part of the temporal bone that encloses the middle and internal sections of the ear. The air sinuses provide lightness and serve as vibrating chambers for the voice.

Bones of the shoulder girdle, upper vertebra, upper arm and chest

The bones of the shoulder girdle allow the arms to move freely. The **clavicle** is more commonly known as the collar bone, and you can feel it in the area where the collar of a shirt or blouse would sit. The **scapula** is commonly referred to as the shoulder blade. The scapula is only secured to the skeleton by muscle, so it is fairly free to move about.

Bones	Girdle
1 Clavicle (2)	Across the front of the chest, going from each shoulder to the breast bone
2 Scapula (2)	At the back of the shoulder girdle, sitting on top of the rib cage
3 Sternum (1)	This is often called the breast bone; it forms part of the rib cage
4 Cervical vertebra (7)	The vertabrae which form the neck; the first two are called the Atlas and Axis, and support and allow free movement of the head
5 Humerus (2)	These bones form the top of each arm; they move in a groove in the clavicle by a joint called a ball and socket

Try it out

Draw your arms back, and look in the mirror. Can you see your scapula? It may be easier to identify this on a partner.

Related anatomy and physiology

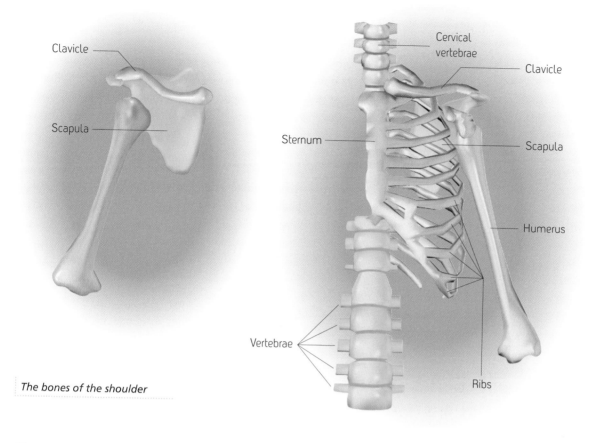

Clavicle

Scapula

Cervical
vertebrae

Clavicle

Sternum

Scapula

Humerus

Vertebrae

Ribs

The bones of the shoulder

Bones of the arm and leg

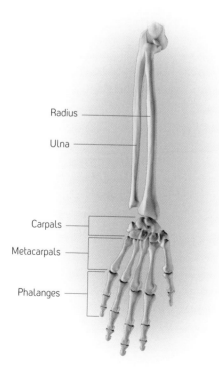

Radius

Ulna

Carpals

Metacarpals

Phalanges

Bones of the forearm and hand

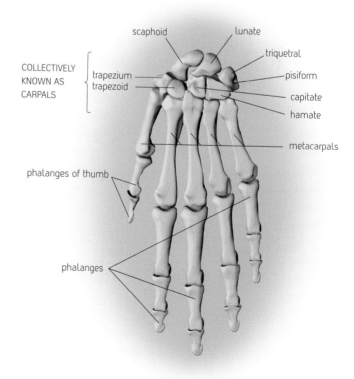

scaphoid

lunate

triquetral

COLLECTIVELY
KNOWN AS
CARPALS

trapezium
trapezoid

pisiform

capitate

hamate

metacarpals

phalanges of thumb

phalanges

Bones of the hand and wrist

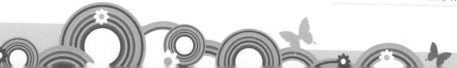

Key terms

Radius – bone on the outer side of the forearm; smaller of the two bones in the lower arm.

Ulna – bone on the inner side of the forearm; larger of the two bones in the lower arm.

Humerus – bone of the upper arm; sometimes called the funny bone.

Ligament – strong bands of fibrous, connective tissue binding bones together.

Carpals – bones that make up the wrist joint, consisting of hamate, capitate, pisiform, triquetral, lunate, scaphoid, trapezium and trapezoid.

Metacarpals – bones that make up the palm of the hand.

Phalanges – bones that make up the fingers.

Pronation – rotation movement of the palm away from you.

Supination – rotation movement of the palm to face you.

The lower arm is made up of two bones: the **radius** and the **ulna**. The ulna is the larger of the two bones.

The radius and ulna form a hinge with the **humerus** (the bone of the upper arm sometimes referred to as the funny bone). This hinge joint enables the arm to flex and extend. The rotation of the hand is made by the radius being able to cross over the ulna. A **ligament** connects the two bones.

The wrist is made up of eight individual bones in two rows. Collectively these bones are known as **carpals**, although they each have individual names.

The palm of the hand is made up of five bones called **metacarpals**, and the fingers are made of three bones called **phalanges**. The thumb contains only two phalanges bones.

Try it out

Have the palm of your right hand facing you. Now rotate your palm so it turns away from you. This rotation movement is known as **pronation**. Now rotate your hand so your palm faces you again. This is called **supination**.

Think about it

A simple way to remember which forearm bone is which: ulna contains the letter 'l' and this bone goes to your little finger.

Bones of the lower leg and foot

The bones that make up the lower leg are the **tibia** and **fibula**. The tibia is often called the shinbone. This bone is the stoutest in the body and transmits body weight directly to the ankle joint. The fibula forms part of the ankle joint.

The foot is constructed in a similar way to the hand. Seven bones, all with individual names, make up the **tarsals** (like the wrist). Five **metatarsals** together support the major arches of the foot.

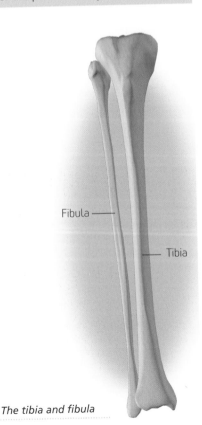

The tibia and fibula

Fibula

Tibia

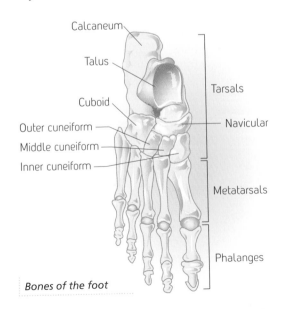

Calcaneum

Talus

Cuboid

Outer cuneiform

Middle cuneiform

Inner cuneiform

Tarsals

Navicular

Metatarsals

Phalanges

Bones of the foot

Key terms

Tibia – shin bone; inner, thicker of the two bones in the lower leg. Articulates with the femur, fibula and talus.

Fibula – a long thin bone on the outer side of the leg; smaller of the two bones in the lower leg.

Tarsals – bones of the foot.

Metarsals – bones supporting the major arches of the foot.

The foot has four arches: two **transverse** (across the foot) and two **longitudinal** (from heel to toe). The function of these arches is to:

○ provide support for the body

○ act as shock absorbers

○ aid posture.

Key terms

Transverse – running sideways, that is across a bone or muscle from one side to the other.

Longitudinal – running lengthways, that is the length of a bone or muscle from top to bottom.

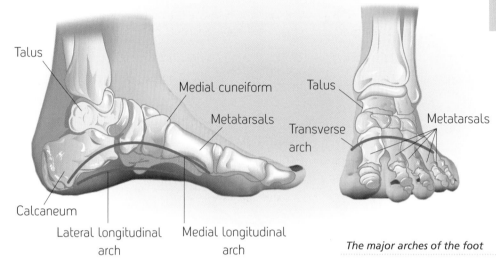

The major arches of the foot

Like the fingers, the toes are made of phalanges. The big toes have two phalanges each and the other toes have three.

The skin – structure and functions

Refer to You and the skin, pages 175–220 for further information on the skin.

The skin's structure

Skin is a remarkable organ that is able to adapt and perform various functions. It can mould to different shapes, stretch and harden, but can also respond to delicate touch, feel pain, pressure, hot and cold, so it is regarded as an effective communicator.

Skin makes up about 12 per cent of an adult's body weight and consists of three layers: the **epidermis**, **dermis** and the **subcutaneous layers**. You can think of these layers like clothing. The epidermis is the outer skin, like a breathable waterproof jacket – this is the skin we see. Our skin, or dermis, is under this and could be thought of as a blouse or shirt with lots of pockets containing many different items. Underneath this is a cushioned soft layer for protection, like a soft thermal vest. This bottom layer (the subcutaneous layer) contains fat which helps to insulate and keep in warmth. The layers vary in thickness over different areas of the body. The thickest layers are over friction and gripping areas, such as the palm of the hand and soles of the feet, and the thinnest are over the eyelids, which must be light and flexible.

Key terms

Epidermis – outer layer of the skin.

Dermis – layer of skin below the epidermis.

Subcutaneous layer – the fatty tissue found beneath the dermis which contains fat cells that act as both insulation against heat being lost and for the protection of the internal organs.

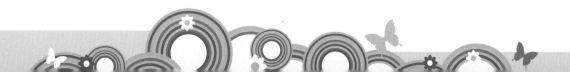

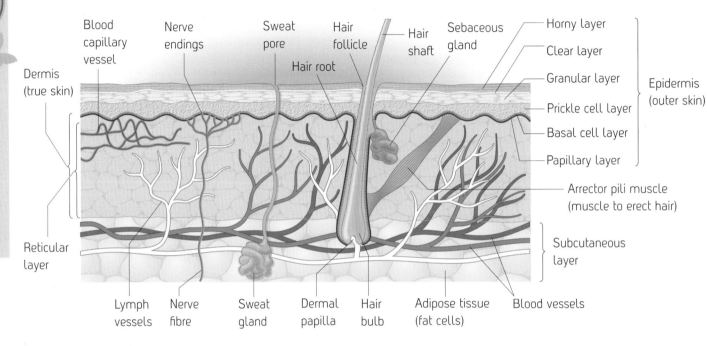

Think about it

Even though on average skin is just 2 mm thick, it receives about one eighth of the blood supply for the whole body. In some areas, such as the soles of the feet, the skin can be 6 mm thick while on the eyelids, it's just 0.5 mm thick.

Blood capillary vessel

Nerve endings

Sweat pore

Hair follicle

Hair shaft

Hair root

Sebaceous gland

Horny layer

Clear layer

Granular layer

Prickle cell layer

Basal cell layer

Papillary layer

Epidermis (outer skin)

Dermis (true skin)

Reticular layer

Arrector pili muscle (muscle to erect hair)

Subcutaneous layer

Lymph vessels

Nerve fibre

Sweat gland

Dermal papilla

Hair bulb

Adipose tissue (fat cells)

Blood vessels

The structure of the skin

Key terms

Horny layer – top layer of skin.

Clear layer – layer of skin beneath the horny layer.

Granular layer – layer of skin between the clear and prickle cell layers.

Prickle cell layer – layer of skin between the granular and basal layers.

Basal cell layer – bottom layer of skin.

The epidermis

The epidermis is the outermost layer of the skin. It is made up of five layers.

1 **Horny layer** (*Stratum corneum*)

2 **Clear layer** (*Stratum lucidum*)

3 **Granular layer** (*Stratum granulosum*)

4 **Prickle cell layer** (*Stratum spinosum*)

5 **Basal cell layer** (*Stratum germativum*)

Layers 1 to 3 – the horny, clear and granular layers – are dead and are constantly being shed. But the prickle cell and basal cell layers – layers 4 and 5 – are still living because the cells contain a nucleus and can therefore reproduce. Skin renews itself every 28 days.

For assessment purposes you are only required to learn the English names for the epidermis. In some books you will find Latin names for the layers (shown in brackets above).

The layers of the epidermis need to be looked at in order of formation.

The five layers of the epidermis, or our outer skin, begin at the basal cell or bottom layer (5). This skin is constantly being reproduced, as the cells contain a nucleus or seed. As the cells reproduce the layers get constantly pushed up into the next layer. Each of the layers has its own specific function.

The prickle cell layer (4) is called this because the cells have spines, which prevent **bacteria** entering the cells and moisture being lost. These cells also have a nucleus and so reproduce.

The next layer is the granular layer (3). The prickle cells lose their spines and become flatter. The nucleus dies and a protein is formed called **keratin**. This protein prevents moisture loss and is found in skin, nails and **hair**.

The next layer is the clear layer (2). This layer is for cushioning and protection and is found only on the palms of the hands and soles of the feet.

The final layer is the horny layer (1), where the cells are dead and ready to be shed. If you look at flakes of skin under a microscope they would resemble flakes of almond. The name for the shedding of the skin is **desquamation** (refer to You and the skin, page 183). This process speeds up as we age.

Layer	Function
1 Horny layer	Made up of many flattened dead skin cells which contain the tough keratin This is the final top layer of skin. These cells are shed continuously to allow the new cells through.
2 Clear layer	3 to 4 rows thick of dead flattened cells Only found on the palms of the hands and the soles of the feet, above the granular layer. These cells act as protectors in areas of friction.
3 Granular layer	2 to 4 layers thick, the cells begin to die and flatten The middle layer of the epidermis Waste and other substances from the cell get squashed together and harden.
4 Prickle cell layer	10 to 20 cells thick, with spines that connect with other cells. Sits on top of the basal layer. This layer of cells, called **melanocytes**, starts to harden and produce keratin. **Melanin** is also produced here which determines our colouring and helps protect against ultraviolet light.
5 Basal cell layer	A single layer of column-shaped cells The deepest layer of epidermis Continuously produces new cells

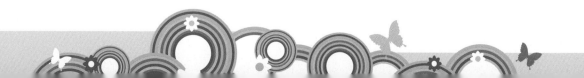

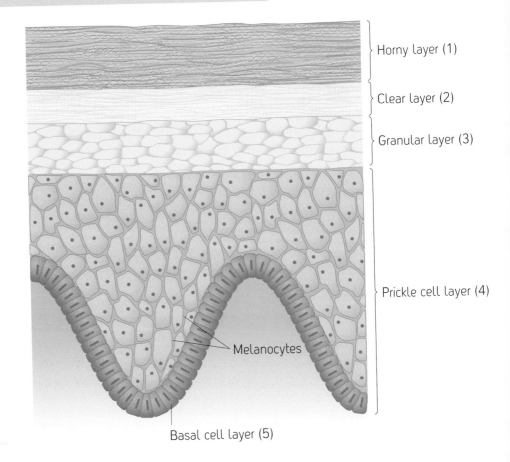

Horny layer (1)

Clear layer (2)

Granular layer (3)

Prickle cell layer (4)

Melanocytes

Basal cell layer (5)

The layers of the epidermis

Key terms

Hair follicle – threadlike growth of the epidermis.

Regulation – control.

Papillary layer – connected to the underside of the epidermis; a connective tissue that contains nerve endings and a network of blood and lymphatic capillaries.

Reticular layer – situated below the papillary layer; formed of tough, dense, fibrous connective tissue which contains collagen, elastic and reticular fibres for support and elasticity within the skin.

Collagen – protein found in white, fibrous connective tissue. In the skin it provides strength and resilience.

Elastin – allows the skin to stretch easily, and then regain its original shape.

You may be required to label this diagram for a written skin assessment.

The dermis

The dermis or true skin contains many structures. It can be subdivided into two parts.

1   Papillary layer
2   Reticular layer

The dermis contains the main components of the skin such as nerve endings (for pain, pressure, hot and cold), the blood supply and the lymph vessels, **hair follicles** and our sweat glands for temperature **regulation**.

Papillary layer

O   Undulating wavy tissue, rich in blood and lymph vessels and nerve endings.

O   Joins the dermis to the epidermis.

O   Area of cell reproduction provides lots of nourishment and aids waste removal via lymph system.

Reticular layer

O   Dense and fibrous, contains main components of dermis.

O   Found beneath the papillary layer.

O   Protects and repairs injured tissue, contains **collagen**, **elastin** and reticulin tissue.

The subcutaneous tissue

This is the fatty layer of the skin, underneath the dermis. Cells called lipocytes produce lipids, which are the fat cells from which we form subcutaneous tissue.

The job of the subcutaneous tissue is to:

○ protect the muscles, bones and internal organs from being damaged

○ provide insulation against the cold and provide a source of energy if the body should need it.

Functions of the skin

You can help yourself to remember the functions of the skin by the word 'shapes'.

S = Sensitivity
There are five types of nerve ending within the skin to help identify pain, touch, heat, cold and light pressure.

H = Heat regulation
The skin helps regulate the body's temperature by sweating to cool the body down when it overheats and shivering when it is cold. Shivering closes the pores. The tiny hairs that cover the body stand on end to trap warm air next to the skin and therefore prevent heat loss, when cold.

A = Absorption
Absorption of ultraviolet (UV) rays, from the sun. The skin synthesises vitamin D when exposed to UV light: modified cholesterol molecules in the skin are converted by the UV to vitamin D. The body needs vitamin D for the formation of strong bones and good eyesight. However, the skin has limited absorption properties. Only fat-soluble substances, such as oxygen, carbon dioxide, fat-soluble vitamins and steroids, along with small amounts of water are allowed through. Some creams, essential oils and some medication may be absorbed through the skin.

P = Protection
Too much UV light may harm the skin, so the skin protects itself by producing a pigment, seen as a tan, called melanin. Bacteria and germs are prevented from entering the skin by a protective barrier called the acid mantle. This barrier also helps protect against moisture loss. (Refer to You and the skin, page 182, for more information on the acid mantle and the pH of the skin.)

E = Excretion
Waste products and toxins are eliminated from the body through the sweat glands.

S = Secretion
Sebum and sweat are secreted on to the skin's surface. The sebum keeps the skin lubricated and soft, and the sweat combines with the sebum to form the acid mantle.

For your portfolio

Try these activities and think about your skin or that of your partner.

1 Look in the mirror and see if you have any pigmentation marks, for example freckles. Do they appear more in the summer?

2 What causes your skin to change colour?

3 Feel the texture of your skin with the side of your little finger, is it smooth, oily, dry, or uneven, does it change on different areas?

4 Pull the skin up on the back of your hand – does it spring back quickly, or does the skin take a while to return to its place?

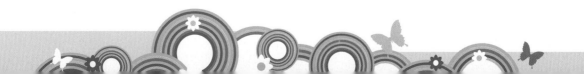

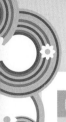

Related anatomy and physiology

Key terms

Sudoriferous glands – found in the dermis; excrete waste products through sweat and help to control body temperature; classified as apocrine and eccrine.

Apocrine glands – sweat glands that occur on hairy parts of the body, especially armpits and groin. They develop during puberty and produce sweat that contains fatty materials. It is the activity of these glands that causes body odour due to bacteria breaking down the organic compounds in the sweat.

Eccrine glands – sweat glands with ducts opening directly on to the surface of the skin; linked to the sympathetic nervous system, they help to regulate body temperature and are found all over the body, but more abundantly on the soles of the feet, palms of the hands and forehead. They produce sweat that is composed mainly of water and salts.

Sebaceous glands – exocrine glands found all over the body, in the dermis, apart from the soles of the feet and palms of the hands; secrete sebum and are situated adjacent to hair follicles.

Arrector pili muscle – fan-shaped, smooth muscle in the dermis attached to the base of each hair that contracts when the body surface is chilled causing the hair to stand erect.

Blood vessels – arteries, veins and capillaries that carry blood to and from the heart and body tissues.

Arteries – the largest blood vessels with thick muscular walls that carry blood away from the heart.

Capillaries – the smallest blood vessel in the body; has thin walls and is located between an arteriole and venule. A capillary is one cell thick, allowing the exchange of substances, such as oxygen, water and lipids, between blood and body cells.

Veins – blood vessels conveying blood towards the heart.

Structure	Location	Function
Sudoriferous glands There are two types: 1 **Eccrine glands** (sweat glands) 2 **Apocrine glands** (post-puberty sweat glands)	Eccrine glands are found all over the body but dense on the palms of the hands and soles of the feet. Apocrine glands are fewer in number and larger than eccrine. Only found in hairy parts of the body, i.e. armpits, nipples, anal and genital areas.	Eccrine glands produce sweat, water and urea, so help to regulate body temperature, remove toxin accumulations and help with the acid mantle. Apocrine glands are under the control of the nervous sysyem and respond to sexual attraction, emotional demands and psychological factors.
Hair follicle A threadlike outgrowth of the epidermis	Found in the dermis but not present on the soles of the feet or the palms of the hands or lips.	Produces and contains the hair during its life cycle.
Hair Not present on the soles of the feet and the palms of the hand or on the lips	Grows in the follicles in the dermis and is then seen growing out through the epidermis.	Believed to be connected to the production of body warmth. It is also a sexual characteristic.
Sebaceous glands Not found where there are no follicles present – see hair follicles	In the dermis, adjacent to hair follicles.	Produces sebum to lubricate the hair and the skin. Combines with sweat to form the acid mantle. Helps to waterproof the skin.
Arrector pili muscle (also spelt erector) Muscle tissue	Attached to the hair follicle at the base of the epidermis.	Raises the hair follicle to close the pore and so trap warmth in the body. Gives that goose pimple look to the skin.
Nerves Sensory nerve endings	Found on the dermis and subcutaneous tissue.	Responds to pain, pressure, heat, cold and touch. The nerves carry impulses to the brain for response by the body for protection.
Blood vessels These consist of **arteries**, **veins** and **capillaries**	Found in the dermis and subcutaneous layer.	Arteries carry nutrients and oxygen to the skin via capillaries. Veins remove waste products. Capillaries also help with heat regulation.
Lymph vessels	Found in the dermis and subcutaneous layer.	The body's secondary circulation system, they collect germs, bacteria and waste from the system that the blood supply cannot take. The lymph is filtered and returned to the bloodstream.

Location and function of structures found in the dermis and subcutaneous layer

Additional knowledge
Cells

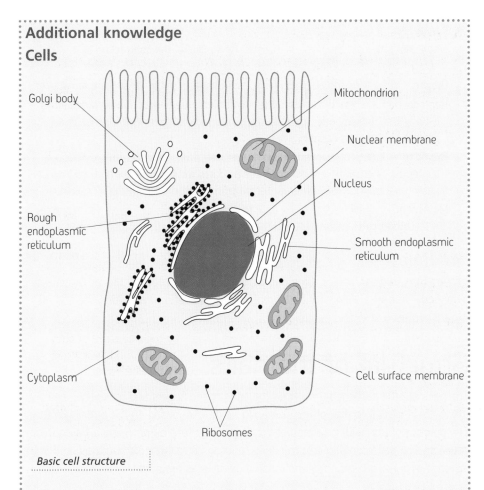

Golgi body

Mitochondrion

Nuclear membrane

Nucleus

Rough endoplasmic reticulum

Smooth endoplasmic reticulum

Cytoplasm

Cell surface membrane

Ribosomes

Basic cell structure

Cells are the basic building blocks of the body. There are about 200 different types of cells. Cells that group together form tissue, and several tissues grouped together form the organs of the body.

A cell is a parcel of complex chemicals that have a basic structure.

- **Cell membrane** – this is the outer wall of the cell. It consists of two layers of membrane with a thin fatty layer between. The membrane is slightly elastic and **porous** to allow nutrients in to feed the cell and waste products to be removed.
- **Cytoplasm** – this is a semi-solid, jelly-like substance that is made of approximately 70 per cent water.
- **Nucleus** – this is located in the middle of the cell. This is where the genetic information about the cell is interpreted.
- **Nucleolus** – this the control centre of the cell. It provides the genetic information.

Cells are living structures; therefore they exhibit the properties of all living things. In order for a cell to function it must have the following properties.

- **Metabolisation** – this is essential for life. Metabolism involves taking in and using nourishment. The cell receives nourishment from the bloodstream, which passes through the porous membrane walls. Metabolism refers to the basic working of the body's cells and concerns the continuous chemical changes that occur to sustain life. Energy released is a by-product of the reactions within the cells.
- **Respiration** – this process allows oxygen and nutrients to pass into the cell and waste products to pass out of the cell.

Key terms

Porous – allowing substances to pass in and out.

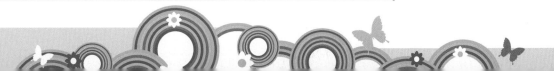

Key terms

Contraction – tightening.

Mitosis – a complicated method of cell division occurring in specialist cells; process involves four stages: prophase, metaphase, anaphase and telophase.

Blood cells – known as corpuscles; they are of two types: red cells called erythrocytes and white cells called leukocytes.

Think about it

Some facts about cells – red blood cells are some of the smallest cells in the body; they have no nucleus and are just 0.0075 mm across.

- **Sensitivity** – this means that the cell is able to respond to a stimulus, which could be either physical, chemical or thermal: for example, the **contraction** of a muscle fibre when it is stimulated by a nerve impulse would cause movement.
- **Growth** – cells have the ability to grow until they are mature enough to reproduce.
- **Reproduction** – when growth in a cell is complete, reproduction takes place. The cells of the human body reproduce by division, making identical copies. This process is known as **mitosis**.
- **Excretion** – during metabolism the cell produces waste products that it can no longer use. If allowed to build up, these products will become harmful, so they are passed out through the cell wall via the porous cell membrane to be excreted.
- **Movement** – the cell needs to be able to move either fully or in part: for example, white **blood cells** move freely so that they are able to move quickly to the site of an infection.

Nerve cells are some of the biggest cells as they have tails that can be up to a metre long and can be seen without the aid of a microscope. Unlike other cells in the body that are continually being replaced, nerve cells have a long life and are rarely replaced.

Structure of the nails

The nails are the hardened growth on the ends of the fingers and toes. Their cell formation is similar to that of the skin and hair follicle, based on the protein keratin. The purpose of the nails is to protect the fingers and toes by providing a hardened covering. The nails contribute to the daily functions of the fingers and toes, and in the instance of finger nails many people use their nails as tools.

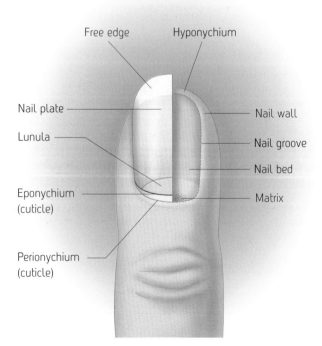
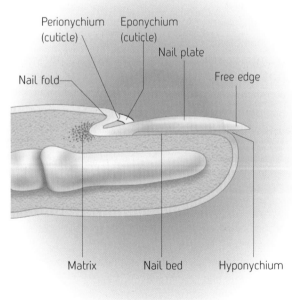

Structure of the nail unit

Structure	Location	Function
Matrix	Situated in the dermis in an area of dense fibrous tissue called the mantle.	The reproductive part of the nail, where new cells are formed. It contains nerves, blood and lymph vessels. The continual process of cell renewal is called mitosis. If the matrix does not get enough nutrients, the nail may not grow correctly.
Mantle	An area of tissue that contains the matrix.	Helps protect the matrix cells from damage.
Nail bed	Underneath the nail plate.	Continuation of the matrix, similar to ordinary skin, with a good nerve supply and blood vessels. The nail bed gives a healthy nail its pink appearance.
Lunula (half moon)	At the base of the nail, linked to the nail plate. Sometimes hidden by the cuticle.	Visible part of the matrix. It is crescent-shaped with translucent appearance.
Lateral nail fold	An extension of the cuticle.	To prevent bacteria entering the matrix.
Nail groove	These are deep ridges like train tracks that run under the sides of the nail.	As the nail grows it runs along the grooves which help the nail to grow straight.
Nail plate	Lies on top of the nail bed.	The compressed keratinised cells produced by the matrix form the nail. They lie in three layers and are held together by moisture and fat.
Nail wall	Around the three sides of the visible nail plate.	The framework of skin to support the nail plate.
*Cuticle	The barrier that protects the matrix by preventing bacteria entering the nail.	The horny layer of epidermis around the nail. It is constantly discarding old cells and producing new ones.
*Eponychium (pronounced ep-on-nik-ee-um)	The extension of the cuticle around the nail.	To prevent bacteria entering.
*Perionychium (pronounced peri-on-nik-ee-um)	Surrounds the entire nail border.	A framework of skin to support the nail plate.
Hyponichium (Pronounced hy-po-nik-ee-um)	Underneath the nail plate where the free edge is formed.	A horny layer of the epidermis for protection.
Free edge	An extension of the nail plate which grows over and beyond the finger tip. It does not adhere to the nail bed, so therefore it lacks the colour of the nail plate.	For protection of the nerves at the fingertip. This is what we shape during a manicure. It is the hardest part of the nail. The nail plate and therefore the free edge are dead so there is no pain when they are cut and shaped.

* These are often collectively referred to as the cuticle rather than by their individual names. The cuticle is an extension of the horny layer of the epidermis.

Related anatomy and physiology

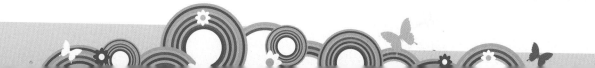

Try it out

1 Look at your hands and finger nails. Can you identify your lunula? Do your cuticles overgrow your nail plate and is your free edge growing over your finger tip?

2 How much does a healthy nail grow each month and what should your nails look like?

3 Are your nails healthy? For further information on the skin and nails, refer to You and the skin, pages 175–219.

Key terms

Matrix – root of the nail; produces cells that form the nail plate.

Mantle – the area of tissue that contains the matrix.

Nail bed – underneath the nail plate.

Lunula – often called the 'half moon' as that is what it looks like; found at the base of the nail, often hidden by the cuticle.

Lateral nail fold – the flap of skin which cushions the cuticle and covers the matrix.

Nail groove – the border of the nail bed which allows the nail plate to grow upwards.

Nail plate – the tough protective coating of cells on top of the nail bed, which grows up, and we then paint with nail varnish!

Nail wall – around the nail plate along the three edges of skin.

Cuticle – a barrier around the nail plate to protect the matrix and prevent bacteria from entering.

Eponychium – extension of cuticle around the nail to prevent bacteria from entering under the cuticle.

Peronychium – surrounds the entire edge of the cuticle, to support the nail plate.

Hyponychium – under the free edge.

Free edge – the white part of the nail plate which grows up and is seen over the top of the finger when the palm is facing you.

Key terms

Keratinisation – the process of cells hardening.

Nail growth

The cells in the matrix reproduce to form the nail plate. As the cells multiply they are gradually pushed up, before they die and harden. This process is called **keratinisation**. For cells to reproduce, the matrix needs a good supply of oxygen and nutrients.

The growth of the nail can be influenced by:

○ poor diet – through lack of vitamins and minerals

○ illness – provide medical professionals with indications of general health and certain diseases

○ medication – some medication can enhance or slow down growth rates

○ age – cellular regeneration declines with age

○ time of year (more growth in summer)

○ injury to the matrix or nail bed

○ neglect – if nails are looked after, their growth rate and appearance can be enhanced

○ pregnancy – increases nail growth by up to 20 per cent

○ poor circulation – affects the blood supply to the matrix, restricting cellular regeneration, which will affect growth.

If the cells in the matrix are damaged by illness or injury, the thickness of the nail plate can vary, showing itself as a furrow ridge or overgrowth of the nail plate.

For your portfolio

Nail growth does not follow a cycle. It is a continuous process throughout life. Nails start to grow on a foetus before the fourth month of pregnancy, and the nail on the index finger grows the fastest.

A healthy nail grows at an average of 1 mm per week for finger nails, and 0.5 mm for toe nails, so it takes approximately six months for the nail to grow from matrix to free edge.

A healthy nail should have:

- supple unbroken cuticle
- no inflammation
- a natural sheen
- a pink glow from beneath the nail bed
- no ridges or spots
- an unbroken free edge.

Muscles of the face, neck and shoulder area

Muscles

The body is made up of more than 600 **voluntary muscles** (that is muscles we can control). They make up 40 per cent of a person's body weight. The contraction (or tightening) of these muscles causes body movement: it can be a large movement, for bending or running, or a small movement which brings about a change in facial expression.

Most muscles are arranged in pairs because, although muscles can shorten themselves, they cannot make themselves longer, so a muscle known as a **flexor** works with a muscle called an **extensor**: the flexor shortens the muscles and the extensor straightens the muscle out again, for example doing a bicep curl.

All practical units require knowledge of muscular structures and functions for underpinning knowledge, so an understanding of the position and the action of these muscles is vital for beauty therapists.

Facial muscles

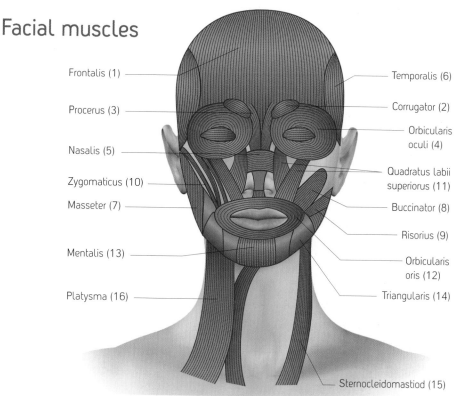

Frontalis (1)
Procerus (3)
Nasalis (5)
Zygomaticus (10)
Masseter (7)
Mentalis (13)
Platysma (16)

Temporalis (6)
Corrugator (2)
Orbicularis oculi (4)
Quadratus labii superiorus (11)
Buccinator (8)
Risorius (9)
Orbicularis oris (12)
Triangularis (14)

Sternocleidomastiod (15)

> ### Key terms
>
> **Voluntary muscles** – muscle we can control with conscious thought such as skeletal muscles for movement.
>
> **Involuntary muscles** – muscles we do not control with conscious thought such as digestion and respiration.
>
> **Extensor** – straightens the muscle, or increases the angle between the joint, e.g. when the hand touching the shoulder then moves out so the arm is in a straight line.
>
> **Flexor** – shortens the muscle, or decreases the angle between the joint, e.g. when the hand comes up towards the shoulder, the elbow joint is made smaller.

Related anatomy and physiology

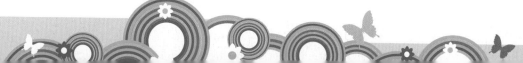

Forehead muscles

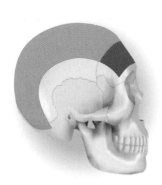

1 Frontalis
- Upper part of the cranium
- Scalp moves forward, raises eyebrow

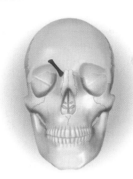

2 Corrugator
- Inner corners of the eyebrows
- Draws eyebrows together — as in frowning

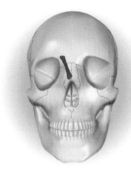

3 Procerus
- Top of nose between eyebrows
- Depresses the eyebrows, forming wrinkles over the bridge of the nose

Eye and nose muscles

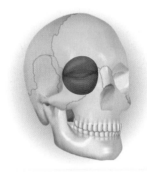

4 Orbicularis oculi
- Surround the eye
- Closes eyes, blinking

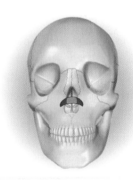

5 Nasalis
- Over the front of the nose
- Compresses nose, causing wrinkles

Side of face muscles

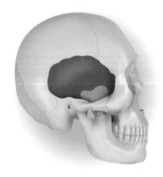

6 Temporalis
- Runs down side of face towards upper jaw
- Aids chewing and closing mouth

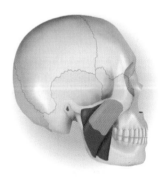

7 Masseter
- Runs down and back to the angle of the jaw
- Lifts the jaw and gives the teeth strength for biting

Cheek muscles

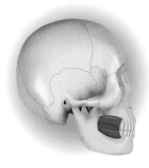

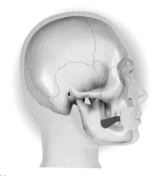

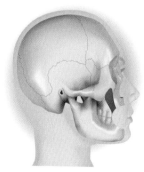

8 Buccinator
- Forms most of the cheek and gives it shape
- Puffs out cheeks when blowing, keeps food in mouth when chewing

9 Risorius
- In the lower cheek. It joins to the corner of the mouth
- Pulls back angles of the mouth — smiling and in grimace

10 Zygomaticus
- Runs down the cheek towards the corner of the mouth
- Pulls the corner of the mouth upwards and sideways

Mouth muscles

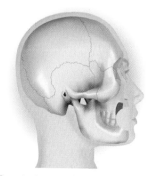

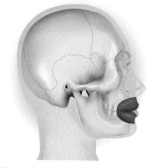

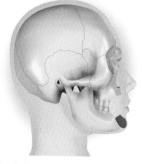

11 Quadratus labii superiorus
- Runs upward from the upper lip
- Lifts the upper lip and helps open the mouth
- The collective term is levators labatis

12 Orbicularis oris
- Surrounds the lips and forms the mouth
- Closes mouth, pushes lips forward. Pulls the corner of the chin down

13 Mentalis
- Forms the chin
- Lifts the chin and moves the lower lips outwards

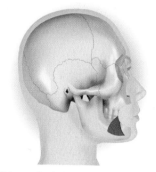

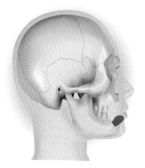

14 Triangularis
- Corner of the lower lip, extends over the chin
- Pulls the corner of the chin down

15a Depressor labii inferioris
- Runs from the outer surface of the mandible to the lower lip
- Pulls lower lip downwards and laterally

15b Depressor anguli oris
- Runs from the platysma to the corner of the mouth
- Pulls the corners of the mouth downwards, when sad or frowning

Neck muscles

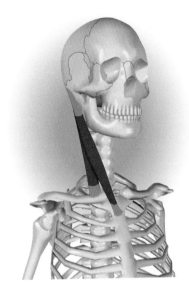

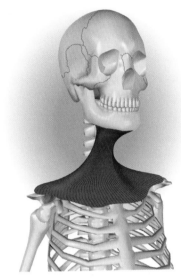

15 Sternocleidomastoid
- Either side of the neck
- Pulls head down to shoulder, rotates head to side and pulls chin onto chest

16 Platysma
- Front of throat
- Pulls down the lower jaw and angles of the mouth

Upper body or trunk muscles

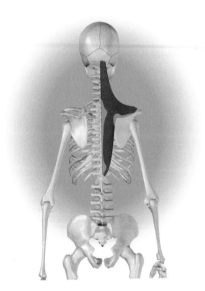

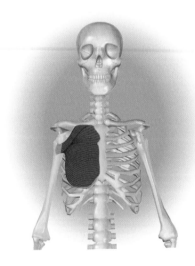

17 Trapezius
- The upper back and sides of the neck
- Rotation of shoulders, draws back the scapula bones, pulls head back, assists in rotation of head

18 Pectoralis
- Front of chest, under the breast
- Pulls arms forwards and assists rotation of the arm

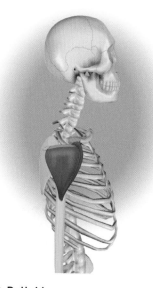

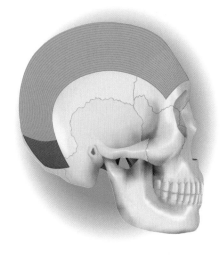

Think about it

The occipitalis is linked to the frontalis by a tendon called the epicranial aponeurosis which covers the skull like a tight swimming cap. A tendon joins muscle to bone.

Think about it

It takes less effort to smile than frown: 17 muscles are involved in smiling while over 40 can be used in a frown.

19 Deltoid

- Caps the shoulder
- Raises arm from the side, pulls it back and forward

20 Occipitalis

- At the back of the skull
- Helps with the movement of the head

Muscles of the arm and leg

Muscles of the forearm and hand

There are 12 muscles that allow us to move our forearms, hands and fingers, and they are referred to as flexors and extensors. These muscles allow us to **supinate** and **pronate** the hand and arm, and flex and extend the fingers, thumb and wrist. The muscles allow the fingers to be spread apart (**abduction**) and to close together (**adduction**). A band of tendons holds all these muscles together at the wrist.

Key terms

Supinate – palm up.

Pronate – palm down.

Abduction – to take away.

Adduction – to bring together.

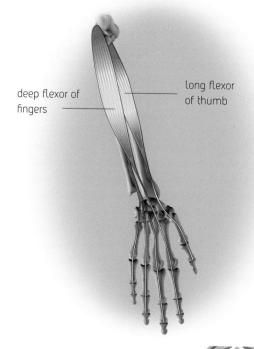

deep flexor of fingers

long flexor of thumb

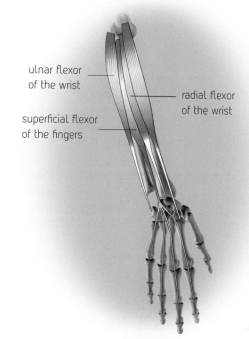

ulnar flexor of the wrist

radial flexor of the wrist

superficial flexor of the fingers

Flexors of the forearm

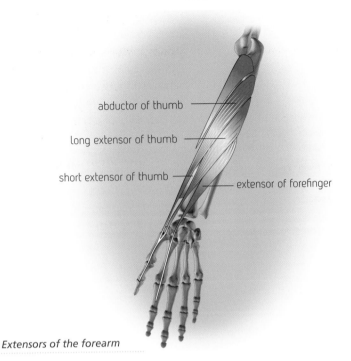

abductor of thumb

long extensor of thumb

short extensor of thumb

extensor of forefinger

Extensors of the forearm

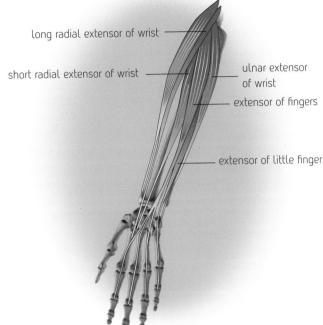

long radial extensor of wrist

short radial extensor of wrist

ulnar extensor of wrist

extensor of fingers

extensor of little finger

Muscles of the lower leg and foot

There are four main superficial muscles of the lower leg that you will be concerned with when carrying out a leg massage. Many more muscles also work to move the leg. Two of the main superficial muscles are at the back of the leg: the gastrocnemius (often referred to as the calf muscle) and the soleus, which sits slightly underneath the gastrocnemius. The third muscle of the lower leg is the tibialis posterior and acts in conjunction with the tibialis anterior at the front of the leg. They act to flex and extend the foot, and are often referred to as flexors and extensor muscles, and work in harmony when we move.

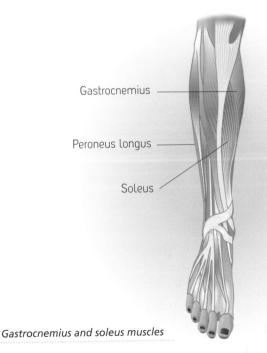

Gastrocnemius

Peroneus longus

Soleus

Gastrocnemius and soleus muscles

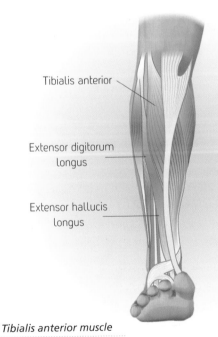

Tibialis anterior

Extensor digitorum longus

Extensor hallucis longus

Tibialis anterior muscle

Name of muscle	Action of muscle
Gastrocnemius	**Plantar flexes** the foot (points toes), pushes body forward when in motion
Soleus	Plantar flexes the foot, maintains standing position
Tibialis anterior	**Dorsi flexes** the foot (bends ankle) and inverts the foot (turns sole inwards)

The muscles of the lower leg and foot are also held in place by a band of tendons at the ankle – known as the **Achilles tendon** – like those of the wrist. A tendon is made up of white fibrous connective tissue which attaches muscle to bone.

Key terms

Plantar flex – the action of the gastrocnemius muscle that helps to point the foot down.

Dorsi flex – the action of the tibialis anterior that makes the heel go down and the toes point up.

Achilles tendon – band of tendons in the ankle.

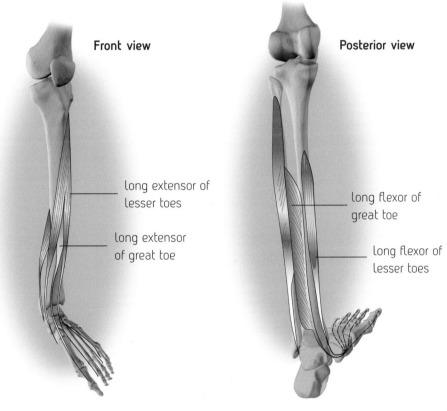

Front view

long extensor of lesser toes

long extensor of great toe

Posterior view

long flexor of great toe

long flexor of lesser toes

Flexors and extensors of the foot

Hair

Humans are one of the few land mammals with almost bare skin, but we have a coating of downy hair all over the body, and in certain places the hair grows thicker and more densely. The average human head has approximately 120,000 hairs, which grow about 3 mm per week.

The colour of hair is dictated by the pigments melanin and **carotene**. Black, brown and blond hairs get their colour from melanin, while red or auburn gets its colour from the pigment carotene.

Key terms

Carotene – a pigment found in the granular layer of the epidermis.

Related anatomy and physiology

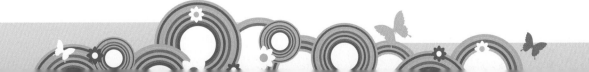

Types of hair found on the body

Hair is found all over the body except on the lips, palms of the hands and soles of the feet. Before birth the body is covered in a soft, downy hair called **lanugo**. This has mostly disappeared at birth.

Different areas of the body have different types of hair growth. These can be divided into two types:

- vellus
- terminal.

Vellus

This is soft, downy hair, covering most of the body. Normally without colour, it rarely grows longer than about 2 centimetres in length. Regardless of ethnic origin, vellus hair is usually straight due to the fact that the follicles are not very deep.

Terminal

Terminal hair grows from deep follicles which go down to the subcutaneous layer of the skin. They are strong hairs, which contain pigment, and grow on the scalp, eyebrows, under the arms and pubic areas.

Terminal hair can be curly, wavy or straight depending on ethnic origin, hereditary factors and chemical hair treatments, such as perms. If a cross-section was taken of a terminal hair for Europeans, the hair would be oval in shape, and would tend to be wavy. Asian hair would appear round in shape and tend to be straight, and African-Caribbean hair would appear flattened and tend to be very curly.

Key terms

Lanugo – soft, downy hair covering most of the body before birth.

Vellus – soft, downy hair covering most of the body.

Terminal – strong hairs which contain pigment; found on the scalp, eyebrows, under the arms and pubic areas.

Key terms

Outer root sheath – the outer lining of the hair shaft.

Inner root sheath – the inner lining of the hair shaft.

Dermal papilla – a projection of the papillary layer of the dermis that contains blood vessels or nerve endings; the blood supply that provides nourishment to the hair follicle.

Cortex – middle layer of tightly packed, keratinised cells that contain pigment.

Medulla – the middle of the hair shaft.

Structure	Function
Connective tissue sheath	Surrounds the hair follicle and sebaceous gland. It has a rich blood and nerve supply to feed the hair.
Outer root sheath	Forms the hair follicle wall – made of basal cells.
Inner root sheath	The cells in the inner root sheath run in the opposite direction to the cells in the outer root sheath, acting like Velcro™ to anchor the hair into the follicle. They grow upwards with the hair. The outer root sheath stops where it meets the sebaceous gland.
Dermal papilla	This is the vital blood supply for the hair cells providing food and oxygen.
Hair bulb	The hair bulb is where the cells grow and divide by mitosis.
Matrix	The lowest part of the hair bulb where the cells grow.
Sebaceous gland	Produces sebum which lubricates both the hair and skin.
Arrector pili muscle	Attached to the hair to trap warm air next to the body when we are cold.

Cuticle	Gives the hair its elasticity. Made of transparent scales that interlock with each other like roof tiles. The cuticle protects the cortex.
Cortex	The middle layer of tightly packed keratinised cells that contain the pigment. The cortex gives hair strength.
Medulla	The middle of the hair consists of loosely connected keratinised cells and tiny pockets of air. The air spaces allow light to be reflected through them, giving the hair both colour and sheen.

Structure and function of hair

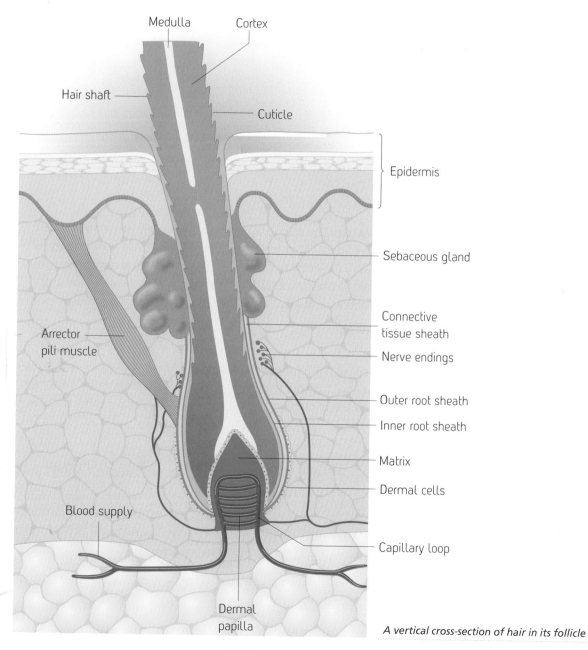

A vertical cross-section of hair in its follicle

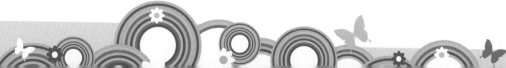

Key terms

Anagen – a stage of growth in the life of a hair: the growing phase.

Catagen – a stage of growth in the life of a hair: the changing phase.

Telogen – a stage of growth in the life of a hair: the resting phase.

Think about it

Here is an easy way to remember the different stages of hair growth:

A – active (anagen)

C – change (catagen)

T – tired (telogen).

Hair growth

A normal hair in the body is contained in a tube-shaped pocket called a follicle. These follicles consist of an inner sheath and an outer sheath which are similar in structure to the cells of the epidermis.

The hair is made of hardened protein called keratin. The outside of the hair is a scaly layer called the cuticle. The hair grows from the bottom of its follicle by cell division, being fed by a good blood supply from the dermal papilla.

Hair growth is a continuous cycle of events that is repeated as long as nourishment is available, or until the hair follicle is damaged through illness or the ageing process. Hair does become thinner in old age due to hormonal changes which occur within the body.

The life of a normal hair is divided into three stages of hair growth:

○ **anagen** – the growing phase

○ **catagen** – the changing (transition) phase

○ **telogen** – the resting phase.

Anagen

In the anagen stage the hair receives its nourishment via the blood supply from the dermal papilla. This enables the cells to reproduce. The cells move upwards and form the different structures of the hair shaft. Melanin cells are also produced and this forms the hair colouring.

Catagen

This is the resting or transition stage of hair growth. During this stage the dermal papilla breaks away and the lower end of the hair becomes loose from the base of the follicle. The hair is still being fed from the follicle wall and is sometimes known as a club-ended hair. The hair gradually becomes drier and continues to move up to just below the sebaceous gland. Here it is very vulnerable and can easily be brushed out.

Telogen

This is the final stage of hair growth and is the resting period. The follicle rests until stimulated by hormones to return to the anagen phase. Telogen lasts for a few weeks, with the club hair often being retained until new hair is produced – pushing the club hair out.

Think about it

- We lose between 50 and 100 hairs a day!
- People with blond hair have more hairs per square centimetre than people who have other hair colours, although no one knows why.
- One eyebrow contains approximately 900 individual hairs.

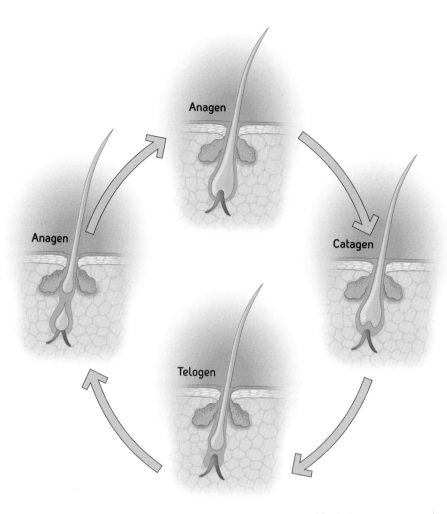

The hair growth cycle

Blood

Blood is the transport system for the body to deliver and remove vital ingredients needed by the cells in the body. It is pumped around the body by the heart. (You may want to read the additional section about the structure of the heart to aid your understanding.) Arteries, veins and capillaries are the vessels that carry the blood to their destination.

Composition of the blood

Oxygenated blood flows from the heart through the arteries and deoxygenated blood flows back to the heart through the veins. Capillaries are very small vessels which form a network to get into tiny cell spaces to allow delivery (of oxygenated blood) and removal (of deoxygenated blood) to take place.

Blood is a slightly sticky fluid that is composed of:

○ 55 per cent **plasma**

○ 45 per cent blood cells.

> **Key terms**
>
> **Plasma** – yellow, transparent fluid which makes up 55 per cent of blood; the liquid part of blood in which cells are suspended. It contains vital proteins, including: fibrinogen which helps with blood clotting; globulins such as haemoglobin to help transport oxygen; and serum albumin. It is essentially a transporter for glucose, lipids, amino acids, hormones, metabolic end products, carbon dioxide and oxygen.

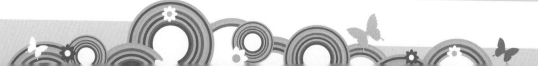

Key terms

Platelets – type of blood cell. They are irregularly shaped, colourless bodies present in blood to aid clotting and reduce blood loss.

Plasma is a yellow, transparent fluid made up of mostly water, with a small amount of protein present. There are three types of blood cells.

1 Red blood cells transport oxygen to the cells and take away carbon dioxide.

2 White blood cells protect the body against invading bacteria and help form the immune system.

3 **Platelets** play an important role in blood clotting.

Functions of the blood

The blood has three main functions in the body:

- transport
- regulation
- protection.

Transport

Blood transports or carries:

- oxygen from the lungs to the body cells
- carbon dioxide from the cells to the lungs
- nutrients from digestion to the cells
- waste products from the cells to be excreted
- hormones sent from the endocrine gland to regulate the cells
- medication, which can be passed into the cells.

Regulation

Blood regulates:

- water content of cells
- body heat.

Protection

Blood protects against:

- infection and disease
- blood loss by clotting.

Blood circulation to the lower arm and hand, and lower leg and foot

After picking up oxygen in the lungs, oxygenated blood is pumped from the heart via the arteries, which work under pressure to supply all the extremities (the fingers and toes). Once the blood has delivered food and oxygen to the cells, the veins return waste matter and carbon dioxide. The veins do not have the same pressure as the arteries, so it is the pressure of the muscles on the veins in the hands and feet which aids the blood's return. Veins have valves to prevent the blood flowing back, and they can become enlarged, as in varicose veins.

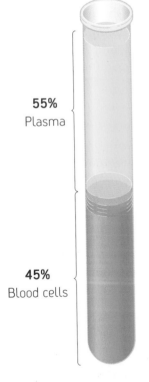

55%
Plasma

45%
Blood cells

The structure of blood

All clients benefit from massage to the hands and feet: it stimulates blood flow and enables oxygen and nutrients to get into the area more quickly, the blood warms the tissues and muscles, so muscles relax and circulation is improved. When massaging, remember that you must always work towards the heart, so that you work with the natural flow of the blood, instead of against it.

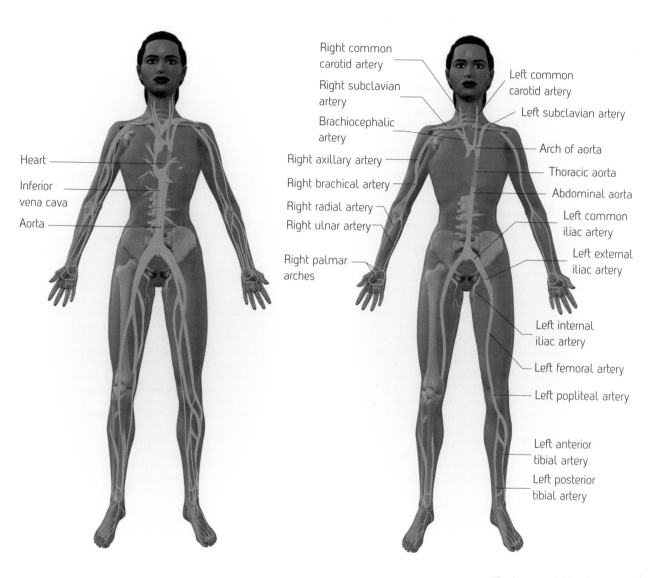

The heart and blood vessels

The effects of massage on blood circulation

Massage increases the amount of blood flow into the area, which is seen as an **erythema** or reddening of the skin. It has a number of beneficial effects.

- It speeds up the flow of blood through the veins and therefore helps with the metabolic waste being carried away.
- It increases the fresh blood to the area, bringing oxygen and nutrients to the cells and so helping with cell growth and repair.
- Warmth is created by the increase in blood flow, which is relaxing to the client.

Key terms

Erythema – vasodilation of the blood capillaries, causing surface reddening of the skin.

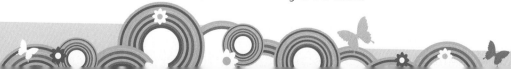

1 Test your pulse rate. First take your pulse for 15 seconds and multiply by 4. This tells you your pulse rate at rest (multiplying by 4 gives you the rate per minute). Do this again after jogging on the spot for two minutes.

2 Has your skin developed any reddening?

3 What is this reddening called?

○ Because of the increase to the cells of oxygen and nutrients the skin will look and feel softer.

○ Muscle efficiency and response is improved due to the increased oxygen and nutrients.

○ The removal of waste products gives a more toned appearance to the muscles and makes them more relaxed.

Blood flow to the face and head

Arteries of the head

The blood is pumped to the head via the common carotid artery, which has two branches. The internal carotid artery passes through the temporal bone of the skull behind the ear and takes blood to the brain. The external carotid artery remains outside the skull and divides into facial, temporal and occipital arteries which supply the skin and muscles of the face, side and back of the head.

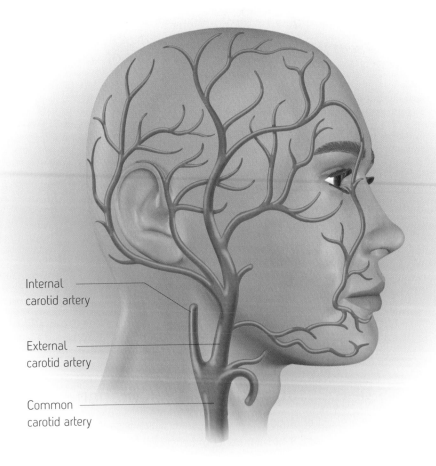

Internal carotid artery

External carotid artery

Common carotid artery

Arteries of the head

Veins of the head

Blood is collected up from the scalp capillaries by the facial, occipital and posterior veins, which run alongside the similarly named arteries. These join to form an external jugular vein behind and below the ear on both sides.

The external jugular veins go down the neck and enter the **subclavian veins**. An internal jugular vein brings blood from the brain, goes down on either side of the neck and enters the subclavian vein. The subclavian veins carry on towards the heart and eventually the blood enters the superior venae cavae.

Key terms

Subclavian veins and arteries – these are the blood vessels beneath the clavicle.

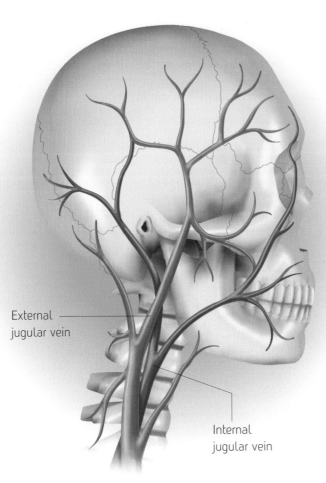

External jugular vein

Internal jugular vein

Veins of the head

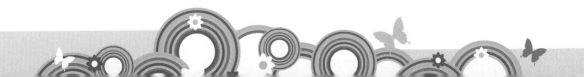

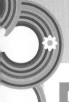

Key terms

Cardiac – of the heart.

Atrium – the top smaller chambers of the heart.

Ventricles – the bottom larger chambers of the heart.

Septum – division or separation.

Think about it

- Arteries carry oxygenated blood away from the heart – except the pulmonary artery, which carries deoxygenated blood.

- Veins carry deoxygenated blood to the heart – except the pulmonary vein, which carries oxygenated blood.

- Arteries always *leave* the heart and veins always *go* to the heart.

Additional knowledge

The heart

The heart is the size of a clenched fist. It has a lung each side of it and is protected by the rib cage. It is made of **cardiac** muscle – unlike normal muscle, cardiac muscle continually contracts. These contractions occur approximately 70 times a minute and throughout the average life span contract roughly three billion times.

The heart has four chambers: two smaller **atrium** at the top of the heart and two larger **ventricles** at the bottom of the heart. The heart is divided into two sections by a muscular wall called the **septum**.

To prevent blood flowing back into the other chambers, the heart contains four valves – tricuspid, bicuspid or mitral, aortic and pulmonary. The bicuspid and tricuspid valves help maintain the direction of the blood flow through the heart by allowing blood to flow into the ventricles but prevent it from returning to the atrium. The aortic and pulmonary valves are semi-lunar, that is divided into halves. They control the blood flow out of the ventricles into the aorta and pulmonary arteries respectively without any back flow into the ventricles.

Each of the four chambers of the heart ejects about 70 ml of blood with each beat.

The left ventricle wall is thicker than the right because it pumps blood all round the body – the right ventricle only pumps blood as far as the lungs.

Deoxygenated blood is brought back to the heart by the veins and enters the heart via two larger vessels – the superior and inferior vena cava – which flow into the right atrium. The blood then passes into the larger right ventricle and is pushed into the pulmonary artery, which takes the blood to the lungs where the exchange of carbon dioxide and oxygen takes place.

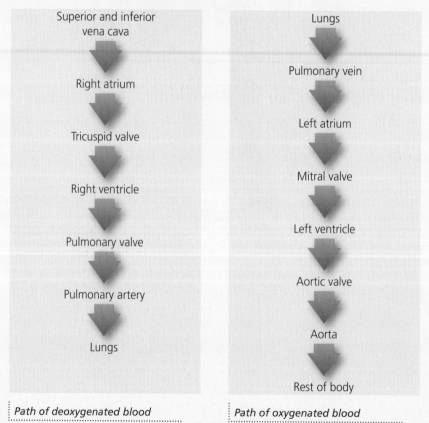

Path of deoxygenated blood   *Path of oxygenated blood*

Blood then re-enters the heart via the pulmonary vein into the left atrium. It passes to the left ventricle and is then pushed into the aorta. From here the blood is carried into the arteries of the body, and so the cycle continues.

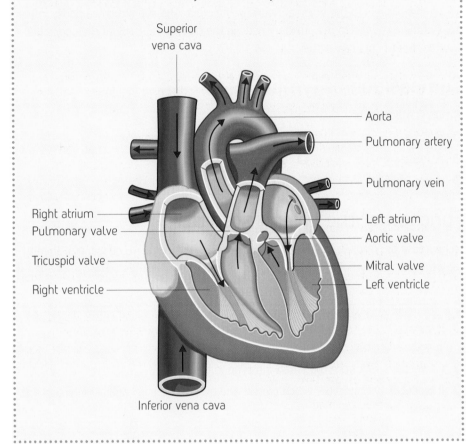

Superior vena cava

Aorta

Pulmonary artery

Pulmonary vein

Right atrium
Pulmonary valve

Left atrium
Aortic valve

Tricuspid valve

Mitral valve

Right ventricle

Left ventricle

Inferior vena cava

The lymphatic system

The **lymphatic system** is the body's second circulation system for collecting waste products. It carries away waste from the tissues that the blood cannot manage to take. For example, you could think of it as a second bus that collects all the passengers the first bus left behind.

The fluid that is left behind is known as lymph and is straw coloured. It is emptied back into the blood system via the subclavian vein, which is in the upper chest. The removal of the lymph from around the body prevents the tissues from becoming clogged and swollen. If **tissue fluid** builds up, swelling occurs and this is called **oedema**. People who are pregnant, ill or have very sedentary life styles can suffer from oedema. Gentle massage can aid the removal of the stagnant fluid. Lymph, like blood in veins, relies on muscular movement to push it around the body, so the healthier and fitter a person, the better their lymphatic system is at dealing with waste.

The lymphatic system also plays an important role in protecting the body against infection. At various stages along the route that the lymph travels are glands or nodes; you could think of these as bus stops. It is here that the lymph is filtered of bacteria and germs, and **antibodies** are produced to fight infection. When someone is ill the doctor often feels the glands in the neck and looks in the mouth. This is to

> **Key terms**
>
> **Lymphatic system** – a separate system of vessels that comes from the blood stream to filter toxins and waste by passing lymph fluid through a series of glands.
>
> **Lymph** – fluid in the lymphatic system derived from tissue fluids; circulates around the lymphatic system removing bacteria and certain proteins from the tissues.
>
> **Oedema** – a build-up of fluid in the tissues causing the area to become swollen.
>
> **Antibodies** – proteins produced by the body to fight an infection.

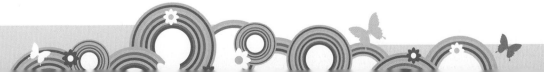

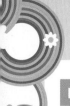

Key terms

Lymph nodes – small structures made of lymph tissue, located at intervals along the lymphatic system particularly at the neck, under the arm and in the groin. They filter bacteria and foreign particles from lymph fluid. When the body is fighting infection lymph nodes may become swollen with activated lymphocytes.

Think about it

By the time your lymph glands become swollen and sore, your body is already fighting the infection and filtering harmful bacteria, so this would be a contra-indication to any treatment.

find out if the glands are filtering the bacteria properly. If the glands are very swollen, antibiotics may be needed to help the **lymph nodes** and antibodies fight infection.

The main lymph nodes in the leg are the popliteal, at the back of the knee. The lymph then travels to the inguinal nodes in the groin. The supratrochlea nodes in the crook of the arm lead to the auxillary node in the underarm. If any of the nodes are swollen, treatments can be painful.

Composition of lymph

Lymph is made up of:

- plasma
- proteins
- waste products
- toxins
- fats
- oxygen
- carbon dioxide
- urea
- lymphocytes.

Function of the lymph system

The purpose of lymph is to collect germs, bacteria and waste in the system, then to carry these to the lymph glands to be filtered and made harmless. The lymphatic system uses different methods to do this.

- The lymphatic system drains tissue fluid from the spaces between the cells.
- It transports the tissue fluid and proteins back to the bloodstream via the subclavian vein.
- It transports fats from the small intestine to the blood.
- It produces lymphocytes which protect and defend the body against infection and disease.

Benefits of treatments on the lymph system

As a therapist the treatments that you can perform can greatly assist the lymphatic flow. This is because:

- massage stimulates the flow of lymph, so removing the toxins and fluid from the area faster
- general swelling can be reduced
- absorption of waste matter can be speeded up
- skin will be smoother and softer because cell renewal is helped
- muscles will be relaxed and work more efficiently.

Lymphatic flow to the head and neck:

- **Left side** – lymph from this side of the head and neck passes through the thoracic duct and empties into the left subclavian vein (the thoracic duct is situated in the upper chest under the rib cage).
- **Right side** – lymph from this side of the head and neck passes through the right thoracic duct and empties into the right subclavian vein.

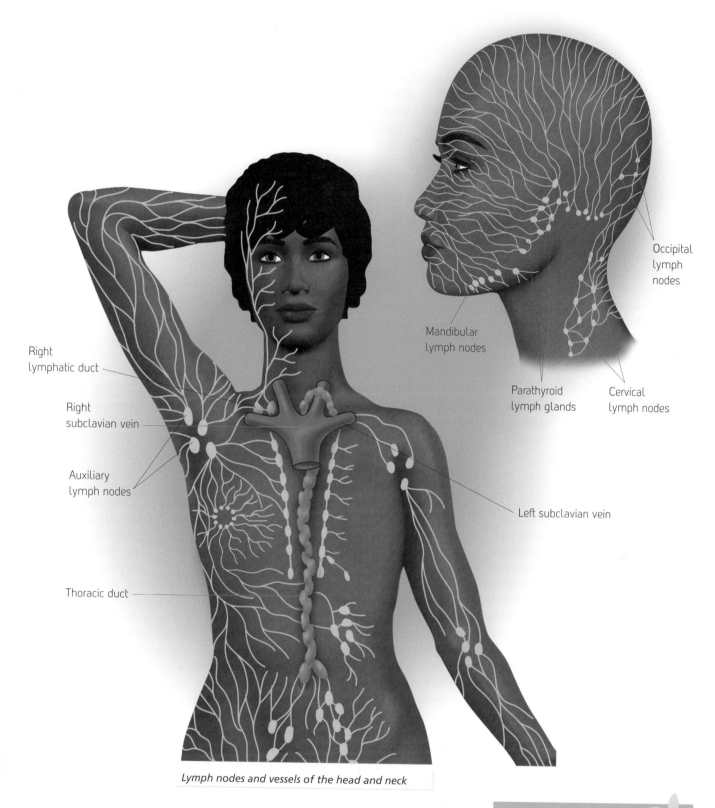

Occipital
lymph
nodes

Mandibular
lymph nodes

Parathyroid
lymph glands

Cervical
lymph nodes

Right
lymphatic duct

Right
subclavian vein

Auxiliary
lymph nodes

Left subclavian vein

Thoracic duct

Lymph nodes and vessels of the head and neck

Try it out

Look in your mouth – can you see
any lymph nodes? What are they
called? Remember not everyone
has these.

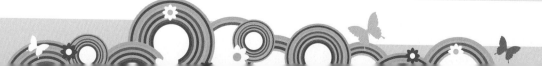

Check your knowledge

Bones

1 How many bones make up the skull?
2 What is the name for the fibrous joints that join the bones of the skull together?
3 What is the clavical commonly called?
4 Where would you find the zygomatic bone?
5 Name the bones of the shoulder girdle.
6 What are the functions of the arches of the foot, and how many are there?
7 Where would you find the tibia?
8 Where would you find carpals?
9 What is the function of a ligament?
10 What is the upper part of the vertebral column called?

Skin

1 Name the five layers of the epidermis.
2 What is the function of the arrector pili muscle?
3 What is desquamation?
4 What is a melanocyte?
5 What is the function of a sebaceous gland?
6 Name the four senses that can be detected by the sense receptors in the dermis.
7 What are sudoriferous glands?
8 Name the hardened protein that is found in the skin?
9 In what layer of the epidermis do cells start to die?
10 Name the two living layers in the epidermis.

Nails

1 What is the reproductive part of the nail called?
2 What is the function of the nail groove?
3 What type of protein is the nail plate made of?
4 How many layers is the nail plate made of?
5 Where would you find the peronychium?
6 Is the nail living or dead?
7 What is the function of the cuticle?
8 State the appearance of a healthy nail.
9 State four factors that can affect nail growth.
10 What is the purpose of finger and toe nails?

Muscles

1 Approximately how many voluntary muscles are there?
2 Where would you find the gastrocnemius?
3 What is the action of the buccinator muscle?
4 Where would you find the platysma muscle?
5 What does supinate mean?
6 State the action of the orbicularis oris.
7 How many muscles make a smile?
8 What is the action and position of the deltoid muscle?
9 Is the triangularis a happy or sad muscle?
10 What action does the masseter muscle have?

Hair

1 What are the two pigments that give hair colour?
2 Name the resting stage of hair growth.
3 Which hair type is found on a foetus?
4 Which type of hair forms the eyebrows?
5 What protein is hair made of?
6 What is the function of the matrix?
7 Where would you find the medulla?
8 How many connective tissue sheaths does a hair have?
9 What type of hair covers the body?
10 Where do humans not have hairs?

Blood

1 What is the function of platelets?
2 Blood is a sticky fluid composed of blood cells and _____?
3 What are the three main functions of blood?
4 What do arteries carry?
5 What do veins carry?
6 When carrying out massage in which direction must you go?
7 List five products that are transported in the blood.
8 Which bone does the internal carotid artery pass through?
9 Which vein does the external jugular vein join?
10 List three effects massage can have on the blood supply.

Lymph

1 What colour is lymph?
2 What important role does lymph play in protecting the body?
3 List three substances that you will find in lymph fluid.
4 State four benefits of massage on the lymphatic system.
5 Name the vein where lymph joins the blood supply.
6 Name the lymph nodes in the mouth.
7 The lymph system is often referred to as the body's _____?
8 Name the lymph node in the back of the knee.
9 Name the lymph node under the arm.
10 If lymph builds up, it will cause swelling in the tissues. What is this called?

Section

4

Practical skills

Provide facial skincare treatment

What you will learn

Maintain safe and effective methods of working when improving and maintaining facial condition

Consult, plan and prepare for facials with clients

Improve and maintain skin condition

Provide aftercare advice

Introduction

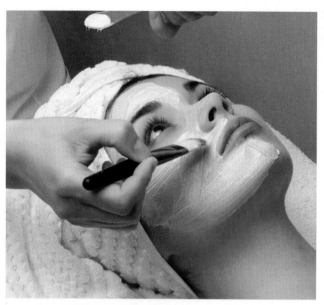

A facial is both relaxing and beneficial

A facial is a lovely treatment to offer any client: it is both extremely relaxing and very beneficial. In fact, for a professional beauty therapist, a facial can be as relaxing to give as it is to receive. The client is cocooned on the couch, wrapped warmly and securely, with the luxury of knowing that expert hands are cleansing, massaging and improving the skin's condition. Many clients fall asleep during a facial, as the relaxation is so deep.

A facial makes a perfect gift, and vouchers for the treatment can be purchased in most salons. For many women a facial is the height of luxury; for a beauty therapist it rates very highly on the scale of favourite treatments to give. Many beauty therapists decide to specialise only in facials and call themselves facialists. The majority of their bookings will be for top-of-the-range facials and little else – and with a celebrity endorsement and/or a write-up in a woman's magazine, the facialist can be booked up months in advance!

This unit is about improving and maintaining facial skin condition using a variety of treatments. All of these treatments will be carried out on a variety of skin types, age groups and conditions. It is also important to remember that you need to maintain your health and safety, along with rigorous hygiene practices throughout.

Maintain safe and effective methods of working when improving and maintaining facial condition

In this outcome you will learn about:

- setting up the work area to meet legal, hygiene and treatment requirements
- ensuring that environmental conditions are suitable for the client and the treatment
- ensuring your personal hygiene, protection and appearance meets accepted industry and organisational requirements
- ensuring all tools and equipment are cleaned using the correct methods
- effectively disinfecting your hands prior to facial treatments
- maintaining accepted industry hygiene and safety practices throughout the treatment
- positioning equipment and materials for ease and safety of use
- ensuring your own posture and position minimises fatigue and the risk of injury while working
- maintaining the client's modesty and privacy at all times
- disposing of waste materials safely and correctly
- ensuring that the treatment is cost-effective and is carried out within a commercially viable time
- leaving the work area in a condition suitable for further treatments
- ensuring the client's records are up to date, accurate, easy to read and signed by the client and practitioner.

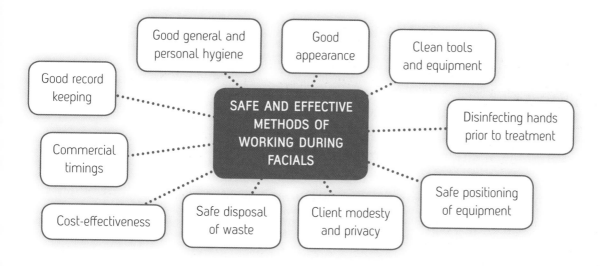

Good general and personal hygiene

Good appearance

Clean tools and equipment

Good record keeping

SAFE AND EFFECTIVE METHODS OF WORKING DURING FACIALS

Disinfecting hands prior to treatment

Commercial timings

Cost-effectiveness

Safe disposal of waste

Client modesty and privacy

Safe positioning of equipment

For facials, as with all other beauty treatments, you must work within the legal, hygiene and treatment requirements as set out by your Awarding Body and to meet industry standards. This will ensure the health and safety of the client and puts them in the centre of your focus – exactly where they should be. Preparation is the key to giving a relaxed and flowing treatment. All aspects of the treatment need to be carefully prepared to enable you to give the client your full attention and a super-pampering treatment.

Setting up the working area

Be fully prepared. This allows you to concentrate on your client and to give a relaxed treatment without the distraction of having to leave the area to get products, equipment or towels. A little preparation time should be built into each appointment slot, so that each client feels special. It is also important to ensure that your working area is kept clean to ensure good health and safety.

Good habits to stay tidy

○ Organise the layout of the trolley in an ordered fashion – have all the labels of products facing you so you can easily see which is needed. Arrange the products in order of use, and replace them back in their slot when you have finished with them. They will always then be at hand, and you will always look tidy and controlled. Have a space for everything and everything in its place. Have a system where all necessary tools are in a jar or pot (even a plastic beaker is easy to clean), the tissues and cotton wool in their own plastic bowl or tub.

○ Tidy as you go along – put used tissues and cotton wool into a small pedal bin (lined with a bin liner) as you finish with them, rather than leaving them on the trolley.

○ If you can, wash up mask brushes and bowls while the mask is setting on the client's face. This may not be possible if you do not have a sink near the workstation, as you should not leave the client unattended.

○ Minimise waste by using only the amount of product required. This is not only cost-effective, but it also means there is very little product left over to clear up.

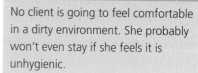

Think about it

No client is going to feel comfortable in a dirty environment. She probably won't even stay if she feels it is unhygienic.

Unit B4 Provide facial skincare treatment

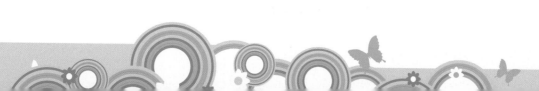

○ Always put lids back on to pots if decanting products. This avoids the possibility of a spillage, which is time-consuming to clear up. It also stops alcohol-based products from evaporating.

○ Mop up spills as they occur and do not allow them to endanger others.

If you follow these hints, you will not need a major tidying session at the end of your treatment. Becoming tidy is a skill that comes with experience.

Risk assessment for facials

Facials have many potential hazards. Remember to complete a risk assessment to minimise risks prior to the client coming in for the treatment.

Here is a risk assessment list for some aspects of facials — how many more points could you add?

Risk assessment for facials

Refer to Unit G20, Make sure your own actions reduce risks to health and safety, pages 71–104, for a complete discussion of risk assessment.

Hazards: look for hazards that you would reasonably expect to result in significant harm under the conditions in your workplace. Use the following examples as a guide.

- **Environmental** risks such as slipping/tripping (e.g. poorly maintained floors or stairs) or spillage of massage oil, creams, etc.

- **Fire** from flammable materials or products (e.g. the magnifying lamp with no cap on it can be considered a fire risk if left by a window — the sun will come through the window, magnify the heat through the lamp and may set the couch cover on fire).

- **Equipment** The height of the couch, trolleys or stools could cause repetitive strain injury or a sore back through poor posture.

- **Reactions** Any products may cause irritation, swelling, redness of the skin, eye irritation or eczema. There may be a reaction between products, e.g. if a client has recently used a home hair colour and then uses her normal cleanser, one may trigger a reaction from the other.

- **Allergies** The most common ones are to nuts in almond-oil based products, cleansers and moisturisers and nickel, which is in some cotton wool as filaments, but clients can develop a sudden sensitivity to any product that they may have been using without problems for years.

- **Noise** Not necessarily a hazard unless the stereo is so loud it affects the eardrums, but certainly a distraction from relaxation if the noise disturbs.

- **Poor lighting** May cause accidents through not seeing a trailing lead or cable, and may cause the wrong products to be applied if the lighting is too low.

- **Low temperature** Not necessarily a hazard but this would certainly make the client uncomfortable and cause shivering, which is hardly relaxing.

Many of the topics in this outcome are covered in the Professional basics, or in Unit G20 Make sure your own actions reduce risks to health and safety.

Topic	Professional basics or Unit G20
Hygiene requirements	pages 39–45
Treatment requirements	pages 21–23
Personal appearance	pages 12–15
Protective clothing	page 53
Environmental conditions	pages 70–104
Client's comfort and safety	pages 45–47
Sanitising hands	page 44

Disposing of waste materials safely and correctly

Important Acts of Parliament to take into consideration are:

- Environmental Protection Act, 1990
- The Controlled Waste Regulations, 1992 (as amended)
- Special Waste Regulations, 1996 (as amended).

All clinical waste must be kept apart from general waste and be disposed of in a licensed incinerator or taken to a landfill site by a licensed company.

This includes:

- waste which consists wholly or partly of animal or human tissue
- blood or other body fluids
- swabs or dressings
- syringes or needles.

Refer back to Professional basics, 'You, your client and the law', pages 48–68, for further information.

The only human tissue you may be required to dispose of as contaminated waste during a facial treatment is the by-product of **extraction** (including milia extraction), or if you have made the client bleed during extraction. This human tissue needs special treatment. The probe should also be treated as contaminated waste, and be put into the sharps box for safe disposal by a registered firm. (Refer to Professional basics, page 58.)

Your legal and personal obligations are all covered in Professional basics, 'You, your client and the law' (pages 48–68). The Health and Safety at Work Act (see pages 49–50) and Unit G20 Make sure your own actions reduce risks to health and safety (pages 70–104) are also important, as the client's safety is a vital aspect of any facial treatment.

> **Key terms**
>
> **Extraction** – the act of drawing or pulling out of the body a foreign body, blackhead or something from the eye.

Leaving the work area suitable for further treatments

The client has left the salon, and you are basking in job satisfaction. Now it is time to go back to your workstation and clear up. Look around you. How much mess have you made? Could you have been tidier as you went along? Unless the client is the last one of the day, you will not have the luxury of time to clean and tidy the area. If your next client is due straight away, you could be in trouble if you have to spend a long time tidying and preparing for your next treatment.

Ensuring the client's records are up to date and accurate

Refer to Professional basics (pages 29–31) for client record keeping. It is important, both for the client and you, that you fill out the skin analysis sheet and any other details accurately. This will avoid any health and safety problems and keep the

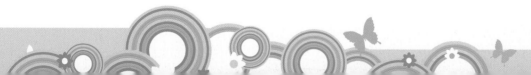

client safe, therefore safeguarding your own professional reputation. Do not return the record card to be filed incomplete, thinking you can do it later — you will not remember and vital information may not be recorded.

Be constructive when filling out the card: remain positive and helpful in what you write and avoid making any negative comments or personal observations about the client. After all, clients are entitled to see their own records under the Data Protection Act. Also avoid leaving the card lying around for anyone to read. Once you have completed the write-up, give it to the person who is responsible for filing.

Consult, plan and prepare for facials with clients

In this outcome you will learn about:

- using consultation techniques in a polite and friendly manner to determine the client's treatment plan
- obtaining signed, written informed consent from the client prior to carrying out the treatment
- ensuring that informed and signed parental or guardian consent is obtained for minors prior to any treatment
- ensuring that a parent or guardian is present throughout the treatment for minors under the age of 16
- asking the client appropriate questions to identify if they have any contra-indications to the treatment
- accurately recording the client's responses to questioning
- encouraging clients to ask questions to clarify any points
- accurately establishing and recording the client's current skincare routine
- helping the client into a comfortable and relaxed position for the treatment

- ensuring your client's clothing, hair and accessories are effectively protected or removed
- effectively cleansing the client's skin prior to skin analysis
- correctly performing a skin analysis on the client and accurately recording the skin type and skin condition
- taking the necessary action in response to any identified contra-indications
- ensuring client advice is given without reference to a specific medical condition and without causing undue alarm and concern
- recommending suitable treatments and products for the client's skin type and condition
- agreeing the service and outcomes that are acceptable to the client and meet their needs
- selecting suitable facial products and equipment for the client's skin type and skin condition based on the results of the skin analysis.

Using consultation techniques to determine the client's treatment plan

A full consultation is vital before the treatment can begin. Refer to Professional basics, pages 31–35, for further information on how to conduct a consultation. Anatomy and physiology relating to the head and neck are covered in Related anatomy and physiology, pages 239–43.

A good skin analysis takes time and practice. Eventually, you will be able to:

- identify the correct **skin type** and **skin condition**
- evaluate and decide which products are most suitable
- evaluate and determine which treatments are most appropriate
- clarify which home care routine to recommend
- recommend a personal skincare régime to retail.

Key terms

Skin type – a means of classifying the skin during skin analysis.

Skin condition – the appearance, texture and state of health of the skin including classification of skin type and any problems.

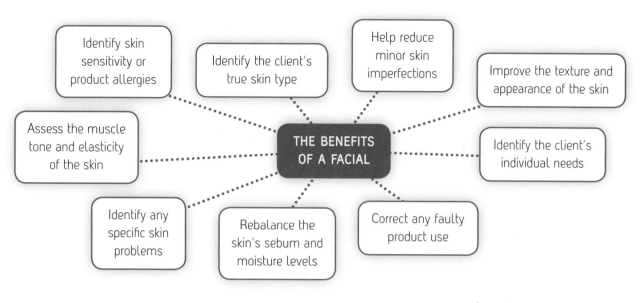

A facial is a treatment that helps the client in a number of ways

Always use a consultation sheet to record all the client details during your analysis.

It should be in three parts:

○ the client's history

○ skin analysis

○ client treatments and retail recommendations.

Think about it

Product houses or companies have their own facial diagnosis and consultation techniques. Therapists working for them are trained to use these techniques: for example, one company may start with a back **massage** and diagnosis, then turn the client over and diagnose any facial problems; another company may include a hand and foot massage in the facial, which is carried out while the mask is on! So, once you are qualified be prepared to learn new techniques, but first you need to learn the basics!

When examining the face and neck it is important to consider the following:

○ **Contra-indications** – check the skin prior to the treatment for any condition present that would prevent treatment or any adaptation that may be necessary. For more information on contra-indications see below, pages 274–75, and You and the skin, pages 199–203.

○ **Client's skin type** – identify the client's skin type correctly. This is essential, both to enable the therapist to give the right treatment, and to recommend the most suitable products.

○ **Minor skin problems** – look for any problems that can be given specific treatment for improvement.

For your portfolio

Many salons provide skin analysis as a free service prior to the facial. Specialist facial therapists offer a one-hour service, which is chargeable. Do some research and find out which large commercial companies offer a stand-alone skin analysis and how much they charge. Compare prices and find out what the process involves. You may even decide to have one done yourself as a hands-on investigation!

Key terms

Massage – manual manipulation of the skin and muscles for a therapeutic purpose using different massage techniques

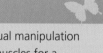

Unit B4 Provide facial skincare treatment

- **Client work/life balance** – take into account the client's age, lifestyle, nutrition and general health. These will be reflected in the colour and texture of the skin, muscle tone in the face, elasticity, the number of wrinkles present and skin discoloration. Stress, alcohol, dehydration, smoking and central heating are also reflected in the skin's condition. Record the client's colouring and pigmentation, as well as any other facial features: this will help with a make-up application and when recommending other treatments such as eyebrow shaping.

- **Medication** – if the client is taking regular medication, has been under a consultant within the last year or has had surgery in the last nine months, this should be noted. Many different types of drugs affect the skin and need to be taken into account.

- **Hormone levels** – the client's age will give a good indication of her hormone levels. Teenagers' hormone levels may be erratic and unsettled causing acne and breakouts, pregnancy will have an effect on the skin, and older women going through the menopause may be lacking in the vital hormones that help the skin's collagen and elastin levels, which support underlying structures (refer to Related anatomy and physiology, pages 229–36).

Facial examination techniques

There are four techniques to a facial examination:

- questioning
- visual
- manual examination
- reference to client records.

Key terms

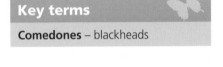

Comedones – blackheads

Questioning

Follow your consultation form when questioning the client before their facial. This will establish the factors that contribute to the skin's condition. Gentle questioning should help identify the client's normal skincare routine and products used as well as the client's expectation of the treatment – clients do need to be realistic. Encourage the client to ask questions to clarify any points they do not understand. It is important that the client understands that a skin condition may take several treatments to clear. A realistic treatment plan, with both time-scale and cost, should be discussed prior to the treatment taking place.

Visual

Visual examination should be done under a strong light with a magnifying glass to determine the client's skin type and condition. The skin should be clean and free of make-up. Any areas of sensitivity, problem areas such as **comedones** or an oily T-zone can be recorded on a facial record card.

Look at the colour of the skin, so that you can see pigmentation levels and patches, sun damage, capillary damage and the circulation of the skin. The efficiency of the skin cells for respiration, elimination of waste products

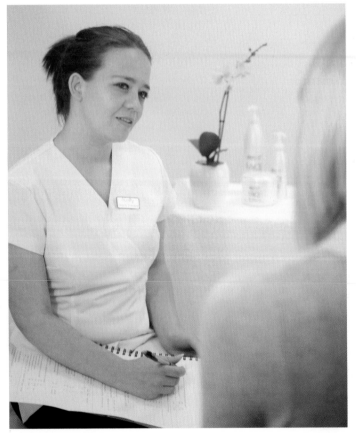

Fill out the record card prior to treatment

and blood flow to the epidermis are all indicated by skin colour (see You and the skin, page 196). Colour changes are also caused by fluctuating hormone levels, exposure to chemicals, allergic reactions, some skin conditions such as eczema, certain drugs and extremes of temperature. It may also be something which is inherited – a client with high colour and a tendency to blush or have a flushed appearance may have just been given that in the gene pool with their DNA! You will also be able to look at the skin and see if it looks naturally oily or has a drier or irritated appearance.

Manual examination

This should be gentle, and will give some indication about the elasticity of the skin, its warmth and texture. After a gentle pinch of the skin in the main facial areas the skin should spring back to its original shape. Poor elasticity of the fibres will mean that the skin takes longer to recover from the pinch test and this could be due to age. The warmth of the skin will indicate how good the circulation is, and the texture will be felt as smooth, coarse or rough. Lumps under the skin may need further investigation.

There are some excellent skin diagnosis devices available which can be incorporated into the skin analysis. Until recently, the woods lamp was the prime diagnostic equipment, but there are also skin scanners and skin analysers which measure hydration levels, fat content, melanin levels and erythema levels of the skin. These are all tools for an experienced therapist once you have developed a trained eye! (Refer to You and the skin, pages 195–97, for a full explanation of woods lamp and skin scanners.)

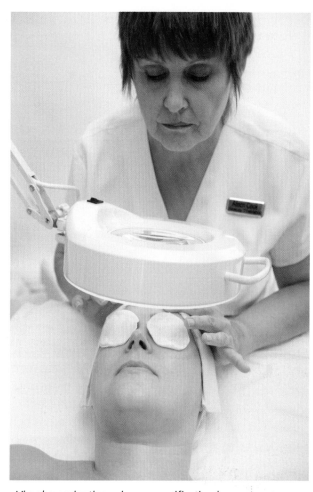

Visual examination using a magnification lamp

Referring to client records

If the client is a regular customer, always have the record card with you so that you can view previous treatments, talk about how successful they are/were, if there were any contra-actions, allergies, anything the client was particularly pleased with, or anything she did not particularly like. Not only is this a good ice breaker if the client is new to you, it is also important to continue the good work that the previous therapist has done. For more information on record cards, refer to Professional basics, pages 29–31.

Additional knowledge

Some skin scanners are able to measure the density of the skin, the pH of the skin and pigmentation levels. These are very good tools and valid for a clinical examination of the skin. However, there is no substitute for touch, looking under the magnification lamp and massaging the skin, to feel texture and depth. All leading commercial companies agree that the scanners, even in the hands of experts, will never replace the touch of an experienced therapist!

Unit B4 Provide facial skincare treatment

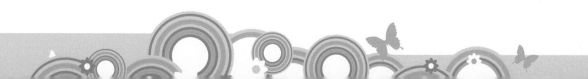

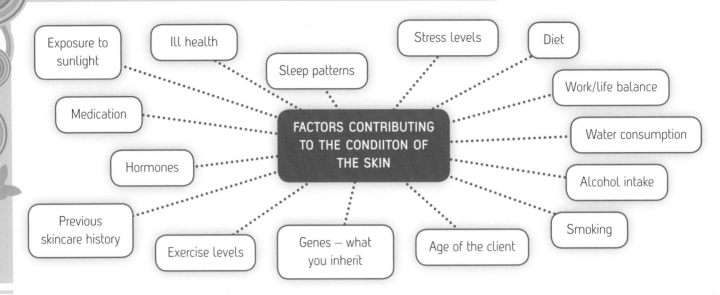

Think about it

You should never diagnose a contra-indication as you are not qualified to do so. You can give advice without referring to a specific medical condition and always advise the client to see their GP for a diagnosis.

Preparing the client for examination

Initial discussion with the client will take place while the client is still clothed and sitting with you. The discussion will cover contra-indications, her expectations of the treatment and your treatment plan. Obviously, a full treatment plan cannot be given until you have closely examined the skin, but you may not get that far if the client has an infectious condition and the treatment cannot go any further. It is much better to terminate the treatment with the client at that point, rather than place her on the couch and remove the make-up, if appropriate, only to find that the treatment cannot go ahead as a contra-indication is present.

Think about it

Male grooming is big business and more men are booking facials. Ask male clients to have a close shave prior to their appointment. This stops the tissues or cotton wool dragging on the skin and the skin gets maximum benefit of the massage, mask and products used.

Examining the face and neck

When examining the face and neck there are many points to consider:

○ A full picture of the skin can only be done in a good light, with the skin free of make-up, which may mask the skin's true condition. The client is usually laid on the couch, wrapped up and then eye make-up and lipstick removal and a full cleanse takes place. Only then can you look at the skin in detail, under a magnifying lamp with the light on. However, that is an unnatural position for the client to be in – the human body is usually upright (vertical) and you should look at the client's skin when they are standing or sitting too so that you can allow gravity to show how the skin behaves naturally. This shows what muscle tone is like and how the contours of the face dictate the face shape, how lined the skin is and the firmness of the jaw line.

○ Do carry out the first part of the client's history when you are sitting face to face with the client. The eye contact you have gives the client the feeling that you are interested in her, that you are listening and she can see exactly what you are writing on her card.

○ Try not to be too judgemental when talking to your client about skincare and their existing routine. They will not want to be made to feel like a naughty child who has not used the correct products.

○ Skin conditions may not be what they at first appear. You may have to dig slightly deeper than your initial skin-type judgement. There are lots of factors which may lead you to make an incorrect diagnosis. Skincare products used wrongly and which may not be appropriate for the skin type can mislead the client into damaging the skin. For example, if strong products are used on an oily skin, it can look very dry on the top of the epidermis, with lots of sebum still being produced by the sebaceous glands. The client then adds more oil-based moisturiser as she thinks her skin is dry, and the problem gets worse. A dry skin with a rich moisturiser applied can appear to be greasy and redness can be caused by an irritation or allergy to a food, product or chemicals. All of these mask the true condition of the skin.

1 Couch and working area tidied and prepared:
- Couch prepared with blanket and towels
- Couch roll on headrest and foot area and on the floor for client to stand on

2 Trolley prepared with:
- products
- spatulas
- tissues
- wet and dry cotton wool
- sponges (if preferred)
- jewellery bowl for client
- headband

3 Ensure client record card (and client record number if known) and pen are to hand

4 Make sure there are two chairs, a magnifying mirror and a bin with a bin liner

5 Ensure your nails are short and you are not wearing jewellery

6 Greet your client

7 Carry out a full consultation and contra-indication check

8 Position client on couch with headband on and jewellery off

9 Wash hands prior to treatment

Preparation for full facial, including massage

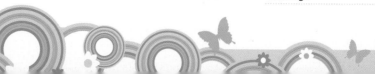

Before beginning the examination, remember the following.

○ Wash your hands thoroughly.

○ Remove any make-up a client may be wearing, and cleanse, deep cleanse, tone and pat dry the skin using a tissue.

○ Ideally, a male client will have had a clean shave prior to the facial examination – otherwise the cotton wool may stick to the beard growth or stubble. Also the state of the skin may be camouflaged behind a day's growth of hair, and a true picture of the skin's condition may not be seen.

○ The texture of the skin and the muscle tone will be felt as the cleansing movements are made.

○ The warmth of the skin will indicate how good the circulation is.

○ You need a pen and your record card so you can fill in all the client's details.

○ Remember to include on the record card the client's current skincare routine and how successful it is (refer to You and the skin, page 30, for a sample record card).

Think about it

Obtain a signed, written consent form from the client prior to carrying out the treatment. If the client is under the age of 16, a signed parental or guardian consent is essential prior to treatment and a parent should be present.

Think about it

Facials make the skin look cleaner, refreshed and are relaxing for the client. However, many long-term skin conditions will need more than one treatment before you see a good result, so you must explain that to the client and manage her expectations of the results after only one facial.

The client treatment plan

For further information, refer to Professional basics, pages 31–35. Revisiting these pages will remind you of assessment techniques and questioning techniques, along with treatment, services and product advice and, most importantly, client expectations.

If the client is suitable for treatment, with no contra-indications, you can go ahead and prepare the client for the beginning of the facial and the full skin analysis.

The treatment plan should be agreed with the client and recorded on the personal record card, along with a suitable time frame for a course of treatments, a price and budget structure (payment planning or perhaps a discount for payment in full) and details of recommended treatments and products. Remember that if you are off sick, another therapist will not know what you have agreed with your client if you have not written it down fully on the record card.

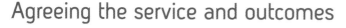

My story

Practice makes perfect

Hi, my name is Safia. My parents originally came from Pakistan, but I was born in the UK. I have been a qualified therapist for two years now, and the thing I found most difficult with facial diagnosis and talking to older clients was my age. Being young I felt shy and I had no personal knowledge of lines, wrinkles or pigmentation problems that older clients suffer from. Also, my mother and grandmother have lovely skin and we don't suffer from many problems — so I am lucky with my genes. I felt at first that I wasn't taken very seriously, and one client actually said to me, 'Well it's all right for you, dear, you haven't got a line or a blemish on your face!' Even so, I persevered with my facial diagnoses and my regular client base began to build. The more skin analyses I did, the better I felt about what I was doing — I wasn't going to let age be a hindrance to enjoying giving facials.

Then I began working for a commercial company that does face mapping, where the face is divided up into zones and each section is analysed so as to get a clear picture of what's happening under the skin's surface. I carried out as many as I could. Gradually, clients began to say that my clear skin was a good advert for the salon and our treatments, so it did slowly begin to feel as though I was being thought of as a genuine professional.

My advice to all beauty therapy students would be: keep practising — the more skin diagnoses and talking to people about their skin that you do, the better your judgement will be and you will feel confident about recommending the correct products. Clients will also have confidence in you — they will appreciate that you are well trained and that you know what you are doing.

Agreeing the service and outcomes

This combines very well with Unit G18 Promote additional products or services to clients, pages 105–22, so revisit this unit and remind yourself how to agree services and treatment outcomes with the client. Above all, you want the client to be happy with your recommendations — your client is a valued customer, who you want to keep for a long time, and your professionalism and integrity will ensure this.

Your final treatment plan should be suitable for the client's skin type and condition and she must be happy with what you are planning to do.

Ensuring the client's clothing, hair and accessories are protected or removed

The client's modesty and privacy must be preserved. In a closed cubicle ask the client to remove all outdoor and top clothes and put on a gown.

The client should remove all jewellery, accessories, wig, if worn, and glasses. Clients wearing contact lenses may prefer to remove them during the written consultation stage if they have suitable storage for them. Some clients prefer to keep them in, even though make-up will be removed and the eye area will be massaged. Be guided by the client's choice, as only the client will know which is most comfortable.

A headband or turban should be used to remove all hair from the face.

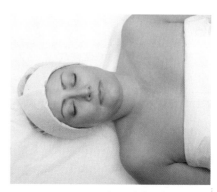

Preparation of the client

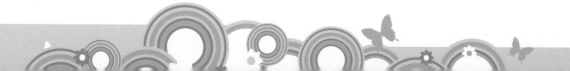

273

Think about it

During a facial treatment the client should feel warm and cosy under either a blanket and towels, or a quilt – often clients fall asleep when the mask is on. However, check with the client that they are not claustrophobic and are happy to be cocooned. It will detract from the treatment and add to their stress if they feel trapped and hot and bothered.

For the female client	Tights and half-slip may be kept on, but shoes should be removed. Bra straps may get oily and should be dropped off the shoulder, or the bra may be taken off altogether, depending on client preference. If the client chooses to push her straps down on to the top of her arms, there is still a danger they will get massage medium on them, as you will be going halfway down the upper arm with your movements. Above all, you want the client to be comfortable and she will not be if she has a bra clasp digging into her.
For the male client	Facial massage includes the upper back and shoulders, and these therefore need to be free of clothing. The shirt or T-shirt of the male client should be removed, and his chest covered with towels and/or blankets to prevent his upper body getting cold.
For all clients	Assist the client on to the couch and remove the gown. Depending upon the time of year, wrap the client in either a blanket with towels or just towels, so that he or she is comfortable and warm. There is nothing more distracting than clients feeling insecure or cold – they need to unwind and feel relaxed.

Taking the necessary action in response to identified contra-indications

Contra-indications to a facial treatment

- Cuts and abrasion of the skin's surface
- Scar tissue less than six months old
- Recent sunburn
- Any undiagnosed lumps or swellings
- Severe eye infections
- Any bacterial, fungal or viral infections
- Conjunctivitis
- Bruising to the area
- A known allergic reaction
- Any loss of sensation in the face, dropped muscle contour or speech impediments

For a visual reminder of the various contra-indications, refer to You and the skin, pages 36–37.

Other skin conditions

Although not commonly seen, you need to be aware of these skin conditions.

Pseudo folliculitis

Folliculitis is an inflammation of a follicle: usually referring to infection around the hair follicle as in *barae*, which is an infection of the hair follicle of the beard. *Pseudo* means false or a deceptive resemblance, or an illusion. So, pseudo folliculitis means the follicle is inflamed, but there may not always be an infection present.

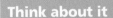

Keloids

A keloid is a scar which has overgrown and developed into a shiny, firm, usually raised, benign (non-malignant), thickened mass of fibrous tissue. It is often seen at the site of a burn, skin wound or surgical incision, and is mostly found on the trunk or face. It is more common in pigmented skin.

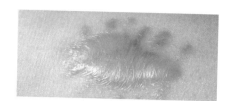

Ingrowing hair

An ingrowing hair is one that grows abnormally under the skin having been covered by an overgrowth of skin cells. There are several reasons for this: some people are genetically predisposed towards them; waxing or tweezing often causes them when the hair breaks at the weakest point just below the surface of the skin. If the hair continues to grow under the skin, it can often been seen and may develop into an infection. If not infected, the hair can be freed using a sterile microlance and an antibacterial wipe.

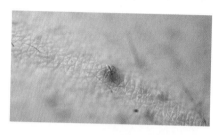

Papule

A papule is a small, solid, round, rising of the skin — in other words, a pimple. It can be quite large and sore.

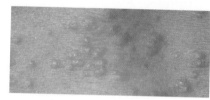

Pustule

A pustule is a papule with an infection present as in acne, eczema, smallpox, chicken pox or impetigo. Pus forms and will need to be treated with antibiotics. If the papule becomes infected and red, then pus is present.

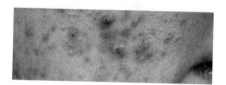

Taking action if a contra-indication is found

Treating a client with a known contra-indication has consequences. The client could experience pain and discomfort if the treatment went ahead and the condition could be made worse, or spread to other parts of the body. The therapist could be found to be negligent, both by her insurance company and by her professional body, and the expected support may not be forthcoming should the client decide to take legal action. Any client with a suspected infection should be referred to her GP. But be careful — it is not a therapist's job role to give a medical diagnosis.

If no contra-indications are present, continue the skin analysis.

Recording the client's current skincare routine

All the findings from your consultation and skin analysis should be recorded on the client's personal chart. The style of the chart may vary from salon to salon, but the basic information recorded is the same (see Professional basics pages 30–31).

Refer to You and the skin pages 184–97, to refresh your knowledge of skin types and how to recognise them.

It is important that all information is recorded — the client may not be booked in with the same therapist every treatment, and records of any allergies, reactions and favourite products will help keep the client safe and avoid duplication.

Think about it

Never be persuaded to carry out a treatment on a client with any contra-indications present. They are asking you to compromise your professional standing and there could be serious consequences. There is both a risk of cross-infection and of cross-contamination. If the client then decides that you have caused further skin damage or made an existing condition worse, she could sue you, your insurance may be void, and you might be proven to be negligent in a court of law. It really is not worth risking your whole career to keep a client happy. Just say no.

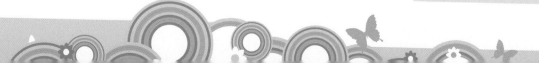

Cleansing the client's skin prior to skin analysis

Step-by-step facial cleanse

1 Using damp cotton wool apply eye make-up remover, working around the eye, over lid, underneath and over lashes. Work from inner to outer area. Remove with damp cotton wool. Follow the same routine with the other eye. Be careful to support the eye area, and do not drag, or apply any pressure.

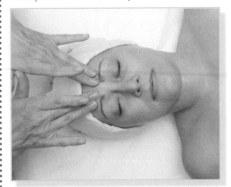

2 Apply a small amount of cleanser, using damp cotton wool, and remove the lipstick in small circular motions.

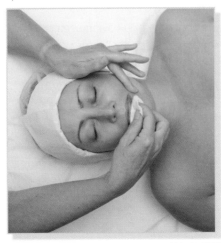

3 Apply dots of cleanser over the entire face and warm some in the palms of your hands. Working from the neck upwards, use upward movements towards the jaw line.

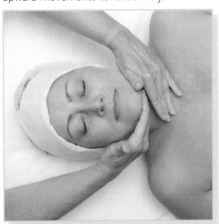

4 Work from the jaw line; use alternate hand movements to cover the entire cheek area.

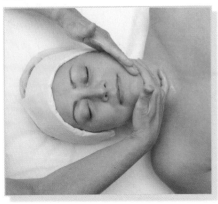

5 Using the index fingers, work into the nose, with small circular motions, without blocking the nostrils in! Use light pressure only.

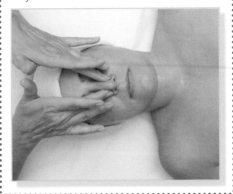

6 Travel over the bridge of the nose, on to the forehead working out towards the temple areas. Using index fingers, apply a little pressure to the temples.

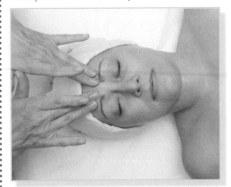

7 Sweep back down to the chin, working over the jaw line with alternate hand movements, to finish the cleanse routine.

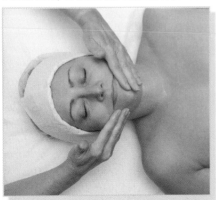

8 Remove cleanser, following the same routine direction as for the application of cleanser, with tissues, damp cotton wool or sponges.

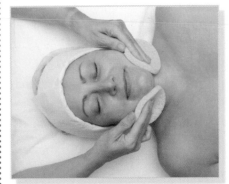

9 Blot the face with the tissue folded in a triangle. Pat gently with the hand, turn tissue over and repeat on the other side of the face.

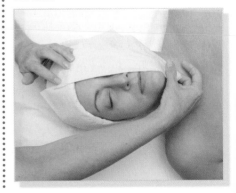

How did you do?

You can check your facial cleansing techniques quite easily. To ensure that the eyes are grease free, go back to the eyelashes and run a dry cotton bud along the length of the lash. If the cotton bud is dirty, you will know you have not cleaned thoroughly enough.

You can repeat the exercise for the skin by running a dry cotton bud along the cheek bones.

Do not be disappointed if you haven't got it right the first time. Your technique will improve with practice.

Performing a skin analysis

Refer to You and the skin for information on skin analysis (page 195), how to identify skin types (pages 184–86), skin conditions (pages 186–88) and any contra-indications (pages 199–203).

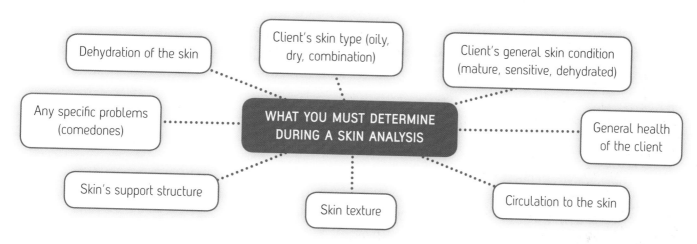

- Dehydration of the skin
- Client's skin type (oily, dry, combination)
- Client's general skin condition (mature, sensitive, dehydrated)
- Any specific problems (comedones)
- **WHAT YOU MUST DETERMINE DURING A SKIN ANALYSIS**
- General health of the client
- Skin's support structure
- Skin texture
- Circulation to the skin

Selecting suitable treatments, products and equipment for the client's skin type and condition

Before you can decide on any treatment plan or recommend suitable products, you have to know the treatments and products thoroughly. You should have experience of the treatments yourself, so you can talk about the sensations as well as the effects.

You need to have a full knowledge of products and treatments before you go on to facial massage techniques. This is so you can decide upon oil or cream, which massage medium and movements are most suitable for the skin type. You will need to refer back regularly to the planning section as you work through the massage techniques.

Facial products

To improve the facial skin condition, there are many **facial products** available on the market that can be used to good effect within the facial treatment:

- ○ eye make-up remover
- ○ cleansers

> **For your portfolio**
>
> Most large product houses (e.g. Dermalogica, Decleor and Clarins) produce their own skin analysis and record cards. Investigate two of them and see how they differ from the one you use at college – which one is best and why? Should you devise one of your own?

> **Key terms**
>
> **Facial products** – therapeutic beauty treatments using manual techniques and a variety of cleansers, toners, moisturisers and masks designed to improve all skin conditions.

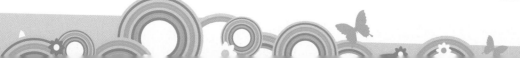

Unit B4 Provide facial skincare treatment

- ○ toners
- ○ moisturisers
- ○ exfoliants
- ○ masks
- ○ specialist skin preparations
- ○ massage mediums – usually oil or cream.

The cosmetic and skincare preparation market is huge. The range of manufacturers producing good-quality products both for salon use and for retailing is ever-growing. Your salon or teaching establishment may have their own particular favourite which, from experience, they prefer.

For your portfolio

Do some research to discover the latest trends in techniques. Today's discerning skincare and massage clients are often quite knowledgeable and expect the latest massage techniques and anti-ageing preparations. The eastern-influenced Ayurveda treatments are also very popular and skincare companies are trying to match the trends. Many clients will be interested in Fairtrade and organic products, so research the best ones to offer.

Think about it

Skincare products must, by law, display their ingredients on the outside of the package, with the ingredient with the highest percentage of content appearing first. Check for products which may prove to be allergic to your client. There may also be a rabbit sign which means the product has not been tested on animals – but be careful, as although the finished product might not have been tested on animals, individual ingredients might have been. This may be important to your client.

Reasons for skin damage	Signs or symptoms
Ultraviolet radiation – excessive exposure to the sun or artificial sunlight (sunbeds)	The skin ages prematurely because of free radicals (highly reactive chemicals that attack molecules by capturing electrons and thus changing chemical structure) causing breakdown of collagen and elastin that supports the skin Uneven pigmentation – either brown spots (hyperpigmentation) or loss of pigmentation (hypopigmentation) Blood and lymphatic flow to the skin cells may be impaired due to loss of structural support of the connective tissue Cellular reproduction is slowed down through damage to the DNA in each cell Loss of strength and resilience in the skin Skin looks lined and wrinkles appear prematurely Skin feels thick and may be dry to the touch
Insufficient fluid intake	Poor blood flow and sluggish lymph drainage to the skin resulting in lack of oxygen to the skin cells and reduced removal of water products Impaired epidermis enzyme activity resulting in loss of strength in the skin's fibres
A fat-free diet and/or general poor nutrition	Lack of essential fatty acids in the diet weakens the acid mantle resulting in slow healing and poor nerve reactions to stimulus Impaired defence against disease and infection Poor cell division for healing and a higher likelihood of scar tissue forming because of lack of vitamins Hyperpigmentation Vascular conditions forming and developing earlier such as spider naevus or couperose conditions Reactive skin conditions more likely, e.g. acne rosacea
Excessive lines and wrinkles from alcohol intake and smoking	Contamination of skin, clogged and blocked pores, irritations occur and a tendency to comedones. Skin is more prone to allergic reactions. Lack of oxygen makes the skin yellow with sallow tones often with nicotine residue left on the skin
Pollution from chemicals, traffic and thinning of the protective ozone layer	Leads to dehydration and overactivity of the sebaceous glands causing congestion problems

Reasons for skin damage	Signs or symptoms
Heat and steam	Overstretches the skin, causing damage such as permanent open pores
Incorrect use of skincare products	Inappropriate products can cause comedones to form or skin becomes oversensitive. Using products with a high alcohol content will dry out the surface but with sebum coming through from the sebaceous glands, so greasy skin has dry patches The acid mantle may be disturbed as it trys to rectify the damage caused by incorrect skincare

How to recognise skin damage

Think about it

In a salon you will need to have all equipment to hand while talking through the client's needs. You will choose the equipment you need according to the results of your skin analysis. So, while you may think you do not need equipment information at this stage in your training (as you have yet to learn a facial cleanse routine), you will need the information to make an informed decision at the consultation stage in a proper client situation.

For your portfolio

All beauty therapists need to use a variety of different products until they find their own personal preference. You should attend the various trade shows and exhibitions to experiment and try the vast range available. Go to your nearest large perfumery and approach the various cosmetic houses for free samples of products, until you find one you most like. Try at least three each of cleansers, toners and moisturisers. Collect price lists and advertising leaflets for your portfolio.

Procedure	Action on the skin	Products available
Pre-cleanse – am and pm	Part of a double cleanse – mixed with water this liquefies sebum on the skin and helps dissolve make-up making the second cleanse more effective and deep	Emulsifying cleansing oil Facial washes
Cleanse – am and pm	Removes dirt, sweat, sebum and make-up from the skin's surface and freshens the skin after sleep	Cleansing creams, lotions and milks, facial wash-off bars, gels Water-soluble creams with muslin cloths to remove
Tone – am and pm	Tightens the skin, stimulates the circulation and eliminates any trace of remaining cleanser from the skin	Toning lotion astringent, skin tonic bracers and fresheners
Exfoliate – once a week (some product houses produce a mild exfoliant which can be used daily)	Sloughs off the dead cells from the top layer of the epidermis to improve texture and colour while stimulating circulation	Cleansing grains that form a paste when mixed with water, ready-mixed granular paste, fruit acid peels
Day cream – am	A protective film to keep the skin soft and supple – it restores the oils to the skin after toning, helping to keep the outer layers hydrated – also forms a seal and a good surface for make-up	Moisturiser creams or milks and lotions
Night cream – pm	An absorbent, intensive, rich cream to restore the skin's well-being without leaving the skin feeling oily	Rich moisturisers, usually in cream form

Unit B4 Provide facial skincare treatment

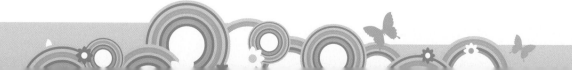

Procedure	Action on the skin	Products available
Face mask – once a week	Deep cleanses, soothes and balances the skin	Clay masks, peel-off masks, thermal masks, fruit masks, biological masks
Eye make-up remover – pm	A very gentle eye make-up remover, finer than a cleanser for the delicate eye area	Lotions and creams, wash-off gels
Eye balm	A delicate balm for upper and lower lid area when needed – soothing, refreshing, reduces puffiness	Moisturising lightweight creams or lotions

A good skincare routine

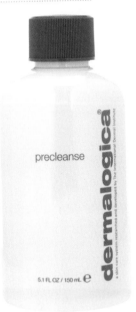

Pre-cleansers help to dissolve make-up

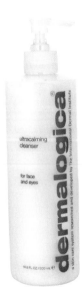

Cleansers leave skin smooth and supple

Pre-cleanser wash/emulsifier

Key ingredients

- Oils – olive, apricot kernel and nut oils
- Vitamin E
- Caprylic/capric triglyceride emulsifier

What they do

- Olive oil acts as a rich emollient to smooth and soften.
- Vitamin E is a rich, antioxidant vitamin to soothe.
- Capric triglyceride is an emulsifier which releases bonds into the skin when mixed with water.

Summary of action

- Liquefies sebum deposits from the skin's surface.
- Forms part of a double cleanse for a clean skin.
- Dissolves make-up.
- Removes grime and pollution without affecting the acid mantle.
- Helps smooth and nourish skin.

Method of use

- Mix with water in the palms of the hands and spread evenly over the face and neck, avoiding the eye areas.
- Lather up and massage in, using small circular motions, then rinse off with wet sponges and warm water.

Cleansing creams

Key ingredients

- An emulsion of oils, usually mineral oil or olive oil
- Waxes, usually beeswax or paraffin
- Water and water-soluble ingredients
- Emulsifiers
- Fragrance
- Preservatives

What they do

- A mineral oil will dissolve grease and oil-based products on the skin, i.e. make-up.
- Waxes provide a creamy firm texture to the product.
- The water content cools the skin and provides slip to allow easier spreading.
- Emulsifiers prevent the ingredients separating, i.e. oil and water.
- Fragrance makes the cream more appealing.
- Preservatives provide the product with a good shelf life and prevent deterioration.

Summary of action

- A deep efficient cleansing action, removes even heavy make-up.
- Leaves skin smooth and supple.
- Ideal for dry or normal skin types; too rich for an oily skin.

Method of use

- Decant a small amount onto a spatula, close lid, spread from spatula onto fingertips and massage over face and neck area using upward circular movements.
- Remove with tissues or damp cotton wool.

Cleansing milks

Key ingredients

- An emulsion of oils, usually mineral oil
- A smaller proportion of waxes than in a cleansing cream
- A higher proportion of water and water-soluble ingredients than creams
- Detergent
- Emulsifiers
- Fragrance
- Preservatives

What they do

- Detergent will act as a surface-active agent, which helps emulsify and create foaming action.
- For other ingredients, see above.

Summary of action

- A light cleansing lotion, which is easier to remove than a cleansing cream.
- Some cleansing milks can be worked into lather with water to wash off the skin.
- Ideal for most skin types except the very dry.
- Preferred by people who like a lighter feel to their cleanser.
- Also ideal for younger or greasier than normal skins.

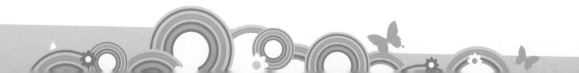

Method of use

- Either apply directly on to the skin on damp cotton wool pads stroking in an upward motion, or apply with the fingertips in small circular movements.
- Remove with tissues or damp cotton wool.

Cleansing lotions

Key ingredients

- Detergent solution in water
- Emulsifiers
- Fragrance
- Preservatives
- Anti-bacterial ingredients

What they do

- Anti-bacterial ingredients help a greasy or problem skin.
- For other ingredients, see above.

Summary of action

- A light cleansing lotion, which can be applied on cotton wool pads.
- Ideal for most young skins, especially problem or blemished skins.

Method of use

- Apply directly on to the skin on damp cotton wool pads, stroking in an upward motion.

Facial washes and gels

Key ingredients

- A mixture of cleansing and wetting agents (often derived from palm oil)
- Water and water-soluble ingredients
- Fragrance and foaming agents
- Preservatives
- Conditioners and colour

What they do

- Cleansing agents will absorb the oil particles of dirt.
- Conditioners will match and balance the natural pH of skin.
- Colour and fragrance will give appeal: for example, tea-tree may be added to give an anti-bacterial, healing property to a wash that is enhanced with a colour additive.
- For other ingredients, see above.

Summary of action

- Use a small amount on a moist skin, massage lightly over face and neck, and rinse off with water.
- Foaming properties will vary depending on hardness or softness of water.
- This method of cleansing can be used with a facial soft bristle brush for added stimulation.

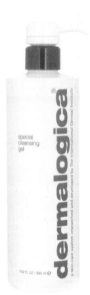

Encourage clients who like to wash their face to use a cleansing gel rather than soap and water

- This is ideal for use with a brush cleanser unit (a small motor rotates the brush) and can be applied to the chest and back. This makes a very good salon treatment for a congested skin, and is very popular with male clients who suffer with problem skin.

- Some gels can also be used as shaving foam, cleansing at the same time. Check individual manufacturer's instructions for use — there are many preparations that can be bought over the counter.

Method of use

- Apply directly onto moist skin in circular motions, avoiding contact with the eyes.
- Rinse off.

Toners and skin fresheners
Key ingredients

- Alcohol, usually ethanol
- Astringents, such as witch hazel
- Antiseptic, such as hexachlorophene
- Humectants, such as glycerine
- Additives, such as cucumber, althea extract (from plants)
- Preservatives and perfume

What they do

- The alcohol removes traces of grease on the skin and helps with the drying action.
- The water content cools the skin and dilutes the alcohol content.
- Fragrance makes the toner more attractive and hides the alcohol smell!
- Antiseptic properties help heal a congested skin.
- An astringent tightens the skin and makes pores appear smaller.
- Additives such as cucumber and plant extracts soothe and soften skin.
- Humectants attract water and help rehydrate the skin.
- Colour and fragrance give appeal: for example, cucumber may be added to give a soothing property to the toner and it may be enhanced with a colour additive — blue or green are associated with cooling and calming properties.

Summary of action

- Toners cool and refresh the skin, and are available in differing strengths depending upon skin type.
- Strong toners for oily skins contain more alcohol, which dissolves grease; the astringent properties tighten the skin.
- All toners contain mostly water and humectants, which help with moisture retention.
- Fresheners are available which contain only soothing agents, such as azulene or camomile. As no alcohol is present, they are not as good at removing grease from the skin but are ideal on a sensitive skin.

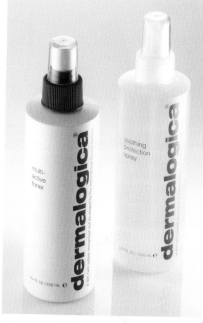

Toners and skin fresheners cool and refresh the skin

Provide facial skincare treatment Unit B4

Think about it

Skin toners contain 20–60 per cent alcohol.

Skin fresheners contain up to 20 per cent alcohol.

Some gentle toners for use on dry or sensitive skins do not contain any alcohol.

Skin toners with more than 25 per cent alcohol can only be used on an oily skin.

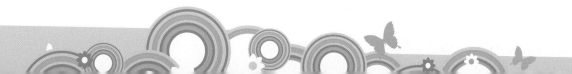

Method of use

- Apply to the skin with damp cotton wool pads, stroking in a firm but gentle rhythm all over the face and neck.
- Toners can help smooth, soften and heal skin, increasing cell regeneration.
- They prepare the skin to receive a moisturiser by removing any trace of grease left by the cleanser.

Exfoliants

Key ingredients

- Abrasive powders such as finely ground olive stones, nuts, oatmeal, corn-cob powder or synthetic micro-beads
- Detergent
- Water and water-soluble ingredients
- Kaolin, or other clay-based ingredients
- Sodium lactate
- Added moisturisers and vitamins

What they do

- An abrasive will act as a gentle buffer to remove the dead skin cells, felt as small grains on the skin.
- Detergent continues the cleansing process.
- Water and water-soluble ingredients help provide slip so that the cream or paste flows over the skin easily and does not pull or drag the skin.
- Kaolin or other clays will absorb grease and dirt particles, gently cleansing and bleaching the skin slightly.
- Sodium lactate is an excellent humectant to regulate moisture content within the skin.
- Added moisturisers and vitamins impart a light, smooth feel to the exfoliant without being sticky or greasy.

Summary of action

- The definition of exfoliate is to peel, flake or scale, in this case the skin's cells.
- As the top layer of the epidermis is constantly shedding, an exfoliant helps the process along.
- Helping the skin clear the accumulation of dead cells brightens the complexion, softens the skin and makes the skin very receptive to receiving moisture.
- Exfoliants come in many commercial forms: a powder, which must be mixed with water, a ready-made paste, or in a suspension (with water) that can also be left on to form a face mask.
- Exfoliating face masks usually have a higher proportion of clay to make the mask dry and set on the face.
- All skin types benefit from **exfoliation** providing care is taken.

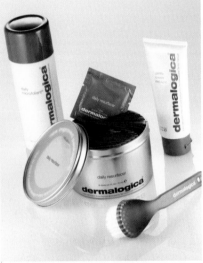

Exfoliants help to brighten the complexion and soften the skin

Think about it

Exfoliation can be done in the shower over the whole body and is an ideal pick-me-up for the skin, for a special evening occasion, make-up application or fake-tan application. Because exfoliants remove old skin cells, other skin preparations will be able to penetrate more effectively. Many salons use exfoliants instead of steamers as they are quicker, take up less space and are economical to purchase.

Key terms

Exfoliation – the manual or mechanical method of removing dead skin cells from the epidermis.

Method of use

○ Apply a thin layer onto damp, cleansed skin in circular motions, avoiding the eyes. Work upwards with light pressure. Care must be taken over the delicate cheek area; if sticking or dragging of the skin occurs, add more water without soaking the client.

○ Rinse off.

○ Follow manufacturer's instructions. Some exfoliants can also be left on the skin as a face mask, which is left to dry and then rinsed off.

○ Some face masks double as a peel, and the mask is removed by using dry fingers in a circular motion to slough off the remaining cream before rinsing.

Fruit acid peels

Key ingredients

○ Available as lotions or masks containing alpha hydroxy acids (AHA)

○ AHAs are fruit acids from citrus fruits, bilberries and sugar cane

What they do

○ The fruit acids help dissolve the surface skin cells while stimulating the blood supply.

○ They soften the skin cells and give the skin an appearance of being smoother and brighter.

Method of use

○ The products come as a mask or a lotion to be applied to the skin in an upward smooth motion.

○ They are ideal for a dry, mature skin.

Summary of action

○ AHA treatments can cause a slight contra-action after treatment. The skin may go pink, with a tingling sensation and mild itching. This is a normal reaction and the client should be advised to expect it.

Moisturising creams can be used morning and evening

Key ingredients

○ An emulsion of oils and waxes such as coconut or jojoba oil

○ Water and water-soluble ingredients

○ Fragrance

○ Preservatives

○ Emulsifier

○ Humectants such as glycerine or sorbitol

What they do

○ Creams contain approximately 60 per cent water, which rehydrates the skin.

○ Oils and waxes condition and improve the skin's natural water barrier; some oils such as jojoba oil prevent water loss so are ideal to add to a cream.

Think about it

There are many moisturisers on the market, with different prices and varying promises to work wonders on the skin. The brand name, the packaging and the promotional skills that go with the cream can dictate the price as well as the quality of oil used and whether other key selling ingredients are included, such as vitamins.

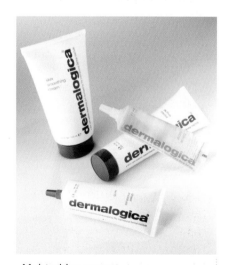

Moisturising creams

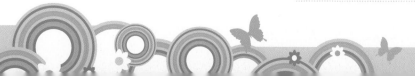

○ Emulsifiers prevent the ingredients separating, i.e. oil and water.

○ Preservatives provide the product with a good shelf life and prevent deterioration.

○ Colour and fragrance will give appeal: for example, coconut oil has a very distinctive smell which appeals to most people.

Summary of action

○ Moisturising creams can be used morning and evening depending upon skin type and cream used.

○ Moisturising creams are recommended for dry skins that need the softening effects of the oil and waxes.

○ Cream is especially good for skin in dry conditions, such as hot sun or central heating, and in very cold weather.

○ Make-up application is made easier with a moisturiser underneath it. Be careful about applying cream too near the delicate eye area, which may absorb the cream and become puffy. Only eye cream should be used in the eye area.

Method of use

○ Apply a light film to create a natural protective layer and prevent dehydration of the skin.

○ To avoid too much cream sitting on the skin surface, check the amount applied by pressing a clean tissue to the face one minute after application. If grease is present on the tissue, too much cream has been applied, or the cream is too rich for the skin type.

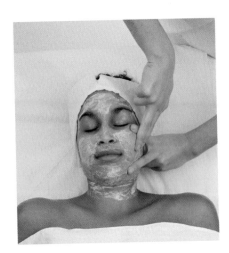

Face masks

Key ingredients

○ Varies depending upon type of mask used. Refer to pages 314–21 where all the products are discussed.

What they do

○ Masks are deep-cleansing and draw any impurity to the surface of the skin.

○ They may be slightly astringent to help dry up an oily skin, or rehydrating for a dry skin.

○ Refer to specific mask information.

Summary of action

○ Refer to specific mask information.

Method of use

○ Refer to specific mask information.

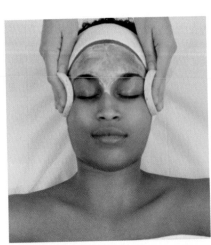

COSHH considerations

○ Health hazard: inhalation of fine particles can cause irritation when mixing powder.

○ If inhaled, move to fresh air; if coughing persists seek medical advice.

○ If mixing large quantities, a face guard is advisable.

- Store in a cool, dry place in a closed container.
- If in contact with eyes, rinse with plenty of water; if irritation continues, seek medical advice.
- If ingested, seek medical advice immediately.

Eye make-up removers

Key ingredients

- Varies depending upon whether oil, gel, or lotion preparation.
- Most are prepared from a mild cleaning agent in a cosmetic base.

Typical ingredients may include:

- horse chestnut extract
- hydrolysed wheat proteins
- vitamins
- organic alcohol, e.g. PEG 200.

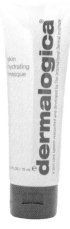

Face masks draw impurities from the skin

What they do

- Horse chestnut is used to decrease swelling and reduces puffiness in the eye area.
- Wheat proteins moisturise lids and lashes.
- Vitamins such as B5 increase cell regeneration.
- Organic alcohol is a solvent, which cleanses water and oil-based dirt.

Summary of action

- Eye make-up remover should be light, non-greasy and easily used without dragging the skin.
- Always ask the client if she is wearing contact lenses or false eyelash extensions. Both may require specialist removers, certainly one that is non-oily.
- Nothing is more irritating to the client than having a film left over the eye after removal of eye make-up. It must be thoroughly removed and not leaked into the client's eye.

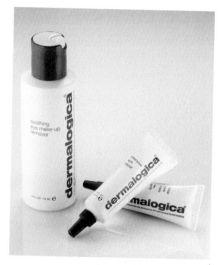

Eye-make-up removers can be oils, gels or lotions

Method of use

- Pre-soaked pads bought over the counter are usually lint pads soaked in remover.
- In a salon damp cotton wool pads are normally used. Gently move over the eye area with an upward and inward movement while supporting the eye area.
- Be careful to check that the client is not allergic to the metallic fibres present in cotton wool before commencing the treatment.
- A good eye make-up remover dissolves make-up immediately. Specialist oil-based remover may be needed to remove waterproof mascara.

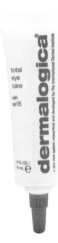

Eye cream should be used to delay the formation of wrinkles and lines

Eye creams, balms and gels

Key ingredients

Varies depending upon whether a cream or gel; may include:

- oil-in-water emulsions
- vitamins
- methyl cellulose
- collagen
- plant and herb extracts
- essential oils
- azulene, witch hazel, cucumber and camomile.

What they do

- Oil-in-water emulsion is easily absorbed by the skin so it moisturises and forms a good base for a daytime cream under make-up.
- Water-in-oil is a heavier solution and therefore only really good for the eye at night.
- Vitamins help with cell regeneration.
- Methyl cellulose thickens the suspension to give it a gel-like consistency, which dries on the delicate eye area firming and tightening the skin.
- Witch hazel and cucumber are mildly astringent and cooling to the eye, usually found in eye lotions.

Summary of action

- Eye creams should be used regularly to delay the formation of fine wrinkles and lines appearing with age.
- Prevention is better than cure, so eye protection should begin prior to lines forming.
- Lotions are better for oily skins and the richer, thicker-textured creams are suitable for drier, lined skin.

Applying eye cream

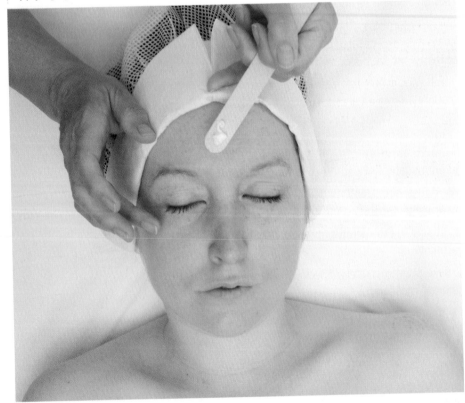

Method of use

- Less is more with eye creams. Application of too much is a waste of product and may cause swelling in the eye area if the soft tissue around the eye area has absorbed it.
- A small blob of cream should be warmed between your fingers before gently massaging the cream around the eye area. The ring fingers, i.e. the third fingers of each hand, have the lightest pressure and will avoid damage to the area.
- Work in small, circular motions from the bridge of the nose outward to the temples, across the top of the eye just under the eyebrow, and then underneath the eye towards the nose.
- Any excess can be blotted, but do try not to waste any of it.

COSHH considerations

For cleansing creams, milks and lotions; facial washes and gels; toners and skin fresheners; exfoliants; fruit acid peels; eye make-up removers; and eye creams, balms and gels:

○ Non-hazardous, non-inflammable if less than 10 per cent alcohol.

○ If ingested, drink milk or water.

○ If in contact with the eyes, wash well with water; if irritation occurs, seek medical advice.

○ If spilled, use absorbent towels to clean the area, wash with detergent and water to avoid slippery floors.

○ No special handling and storage precautions are necessary.

Neck creams

While a lot of attention is given to the face, the neck area is a very clear mirror reflecting age and/or neglect of the skin. All facials should include the neck area, and some very good preparations are available.

Unfortunately, many clients do not bother with their necks – it is worth encouraging younger clients to pamper the neck area to prevent damage occurring.

Most neck preparations are very rich in formula, with high oil content to nourish and moisturise.

Hydrolysed collagen, elastin and vitamin E are common ingredients, which will moisturise, increase suppleness and firm the neck.

Instruct the client to apply a light film after toning at night. Encourage her to include the neck area in the morning routine of cleanse, tone and moisturise, even though make-up application will not go on to the neck. The neck still needs protection from pollution, the environment and the sun, and from the danger of dehydration.

Hand care

Hands often show the first signs of ageing (like the neck area), especially if neglected or unprotected.

Encourage the use of hand creams – again, prevention and protection are better than cure!

The client should rub in any excess moisturiser into her hands, rather than waste the product, and a hand cream should become part of a night-time routine.

Refer to Unit N2/N3 Provide manicure and pedicure services, pages 455–94, for further information.

Lip care

Lips can be sadly neglected, until cold sores and chapped lips become a problem.

When you are removing the client's eye make-up the lipstick can also be removed, and the cleansing medium and massage motion will help keep the lips moist.

Lip balms, flavoured lip-gloss and lip creams are available to help dry or sore lips. Remember, the lips need protection against the sun, as they have no melanin of their own. While most lipsticks contain a sunscreen, naked lips will not be protected.

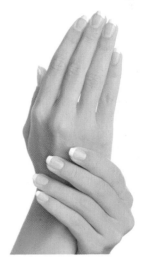

Keep hands well moisturised to delay the signs of ageing

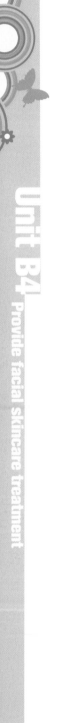

Skin type	Products most suitable
Normal	Eye make-up remover lotion Light cleansing cream or lotion Facial wash if preferred Toner with 10–20 per cent alcohol content Light moisturiser cream or lotion Eye lotion
Dry	Eye make-up remover oil or cream Cream cleanser Low-alcohol-content toner, or no-alcohol if sensitive too Paraffin wax mask Non-setting (hydrating) mask Eye cream Cream moisturiser
Greasy	Eye make-up remover lotion Cleansing lotion or cleansing milk Facial wash or foaming gel Toner with 2–50 per cent alcohol content Cleansing grains or peel Clay-based masks Moisturiser milk Light eye gel
Combination	T-zone – follow greasy skin recommendations Dry cheek areas – follow dry skin recommendations Normal cheek areas – follow normal skin recommendations Young congested T-zone – follow congested skin recommendations with normal skin recommendations on cheeks Exfoliating cream/gel Balancing mask (two masks can be used, one on the T-zone and one on the cheeks)
Sensitive	As for dry skin Specialist products are available for hypersensitive skin Check for known allergies to products Check for allergies to cotton wool
Dehydrated	As for dry skin Specialist treatments are available in most salons using advanced techniques such as a galvanic facial (NVQ Level 3 work). Be aware and read the salon price list. Another therapist may be able to help the client's skin.
Congested	Eye make-up lotion Cleansing lotion or cleansing milk Facial wash or foaming gel Toner with 25–50 per cent alcohol content Cleansing grains or peel Clay-based masks Moisturiser milk Light eye gel

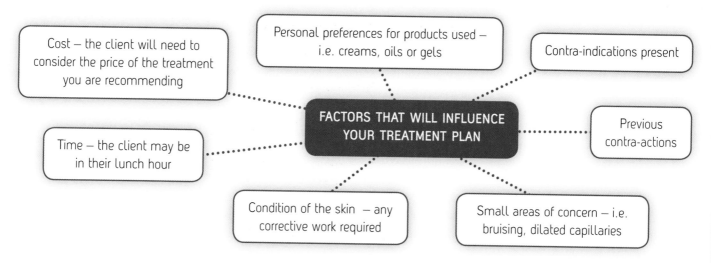

Cost – the client will need to consider the price of the treatment you are recommending

Personal preferences for products used – i.e. creams, oils or gels

Contra-indications present

FACTORS THAT WILL INFLUENCE YOUR TREATMENT PLAN

Time – the client may be in their lunch hour

Previous contra-actions

Condition of the skin – any corrective work required

Small areas of concern – i.e. bruising, dilated capillaries

Suggesting a treatment plan

This will depend partly on the personal product preferences of the client. Some clients like the feel of water on the face, others do not; some like a cream, others prefer a lighter texture. Investigate different product houses – most produce specific lines for each skin type, and you can recommend a whole range which work together.

Equipment and materials

As well as deciding on the type of products that will meet your client's needs when planning her treatment, you should give some thought to the equipment and supporting materials required – such as magnifying lamp, skin warming devices, for example hot towels, and consumables – before beginning the facial. Refer to skin-warming technique below.

Specific preparation of the client

This will depend on the equipment used. You need to consider each piece of equipment as well as the manufacturer's recommendations.

Improve and maintain skin condition

In this outcome you will learn about:

- using facial products and equipment correctly and following manufacturers' instructions
- leaving the skin clean and free of all traces of make-up using suitable deep-cleansing techniques
- using suitable exfoliation techniques, minimising discomfort to the client
- leaving the skin smooth, free of any surface debris and products using an exfoliation technique suitable for the client's skin type and skin condition
- using a suitable skin-warming technique relevant to the client's needs
- carrying out any necessary comedone extraction, when required, minimising discomfort to the client and with minimal damage to the skin

- using a suitable massage medium for the client's skin type and skin condition using and adapting massage techniques to meet the needs of the client and agreed treatment
- using and adapting massage techniques to meet the needs of the client and agreed treatment
- applying mask treatments evenly and neatly, ensuring that the area to be treated is covered
- removing masks after a recommended time and without discomfort to the client
- ensuring that the skin is left clean, toned and suitably moisturised
- ensuring the finished result is to the client's satisfaction and meets the agreed treatment plan.

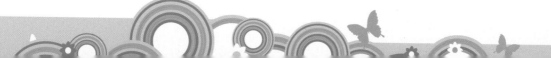

Unit B4 Provide facial skincare treatment

This outcome is all about performing the facial treatments: you have completed your skin analysis in a hygienic manner, you have prepared your products and equipment and the treatment plan is agreed with the client. The client is in a safe and comfortable position, with the skin cleansed and ready to receive your attention.

Using a suitable skin-warming technique

Warmth applied to the face is a very good way of helping to maximise the effects of the treatment. Warmth will help relax the muscles, open the pores and soften the skin in preparation for further treatments. Extraction and nourishing the skin are extremely effective after warming.

There are several ways to warm the skin:

○ hot towels

○ facial steaming

○ self-heating products such as thermal masks.

Hot towels

Hot towels are a very convenient method of warming the skin. They can be applied without equipment and are ideal for the mobile therapist who does not have access to a facial steaming unit.

Hot towels were always used in the old-fashioned barbershop when a close shave was offered with the haircut. A hot flannel would have the same effect but may make the client feel claustrophobic.

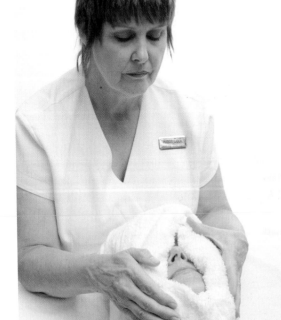

Hot towels can be used to apply heat to the skin

How do I do it?

○ Fold a hand towel into four and immerse in hot water leaving an edge for the hands to grip.

○ Alternatively, if you have a hot-towel steaming unit (a small oven that looks like a microwave), put in a damp towel and the heater will warm it up for you.

○ Remember health and safety – if the towel is too hot to wring out with the hands, it is too hot to go on the face. It needs to be hand hot.

○ Wring out and fold over the client's face, with the towel ends at the forehead. This will allow the nose to remain uncovered for claustrophobic clients.

○ Press gently into the contours of the face until the towel cools. Do not allow the face to become cold again as this will negate the benefits of the treatment.

The hot-towel procedure can be repeated if needed.

Treatments can now be carried out on a beautifully clean, receptive skin.

Facial steaming

Face steamers are like big kettles — they boil water to create steam. Steam benefits the skin by opening the pores and allowing deep cleansing. They are nearly always used in conjunction with face masks and are classed as a special treatment.

Most facial steamer machines have the following characteristics:

○ Vapour jets can be swivelled in all directions.

○ Control panel has a warning light.

○ Water capacity is 2 litres.

○ Boiling time with 2 litres of water is nine minutes.

○ Distilled water only must be used to maintain the life of the equipment and avoid limescale build-up on the heating element.

○ Essential oils can be added by applying them to cotton wool, which is placed in the special filter basket located in the filling funnel. Oily liquids must not be poured directly into the steamer.

○ The heater should be de-scaled periodically with acidulated water, following the manufacturer's instructions.

Caution

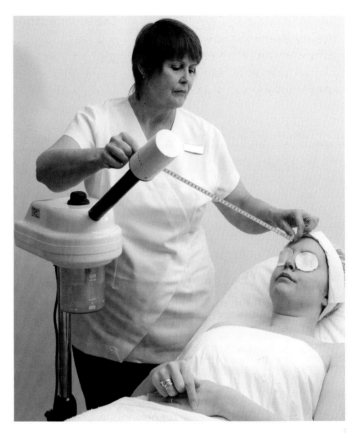

Always measure your steamer's distance from the client's face to avoid scalding the client

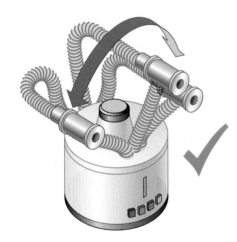

The illustration shows the maximum possible head swivel to prevent the vapour from spraying water during the treatment.

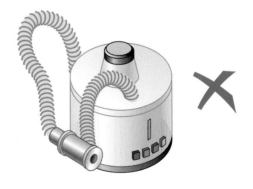

The vaporiser must under no circumstances be used with the head in the position shown on the left. This position stops the condensation returning to the heater and the vaporiser will spray water.

Contra-indications to a steam treatment

○ Hypersensitive skins

○ Open cuts — infection could set in

○ Acne rosacea

○ Split capillaries — increasing the circulation and heat will put extra strain on these delicate blood vessels, and in some cases will worsen them

○ Bad streaming colds or hay fever

○ Severe bronchial conditions or asthma

○ Very high blood pressure or where the client suffers from dizzy spells

○ Any eye infections, such as conjunctivitis, which could spread in the warm conditions

○ Diabetes — the metabolic rate must not be increased

○ Sunburn or previous ultraviolet exposure

○ Claustrophobia

Benefits of steaming

○ The circulation is increased, causing the pores to open; the skin sweats, getting rid of impurities such as dirt, old make-up and dead skin cells, leaving the skin with a fresher, glowing appearance.

○ Stimulates oil glands and improves moisture content in the skin.

○ Comedones are more easily removed with less risk of scarring or marking the skin.

○ Aids the process of shedding old skin cells — called desquamation.

○ Helps with regeneration of skin cells in a dry, mature or dehydrated skin.

○ A relaxing treatment for the client, because of the warmth and the essential oils if used.

Items required

○ Distilled water (required for refilling machine).

○ Cotton wool rounds (damp) for eyes.

○ Tissue (this is used to wipe the client's face during treatment, avoiding drips which can lead to discomfort for the client).

Preparation of couch

○ Check that the couch is stable and will not move during treatment.

○ Place the couch in semi-reclining position.

Preparation of client

○ Prepare the client, as you would do for any facial treatment, paying special attention to the head and ensuring that there are no stray hairs around the face and neck.

○ Ensure the client is comfortable and relaxed and all jewellery has been removed.

○ Lay a towel across the neck area (if treating the neck and face, then lay the towel across the chest). Tuck the towel in at either end.

○ Explain the treatment to the client – this will allay any fears she may have. Commence the treatment with a facial cleanse.

Safety precautions

○ Check the machine, e.g. wires, flex, plug and on/off switch.

○ Check the level of distilled water is correct.

○ Check the machine is functioning correctly and producing ozone (before the client's arrival).

○ Ensure the couch is stable and in the correct position.

○ Ensure that the flex does not trail across the floor, endangering other clients, your colleagues and yourself.

○ When the machine is not in use, make sure it is unplugged and in a safe area away from the main activity in the salon.

○ During treatment the therapist must be in attendance at all times.

○ Eye pads must be used throughout this treatment.

○ While the machine is in use, ensure that it is the correct distance away from the client to avoid scalding.

○ Take care when repositioning the machine, as it gets hot during use.

○ Make sure there is a steady flow of steam coming from the nozzle before placing the steamer arm over the client's face. This will ensure the nozzle does not spit out hot water and burn the client.

Face steaming – application

○ Salon pre-treatment to facial steaming

○ Manual cleanse.

○ Brush cleanse (depending on skin type).

○ Facial vacuum (depending on skin type).

Aftercare to facial steaming

Dry the skin with tissue before commencing other treatments.

Continue with either massage or other electrical equipment that might be recommended for the client's skin type.

A mask must always follow a facial steam treatment.

Steaming procedure

1 Check the tank is full and switch the machine on 5–10 minutes before it is required, to permit water heating to commence. The vapour switch is only required at this stage.

2 Ensure the client is well protected with towels and that her hair is covered.

> ### Think about it
>
> As a safety precaution for steaming, always place the client in a semi-reclining position. Never have the client lying flat with the face up and the steamer directly over the face – if the boiling water spits out or drips, it will fall on to the client and cause burns. If the steamer is parallel to the face, any drips will go on to the floor, which although potentially hazardous, will not harm the client. All spillage must be cleaned up, before an accident occurs.

Unit B4   Provide facial skincare treatment

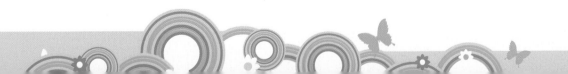

Unit B4 Provide facial skincare treatment

3   Prepare the client for facial treatment by cleansing the skin, and at the same time discuss and explain the treatment and its effects, thus alleviating any fears she might have. Inform her that the machine will make a noise and that an unusual smell will be present – all of which is perfectly normal.

4   Ensure the client is in a semi-reclined position.

5   Place eye pads (damp) over the client's eyes. This will avoid irritation.

When the client is fully prepared, position the steamer approximately 30–45 cm from the client's face, using at this stage only vapour.

6   Once the client is settled, inform her you are switching over to ozone, then switch on the ozone control. The steam changes its consistency, becomes ionised, cloud-like and very fine in appearance.

(Refer to your professional body for directives about using ozone.)

7   Stay in attendance at all times and regularly check the client's skin reaction. Points to note are hot spots, erythema or client's discomfort – if any of these occur, discontinue treatment. Cool the skin with the application of a cool compress – not too cold as this will make the client jump.

8   Remember to wipe away with tissue any drips that might cause client discomfort.

9   Do not exceed the treatment time. This will vary between 10 and 20 minutes depending on skin type.

10   On completion of the treatment return to vapour, then switch the machine off completely.

11   Unplug the machine and place it in a safe area of the salon.

12   Remember to remove all surface moisture with a tissue.

13   If necessary, use your metal eradicator (comedone extractor) for blackheads.

14   Complete the treatment with a massage and face mask or continue with another electrical apparatus depending on the client's skin type or treatment plan.

General cleanse and tone	5 minutes on lower neck 5 minutes on lower face 4–5 minutes on full face
Disinfecting and antibacterial effect on oily and blemished skin	10 minutes on lower face and neck 10 minutes on full face
Regenerating effect on dry/dehydrated mature skin	2–3 minutes on lower face and neck 1–3 minutes on full face to achieve erythema

Recommended application time and treatments

Conclude this treatment with a nourishing massage to prevent irritation and overdryness.

Note: After treatment, surface moisture should be removed, then other treatments or a mask should be applied.

Risk assessment for steaming equipment

Refer to Unit G20, Make sure your own actions reduce risks to health and safety, pages 71–86, for a complete discussion on risk assessment.

Hazard: only look for hazards that you could reasonably expect to result in significant harm under the conditions in your workplace. Use the following examples as a guide.

- **Fire** (e.g. from electrical flex or lead)
- **Burning of equipment** (through low water level in the tank)
- **Moving parts of machinery** (e.g. casing gets hot — use towel to protect hands)
- **Ejection of materials** (spitting hot water)
- **Electricity** (e.g. poor wiring)
- **Fumes** (e.g. from added aromatherapy chemicals)
- **Manual handling** (hot casing)
- **Falling machinery** (if not securely attached to base when moving steamer)

Salon after-treatment

- Extraction of blackheads — if required on oily skin. (Refer to page 298 for the procedure to use for comedone extraction.)
- Massage — all skin types.
- Massage including audio sonic — dry or dehydrated skin.
- Mask — use appropriate mask for client's skin type.
- High frequency: direct — oily skin; indirect — dry or sluggish skin.
- Galvanic-iontophoresis — dry or dehydrated skin.

From this list and from the salon pre-treatment list for facial steaming, a treatment plan with variety can be compiled, offering maximum benefit to the client.

Face steaming – suggested routines

A	B	C	D
Cleanse Facial steam Manual massage – either normal/dry or oily skin Mask Tone, moisturiser	Cleanse Brush cleanse Facial steam Use of comedone extractor – oily/blemished skin Mask Tone, moisturiser	Cleanse Facial steam Massage including audio-sonic – dry/dehydrated skin Mask Tone, moisturiser	Cleanse Brush cleanse Facial vacuum Facial steam – oily/blemished skin Mask Tone, moisturiser

E	F	G	H
Cleanse Facial steam Direct high frequency	Cleanse Facial steam Massage Galvanic iontophoresis – dry/dehydrated skin	Cleanse Facial vacuum Facial steam Indirect high – dry/dehydrated skin Cleanse	Cleanse Facial steam Non-surgical face lifting Galvanic cleanse Balancing programme Lifting Iontophoresis

Awarding Body code of ethics on the use of ozone

The use of ozone can be very beneficial when administered in small quantities and under supervision, but it may also be destructive when used incorrectly.

Some public health authorities and beauty examination boards believe that the use of ozone can be bad for your health. Inhaling it in great strength can lead to respiratory infections.

Most Awarding Bodies do not recommend that ozone is used under any circumstances.

Self-heating products such as thermal masks

Refer to **mask treatments** (on pages 314–21) for the use of thermal masks to pre-heat the skin.

Carrying out comedone extraction

Some salons offer milia extraction during a facial, using a sterile probe to pierce the skin at the site of the milia. The milia are then safely squeezed out. Tissues should be used to protect the hands, and gloves should also be worn. There is often a small amount of blood spotting.

Using a sterilised comedone extractor, gently apply pressure to the comedone centre and ease the comedone out. Do not apply too much pressure, or squeeze, as this can cause scarring. Using suitable exfoliation techniques

If a metal comedone extractor is not available, cover the fingertips with tissue and gently roll the skin around the comedone, to ease it out.

> **Key terms**
>
> **Mask treatment** – preparation applied to the skin as part of a facial to reinforce cleansing of the facial skin.

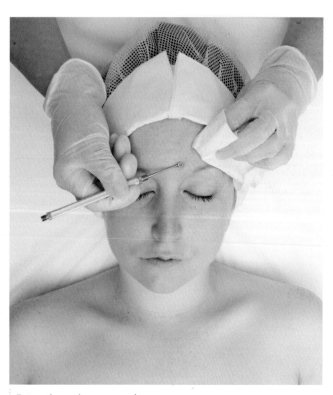

Extraction using a comedone extractor

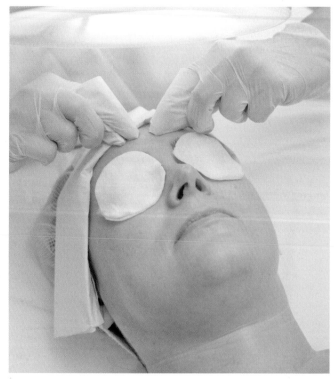

Manual comedone extraction

Brush cleansing

Brush cleansing is designed to give deep cleansing and a stimulating massage. It can be used to remove a mask or peel from the skin. It is essential to follow the individual manufacturer's instructions.

Most brush systems are supplied with a complete range of brush, sponge and pumice heads, which ensures perfect treatment on most skin types, providing no contra-indications are present.

To ensure there is no unnecessary pulling of the delicate facial or neck tissue, most machines have variable speed control and directional change for the heads.

Pumice stone head (small 20 mm)

This pumice stone head will remove film or gel masks with a slightly abrasive action yet will cause very little skin drag. It can also be used for desquamation and treatment on scarred or pigmented tissue. It can be incorporated into a pedicure treatment for the removal of hard skin on the heel.

Sponges (small 20 mm, medium 40 mm)

When dampened, these very versatile heads can be used on the most delicate and sensitive skin types. For best results, they should be used in conjunction with a foaming, deep-cleansing product.

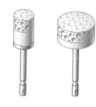

Brushes (small 20 mm, medium 40 mm)

Soft brushes can be used for all types of deep-cleansing treatments and stimulation massage on most areas of the face or body. The small head will easily treat areas around the ears, nose and eyes, while the larger head can be most successfully used on foreheads and cheeks.

Brush – bristle (medium 40 mm)

This bristle head gives a very stimulating treatment while desquamating the skin and cleansing blocked pores. It is a suitable treatment for those clients with firmer tissue, especially men.

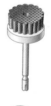

Brush – medium goat hair (cylindrical 60 x 40 mm)

Used in conjunction with a foaming cleanser or any desquamating product, this cylindrical body brush will deep cleanse the back, arms or legs. As well as cleansing, the action provides a gentle, stimulating massage, increasing circulation and therefore improving skin texture and colour.

Contra-indications to a brush cleanse

- Broken skin
- Skin diseases or infections
- Hypersensitive skins
- Extremely loose tissue
- Broken veins
- Inflammation or irritation of the skin
- Diabetes

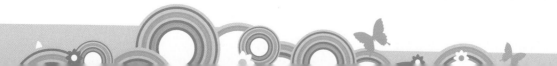

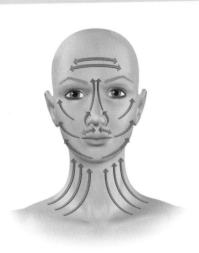

The direction of strokes when giving a skin brushing treatment

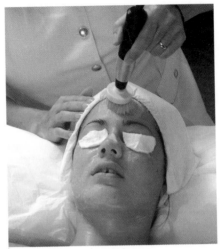

Brush cleansing of the face

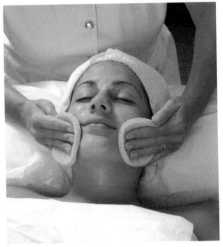

Removal of gel for brush cleanse

Effects of a brush cleanse

○ Aids desquamation.

○ Stimulates deeper cell renewal.

○ Removes surface cellular matter.

○ Deep cleanses and refines skin tissue.

○ Relaxes muscle fibres.

○ Stimulates superficial and deeper tissues.

○ Improves cellular function and regeneration.

○ Aids the removal of waste products from the area.

○ Increases blood and lymph circulation.

How do I do it?

1 Prepare the client for a normal facial procedure.

2 Remove eye make-up.

3 Give a superficial manual cleanse to the face and neck, using skin cleanser suitable for the skin type.

4 Select the recommended product suitable for the skin type to the face and neck. Decant a sufficient amount into a plastic bowl and replace the lid of the product. Application can be done with the brush head, mask brush, damp sponges or hands, depending upon recommendations. The product will either be a foaming cleanser or facial scrub, depending upon client needs.

5 Select the brushing head required, wet it in warm water (without it dripping) and insert it firmly into the black handle. Turn on the machine.

6 Make contact with the back of your own hand and ensure speed control is at minimum – always test the machine on yourself prior to using it on the client. Now switch on to confirm the machine is in good working order. Demonstrate the action to the client – she needs to be aware of the noise before the machine makes contact with the face.

7 Switch off, and remove from your hand. Cleanse the head and start the process again, making contact with the client's skin.

8 Eye pads can be placed over the eyes if the client prefers — it does prevent any product getting into them.

9 Place the applicator head on to the neck and gently increase speed control until the desired action is achieved, ensuring client comfort.

10 Work upwards on the neck and face in straight lines (as in the diagram above) and avoid the delicate skin around the eyes.

11 Work over the area for 5—7 minutes.

12 Reduce speed control to a minimum, turn off the machine and remove the brush from the skin.

13 Remove any remaining product with damp sponges and continue the facial routine.

Risk assessment for brush cleansing equipment

Refer to Unit G20, Make sure your own actions reduce risks to health and safety, pages 71–86, for a complete discussion of risk assessment.

Hazard: only look for hazards that you could reasonably expect to result in significant harm under the conditions in your workplace. Use the following examples as a guide.

- **Fire** (e.g. from electrical flex or lead)
- **Burning of equipment** (through motor running too fast)
- **Moving parts of machinery** (e.g. dropping heads on to client's face when removing them)
- **Ejection of materials** (spitting products into client's eyes)
- **Spillage** (e.g. from too much product applied to heads)
- **Electricity** (e.g. poor wiring)
- **Manual handling** (lifting machine)
- **Loose heads** (if not inserted into handle firmly enough)

Steaming with a brush cleanse

If a steam treatment is indicated for the type of skin being treated, it should be given either before brushing (to soften dead cells and open pores) or in conjunction with brushing — this ensures the area is also kept moist throughout the treatment. It will depend upon the skin texture — too much stimulation will not be good for a delicate skin type. Be guided by your particular manufacturer's instructions.

Care and maintenance of brush heads

After use, clean the brush head thoroughly in hot, soapy water. Rinse and dry. Place in a sanitiser between clients to avoid the risk of cross-infection. Be guided by your particular manufacturer's instructions.

Product exfoliators

If the client is restricted for time, steaming and brush cleansing may be too time-consuming. Exfoliators are now very popular in salons. In this situation the use of a product exfoliator is very effective: it can be applied easily, and is quickly removed after priming the skin to be receptive for massage and mask therapy.

The exfoliator may take the form of granules in a dry form, which you mix into a paste with warm water and massage into the skin. Product houses also make exfoliants which are pre-mixed in tubes and are so gentle some of them can be used daily. Dead skin cells are removed by abrasive powders, such as finely ground olive stones, nuts, oatmeal, corn-cob powder or synthetic micro-beads, buffing the skin. (Refer back to the product information on exfoliant use, page 284.)

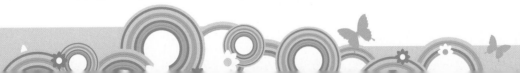

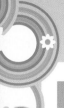

Think about it

Some exfoliants can cause extreme irritation and redness; in these cases, you should carry out a patch test – always follow manufacturer's instructions.

A **patch test** involves applying a small amount of product to an area, behind the ear, 24 hours prior to use, and then checking for a reaction. Any inflammation or irritation means the product is not suitable for use.

Never give professional exfoliant ingredients to clients to use at home – they might not carry out the instructions correctly, which could cause skin irritation.

Think about it

Do not perform exfoliant treatments on people with skin that is already irritated, such as sunburn, or on skin that has been waxed. Clients on strong medication for acne, such as Accutane, should not be given strong exfoliants for six months after the drug has been stopped. Clients using Retin-A for the medical treatment of acne should stop the drug two weeks prior to exfoliation taking place – this is a vitamin A derivative and is available in five strengths of cream, gel or liquid form. It increases cell turnover, so more exfoliation is not good! Always follow manufacturer's instructions and be guided by them.

There is a difference between exfoliants professionally applied in the salon and those sold to clients for use at home. Professional exfoliants have slightly stronger ingredients and require training for application; they also have activators and accelerators which need to be mixed in proportions suitable for each skin type.

The only drawback with using exfoliating products is that they can get a bit messy! Make sure the client's turban is protected with an extra layer of tissue, and put a double thickness of couch roll under the client's neck and shoulders to catch any fallen product. This can then be removed prior to the massage starting. It would be very uncomfortable for the client to be lying on granules throughout the rest of the treatment. Your fingers will also tend to pick them up, especially if you are using an oil medium, and you will drag them over the face – which will be scratchy.

The client may prefer to use eye pads to avoid getting any granules in the eye. Remember also to check the client's ears – and chest area (and in the bra!) – when removing the product, and certainly before she leaves the salon, as granules tend to fall in and look unsightly. The more you have to work with, the harder it is to remove and the messier it seems to get. Practice makes perfect, and in time you will be able to judge the amount of product needed quite effectively.

Using and adapting massage techniques

Facial massage

All massage is extremely therapeutic, whether of the face, scalp or body. It is very relaxing both to give a facial massage and to receive one. A good therapist knows her massage movements so well that she doesn't have to think about where her hands go next, and she can also enjoy the experience.

Massage movements can also be incorporated into a cleansing routine, and most other facial and cleansing treatments.

To be truly relaxing, a good massage has continuity, rhythm and the correct depth, appropriate to the area and the needs of the client.

Facial massage has several benefits.

○ It helps dead surface cells to loosen and be shed. This helps the natural exfoliation process and produces a clean-looking, fresh complexion.

○ Facial muscles are relaxed, and they receive more blood supply because of the stimulation to the circulation. This improves the tone and strength of the muscles, giving a firmer facial appearance.

○ As the blood circulation is improved the face area is warmed. This is very relaxing if muscles are clenched and tense in the jaw and forehead.

○ An increase in lymphatic drainage to the face (massage always flows in the direction of the lymph nodes) produces an increase in cellular activity and the removal of toxins. The sebaceous glands are stimulated to increase sebum production, and this keeps the skin protected and supple.

To make the treatment doubly effective, and help the massage medium penetrate deeper into the skin, try the application of heat on to the skin with either hot towels, steaming or exfoliation by brush cleansing.

Psychologically, massage is very beneficial. It is so relaxing that some clients drift off to sleep! The gentle rhythm is soothing and calming. The atmosphere in your working area should enhance this; relaxing music helps the process along and encourages the client to let go of conscious thought and drift away.

Your massage movements may need adapting for the different skin types, conditions and mediums, as well as muscular tension present and the client choice of medium. You should ask the client if she prefers oil or cream. Oily skin is best massaged with cream to avoid adding oil to the skin. Dry skin soaks up oil (although the client may prefer cream) – make sure you have enough medium on at the beginning so the massage is not disturbed by you breaking contact to apply more.

Minor contra-indications, such as a bruise, can be avoided and muscular tension in the upper back will require firmer movements. Check with the client if she prefers a firm massage or more gentle massage – ideally, facial massage will relax the client to such an extent that she goes to sleep, so avoid vigorous movements.

Massage mediums

Some product houses supply their own massage medium in their treatment range which has the same active ingredients as their face masks and cleansers. Some mediums have aromatherapy oils already added – such as Decleor products. Always follow manufacturer's instructions and remember to check if your client has a nut allergy before using almond oil or any other nut-based oil.

Facial massage movements

Massage movements are performed with the hands over the neck, shoulders and chest, as well as the facial area. The movements require practice in order to perfect the skills and outcomes required.

Movements are adapted according to the client's needs and relate directly to the facial analysis or the consultation. It may be that your client has specific areas of tension, or that her skin is particularly dry and therefore needs an oil, rather than a cream.

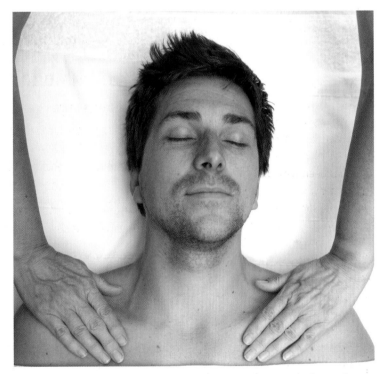

A good massage is very relaxing and therapeutic

The basic massage movements are classified by their names (in French) and their particular effects and benefits to the skin. These are:

○ effleurage   ○ tapotement   ○ petrissage   ○ frictions   ○ vibrations.

There are two types of effleurage: superficial and deep.

Superficial effleurage
This is a light, flowing pressure used at the beginning and the end of most treatments. It introduces your hands on to the client, spreads the massage medium and can be a great linking movement to help the massage flow.

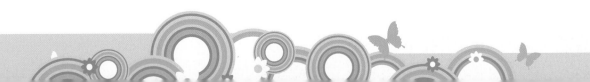

How do I do it?

Use the entire palmar surface of the hands, keeping the fingers together and the thumb either close into the side of the hand, or open and out of the way. The area being massaged is covered by all or part of the palmar surface. Pressure should be light and even, with good contact with the skin, and the hands should be warm and relaxed.

Superficial effleurage does not normally affect the circulation as it is not a deep movement, so it can be used in any direction.

The benefits of superficial effleurage are:

- relaxation of tense muscle fibres
- a general feeling of relaxation
- stimulation of sensory nerve ending and a feeling of pleasure
- introduction of the massage medium and cream on to the skin
- a soothing and calming sensation.

Think about it

How you approach massage also affects your client and the mood of the treatment. If you are rushed and hurried, no benefit will be gained by your client. Be calm, fully prepared and collect your thoughts before you begin. Giving a massage should be a little like meditation for the therapist – a quiet, soothing time for you both.

Deep effleurage

This is the same type of movement as superficial effleurage but with more pressure applied – not too much to make the sensation uncomfortable, but enough to encourage muscular relaxation and for you to feel the tension knots.

Maintaining contact with the skin helps avoid overstimulation of the nerve endings. This is because when contact is broken and then re-established, it sets up a reflex response in the nerve endings, which prevents the muscles from relaxing.

The benefits of deep effleurage are that it aids:

- venous return
- arterial circulation by removal of congestion from veins
- desquamation.

Petrissage

There are four different categories:

- kneading
- wringing – mostly used on body
- rolling – mostly used on body
- picking up.

Petrissage always follows effleurage. It is a compression movement performed using intermittent pressure with either one or both hands, using the hands in different positions. Most petrissage movements work on all or part of a muscle and it is important that, as a muscle is slowly released from application, pressure is reduced.

Petrissage movements must be applied rhythmically and not in a hurried way. Too much pressure may result in damage to the skin – adaptation to the client's needs is vital.

Petrissage has several benefits.

- Aching, hard muscles are relaxed, helping to prevent the formation of tension modules.
- Skin regeneration is stimulated.
- It has a toning effect on muscle tissue.
- It helps eliminate muscular fatigue by aiding in the removal of lactic acid.
- It helps the removal of waste products and lymphatic flow.

Frictions

Frictions are classified within the petrissage group, but their purpose differs. Friction movements will loosen adherent skin, loosen scars, and aid in absorption of fluid around the joints. The pressure is firm and the movement is usually applied in circular directions on the face. Fingertips or thumbs are mostly used in small areas.

Frictions have two main benefits.

- Adhesions and loose skin are freed.
- Scar tissue can be stretched and loosened.

Tapotement

Tapotement is a percussion movement and involves what its name implies — tapping. The tips of the fingers are used over the face to create very light tapping movements, which stimulate the skin.

It is very important that sufficient adipose tissue is present to perform the treatment. It is not used on sensitive skin to avoid possible overreaction and skin damage.

Tapotement has two main benefits.

- It increases localised blood supply.
- It increases nervous response due to stimulation.

Vibrations

Vibrations are fine, trembling movements performed on or along a nerve path by the fingers. The muscles of the operator's forearm are continually contracted and relaxed to produce a fine tremble or vibration, which runs to the fingertips. It is used at the occipital region in facial massage.

The benefits of vibrations are:

- it can relieve pain
- it can relax the client due to its sedative effect.

Think about it

Always use effleurage to link petrissage movements.

Think about it

Make sure you have enough of the massage medium on the skin. If you have too little, the hands become sticky and the movements will not flow. If you have too much, it will run down the client's face! If in the first application you can judge that the client's skin is dry and is soaking up the cream or oil, then apply a little more at the beginning of the second application, rather than having to stop the massage to apply more.

Salon life

My story

My name is Candice and I really wanted to go on to Level 3 but I was having trouble remembering all the information about products, massage movements and skin types for facials at Level 2. I asked my mum and sisters to have facials at home for me to practise my skills and then they started coming into college to model too. It has really made a difference to my confidence — I can now complete my massage without having to refer to my sheet. I would say to anyone just starting that you need to keep practising your skills — it really does make you perfect!

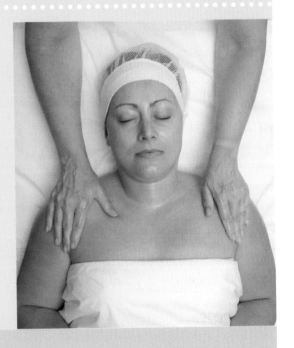

Effects of facials

Benefits of a facial for the client:

- Professional skin analysis for correct diagnosis of skin type
- Healthier looking skin and general health benefits due to better circulation of lymph and blood
- Mental and physical relaxation
- Aftercare advice and product recommendations

Benefits of a facial for the therapist:

- Excellent retail opportunities in recommending products
- Diversity of treatments and clients keeps the day interesting
- Good recommendations and treatments can improve client's confidence as well as their skin — this can be very rewarding

ASK THE EXPERTS

Q *What is the most important part of a facial?*

A The consultation. You need to understand the client's needs before you begin so you can choose the right products and give the correct aftercare advice.

Q *What if a man wants a facial? What should I do?*

A Male skin is slightly thicker but you can follow the basic routine, just as you would for a female client. You will have no make-up to remove but cleansing is still important. For comfort, ensure your movements go downwards with the hair growth pattern rather than against it. Use clean sponges when removing products as cotton wool may get stuck in beard hair.

Top tips

- Practice, practice, practice until facials are routine to you. This allows you to concentrate on the client and their needs rather than focusing on what you are doing.
- Don't be afraid to try new products — the more knowledge you have, the more you can offer your clients.
- Be flexible. Product houses have different methods and procedures and your massage movements will evolve and develop as your confidence grows. When you have qualified you may change and adapt your massage routines according to who you are working with — sharing good practice and picking up tips from more experienced therapists is a great way to learn.

Step-by-step facial massage routine

Female client

All movements should be carried out six times. The massage should last for 20 minutes.

1 Apply massage medium all over the face, neck and shoulders and spread evenly. With both hands together, start at chin, and move down either side of neck towards shoulders.

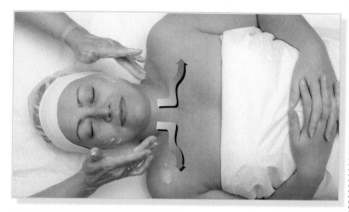

2 Apply pressure over the chest and go over the shoulders, working along the upper back towards the spine.

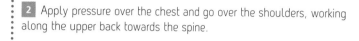

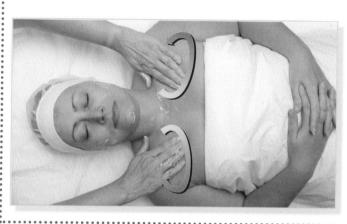

3 When your hands reach either side of the spine, work upwards and gently stretch the neck, lifting the head slightly off the couch.

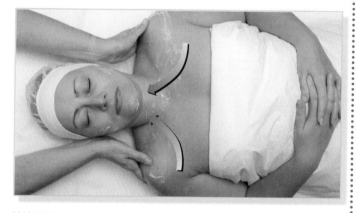

4 Face brace: with hands in an upside-down prayer position, begin under the chin, with heels of the hands resting lightly on the chin. Work upwards, over the cheeks, lifting quite firmly The cheeks will move slightly, as the client is relaxed.

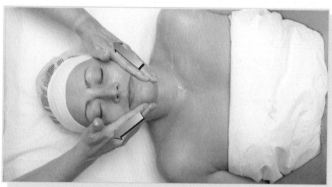

5 Finish with a firm, lifting movement on the forehead.

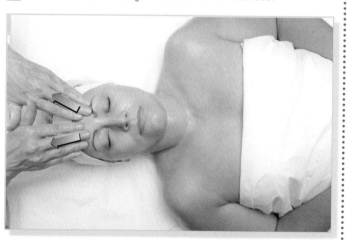

6 From the forehead, gently slide the hands back to the jawline.

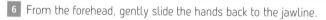

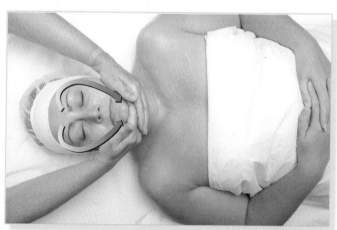

7 Perform rotaries of petrissage, starting from the chin and moving down either side of the neck towards the shoulders and beyond, paying special attention to the arm and deltoid muscle. Use small circular motions across all of the chest area. You may only be able to use your fingertips if the client is small – no long nails!

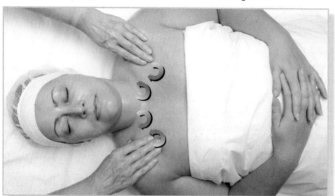

8 Continue your circular massage up the sides of the neck, ready to begin another movement.

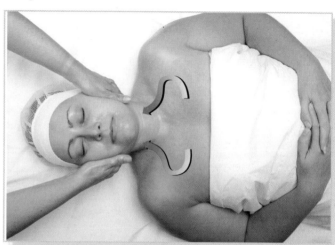

9 Turn your hands into loose fists and rotate your fingers to form knuckling. Come down from the neck and across the chest, over shoulders and back to the occipital cavity.

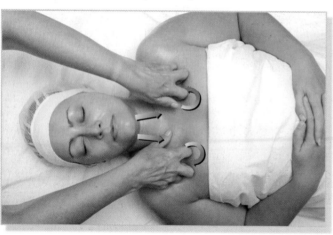

10 Finish the movement at the jawline ready to begin alternate triangular sweeping.

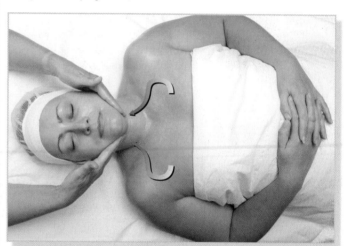

11 Support the jaw with your left hand; with the right hand, stroke down the right side, to the shoulder. Stroke across the chest to the other shoulder.

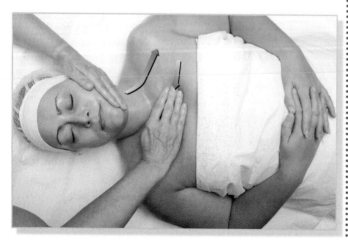

12 Take your right hand behind the shoulder.

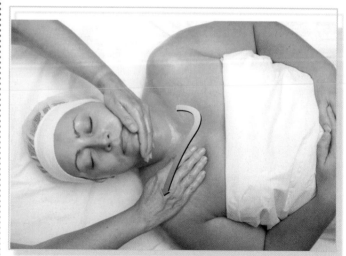

13 Stroke your left hand across the chest to meet the right hand at the right shoulder.

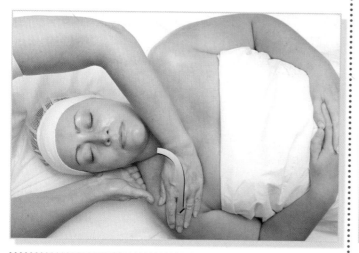

14 Bring the right hand back up to the jaw and left hand back across the chest.

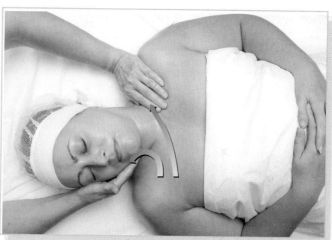

15 Bring the left hand back up to meet at the jaw.

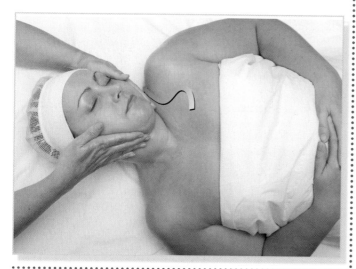

16 Bring the right hand back down at the shoulder.

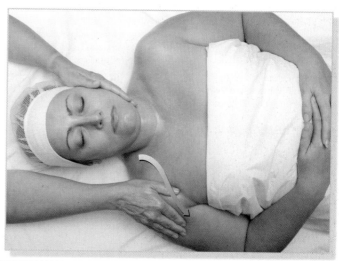

17 Perform trapezius rolling — work hands together on one side, then the other.

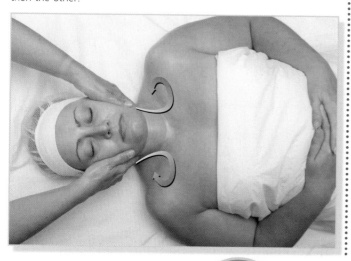

18 Cheek lift — index finger to little finger — turn and twist off.

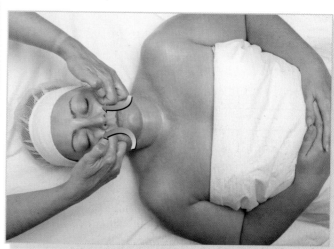

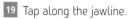

19 Tap along the jawline.

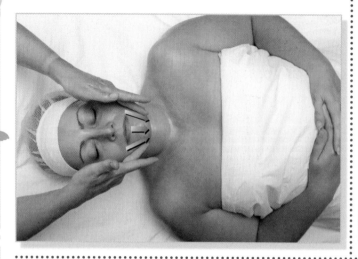

20 Perform rotaries along jawline — thumbs abducted — centre outwards.

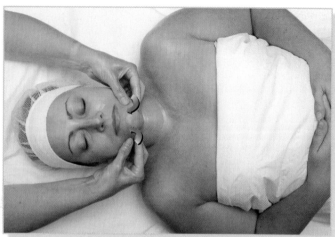

21 Knuckle over chin and cheeks.

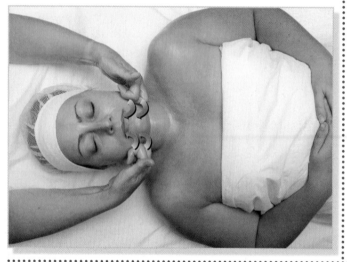

22 Facial lift — work hands along each side of the face — lift and join hands together over the forehead, then divide off.

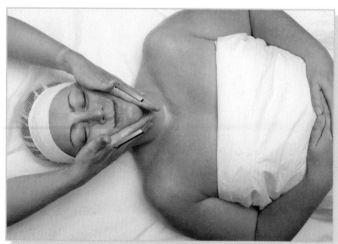

23 Forehead brace — both hands lift up the eyebrows to the hairline.

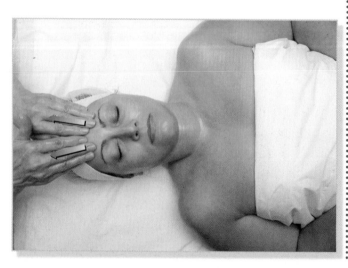

24 Turn hands sideways and gently pull the forehead from the centre, smoothing out the temples.

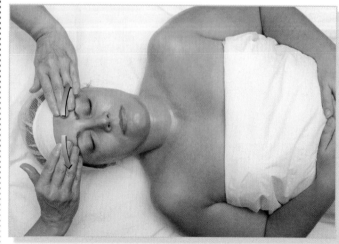

25 Finish with slight finger rotation pressure at the temples.

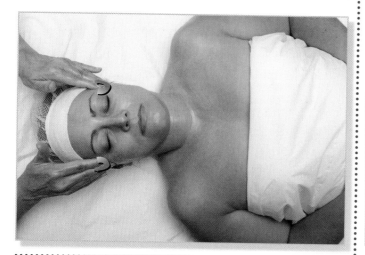

26 Slide hands down to the jaw. Pinch along the jawline, using thumb and forefinger.

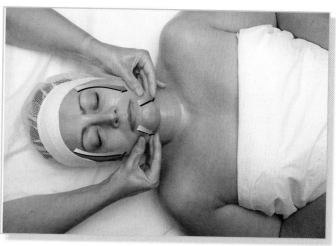

27 Using alternate hand movements, begin roll patting over cheeks and forehead. Repeat this movement over both sides of the face.

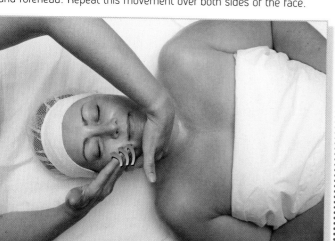

28 Tap over cheeks, using light pressure – fingertips only.

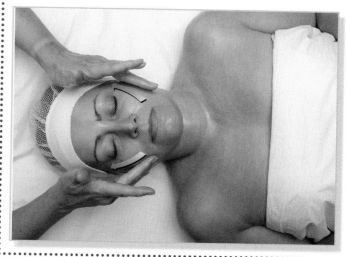

29 Apply frictions, using index fingers, around mouth and chin.

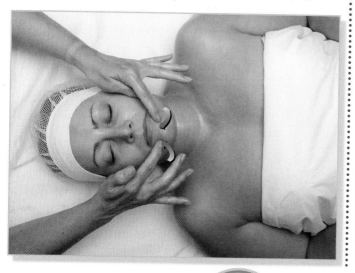

30 Apply frictions, using index fingers, around nostrils.

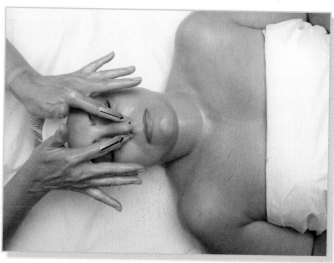

31 Work up nose with index fingers.

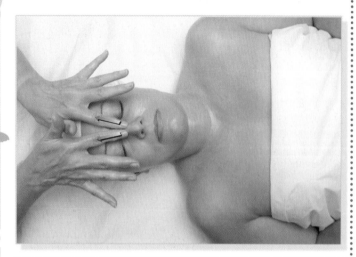

32 Zigzag with middle fingers going into a V created by the other hand over forehead.

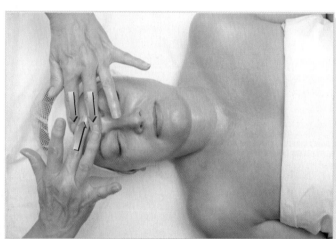

33 Working right across and down the forehead, cover all areas — this movement is especially appreciated by clients who suffer from headaches.

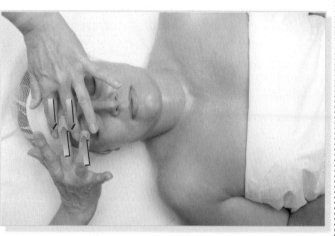

34 Do small circular pinching movements along the length of the eyebrows.

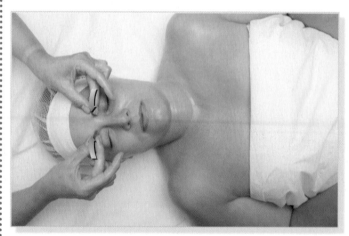

35 Piano playing across brow: circle eyes and bring all fingers across the brow. Start with little finger and finish with index finger.

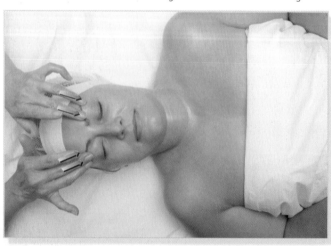

36 Pinch brows — centre to sides. Slide back and repeat.

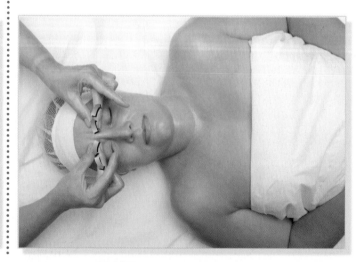

37 Come back to jawline and begin superficial effleurage down either side of the neck.

38 Perform superficial effleurage over shoulder area, gradually slowing down as you finish the massage.

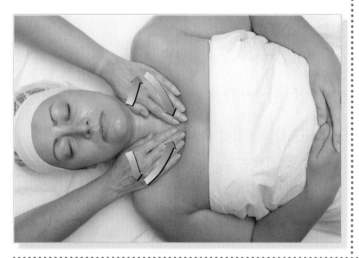

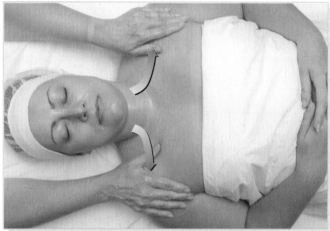

Male client

1 Cleanse as per a female client, making sure to treat the entire forehead. Long hair may still require a headband.

2 Use sponges and warm water to remove cleanser rather than cotton wool, which tends to break up over facial hair causing fluff.

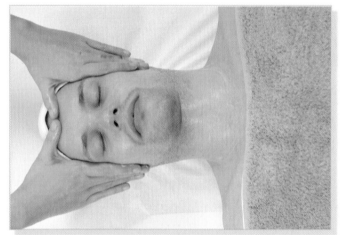

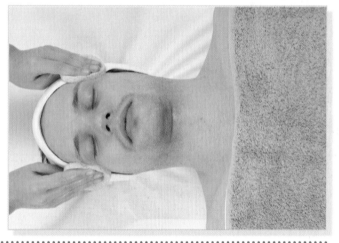

3 A facial scrub or mask will exfoliate and deep cleanse the pores, especially if the client isn't shaving.

4 Remove scrub or mask with warm water and sponges. Pat dry, tone and moisturise.

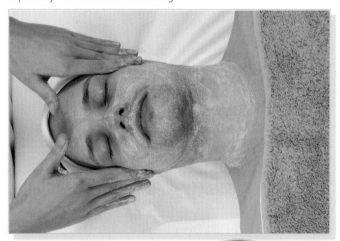

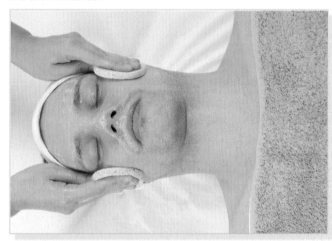

Provide facial skincare treatment **Unit B4**

Think about it

Different product houses have different massage routines and you will be taught various movements when you do your training for them. Over time and with lots of experience, you will find your massage routine grows and evolves – you will leave out some movements and put in others. Remember, movements for your assessments need to be recognisable to your assessor – so stick with the routine in the book until you have passed this unit and then you can adapt your massage to suit you and your client.

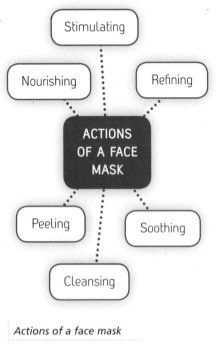

Actions of a face mask

Applying mask treatments evenly and neatly

A large variety of face masks are available, both over the counter and in salons. Face masks can be made out of many different natural ingredients, and there is a huge choice of prepared or ready-mixed masks. They can be divided into two categories.

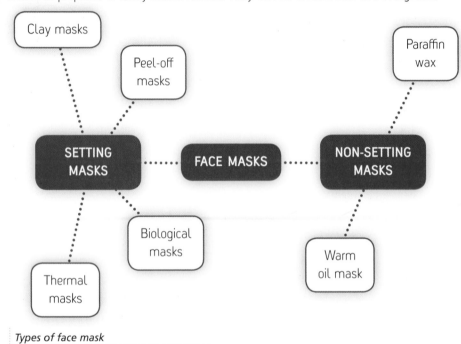

Types of face mask

Masks can have different actions depending upon their formulation.

The choice of mask depends on accurate skin analysis and knowledge of the effects of the basic mask ingredients.

Some masks come already mixed and some need mixing – generally the pre-prepared types tend to be more expensive. The ones that need mixing require more skill and knowledge of the ingredients and proportions, but the basic ingredients can be purchased in bulk and stored.

Natural ingredients can also be used as a face mask and provide great variety and fun!

Properties of face masks

○ They should be smooth and free from gritty particles and unpleasant odours. In powder form, they should be easily dispersed in water to produce a paste.

○ They should be easily removed from the face after use without causing discomfort.

○ They must be harmless to the skin and non-toxic.

Contra-indications to the application of face masks include:

- skin disorders and diseases
- excessively dry or sensitive skin
- loose, crepey skin
- cuts and abrasions
- recent scar tissue.

Note: Clients who suffer from claustrophobia may prefer a non-setting mask.

Materials required for a face mask treatment include:

- bowls
- spatulas
- mask brush – flat and sanitised
- damp cotton wool
- headband
- tissues
- skin tonic
- moisturiser
- couch roll
- client record card
- scissors for eye pads.

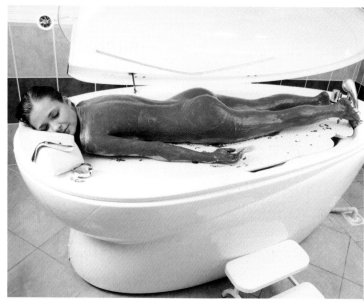

Masks can be used on the body too

Clay masks

Clays can be classed as natural ingredients because they are found in the earth. They are good at drawing out impurities and deep cleansing. Some can be quite stimulating and are good for improving the circulation; others are mild and soothing on the skin. The key is to know which ingredients are suitable for which skin type.

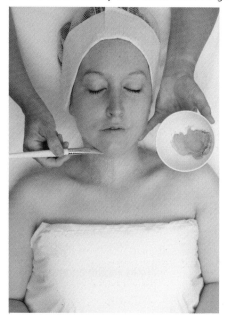

Fuller's earth face mask application

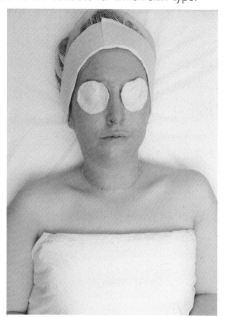

Fuller's earth face mask

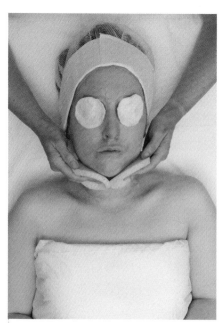

Removing a Fuller's earth face mask

Provide facial skincare treatment **Unit B4**

315

Skin type	Clay powder	Benefits	Mixed with
Dry	Calamine (a pink powder)	Contains zinc carbonate to soothe the skin and calm down a high colour	Rose water, orange flower water (or distilled water for sensitive skin)
	Magnesium carbonate (a white powder)	Refines and softens the skin, mildly astringent	A couple of drops of vegetable oil, almond oil or glycerol can be added
Greasy	Fuller's earth (a grey/green powder)	Deep cleansing	Distilled water with a drop of witch hazel if required Witch hazel is not suitable for a sensitive, greasy skin as it can be quite stimulating
	Sulphur (a pale yellow powder)	Drying action so can be used on individual blemishes	Distilled water with a drop of witch hazel if required
Normal (balanced)	Magnesium carbonate (a white powder)	Refines and softens the skin, mildly astringent	Mix with equal proportions of rose water, orange flower water or witch hazel
	Calamine (a pink powder)	Contains zinc carbonate to soothe the skin and calm down a high colour	Mix with equal proportions of rose water, orange flower water or witch hazel
	Fuller's earth (a grey/green powder)	Deep cleansing; not suitable for sensitive skin as it can be quite stimulating	Mix with equal proportions of rose water, orange flower water or witch hazel
Combination	Follow the dry/normal skin for cheek areas and greasy skin for T-zone skin, depending upon the severity of each area		

Active ingredients

A clay mask needs to be mixed with active ingredients to turn the powder into a liquid paste. The liquids are selected to complement the skin type and mask to be used – they reinforce the action of the mask.

- **Rose water** gives a mild toning effect, which increases the toning action of a mask. Made from rose petals. Recommended for dry, normal and mature skin types.
- **Orange flower water** gives a stimulating, tonic effect. This is natural plant extract from the fruit of the tree.
- **Citrus dulcis** is very fragrant. Recommended for normal, dry and mature skin types.
- **Witch hazel** has a drying, stimulating effect, so is contra-indicated on fine sensitive skins; it is much better suited to greasy or combination skins. It is made from the dried leaves and bark of the hamamelis virginiana tree. It has a tissue-firming action on the skin.
- **Almond oil** can be used on dehydrated or neglected younger skins or on the more mature skin. A natural oil obtained from the kernels of the seeds of whole almonds, it improves the condition of the skin.
- **Distilled water** is ordinary water that has had the chemicals, such as magnesium bicarbonate or calcium carbonate, removed from it. These can be removed by boiling the water or chemically removed by water softeners.
- **Calamine lotion** is a liquid which contains zinc carbonate to soothe and heal the skin. Iron oxide produces the pink colouring.

Think about it

Always check your own posture and position for both mask application and massage techniques – your position should minimise fatigue and the risk of injury. If you have been sitting when giving the massage, you may wish to get up and apply the mask from the front, facing the client, instead of stretching over and getting backache.

Skin type	Recipe	Time on face
Normal	1 part kaolin 1 part Fuller's earth Mix with water and a few drops of witch hazel to form a smooth, thin paste	8–12 minutes
Dry	1 part kaolin 1 part magnesium carbonate Mix with rose water or orange flower water to form a smooth, thin paste	10–15 minutes
Oily	Fuller's earth Mix with witch hazel to form a smooth paste	5–15 minutes
Sensitive	1 part calamine 1 part magnesium carbonate Mix with rose water to form a smooth paste	5–10 minutes

Mask type	Recipe	Time on face
Sulphur mask (for acne)	$\frac{1}{2}$ tsp Epsom salts 1 tsp oatmeal 1 tsp magnesium carbonate 1 tsp precipitated sulphur Mix with hot water to form a paste	Apply over gauze, leave for 15 minutes, keeping warm with infrared lamp
Stimulating mask (for open pores, capillaries and contracting the tissues)	6 parts magnesium carbonate 2 parts fuller's earth Mix with rose water or almond oil according to the moisture content of the skin	5–15 minutes
Astringent mask (to dry an oily skin)	6 parts magnesium carbonate 1 part calamine Pinch of alum Mix with witch hazel	Apply over gauze Apply one coat until almost dry, then apply second coat 10 minutes

Think about it

The setting times for all types of masks, including paraffin wax, are to be used as a general guide only, and you should go by the client response and how the skin reacts to the mask ingredients – this is why it is important never to leave the client unattended. Mask setting depends upon many variable factors: how active the ingredients are, how warm the room is, how hot the client is, what skin type the client has, if the skin is particularly sensitive and even hormone fluctuations (which often affect body temperature). Always judge by looking at the skin, asking the client and remove the mask immediately if you think the skin is reacting.

Peel-off masks

Peel-off masks are gel or latex based. (Paraffin wax masks also come into the peel-off category, although they are classed as non-setting.) Because perspiration cannot escape from the skin's surface, moisture is forced back into the epidermis. Some peel-off masks also create heat, so could come under the thermal category.

Provide facial skincare treatment Unit B4

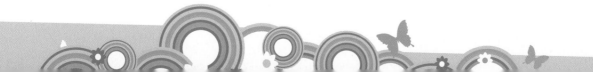

317

Gel masks are purchased as a ready-made suspension containing starches, gums or gelatine, to allow the correct consistency. Synthetic non-biological resins are commonly used as well. The mask is applied over the skin. When it makes contact it immediately begins to dry. It can be peeled off over the face as a whole facial mould when sufficient technique has been mastered. The gel mask can be used on most skin types, depending on the ingredients used, so check with individual manufacturer's instructions.

A latex mask is an emulsion of latex and water. The water evaporates leaving a rubber film to form the mask. Alternatives are synthetic PVC resins. These have a firming, tightening effect on the skin and can be used on a dry or mature skin.

Biological and natural masks

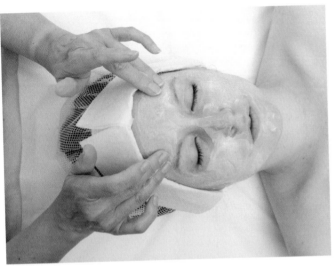

Work an exfoliant mask into the skin using small circular motions

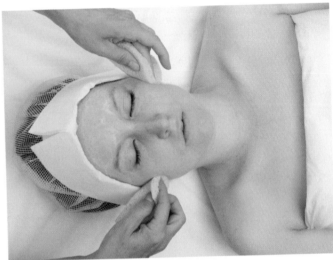

Remove mask thoroughly with warm water and sponges

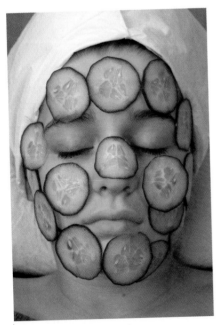

Natural cucumber mask

These include the following:

○ **Fruit extracts**, e.g. avocado mashed to a smooth paste. Action: helps stabilise the skin's pH and acid mantle.

○ **Herbal and vegetable**, e.g. cucumber sliced and placed over the skin. Action: calming or astringent effect.

○ **Biological**, e.g. natural yoghurt applied in bought state. Action: refines the skin's texture, helps rid skin of waste, counteracts possible infection.
Egg mask – with almond oil for dry skin or lemon for oily skin.
Honey mask – has a softening effect on dehydrated or mature skin.

Warm oil masks

The skin is cleansed, and a piece of gauze is soaked in warm olive or almond oil. Eye pads are placed over the eyes, and the gauze is carefully put on to the face. An infrared lamp is placed in position for 10–20 minutes. The distance of the lamp is determined prior to application to suit the client's skin type.

The time of the treatment will depend upon the client's skin tolerance and how hot they get, whether the skin starts to show erythema and client preference.

Risk assessment for warm oil equipment

Refer to Unit G20, Make sure your own actions reduce risks to health and safety, pages 71–86, for a complete discussion of risk assessment.

Hazard: only look for hazards that you could reasonably expect to result in significant harm under the conditions in your workplace. Use the following examples as a guide.

- **Fire** (e.g. from electrical flex or lead)
- **Burning of equipment** (through light bulb burning out)
- **Burns to skin** (lamp too close to skin, left on too long, treatment not timed)
- **Ejection of bulb** (hot bulb falling on to skin, not screwed in properly, lamp should not be directly over skin)
- **Electricity** (e.g. poor wiring)
- **Manual handling** (outer casing is hot and will burn if towel is not used for protection)
- **Falling machinery** (if supporting arm is not screwed in properly)
- **Contamination** (from brushes and equipment not sufficiently sterilised)
- **Cross-infection** (if possible contra-indications are ignored)

Indications for use

- Crepey, finely lined skin
- Premature ageing
- Dehydration or dry skin
- Younger skin as a preventative measure

It is important to prepare the client and couch adequately to protect all areas.

Effects

- It cleanses and aids desquamation.
- It increases smoothness, softness and elasticity.
- As the mask works on heat penetration, the skin will absorb cosmetic preparations more easily, so make-up should be avoided.

Massage oil into the skin after application for maximum benefit. Ensure toning and moisturising is thorough without overstretching or over touching the skin.

The client should be advised that the skin might have an uneven appearance directly after application for 3–4 hours.

Paraffin wax mask treatments

Preparation

A small amount of sterilised paraffin wax should be poured into a small, clean bowl lined with foil. (Wax heaters may be too large to be mobile.) The working temperature is 49°C.

The wax treatment may be applied within the facial routine in place of a setting mask. Disposable paper should cover towels for protection.

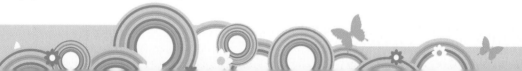

Application

Eye pads are put in place. Wax should be applied in a firm build-up over the neck, cheeks, chin, nose and forehead, using a small brush. The client should have complete confidence in the treatment and your presence so she can relax.

○ Wax must be applied to a clean skin that is free from oil, cream, etc.

○ The protective band should be checked to avoid soiling.

○ The mask is applied as a thin, even film over the face and neck with a brush or spatula.

○ Eyes, nostrils and mouth areas must be avoided.

The application must be accomplished quickly and neatly.

Note: A combination skin condition may require the application of two or more masks to suit the different areas.

Depending upon the skin type, time may vary between 10 and 20 minutes. This will depend upon the skin's reaction and client tolerance to the ingredients – do not let the mask dry on for too long as it will be very difficult to remove.

Remove the eye pads, gently slide the fingers under the edges of the mask, place the hands under the mask at the throat, pulling the mask up a little at a time and taking care that any bits of mask are stuck to the main bulk. Pressure toning with water may be suitable, but usually it is best to leave this.

Risk assessment for paraffin wax equipment

Refer to Unit G20, Make sure your own actions reduce risks to health and safety, pages 71–86, for a complete discussion of risk assessment.

Hazard: only look for hazards that you could reasonably expect to result in significant harm under the conditions in your workplace. Use the following examples as a guide.

- **Fire** (e.g. from electrical flex or lead)
- **Burning of equipment** (through low wax level in the tank)
- **Burns to skin** (from not testing wax temperature first on self)
- **Ejection of materials** (spitting hot wax)
- **Electricity** (e.g. poor wiring)
- **Manual handling** (spillage possible if moving when in liquid form)
- **Falling machinery** (if not securely positioned on a trolley)

Effects

○ Natural perspiration cleans the skin.

○ Circulation is improved.

○ Dead cells are removed and desquamation is improved.

○ Elasticity, smoothness and softness of texture are increased.

○ Removes cellular matter.

○ Moisturises the skin.

○ There is a local increase in temperature.

Indications

- Dry, dehydrated skin
- Mature skin, where regeneration is needed without overstimulation
- Crepey, finely lined skin
- Uneven-textured skin (unstable pH) to promote desquamation and refine texture
- Seborrhoea conditions, to remove oily blockages and surface adhesions

Contra-indications

- Highly nervous, tense clients, or those suffering from claustrophobia
- Extreme vascular conditions
- Sepsis, skin infection and irritation

Client preparation

- The client should be prepared as for cleansing.
- Hair and clothing should be well protected.
- The face should then be cleansed to remove all make-up.
- After deciding on the formula, the powder ingredients are placed in a bowl and mixed to a smooth paste by gradually adding the liquid.

Basic mask formulation

As every facial diagnosis differs slightly, no formulation can be assumed to be suitable for all skin conditions. No rules can apply in mask therapy due to the variety of mask products and the different actions they are capable of producing. Observation and client discussion regarding tolerance to the mask will increase your knowledge of the skin's reaction to certain ingredients.

Final tips for face masks

- Follow the manufacturer's instructions.
- Always use the mask that complements the products being used, e.g. René Guinot or Clarins or whichever range the salon is using.
- Always do a thorough facial analysis to be able to decide the correct mask for the client.

> **Think about it**
>
> When you have finished the client's treatments always check that the client is satisfied with the results and that they meet the agreed treatment plan. Provide a hand mirror so the client can see just how clean and fresh the skin has become.

Provide aftercare advice

In this outcome you will learn about:

- giving advice and recommendations accurately and constructively
- giving the clients suitable advice specific to their individual needs

After a facial it is important to recognise that the immediate aftercare is as important as the long-term aftercare if maximum benefit is to be gained from the salon treatment. Much of this information can be found in Unit G18 Promote additional products or services to clients. Read that unit for tips on how to promote additional services and give accurate information.

Unit B4 **Provide facial skincare treatment**

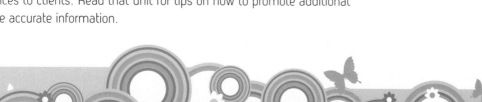

Giving suitable advice and recommendations

Always talk through the aftercare with your client. The client should leave the salon knowing exactly what to do to help the skin and to reinforce the benefits of the salon treatment.

Immediate aftercare to avoid contra-actions

The skin has been deep cleansed, stimulated and nourished. No aftercare is needed except to leave it alone. Avoid picking, squeezing pimples or touching the area.

○ Avoid the temptation to apply make-up for 12 hours, where possible.

○ Evening cleansing is not necessary, but if the client prefers, a light cleanse, tone and moisture may be recommended.

○ Suitable and compatible homecare products should be recommended. These will complement the work of the therapist in the salon.

○ Explain to clients that while it is unlikely that contra-actions will develop after a facial, they should avoid any overstimulation and further heat treatments. If a reaction is going to occur, it will usually be a reaction to a cream used while the facial is going on, not afterwards.

○ Highly perfumed products should be avoided.

○ No depilation (hair removal) should take place after a facial.

○ If any rash, irritation or itching occurs, suggest putting a cool flannel to the area. Remove the offending product from the skin with damp cotton wool, and apply a light calamine lotion to soothe the skin.

Long-term and homecare advice

○ Regular use of homecare products will help the skin.

○ Regular facials will help to regulate a problem skin; timings and intervals are a personal decision between the therapist and client and may depend on cost.

○ Future treatments may be discussed with a view to specialist help for specific problems, such as facial steaming for comedone extraction, or regular paraffin wax mask application for a dry skin condition.

○ Targeting a problem and then giving intensive treatments to help that condition is very rewarding. The client is pleased and the therapist has job satisfaction.

○ A treatment plan should make allowances for timing intervals, the cost involved and how convenient it is for the client to get to the salon.

○ Give the client a price list and all relevant information for present and future treatments with you.

○ Give your client accurate information about additional products and services. Refer to Unit G18, pages 113–15.

Think about it

Your workstation may be shared by other therapists. Most salons have a waxing area, a facial area and a body treatment section, so if your next client is in the waxing room, you have to leave your facial station clean for another therapist to use. Would you like to inherit a messy work area from another therapist?

A client leaving the salon in a relaxed and satisfied state is very rewarding, but your work is not yet over. There are important details to complete, which are as much a part of your job role as everything else that you do. These include completing client records accurately. Take time to fill out all parts of the record card:

○ Were there any reactions during the treatment that will affect the future treatment plan?

○ Did the client express any preferences or dislikes for massage movements, products or mask?

○ Would you leave something out next time?

○ Did the client feel claustrophobic with eye pads on?

○ Were products purchased?

Finally, you must leave the work area and equipment ready for further treatments (see page 265).

Frequently asked questions

Q What instructions should I give to a male client booking in for a facial?

A All treatments are private and confidential whether the client is male or female. Facial massage includes the upper back and shoulders, so upper clothing will be removed but the chest will be covered with a towel to keep the client warm. Advise the client to have as close a shave as possible on the morning of the treatment, to avoid dragging on the facial hair. He should wear loose clothing to aid relaxation, such as a track suit or casual clothing rather than a formal suit.

Q What action should I take if I discover the client has a contra-indication to a facial treatment?

A If the contra-indication is an infection or inflammation, stop the treatment immediately, and suggest that the client sees their GP. You must not make a diagnosis, only a recommendation that the client seek medical attention. If the contra-indication is of a minor nature, simply avoid the area and adapt the treatment accordingly.

Q How would I recognise the signs or symptoms of skin damage?

A The skin ages prematurely causing breakdown of collagen and elastin, which supports the skin, and uneven pigmentation can also occur. There may be contamination of the skin, clogged and blocked pores, irritation and a tendency to comedones and allergic reactions. Skin damage causes dehydration and overactivity of the sebaceous glands resulting in problems. The skin may be overstretched. Inappropriate products can cause comedones to form or an oversensitive skin.

Q Why is it important to complete client records accurately?

A To record relevant details to be able to contact the client if necessary; to provide full and accurate information which will ensure client safety; to ensure consistency of treatment regardless of who performs the treatment; to record the number of treatments in a course and the date of each one; to record changes to the treatment programme or contra-actions if they occur; to record the progress of the condition or treatment success; to safeguard the salon and the therapists against clients taking legal action for damages or negligence.

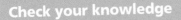

Unit B4 Provide facial skincare treatment

Check your knowledge

1 A skin analysis should be carried out:
   a) after a superficial cleanse
   b) before removing make-up
   c) after the deep cleanse
   d) after the face mask.

2 When in the facial would you use a facial warming treatment such as hot towels or steaming?
   a) After the cleanse
   b) After the mask
   c) After the massage
   d) After extraction

3 The skin type which has oily and dry areas is known as:
   a) unusual skin
   b) problem skin
   c) combination skin
   d) sensitive skin.

4 Facial massage is carried out:
   a) after a deep cleanse
   b) after a face mask
   c) after coffee break
   d) after eye make-up removal.

5 Massage is good for the skin because:
   a) it helps bring oxygen to the skin surface
   b) it soothes the nerve endings
   c) it smoothes out wrinkles
   d) it makes you thinner in the face.

6 The most suitable cleanser for dry skin is:
   a) cream cleanser
   b) milk cleanser
   c) wash-off cleanser
   d) baby lotion.

7 A contra-action to a face mask would be:
   a) milia
   b) a rash or itching
   c) blackheads
   d) keloid tissue.

8 Moisturisers are designed to:
   a) rehydrate the skin
   b) make the skin feel nice
   c) prepare the skin for make-up application
   d) fill up all the wrinkles.

9 Face masks should be of a smooth consistency so that they:
   a) can be applied evenly
   b) look nice on the skin
   c) set quickly
   d) retain moisture.

10 Collagen and elastin are part of:
   a) the epidermis
   b) the dermis
   c) the subcutaneous tissue
   d) the hair follicle.

Getting ready for assessment

- Simulation is not allowed for any performance evidence within this unit.
- You must practically demonstrate in your everyday work that you have met the standard for improving and maintaining facial skin condition.
- Your assessor will observe your performance on at least **three occasions**, **each involving a different client**.
- From the range statement, you must practically demonstrate that you:
  - have used all consultation techniques
  - have carried out at least one of the necessary actions
  - have carried out treatments on two of the three skin conditions
  - have used all types of facial products, massage mediums, massage techniques, masks and provided all types of advice
  - have used all types of equipment.
- It is likely most evidence of your performance will be gathered from the observations made by your assessor, but you may be required to produce other evidence to support your performance if your assessor has not been present.

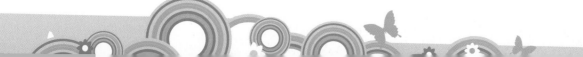

Unit B5

Enhance the appearance of eyebrows and lashes

What you will learn

B5.1   Maintain safe and effective methods of working when enhancing the appearance of eyebrows and eyelashes

B5.2   Consult, plan and prepare for the treatment with clients

B5.3   Shape eyebrows

B5.4   Tint eyebrows and lashes

B5.5   Apply artificial eyelashes

B5.6   Provide aftercare advice

Introduction

This unit focuses on ways to enhance the appearance of eyebrows and lashes by carrying out a range of treatments.

Each of the outcomes can be either combined or carried out independently to meet the requirements of the client.

Some therapists view this section as 'small treatments', but it should not be undervalued. Clients can instantly see an improvement with an eyebrow shape, eyelash tint or application of artificial lashes. Eye treatments can be easily slotted into other treatments: for example, added into the facial while the tint is processing. Remember to include these 'extras' in the cost.

Benefits for the client:

○ fairly quick treatment (depending on the service)

○ immediate result and effect

○ excellent treatment for clients who wear glasses

○ minimum pain from shaping.

Benefits for the therapist

○ easy service to fit into salon day

○ clients find immediate result pleasing

○ excellent opportunity to promote other services

○ enhances wedding, prom and seasonal promotions.

My story

The value of small treatments

My name is Holly. When I first started working in a salon I did not like having only the small eye treatments in my column, especially as my colleagues had larger treatments and could earn more commission from the sale of additional products, for example after a facial. However, my manager encouraged me to use the time with the clients to discuss and introduce other treatments that the salon offered. I found from this that a number of clients booked in not only for further lash and brow maintenance treatments but also for treatments we had discussed. I now value these small treatments as a time to discuss other services with clients.

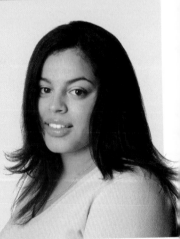

Maintain safe and effective methods of working when enhancing the appearance of eyebrows and eyelashes

In this outcome you will learn about:

- setting up the work area to meet legal, hygiene and treatment requirements
- making sure that environmental conditions are suitable for the client and the treatment
- ensuring your personal hygiene, protection and appearance meets accepted industry and organisational requirements
- ensuring all tools and equipment are cleaned using the correct methods
- effectively disinfecting your hands prior to eyelash and eyebrow treatments
- maintaining accepted industry hygiene and safety practices throughout the treatment
- positioning equipment and materials for ease and safety of use
- ensuring your own posture and position minimises fatigue and the risk of injury while working
- maintaining the client's modesty and privacy at all time
- disposing of waste materials safely and correctly
- ensuring that the treatment is cost-effective and is carried out within a commercially viable time
- leaving the work area in a condition suitable for further treatments
- ensuring the client's records are up to date, accurate, easy to read and signed by the client and practitioner.

For advice on safe and effective methods of working practice, refer to individual treatments:

Shape eyebrows – page 337

Tint eyebrows and lashes – page 339

Apply artificial eyelashes – page 347.

Refer also to Unit B4 Provide facial skincare treatment, and Professional basics, pages 35–47.

Disposing of waste materials safely and correctly

Remember to dispose of all waste materials in the correct bin – if you have drawn blood when eyebrow shaping, the tissue and cotton wool are classed as contaminated material and should be put into a bin liner, which then goes into the yellow bin, to be taken away by your local contractor. Refer to Professional basics, 'You, Your Client and the Law', page 48, for the legal aspects of your actions. Tint brushes, dishes, etc. can be cleaned and ready for use, if reusable. If the tinting brush is a disposable one, put it in a bin with a liner – tint will stain anything it comes into contact with that is porous, including hands and overalls.

Ensuring the treatment is cost-effective

It makes financial sense only to prepare as much product as you are going to use: anything more will oxidise and be thrown away, which is money wasted. Make up the correct quantities of tint, not the whole tube. Be careful with cotton wool and tissues as if you were paying for them out of your own money – wasting products and consumables can cost several pounds each day, so it soon mounts up. Be cost-effective with your time, and remember that you will have other customers waiting for you. Skill is essential, but so is time management: it may be possible for you to fit in, say, enamel application on the same client, while her tint is processing.

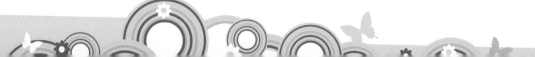

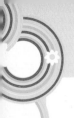

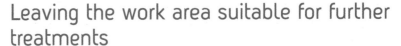

Leaving the work area suitable for further treatments

Always leave your working area as you would wish to find it. Restock tissues or cotton wool, if you have used the last of them, or at least inform the person whose job it is to restock the workstations. Put lids back on pots to prevent products drying out, or oxidising.

Remember that your next client may not be at that couch – you may have to go into the waxing area, or the massage room, and it is not professional to leave a mess for another therapist to tidy up.

Ensuring the client's records are up to date and accurate

While waiting for the tint to develop or the perm to process, you can sit with your client and update her client record card. Although she will have her eyes closed, you can talk to her about aftercare, product use, and caring for her lashes at home, as well as filling in the details of the day's treatments. Now is a good time to check that her address and other personal details are correct, and add any purchases she will be taking home with her.

Consult, plan and prepare for the treatment with clients

In this outcome you will learn about:

- using consultation techniques in a polite and friendly manner to determine the client's treatment plan
- ensuring that informed and signed parental or guardian consent is obtained for minors prior to any treatment
- ensuring that a parent or guardian is present throughout the treatment for minors under the age of 16
- obtaining signed, written informed consent from the client prior to carrying out the treatment
- asking your client appropriate questions to identify if they have any contra-indications to the treatment
- accurately recording your client's responses to questioning
- encouraging clients to ask questions to clarify any points
- helping the client into a safe, comfortable and relaxed position for the treatment

- correctly performing a sensitivity test on a suitable area of the client's skin according to manufacturers' instructions and organisational requirements and recording the results
- ensuring client advice is given without reference to a specific medical condition and without causing undue alarm and concern
- taking the necessary action in response to any identified contra-indications
- informing the client in a tactful way if there is an adverse reaction to the sensitivity test and they cannot be treated
- agreeing the treatment and outcomes that are acceptable to your client and meet their needs
- selecting suitable equipment and materials for the treatment plan based on the outcomes of the sensitivity test
- ensuring your client's clothing, hair and accessories are effectively protected or removed.

Using consultation techniques and obtaining consent

As with all treatments, you will need to carry out a consultation, to check for any contra-indications that may prevent the treatment taking place and to discuss the client's requirements. These contra-indications apply to all eye treatments. (For information on consultation techniques and contra-indications, refer to Professional basics, pages 31 and 35.)

You will need to ensure that the consultation process does not discriminate against clients from different cultures, religious backgrounds or who have disabilities or illness unless any of these areas would deem the treatment unsafe or inappropriate. For example, you should avoid discussing religious topics with clients. You may also need to research illnesses and disabilities to ensure that your client receives the best possible treatment and service.

As with any treatment, if the client is under 16 years of age, signed parental or guardian consent needs to be obtained before treatment can commence and the parent or guardian must be present during the treatment. Every other client would be required to sign to confirm that contra-indications have been checked and that they confirm the treatment plan.

Identifying contra-indications to treatment

During the consultation, you will need to find out if your client has any contra-indications to the treatment by asking her questions and doing a visual check of the area to be treated. Remember to record your client's response to the questions asked. You should also look out for a range of conditions that will contra-indicate treatment. These are the main conditions to look out for:

○ Conjunctivitis – this is a nasty eye condition. The eyelids are red and sore, with itching. Mainly caused by bacteria present. It can be irritated by a virus or an allergy.

○ Stye – this is a small boil at the base of the eyelash follicle. It is raised, sore and red, and there may be considerable swelling in the area.

○ **Blepharitis** – an infection of the lid causing inflammation of the eye, which will look red and sore. Depending on the severity of the condition, you may need to advise the client to see their GP before eye treatments are undertaken.

○ Viral infections – this could include a cold.

○ Bruising to the area.

Reaction to a sensitivity test for tinting, and applying artificial lashes.

You should also be aware of some other conditions:

○ Hypersensitivity – if a client has hypersensitive eyes, it is very important to use hypoallergenic products when cleansing the eyes and ensure a patch test is carried out before the products are used.

○ Active eczema or psoriasis – the area should not be treated, especially if the skin is open or weeping when it is vulnerable to infection and the condition can be spread.

○ Common cold – easily recognised: runny or blocked nose, dry skin around the nose, sneezing, watery eyes, headache.

○ Hay fever – an irritation of the nasal membrane resulting in watery eyes, runny nose and sneezing.

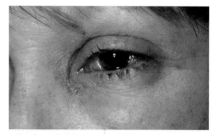
Conjunctivitis

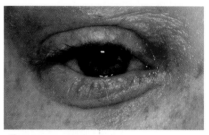
Stye

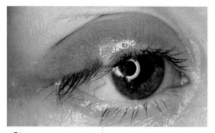
Eczema

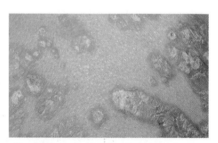
Psoriasis

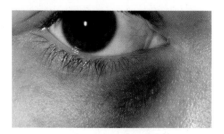
Bruising to the eye area

Key terms

Blepharitis – an infection of the eyelid causing inflammation of the eye.

Enhance the appearance of eyebrows and lashes **Unit B5**

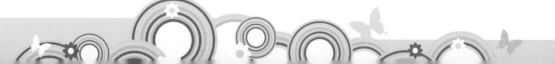

Key terms

Contact dermatitis – a localized rash or irritation of the skin caused by contact with a foreign substance.

Latex – a natural rubber substance often found in protective gloves.

Nitrile – a synthetic rubber substitute that is more durable than latex; can be used as an alternative for therapists or clients with a latex allergy.

Powder-free – some protective gloves contain a powder coating that is used to minimise perspiration and make gloves easier to put on; others contain no such powder and are branded 'powder-free'.

Think about it

It is very easy to cross-infect the eyes, so care must be taken at all times. When carrying out any treatment on the eyes ensure that you use a fresh piece of cotton wool, cotton bud for each eye, and make sure that your tweezers are sterile when transferring from one eye to the next.

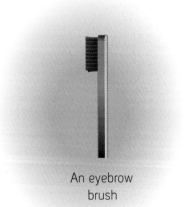

An eyebrow brush

Key term

Terminal hair – strong hair which contains pigment; found on the scalp, eyebrows, under the arms and pubic areas.

○ Watery eyes – an irritating condition, in which the eye area becomes moist, which may make it difficult for the client to have eye treatments.

○ Recent operations – a general rule of thumb is to wait six months before treating an area with scar tissue. However, if it is a minor operation, and you have your client's and her GP's approval, go ahead, but avoid the area itself.

○ Bruising to eye – easy to recognise, a bruise shows as blue/black and yellow skin colouring. Do not treat a bruised eye.

○ **Contact dermatitis** – this condition can affect both the client and the therapist. You will need to check whether the client is allergic to **latex** as gloves are worn in all eye treatments. If the client has an allergy, then **powder-free** vinyl or **nitrile** gloves should be worn. A sensitivity test should be carried out prior to tinting to ensure that allergic reactions and dermatitis do not occur. If therapists have skin contact with tint and peroxide, it is possible that they could develop contact dermatitis, so safe working practices should be adopted.

Remember that it is not your place as a therapist to mention specific conditions to your client as you are not medically trained. You can recommend that your client see their GP over a condition, but do not name the condition, or offer any diagnosis or cure. Ensure advice is given without causing undue alarm or concern to the client.

The client's treatment plan

During the consultation you will gather the information you need to recommend the most appropriate treatment plan for your client. Do make sure that you agree all aspects of the treatment plan with the client before you begin, and encourage them to ask questions to clarify any points they do not fully understand.

Planning the eyebrow shape

Eyebrow shaping is the removal of superfluous hair to enhance the shape of the natural brow. Superfluous hair is the term used if hair growth is normal but the client feels it is unattractive. When shaping the eyebrows you need to plan the treatment carefully, because it cannot be undone. Discuss the needs with your client before commencing the treatment. You may have very different ideas.

Important tools for shaping are a mirror and an eyebrow brush.

Facts about eyebrows

Every natural eyebrow is different in shape, hair type and colour. As well as this, to achieve the most flattering effect, you need to consider both facial and eye types.

Most hairs on the brows are **terminal hairs** (refer to Related anatomy and physiology, page 246). The terminal hairs of the brows, unlike other terminal hairs, are usually

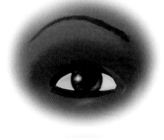
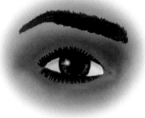

Eyebrows differ in shape, hair type and colour

short in length but are still there for protection. The reason we have hairs on the brows and surrounding the eyes is to stop debris entering the eyes and to keep germs out. The hairs are also there to protect the eyes from excessive light damage.

Eyebrow shapes

It is recommended that the normal eyebrow should look like the wings of a bird in flight: thicker at the inner corner of the eye, tapering to an arch and narrowing at the end of the brow. As the eyebrows frame the face, they should be in balance with the rest of the facial features.

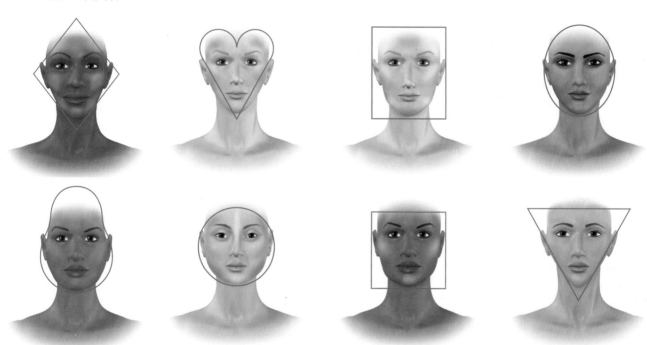

The following indicate the effect of shapes.

Angular shape

This shape can define a round face. Enhance this shape with shading and contouring of the eye make-up for elegance.

Rounded shape

Suitable for clients with large eyes or a wide forehead, a rounded shape can enhance the client's eyes. The eyebrow line should follow the frontal bone and be shaped to a taper.

Arched shape

Sometimes referred to as 'sweeping', this shape is very flattering on most clients. It gives width and expression to the eye. It opens the eye and can help to balance a prominent nose or a large mouth. An arched shape can also be used to detract from a high forehead.

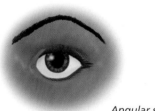

Angular shape

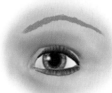

Rounded shape

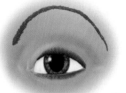

Arched shape

Unit B5   Enhance the appearance of eyebrows and lashes

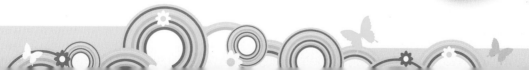

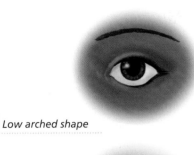

Low arched shape

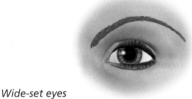

Wide-set eyes

Think about it

You can only work with the eyebrow's natural shape so you may need to discourage your client from expecting unrealistic outcomes.

Low arched shape

This shape works well for a client with a low or small forehead by giving the illusion of more length. It is sometimes referred to as a straight shape.

Wide-set eyes

If a client has wide-set eyes, extend the eyebrow to inside the corner of the eye.

Other factors that may influence the shape of the brows.

○ The natural shape of the brows. If the client has been shaping her own brows, it may be necessary to let them grow for a short time before shaping them professionally; in the meantime, stray hairs can be removed to keep them neat.

○ Client age. More mature clients might have some coarse hairs, which can be long, white or discoloured. These can be removed, provided that doing so does not alter the brow line or leave bald patches. Ideally, the brow should be of medium thickness. Too thick, and it can give an older appearance. Thin eyebrows give a severe appearance.

○ Fashion trends. Each season sees new fashion trends, which have an effect on eyebrow shapes and eye make-up. This should also be considered before shaping the brows.

Other approaches which may be suitable for the client

○ Semi-permanent make-up. This should be applied only by professionals. Pigment is applied to add colour to the brows, e.g. to disguise a bald area.

○ Hair transplants. These are already available in the USA for clients with sparse brows.

○ Artificial individual eyebrow hairs. These are applied in the same way as individual eyelashes and are not permanent.

Measuring the eyebrows to decide length

Once you have carried out the consultation and discussed the client's needs, you need to measure the length of the brows. Here are some points to help you when deciding the correct length and shape for your client.

○ Place an orange stick in a straight line from the side of the nose to the inner corner of the eye. This is where the eyebrow should begin.

○ Place an orange stick from the side of the nose to the outer corner of the eye. This is where the eyebrow should end.

○ Ask the client to look straight ahead. Hold the stick vertically so that it runs through the lateral edge of the eyes. This is where the highest point of the arch should be.

○ Hold the stick horizontally and it should more or less connect the beginning and end of the eyebrow.

These are useful guidelines. With practice you will learn to train your eye.

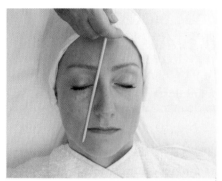

Line up the orange stick with the corner of the mouth and the edge of the nose: the beginning of the eyebrow should start where the orange stick rests on the skin

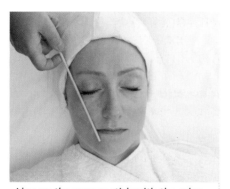

Line up the orange stick with the edge of the mouth and the outer corner of the eye: the end of the eyebrow should be where the orange stick rests on the skin

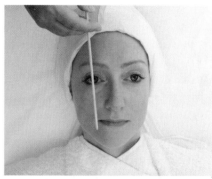

The arch of the eyebrow should match the middle of the pupil. This is your shape guideline; any stray hairs outside the shape can be plucked out.

Selecting suitable equipment and materials

This will depend upon the results of the sensitivity test, consultation and the treatment being undertaken.

Equipment required for eyebrow shaping

- Tweezers (rounded, slanted, pointed)
- Damp cotton wool
- Orange stick
- Antiseptic solution
- Aftercare solution
- Disposable gloves (refer to your professional body for guidance or visit the Habia website)
- Tissues
- Bin and bin liner
- Sterilising dish
- Mirror
- Eyebrow brush

Tweezers

There are two types of tweezers used for eyebrow shaping.

Automatic tweezers

These are designed to remove the bulk of excess hair. They have a spring-loaded action.

Manual

These are used to remove stray hairs and accentuate the shape of the brow. Various ends are available – slanted ends are generally considered to be the best for eyebrow shaping.

For equipment and materials for eyelash and eyebrow tinting, see page 343, and for application of artificial lashes, see page 350.

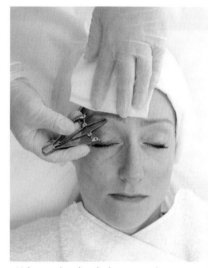

Using spring-loaded automatic tweezers

Think about it

It is important that all tweezers are ready for use, and they should be sterilised between clients, either in an autoclave or in a sterilising solution. It is important that this is carried out as blood and tissue fluids can be drawn during treatment, and these could cause contamination. Any tissue fluid drawn should be disposed of, in accordance with health and safety regulations, to prevent contamination.

Unit B5 Enhance the appearance of eyebrows and lashes

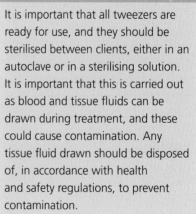
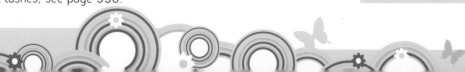

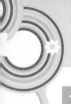

Think about it

If the treatment requires that you use gloves, check with the client before treatment starts whether she has a latex allergy. Any allergy should be recorded on the client record card.

Think about it

Be sure to clarify the shape required with the client before commencing any treatment. If the client is nervous, explain the procedure and reassure her as you progress.

Details of shape, thickness, texture and required shape should all be added to the client record card.

Think about it

All tinting and adhesive products that are used on the eyes are controlled by the Control of Substances Harmful to Health regulations (refer to Professional basics, page 54). These regulations govern the correct use, storage and disposal of products. Be sure that you always refer to the manufacturer's instructions when using these products as incorrect use and storage may harm the client or cause the treatment to be ineffective.

Protecting the client: personal protective equipment for eyebrow and eyelash treatments

It is advisable when carrying out treatments around the eye that you wear gloves, so as to protect you and your client from infection and contamination. Blood spots may be produced when shaping — this is a normal reaction to tweezing or waxing of the brows.

There are several different types of protective gloves available. Traditionally, gloves are made of latex, but a number of people have developed allergies to latex. If you or a client shows signs of redness or irritation when in contact with latex gloves, an alternative made of either vinyl or nitrile that are powder-free should be used.

Care should be taken when putting on and removing gloves to avoid cross-contamination. Gloves should be removed by turning inside out and disposed of in the contaminated waste bin.

Preparing the client

After completing the consultation:

○ Secure client's hair with headband or turban.

○ Place towel or tissue or cape over the client's chest.

○ Position client comfortably; couch or chair should be slightly elevated.

○ Remove all accessories, e.g. earrings. Clients who wear contact lenses may find treatment more comfortable if they remove them prior to treatment.

Risk assessment for eye treatments

Refer to Unit G20, Make sure your own actions reduce risks to health and safety, pages 73–86, for a complete discussion of risk assessment.

Hazards: only look for hazards that you could reasonably expect to result in significant harm under the conditions in your workplace. Use the following examples as a guide.

- **Chemicals** (e.g. eye damage from glue in the eye)
- **Allergies** (allergic reaction to glue or, or tint)
- **Cross-infections** (blood spotting from the eyebrow shape)
- **Contact dermatitis** (continued use of products without the protection of suitable gloves can cause a reaction to the therapist's hands which can be spread to other areas of the body if extreme sensitivity occurs)

Sensitivity testing

For information on how to carry out a sensitivity test, see page 340.

Shape eyebrows

In this outcome you will learn about:

- checking the client's understanding of the treatment prior to commencement and discussing any areas that require clarification
- ensuring the eyebrow area is thoroughly cleansed and suitably prepared prior to the treatment
- keeping the skin taut to minimise discomfort to the client
- ensuring that the hair is removed in the direction of the hair growth
- using suitable soothing products according to the needs of the client and manufacturers' instructions
- ensuring the finished shape is to the client's satisfaction.

Procedure for eyebrow shaping

It is important that the client understands the treatment procedure and the shape is discussed before the treatment commences. The therapist should check the shape at regular intervals.

1 Remove all traces of make-up and clean the area with an appropriate cleanser. Wipe with sanitising solution and prepare the area.

2 Inspect the treatment area to assess the amount of work required. Measure shape (see page 334) and consult the client. A magnifying lamp can be used to give maximum visibility.

3 Brush the brows into shape before you begin.

4 Open pores – it is often suggested that before you begin shaping, you should place warm, damp cotton wool pads over the area. This relaxes hair follicles and softens the eyebrow tissue, making hair removal easier.

5 To remove hairs, gently stretch the skin between your fingers and pluck out the hairs in the direction in which they grow. Begin by removing the stray hairs between the eyes. Hairs below the natural brow shape can then be tackled. The few odd hairs that grow unevenly above the brow may also be removed, provided they do not form part of the main eyebrow growth. If there are any tough, spiky or white hairs, these can sometimes be removed without spoiling the overall shape.

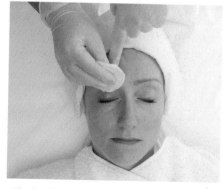

Placing hot cotton wool pads on the brow opens the pores (step 4)

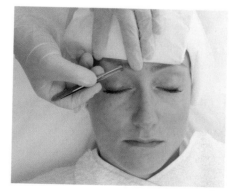

Stretching skin and tweezing near to the root will minimise discomfort

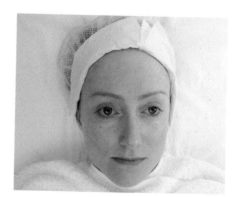

The finished look should be clean and tidy and open up the whole face.

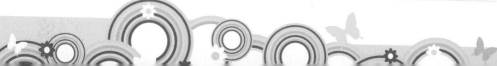

Enhance the appearance of eyebrows and lashes **Unit B5**

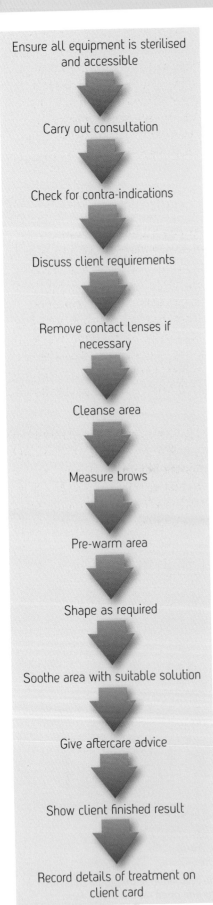

Ensure all equipment is sterilised and accessible

↓

Carry out consultation

↓

Check for contra-indications

↓

Discuss client requirements

↓

Remove contact lenses if necessary

↓

Cleanse area

↓

Measure brows

↓

Pre-warm area

↓

Shape as required

↓

Soothe area with suitable solution

↓

Give aftercare advice

↓

Show client finished result

↓

Record details of treatment on client card

Eyebrow shaping

6 Consult the client as you work, ensure she has a hand mirror and consults with you as you proceed.

7 Place the removed hairs on a tissue placed at the side of the client, or held wrapped around your fingers.

8 Periodically soothe the client's brow with antiseptic, as this helps to remove any stray hairs.

9 When all the shaping is complete, place a dampened cotton wool soaked in witch-hazel over the area to soothe, cool and remove excess erythema (for information on erythema, see page 339).

10 Give aftercare advice and book the client's next appointment.

If blood or tissue fluid is accidentally drawn during the treatment, the following steps should be taken.

1 Apply pressure to the area with clean cotton wool soaked in sanitising solution.

2 Do not panic. Keep calm, and explain to the client so she is aware of the problem.

3 Apply soothing solution to the area.

4 Dispose of waste carefully in accordance with health and safety regulations and local by-laws.

An eyebrow re-shape may take up to half an hour and an eyebrow tidy up to 15 minutes. In all cases it would depend on the density of the hairs, shape required, hair growth and the client requirements. Clients who visit the salon regularly often have an eyebrow tidy as an integral part of their treatment plan. On average, an eyebrow tidy would be carried out every 4–6 weeks.

Aftercare

Clients should be given the following aftercare advice when they have had an eyebrow shape or tidy.

○ Cooling mild antiseptic products, e.g. witch hazel, should be applied.

○ No make-up should be applied to the area for 12 hours, as the follicles are open and infection may occur.

○ Stray regrowth hairs can be removed at intervals to prolong the effect.

Think about it

A nervous client may require eye pads or be advised to keep eyes shut. Heavy brows should be gradually reduced over two or three visits to minimise discomfort and allow the client to become accustomed to her new image.

Trouble-shooting eyebrow problems

Bare sparse brows

Fill in with pencil, using short strokes in the direction of the hair growth, and blend with a brow brush. Ensure that the pencil is sharpened as you move from one eye to the other, to prevent cross-infection.

Stray hairs

Remove any stray hairs with tweezers.

Thin brows

Instead of a pencil, try a shade of powder that matches the brow colour. Apply with a stiff brush, following the natural line, and ensure that you blend in well to prevent the line looking harsh. This will create the illusion of doubling the thickness.

Unruly or thick brows

Long, unruly hairs should be trimmed. Hold the brows straight with a brow comb and trim to the required length. To help the hairs to lie flat, use either a little hair gel or a small amount of hairspray on a comb. Never spray directly on to the face.

Tint eyebrows and lashes

In this outcome you will learn about:

- confirming the client's understanding of the treatment prior to commencement and discussing any areas that require clarification
- ensuring the area is thoroughly cleansed and suitably prepared prior to the treatment
- effectively protecting the skin surrounding the area to be treated
- mixing tints to meet manufacturers' instructions and client requirements
- minimising the spread of colour to the client's skin, clothes and surrounding areas during application
- applying the product evenly and ensuring the product fully covers the hair to be tinted
- promptly removing the tint in the event of any contra-actions and applying a cold water compress to soothe the eye
- accurately timing the product development to meet the colouring characteristics of the client and manufacturers' instructions
- ensuring the treated hair is left free of product
- ensuring finished result is to the client's satisfaction.

The benefits of tinting

- Eyebrows help to emphasise facial expression and eyelashes frame the eyes.
- Tinting may be carried out on clients with light-coloured brows and lashes to define their appearance.
- Brows and lashes can be tinted to complement hair colour.
- Tinting can mean that coloured mascara need not be applied, which is good for those who are allergic to it, or in the summer months when mascara is likely to smudge if it is very hot.
- Tinting is also ideal for clients who wear glasses or contact lenses.

Think about it

Your posture is important when carrying out a shape. Ensure that the client is at the correct height so that you can clearly see the hairs. You may need to use a magnifier to help you if the hairs are fair or white.

Think about it

Contra-actions usually take the form of erythema to the area, but in some cases blood spots occur and sometimes swelling. You should try to reduce the swelling before the client leaves the salon, by applying a soothing antiseptic. In extreme cases, a cold compress or ice should be applied. All contra-actions should be recorded on the client record card.

Key term

Contra-action – an adverse physical reaction during or after the treatment. This should be recorded on the record card.

Unit B5 Enhance the appearance of eyebrows and lashes

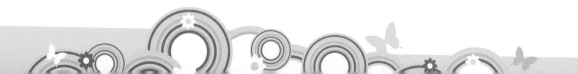

My story

No more smudges

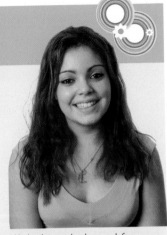

My name is Zaida, and I'm a chef in a busy hotel. Although my working environment is hot and steamy, I like to wear a little make-up. I was finding that whichever brand of mascara I used, by the end of the day it had run. My friend suggested I had my eyelashes tinted. I went to the local salon and I had a tint test to ensure that I was not allergic to the products. Two days later I had my lashes tinted – I was delighted with the results. That was over two years ago. Since then I have had my lashes and brows tinted regularly and for my sister's wedding I had an artificial lash application. I no longer have to put up with smudged mascara!

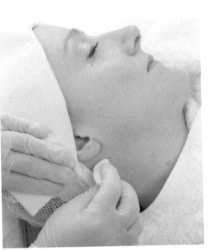

Patch test: cleansing the area first

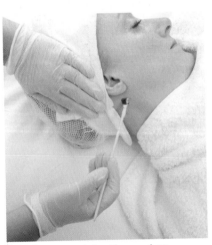

Patch test: applying the product

Performing a sensitivity test

A sensitivity test should be carried out prior to tinting or the application of artificial lashes with the product that you plan to use. A suitable area should be selected, usually behind the ear or the crook of the elbow. An area nearest to the eye would be the most suitable for a more accurate result.

Many professional associations now recommend that this test be carried out 24–48 hours prior to each treatment, even on a client who regularly has the treatment at the salon. The client may have become sensitive to the product, or the salon may have changed products and therefore the ingredients may be slightly different from the ones used previously.

All tests should be recorded on the client record card with the date the test was carried out and the results of the test. An allergic reaction would show as a red, itchy, sore area. Treat with a cold compress and soothing cream. This reaction would mean that the client is unsuitable for the treatment.

If the test is not carried out and a problem does occur, it is possible you could invalidate your insurance policy. A test only takes a few minutes and can easily be performed by the receptionist.

Method

○ Cleanse the area of the skin to be tested (behind the ear or the crook of the arm).

○ Mix the same make and colour of tint to be used with the manufacturer's recommended quantity of 10 per cent volume peroxide.

○ Apply the tint to the area selected with a brush, about the size of a ten pence coin.

○ Allow to dry.

○ Ensure the client is aware that the tint should be left on the skin for 24 hours. If no reaction occurs, then wash off.

- If a reaction occurs, the tint should be removed immediately with water and a soothing lotion applied to the area.
- A reaction will be recognised by an itching, red-hot inflamed area. This should be treated with a soothing substance.

Precautions for lash and brow tinting

- Discuss the client's requirements with her prior to beginning the treatment.
- Ensure all equipment is clean and sterilised.
- Ensure all eye make-up is removed with a non-oily product.
- Check for contra-indications.
- Ensure client has removed contact lenses.
- Ensure area is thoroughly cleansed.
- Apply barrier cream to the skin around the eyes only and not to the hair to be tinted, as the tint will not act. The barrier cream is used to prevent the tint spreading beyond the area being treated.
- Ensure the client keeps her eyes closed at all times when the tint is on the lashes to prevent tint from entering the eyes and causing irritation. As a therapist, you are responsible for giving your client full instructions. This is vital, especially when treating nervous clients.
- Do not leave the client while the tint is processing.
- Complete details of the tint on the record card.
- Ensure that the eyebrows are tinted prior to shaping, to avoid tint seeping into the follicles, resulting in a reaction.

How colour works

The selected dye and hydrogen peroxide are mixed together to produce a chemical reaction. When first applied to the hair, they enter the middle of the hair as small particles, but, because of the chemical reaction, they swell. This swelling prevents the colour from coming out when washed and so becomes permanent. This process is known as **oxidation**. The colour of the hair changes and this will remain until the hair grows or falls out.

Never mix the ingredients until you are ready to use them. Oxidation starts to occur and the tint starts to work as soon as it is mixed, so if you prepare them too early the product will not be able to enter the hair properly, resulting in poor colour.

Always replace caps on the tint and hydrogen peroxide as they will oxidise and future results will be unsuccessful. When using two colours of tint, mix them together and then add peroxide.

Choosing a tint

The skin around the eye is very thin and sensitive, therefore dyes designed for eyelash and brow tinting have been specially formulated to avoid any eye or tissue reactions. Any other type of dye or any hydrogen peroxide solution stronger than 10 per cent dilution should not be used in this area. It is dangerous and may even cause blindness.

Think about it

Always note the date and the results of patch test on the client record card. The details on the card should include:

- date of patch test
- products used
- development time of the treatment
- areas treated
- contra-actions
- aftercare.

For your portfolio

Carry out a skin sensitivity test for tint and the application of eyelash adhesive. Record the date on your client record card and note the result in 24 hours. Make a note of the make of product that you have used.

Key terms

Oxidation – chemical reaction that occurs when peroxide and dye are mixed together.

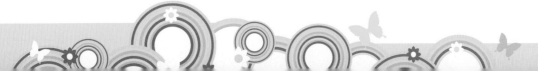

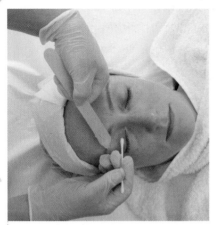

Decant the barrier cream onto a spatula and paint onto the skin surrounding the eyebrow to prevent accidental staining

Unit B5 Enhance the appearance of eyebrows and lashes

Think about it

Although you will not be in contact with blood or tissue fluids during tinting, it may be advisable to wear protective gloves to prevent contact with the tint, which may cause dermatitis. This will also prevent accidental staining of the fingers when applying the tint.

Key terms

Eye shield – used to protect the eyes during a treatment; may be made of paper or cotton wool.

The products used for eyelash and brow tinting are usually available as creams or gels in basic colours of black, blue, brown and grey. These colours are mixed to form variations in tone: for example, blue/black provides a darker colour.

The choice is a matter of personal preference and depends on:

○ the client's overall skin type and hair colouring

○ the type of eye make-up usually worn

○ the age of the client.

As clients grow more mature, they lose a lot of natural colour from hair and eyes. Brown or grey tints are preferable to black for producing a softer, more natural effect. This is an example of when you need to be aware of the fact that the client's expectations may not be realistic. The client may expect a very dark finish or longer eyelashes, where this may not be possible. It is therefore your responsibility to explain to the client that certain expectations cannot or should not be achieved, due to suitability. It is important to provide the client with sufficient professional advice and emphasise that lash and brow treatments are designed to enhance the natural features.

This applies to shaping and artificial lash application too. Expectations are realistic when they can be achieved with success and when the treatment is suitable for the client. The effect of tinting depends on the natural colour of the hair: for example, blond hair colour develops rapidly, usually in 5 minutes; red hair is more resistant and development will take longer, perhaps 10 minutes; white hair will take slightly longer to process, due to the lack of the pigment melanin. Make sure the colour you choose gives a realistic natural effect.

Preparing the client for tinting lashes and brows

○ Help the client into a comfortable, semi-reclined position and protect hair and clothing.

○ Clean and tone the area to ensure that all grease and make-up is removed from lashes and brows. If grease is left on the skin, a barrier will be created and the tint will not take properly.

○ Protect the skin above the eyes with a barrier cream. Take care not to get any barrier product on the lashes or brows that require tinting. Use a tipped orange stick or cotton bud to apply the barrier cream to the skin above the eyes.

○ When applying the cream below the eyes, either stroke it directly onto the skin and position the **eye shields** on top, close to the base of the lashes, or coat the underneath surface of the shields with barrier cream and slide them into position.

Applying lash tint

Precautions should be taken to ensure that neither the tint nor the applicator penetrates the eye. There should not be any problems provided:

○ the eye is well supported by gently holding the area

○ the tint is applied carefully

○ the lashes are not overloaded with tint

○ the client's eyes are kept still.

Tinting – what you will need

- Tinting equipment
- Protective headband and towel
- Couch roll to protect the work area
- Small non-metallic bowl for mixing tint (a metal one would react with the hydrogen peroxide)
- Lined container for waste
- Sterile spatula
- Sterile applicator or tipped orange stick
- Clean water in the event of eye irrigation becoming necessary
- Hand mirror
- Client record card
- Materials
- Damp cotton wool and tissues

- Eye shields made from cotton wool or paper shields
- Selection of coloured tints
- Hydrogen peroxide (usual 10 per cent volume, but always check the manufacturer's instructions)
- Eye make-up remover (non-oily)
- Cleanser and toner
- Gloves
- Barrier cream

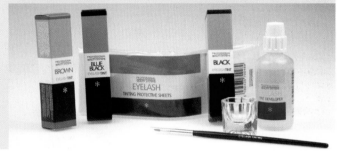

Step by step eyelash tinting

1 After placing shields under the eyes, begin to apply tint to lower lashes, made up to manufacturer's instructions. Ask the client to close her eyes, and apply tint to the top lashes. Cover the eyes

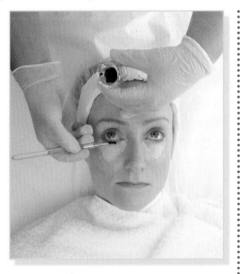

2 While the lash tint is developing you can tint the eyebrows if required

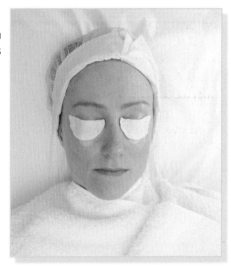

3 When processing time has elapsed, remove all traces of the tint

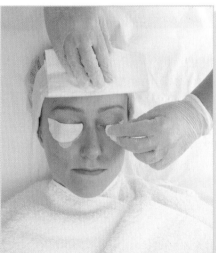

4 The finished eyelash tint defines the lashes and enhances the eyes

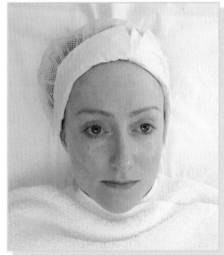

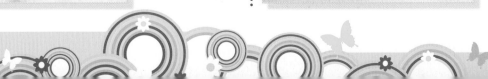

Unit B5 · Enhance the appearance of eyebrows and lashes

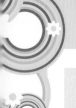

Ensure all equipment is hygienic and close to hand

Carry out a consultation (ensure a patch test has been carried out). Check for contra-indications

Remove contact lenses if required

If shaping is to be carried out always tint first and shape after

Cleanse area with non-oily product

Apply barrier cream and preformed shapes if tinting lashes

Mix tint and apply (never pre-mix the tint). Note processing time on client record card

Remove tint after the required processing time

Show client results. Give aftercare advice

Record details on client record card

Eyebrow and lash tinting

1 Once the client has been correctly positioned and the make-up removed, mix the correct colour of tint according to the manufacturer's instructions. A guide is a 5 mm length of tint with 2–3 drops of hydrogen peroxide, mixed in a tinting bowl with a disposable brush or orange stick to a smooth paste.

2 Remember, before applying the tint a barrier cream should be applied to prevent staining.

3 Ask the client to look upwards and cover the lower lashes with tint (if the client has watery eyes, the lower lashes can be covered with the upper lashes when the eyes are closed, but the result is often not so effective). (See photo 1.) Make sure you do not ask the client to look up into the overhead light as this will over-sensitise the eyes and make them water.

4 Ask the client to close the eyes and apply the tint to the upper lashes.

5 Gently lift the skin to the eyebrows, so the tint can be applied right down to the base of the lashes and include shorter hairs which grow near the inside corner of the eyes.

6 If the client complains of discomfort or the eyes begin to water, remove the tint immediately using damp cotton wool pads, and irrigate the eye.

7 Note the time and allow for the tint to work according to the manufacturer's instructions. The colour should be checked at intervals and the tint reapplied if necessary. As a guide, allow 5–10 minutes, depending on the colour characteristics of the client.

Removal of eyelash tint

If the client experiences irritation, stinging or burning, the tint should be removed immediately before the end of the processing time. Even if a client has not had a negative reaction to a sensitivity test, some clients may find that the process irritates the delicate skin around the eye. The same would apply for the application of eyelash glue.

1 Place a pad of damp cotton wool on each eye. Hold the eye shield and pad of cotton wool together at the base and swiftly remove, enclosing any excess tint.

2 Remove any remaining tint with slightly damp cotton wool, using a gentle downward motion, and remove excess with a cotton bud. (See photo 3.)

3 When both eyes have been cleaned, ask the client to carefully open the eyes.

4 Support the eye and work quickly on the lower lashes with damp cotton wool and a cotton bud.

5 Stand in front of the client to check that all the tint has been removed.

6 Finally, wipe the area over with damp cotton wool to remove traces of the barrier cream.

7 Offer a hand mirror to view the final results.

8 Inform the client of possible contra-actions and aftercare. If irritation occurs, apply a damp cotton wool compress to the area.

9 Enter details on to the client record card. This should include the colour selected and the processing time for the tint, and any contra-actions and other information relevant to the treatment.

The process of eyelash tinting should take about 20 minutes.

Applying eyebrow tint

Step-by-step eyebrow tint

This can be performed after lash tinting, prior to shaping. Many salons and therapists perform this treatment while the lash tint is processing, to ensure they are cost-effective with their time. If shaping is carried out first, the tint will seep into the open pores, causing irritation.

1 Prepare the skin and brows the same way as for treating the lashes. Apply barrier cream around the eyebrows taking care to avoid the hairs.

2 Apply the tint against the hair growth using an orange stick or a fine brush, working gradually from the outer and underneath hairs towards the centre.

3 After one minute, remove a little tint from the inner corners of the eyebrow and check how the colour is developing. Apply more tint and repeat colour checks at one-minute intervals until the desired effect has been achieved. The developing time for tinting brows is much shorter than for lashes, usually 1–3 minutes. Always refer to the manufacturer's instructions for product guidance. Care must be taken to prevent the brows from becoming too dark as this can create an unattractive harsh effect.

4 Remove tint with clean, damp cotton wool.

5 Wipe over the area to remove all traces of barrier cream.

6 Discuss the final effect, possible contra-action and aftercare with the client.

7 Enter details of the treatment on the client record card.

The process of eyebrow tinting should take approximately 15 minutes.

How to irrigate the eye

If tint accidentally enters the eye, do not panic; the client may be feeling discomfort and a slight burning sensation. Calm the client and explain the procedure you are going to follow.

1 Tilt the client's head slightly to one side. Carefully trickle some tepid water into the corner of the eye and allow the eye to be rinsed of the foreign body.

2 Hold some tissue or a small kidney dish to collect the excess water.

3 Apply a damp cotton wool compress to cool and soothe the eye.

It is not acceptable to use an eyebath because of the risk of cross-infection.

Possible causes of eye irritation include:

○ very sensitive eyes

○ too much or incorrect strength of hydrogen peroxide

○ something in the eye

○ inadvertently poking the eye.

Unit B5

Enhance the appearance of eyebrows and lashes

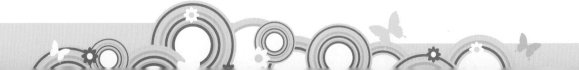

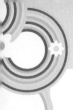

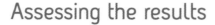

Assessing the results

It is important that the client is shown the results of the treatment to ensure satisfaction before she leaves the treatment room.

○ A successful tinting treatment produces the required colour changes to the lashes and brows without staining the skin.

○ Even the shortest eyelashes should be coloured from the base.

○ The appearance of blond roots after the eyelash tint shows that not enough care was taken. The skin fold of the eyelid was probably not lifted away from the base of the hairs when applying tint.

○ The tint will not have covered the brows successfully if:
 — there was grease or make-up on the hairs
 — old tint was used
 — the hydrogen peroxide had lost strength
 — the tint and peroxide were incorrectly mixed
 — the tint was removed too soon.

Aftercare

As with all treatments, the client should be advised against touching or rubbing the areas immediately after the treatment. If redness or irritation occurs, apply a damp cotton wool compress.

The client should be aware that the effects will last approximately 4–6 weeks as the hairs grow out. Strong sunlight will make the results fade faster.

Product safety data

Product	Description	Ingredients	Hazards	Flammability	First aid procedures	Spillage	Handling and storage
Eye make-up remover	Prepared from mild cleaning agents in a cosmetic base	All ingredients commonly used in cosmetic products and meet accepted standards of purity	Non-hazardous under normal conditions of use	✗	Ingestion: drink milk or water Eye contact: wash well with water; if irritation persists, seek medical advice	Clean using absorbent material, followed by washing with detergent and water to avoid slippery floors	No special precautions
Eyelash tint	Oil/water-emulsion (cream)	Water/cetearyl alcohol/PEG-sorbitan lanolate/sodium cetearyl sulfate/diaminotoluene/aminophenols/dyest. CI 77499 and/or 77007/no preservatives	Non-hazardous on its own. Becomes hazardous when mixed with hydrogen peroxide	✗	Ingestion: drink a lot of water; seek medical attention Skin contact: remove with water; if irritation occurs, seek medical attention Eye contact: avoid by careful observation of the instructions for use; if contact occurs, rinse immediately with warm water	Clean area immediately to prevent. Always wear gloves and avoid contact with skin and eyes. Staining	At least three years, when kept under normal stocking conditions

Product	Description	Ingredients	Hazards	Flammability	First aid procedures	Spillage	Handling and storage
Eyelash tinting peroxide	Mixture of oxidising agents, wetting agents, pH adjusters, fragrance and water Contents: hydrogen peroxide	All ingredients commonly used in cosmetic products and meet accepted standards of purity	Hazardous if precautions are ignored	✗ *Note:* Hydrogen peroxide may react with other chemicals to form explosive mixtures; combustion may occur if hydrogen peroxide is allowed to dry on paper, wood, hair, etc.	Ingestion: seek medical attention immediately. Skin contact: avoid; always wear rubber gloves when using product; if skin contact occurs, wash well with soap and water; if irritation persists, seek medical attention Eye contact: avoid; wash well with water and seek medical attention	Clean area with plenty of water and dispose down drain; do not absorb into flammable material such as tissue or couch roll	Always wear gloves and avoid contact with skin. Store in a cool place away from direct sunlight; store in the original container only and keep closures tightly sealed. Contamination of solutions containing hydrogen peroxide can result in instability with liberation of heat and oxygen
Eyelash tint stain remover	Mixture of ethanol and fragrance oils in solution	All ingredients commonly used in cosmetic products and meet accepted standards of purity	Hazardous unless normal safety precautions followed	✓ Ethanol content: 50 per cent w/w *Note:* In event of a fire, evacuate areas known to contain products and inform fire service of their presence	Ingestion: avoid, drink plenty of milk or water Inhalation: avoid, may cause dizziness, remove to fresh air Skin contact: avoid prolonged contact with skin; if irritation persists, seek medical attention	Clean contaminated area with plenty of water, wash with detergent and water to avoid slippery floors; do not absorb on to combustible material such as tissue or couch roll	Store in a cool place away from direct sunlight; large quantities should be stored in fire-resistant store

Apply artificial eyelashes

In this outcome you will learn about:

- checking the client's understanding of the treatment prior to commencement and discussing any areas that require clarification
- ensuring the area is thoroughly cleansed and suitably prepared prior to the treatment
- positioning and fixing the artificial lashes accurately, leaving the eye area free of excessive products
- identifying and promptly resolving any application problems occurring during the treatment
- promptly removing the artificial lashes with the correct products in the event of any contra-actions and applying a cold water compress to soothe the eye
- ensuring, on completion, that the artificial eyelashes give a balanced and well-proportioned look suitable for the agreed desired effect
- ensuring, on completion, that partial sets are smoothly and evenly graduated into the natural eyelashes
- ensuring finished result is to the client's satisfaction.

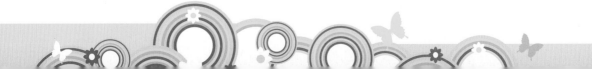

Unit B5 Enhance the appearance of eyebrows and lashes

Artificial lashes can be used to enhance any make-up, but they are especially suitable for evening and photographic applications. Before applying lashes it is important to discuss with the client the effect she wishes to create, be it subtle or dramatic.

This treatment will require a sensitivity test for the adhesive. A check for contra-indications should also be made, as eye infections are easily spread.

The benefits of artificial lashes

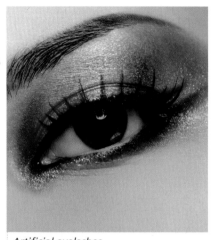

Artificial eyelashes

Artificial lashes are designed to enhance and emphasise the eyes by giving the natural lashes a fuller and more defined appearance. They come in the form of individual lashes or strip lashes. Using artificial lashes can have the following benefits.

- They are a good option for a client who is allergic to mascara and eyelash tint.
- They can be convenient for someone who is going on holiday.
- They make the natural lashes appear longer and thicker.
- They add definition to the eye area.
- They can enhance a photographic make-up.
- They can enhance an evening or fantasy make-up.
- They can complete a corrective make-up.

Effects

- **Deep-set eyes** – fine pointed upper and lower lashes will give added definition to the eye.
- **Round eyes** – individual lashes can be used to thicken the lash line from the centre of the eye outwards.
- **Small eyes** – individual lashes placed at the outer corner will make the eyes look larger.
- **Close-set eyes** – artificial lashes applied to the outer third of the eye will have the effect of widening the eye.

During the consultation, it is important to establish what result the client is expecting to achieve. If expectations are unrealistic, this should be explained to the client. Once a plan has been agreed, treatment can commence.

Factors to consider when choosing artificial eyelashes

- **Client's age.** Artificial lashes create a very bold, dramatic effect, which can make an older client look harsh.
- **Client's natural lashes.** Choose artificial lashes to complement the natural lash.
- **Occasion for wearing artificial eyelashes**. This can determine whether individual or strip lashes are more appropriate, e.g. individual for corrective, strip for fantasy make-up.
- **Maintenance of lashes.** Strip lashes are easily maintained as no special product is needed for removal, and they can be reused. In the case of individual lashes, maintenance may be required to replace lashes due to natural hair loss. Solvent product is required to remove lashes.

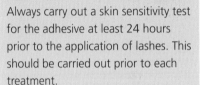

- **Time for lash application.** Strip lashes add 10 minutes to a make-up time. Individual lashes take 20–30 minutes, depending how many are applied.
- **Further appointments.** Strip lashes need to be applied daily. Individual lashes need an appointment in 3–6 weeks for maintenance and to replace lashes lost naturally.

Semi-permanent individual lashes

This type of lash is also known as an eyelash extension. One advantage is that it can be placed on top of the client's own lashes individually. They can therefore be placed independently to create different effects: they can be used sparingly on the outside of the eye to improve the client's eye shape, or placed across the entire upper eye area for a fuller effect.

The lashes are usually available in black or brown and come in four lengths: mini, short, medium and long. Individual lashes also come in single lashes or flared. The flared have two or more strips from one bulb.

Individual lashes may be worn for up to six weeks, and will be lost when the natural lash falls out. These can be replaced each week if the client requires. The client should be made aware of this as part of the aftercare. Individual lashes are usually made from synthetic threads of nylon, although some of the more expensive lashes can be made of real hair. The lashes made of synthetic fibres hold a permanent curl for a longer time than natural hair. Whichever type is applied, they are fixed by using special adhesive which bonds the artificial eyelash to the natural lash. This is available in black or clear.

Performing a sensitivity test on the adhesive

This test is required for individual and strip lashes.

Place a small amount of the adhesive in the crook of the elbow or behind the ear, at least 24 hours prior to the treatment. If a reaction occurs such as swelling, irritation or inflammation, do not proceed with the treatment. It is important to remember that dates of all the tests should be recorded on the client record card.

Preparing the client for application of lashes

- Hold a full consultation checking for contra-indications and ensure a sensitivity test has been carried out.
- Discuss length, colour and type of lash and client expectations.
- Ensure the client has removed contact lenses, and jewellery that may get in the way.
- Place a hairband or turban around the hair.
- Cover client's clothing with a cape, towel or tissue.
- Seat client in a semi-reclined position in a good light or with access to a magnifier lamp.

> **Think about it**
>
> Always carry out a skin sensitivity test for the adhesive at least 24 hours prior to the application of lashes. This should be carried out prior to each treatment.

> **Think about it**
>
> Glue can be an irritant, so always refer to the manufacturer's instructions and COSHH regulations when using this product.

> **Think about it**
>
> If the client wears contact lenses, these should be removed before the treatment commences, as adhesive could damage the lenses.

> **Think about it**
>
> Contra-indications are the same for all eye treatments, so remember to check. Also remember that it is very easy to cross-infect the eyes, so strict hygiene must be followed: for example, use separate cotton wool for each eye.

Unit B5

Enhance the appearance of eyebrows and lashes

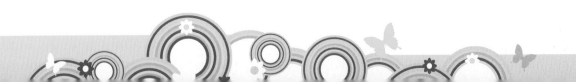

Think about it

Always refer to the manufacturer's instructions when using and applying lashes, using solvents, and adhesives. If the client indicates irritation (contra-action), immediately remove the lashes with the correct products and soothe with a suitable solution. Apply a cool compress to soothe the eye.

Eyelash application – what you will need

- Basic trolley products – tissues, cotton wool, etc.
- Oil-free, eye make-up remover (if oil-based products are used, the adhesive will not adhere to the lashes)
- Magnifier lamp
- Lash kit – containing a selection of lashes, adhesive and adhesive solvent
- Tweezers and orange stick
- Small scissors
- Mirror
- Small bowl of water to irrigate the eye if required – refer to lash and brow tinting for the procedure

Application and maintenance of artificial eyelashes

Step-by-step application of individual lashes

1 Cleanse the eye with oil-free cleanser. Select eyelash – choose a colour and length of lash nearest to the client's lashes for a natural look – and, using tweezers, dip the root into adhesive.

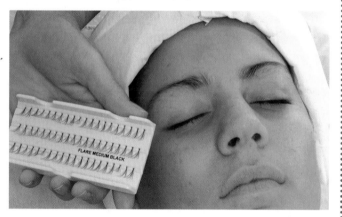

2 Place the lash with bulb at the client's natural eyelash roots. Check with the client's eyes open, then closed, that the lashes follow the natural curve of the eyelid. Apply shorter lashes around the inner/outer eye, and longer ones around the centre.

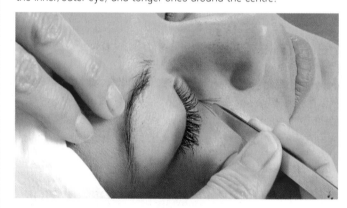

3 Comb through, when the glue is dry, to blend in with the natural eyelashes. Apply eye make-up. The finished result should enhance, but not look too obvious.

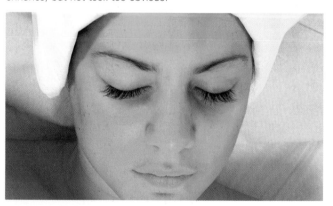

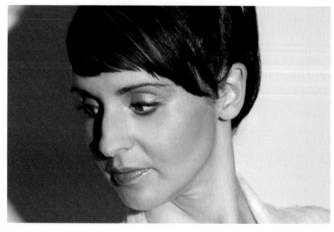

Artificial lashes used to enhance evening make-up

Contra-actions to individual and strip lashes

Eye irritation

○ Always remember to do a sensitivity test for the adhesive. If eyes start to water, blot with a tissue.

○ Never place eyelashes underneath the natural lashes, irritation will occur.

○ Products which are suitable for soothing eye irritation vary but commonly contain witch hazel, calamine and antiseptic.

Adhesive or solvent in the eye

○ If either of these products accidentally enters the eye, irrigate immediately. If serious seek medical advice.

○ Record all details on the client record card.

Maintenance and care of individual lashes

○ As extensions are designed to be worn for some weeks, the adhesive used to fix them is quite strong. It is therefore acceptable to apply eye make-up in the normal way.

○ Eye make-up remover must be oil-free, as oil will dislodge the lashes.

○ The lashes should be touched as little as possible.

○ Mascara will clog the lashes and is difficult to remove.

○ After initial application of lashes, the client should wait several hours before showering.

○ Client should avoid rubbing eyes, as this will loosen the lashes.

○ Client should avoid extremes of temperature, e.g. sauna.

○ You should use the solvent specially designed for the adhesive when removing the lashes. The solvent dissolves the adhesive so that no damage occurs to the natural lashes. A cotton bud soaked in the solvent should be gently rolled down the lashes, on to a tissue, until the lash detaches itself. Always refer to the manufacturer's instructions when using solvents.

Strip lashes

As the name suggests, these synthetic fibres are attached to a fine strip and secured onto the eyelid as near to the natural lashes as possible, with a special adhesive. This enables the lashes to be placed over the entire eye for a full appearance. Strip lashes are manufactured in many colours and shapes, and can include glitter effect and multi-coloured lashes, which can be used in fantasy or photographic make-up. Strip lashes not only add length but also add thickness and texture. When applying strip lashes the client should be advised that they are for short-term wear, unlike individual lashes, for a maximum of a day. As with individual lashes, they also come in a variety of lengths for a realistic appearance.

1   After discussion as to the style and colour of the lash that the client requires, trim to the correct length.

2   Complete the face make-up — foundation, blusher and eye shadow.

3   Seat the client in a semi-reclined position and work from above.

Ensure all materials are to hand and are hygienic

Carry out consultation and ensure an adhesive sensitivity test has been carried out

Contra-indication check

Discuss client requirements (it may be worth taking into consideration the type of event the lashes are being worn to, as this will determine the type most suitable)

Cleanse area using non-oily product

Apply lashes

If lashes require cutting, remember to cut so that they are tapered to avoid an unrealistic appearance

Show client the finished look

Give aftercare advice

Fill out record card. If individual lashes are used remember to include details of the lash number and where they were placed on the eye so that the effect can be recreated

Applying artificial lashes

Enhance the appearance of eyebrows and lashes **Unit B5**

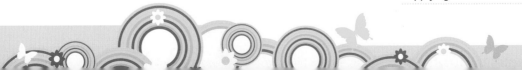

Salon life

My story

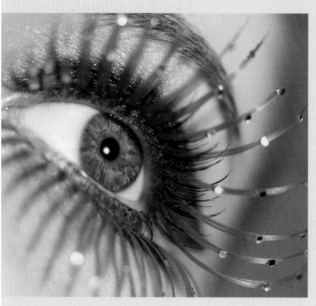

My name is Zena and I finished my Level 2 last year. After my course, I started working in a local salon. One of my clients was attending her sister's wedding and wanted to make her lashes look longer for the occasion. She has fairly short, fair lashes and so I suggested that she had some individual lashes applied to enhance her natural lash line. I performed a sensitivity test prior to application to ensure that she was not allergic to the adhesive that is used and two days later, she had the lashes applied. She was really pleased with the result – it enhanced her natural lashes but still looked natural. Unfortunately a week after the application, the client came back to the salon as more lashes had fallen out than expected. I asked about her daily cleansing routine and found out that she had been using an oil-based cleanser which had dissolved the glue. Luckily, this happened after the wedding and the lashes were ok for her sister's big day but now I make sure that I give my clients really clear aftercare advice.

Benefits for client and therapist

Benefits of using artificial lashes for the client:

- Fairly quick treatment, especially the application of strip lashes
- Instant result that can be tailored to the event
- Strip lashes come in a variety of colours and lengths
- Individual lashes come in a variety of lengths to blend with natural lashes

Benefits of using artificial lashes for the therapist:

- Can be fitted in between other treatments as the service is fairly quick to perform
- Can be linked with other eye treatments
- Can be offered as part of a make-up or bridal package

Q *Why is it important to carry out a skin sensitivity test prior to applying lashes?*

A This should be carried out to ensure that the client is not allergic to the adhesive that is used to apply the lashes. This should be recorded on the client record card and carried out every three months. If the salon starts using new products, a test should be carried out on all clients prior to the use of the new product.

Q *Why should individual lashes be the correct length and colour?*

A The lashes should *enhance* the natural lash appearance. To keep the finished look natural, the artificial lashes should tone in and be of a similar length.

Top tips

- If the artificial lashes do need to be cut, they should be cut on an angle to give a tapered effect, rather than straight across which will give a blunted appearance.

4   Apply a fine film of adhesive to the base of the artificial lash.

5   Using tweezers to hold the eyelash, place them gently on to the skin of the eyelid as close as possible to the client's lashes.

6   With firm careful pressure, use an orange stick to gently press the artificial lash into place from the tear duct outwards.

7   Come round to the front of the client and check fitting, keeping client's eyes closed. Wait for a few seconds before checking the results with the client.

8   Continue with the eye make-up, applying eyeliner to give a professional finish. Mascara should be applied to both natural and artificial lashes to seal them. Use eyelash curlers if necessary.

Maintenance and care of strip lashes

Strip lashes should always be removed at the end of the day — sleeping in them will distort their shape. Their shape will also be distorted by rubbing the eyes as this will loosen the adhesive. To remove the lashes, support the side of the eye and gently pull the lashes from the outer corner to the inner eye.

Clean strip lashes in the following way.

○ **Human hair** – clean with the manufacturer's recommended cleaner or 70 per cent alcohol.

○ **Synthetic lashes** – place in warm, soapy water for a few minutes. Rinse in tepid water.

○ **Re-curling lashes** – after cleaning, lashes should be rolled and secured around a barrel-shaped object, such as a pencil. Keep the base of the lash straight so the whole lash length curls around the object. Once recurled, store in the original container for further use.

Ensuring the client is satisfied with the finished result

Before you pack away your equipment, put tweezers into the steriliser and tidy up, you should always check the client is happy with her treatment. Do not let the client get up from the couch and get dressed before you show her the treatment results – it is then too late to take a little more eyebrow away, or add a little more tint! Give the client a mirror, and ask if she is satisfied with the results. A little more shaping of the eyebrow is possible – time permitting. The tint can be made a little darker next time, if the client requests it. Remind the client that tint only darkens existing lashes – it will not thicken them in the same way that mascara does. You may need to make a note on the record card of the client's opinions, to help you with her next treatment. Never let the client go until you have talked through the treatment with her and she is entirely happy.

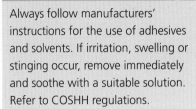

Think about it

Always follow manufacturers' instructions for the use of adhesives and solvents. If irritation, swelling or stinging occur, remove immediately and soothe with a suitable solution. Refer to COSHH regulations.

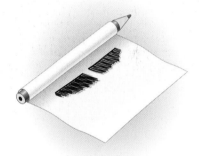

A simple way to restore the shape of strip lashes

Unit B5 Enhance the appearance of eyebrows and lashes

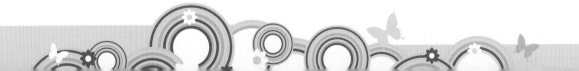

Provide aftercare advice

In this outcome you will learn about:

- giving advice and recommendations accurately and constructively
- giving your clients suitable advice specific to their individual needs.

It is important that you ensure the client receives the correct aftercare advice for the treatment that has been undertaken. You could provide an aftercare leaflet that covers eye treatments highlighting the relevant points for the client to take away.

Frequently asked questions

Q	Why is it important to carry out a sensitivity test?
A	To ensure that the client is not allergic to any of the products used in the treatment. This should be done prior to the first tint or application of lashes.
Q	Why should a sensitivity test be carried out each time the client comes for a treatment?
A	To ensure the client has not become sensitive to the product causing irritation. As a salon you may have changed products. You could invalidate your insurance if a problem arises and this procedure has not been carried out.
Q	Do I have to pre-warm the area prior to shaping?
A	You do not have to pre-warm the area, but this procedure helps to minimise discomfort as the heat opens the hair follicles — making removal easier and less painful for the client.
Q	Why is it important to use a non-oily, eye make-up remover prior to treatment?
A	Oil-based products will form a barrier over the lashes, making the application of artificial lashes or tint non-effective.
Q	Why should a barrier cream be applied prior to tinting lashes and brows?
A	This barrier cream prevents tint seeping onto the surrounding skin, causing unsightly staining of the area.

Check your knowledge

1   What type of condition is blepharitis?
    a) Fungal
    b) Viral
    c) Bacterial

2   How would you minimise discomfort when shaping the brows?

3   What facial features would you use to aid measuring the shape of brows?

4   Name two types of eyebrow tweezers.

5   Why is it important to carry out a sensitivity test before carrying out a tint?

6   How often should you carry out a sensitivity test for tint and adhesive products?

7   Why is it important to mix the tint just before you use it, and not in advance?

8   How long would you leave a tint on the brows?
    a) As long as the client wants
    b) According to the hair type
    c) According to the manufacturer's instructions

9   Why should you tint before carrying out a shape on the client?

10 Which three activities should be avoided after having a brow shape?

11 What is the suggested brow shape for a client?

12 What action would you take if blood spotting occurred when brow shaping?

13 Why should you carry out a patch test for adhesives before applying artificial lashes?

14 What percentage of peroxide is used when carrying out an eyelash or brow tint?
    a) 5 per cent
    b) 15 per cent
    c) 10 per cent

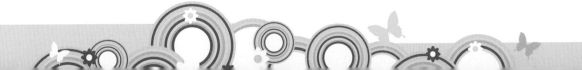

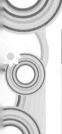

Getting ready for assessment

Your assessor will require you to show competency in the skill areas of shaping, tinting and lash application. However, your assessor will determine whether you need to show competency three times for each skill area, or just show one treatment for each skill area on three different clients. This will depend on what other evidence you can show to cover the ranges as laid down in the criteria. Evidence to support your work may be in the form of photographs or video, employer's or client statements, written papers or project work.

Remember that a client may wish to have all three treatments on the same salon visit. You may also carry out a treatment while the client is having another treatment. An eyelash tint can be performed while the client has a facial mask. These combined treatments maximise salon revenue and save precious salon and client time.

When tinting and applying artificial lashes it is important to remember that the client must have a sensitivity test for the products you are using.

When tinting you only need to show that you have practically covered two colour characteristics (light and dark being more common than white and red). However, your assessor will need you to show that you would be able to treat all colours in the range effectively and will require supporting evidence to prove this. These outstanding ranges may be covered by written work or oral questions.

You must show that you can carry out a total brow re-shape as well as general brow maintenance, and that you can apply both types of artificial lashes and have used adhesive and solvent products.

You must also show that you can carry out a thorough consultation for each treatment, prepare the working area as necessary, give suitable aftercare advice for whichever treatment you have performed, and deal with a contra-action if it arises. This could be by irrigating the eye or identifying a reaction to a patch test or a contra-indication to the treatment.

Unit B8/B9

Provide make-up services and instruct clients in the use and application of skincare products and make-up

What you will learn

8.1 Maintain safe and effective methods of working when providing make-up services

8.2 Consult, plan and prepare for make-up services

8.3 Apply make-up products

8.4 Provide aftercare advice

9.1 Maintain safe and effective methods of working when providing skincare and make-up instruction

9.2 Prepare and plan for skincare and make-up instruction

9.3 Deliver skincare and make-up instruction

9.4 Evaluate the success of skincare and make-up instruction

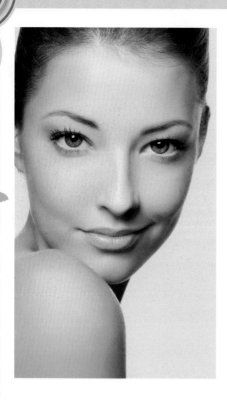

Introduction

These units are presented together as there are many aspects of providing a make-up service where you must also provide the client with valuable skincare information to ensure they gain the most from the service. You may also promote further treatments that can enhance the client's skin and overall appearance.

The subject of make-up application is one that most of you will associate with becoming a beauty therapist. The combined unit focuses on the use of make-up to enhance the appearance, for day, evening and special occasions with the added component of how to instruct clients on the most suitable skincare and selection of products to suit their skin type. This is an important skill if you wish to become a make-up artist, a trainer or pursue a career as a make-up consultant for one of the large cosmetic houses. Most women have used make-up to enhance their appearance and have been pleased with the results — whether it was for hiding a blemish, for a special occasion or just a night out with friends. However, few people know how to use make-up to their best advantage, so it is very rewarding for a therapist to accentuate a client's best features and to enable her to disguise or minimise areas that she is not as happy with. Applying make-up correctly and selecting suitable skincare products can help you do all this: providing the correct base to work on and understanding how to apply make-up to enhance features can boost confidence and self-esteem.

To help with make-up application and selection of skincare products, refer to You and the skin, and Unit B4 Provide facial skincare treatment, pages 266–72, for more information on skin types and how to recognise them, skin conditions that are treatable, and contra-indications that will prevent the treatment or require the therapist to adapt the treatment plan. Although techniques are the same regardless of skin type, a good knowledge of the client's skin is vital if you are going to do the best for the client.

It is also important to ensure that you understand the client's needs, including the time she may have available to spend on applying products and her budget.

Benefits of skincare and make-up session for the client:

- one-to-one, non-intimidating personalised service to suit individual requirements
- individual demonstration and trial
- tailored skincare/make-up planning.

Benefits of skincare and make-up instructional sessions for the therapist:

- one-to-one, personalised service to the client
- opportunity to promote salon products and treatments
- increase in clientele and commission for the therapist
- promotes salon or own business.

Benefits of group demonstration for the client:

- fun activity to do with friends
- informative without the focus just on you — good for people who don't know what to expect!

Benefits of a group demonstration for the therapist:

- ○ targets a larger audience
- ○ as well as all of the above.

Maintain safe and effective methods of working

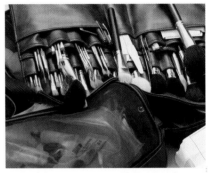

Always ensure your make-up brushes are clean before you put them away

In this outcome you will learn about:

- setting up the work area to meet legal, hygiene and treatment requirements
- making sure that environmental conditions are suitable for the client and the service
- ensuring your personal hygiene, protection and appearance meets accepted industry and organisational requirements
- ensuring all tools and equipment are cleaned using the correct methods
- effectively disinfecting your hands prior to skincare and make-up services
- maintaining accepted industry hygiene and safety practices throughout the service to minimise the risk of cross-infection
- positioning equipment and materials for ease and safety of use
- ensuring your own posture and position minimises fatigue and the risk of injury while working
- respecting a client's modesty and privacy and any sensitivities to their own appearance
- disposing of waste materials safely and correctly
- ensuring that the instruction and service are cost-effective and are carried out within a commercially viable time
- leaving the work area in a condition suitable for further services
- ensuring the client's records are up to date, accurate, easy to read and signed by the client and practitioner.

For advice on safe and effective methods of working practice, refer to individual services. Refer also to Unit B4 Provide facial skincare treatment, pages 262–66, and Professional basics.

Ensuring all tools and equipment are cleaned

As with all salon treatments, hygiene is paramount and make-up services are no exception. The equipment and products should be cleaned after each treatment and the **cut-out method**, where products are **decanted**, should be used, to prevent contamination of the product and cross-contamination from client to client.

Brushes and sponges

These need to be cleaned in hot, soapy water, which should be worked into the fibres before rinsing under running water. Brushes should then be given a final clean in an alcohol solution or suitable brush cleaner before drying naturally — this will prevent the bristles from becoming misshapen. Sponges require soaking for at least one hour in a suitable disinfectant, and should then be rinsed thoroughly.

Key terms

Decant – removing a product from a larger container to a smaller container.

Cut-out method – decanting a product from a larger container onto a spatula or into a bowl for use during a treatment.

For your portfolio

Investigate the type of brushes that are available on the market.

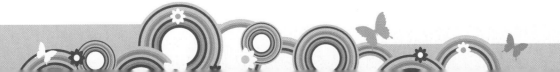

Palettes

These should be scrubbed to remove waxy deposits, then dried thoroughly.

Maintaining industry hygiene and safety practices

There is little risk of products becoming infected if good hygiene procedures are followed. However, to prevent infection by products which are normally applied directly to the face, these simple rules should be followed.

- Eye and lip pencils – sharpen before use to expose a new surface.
- Lipsticks – transfer a small amount on to a spatula before applying. Use a disposable lip brush.
- Pressed powders (eyeshadow and blushers) – either transfer products on to a palette or have a good supply of clean brushes.
- Mascara – use a disposable mascara wand for each eye.
- Wash and disinfect hands before you begin the service.

For information on facial treatments refer to Unit B4, pages 261–323, and for the difference between sanitisation and sterilisation refer to Professional basics, page 43.

Leaving the work area in a condition suitable for further services

It is important to leave the working area clean and tidy. Ensure that all products are put away and that brushes and sponges are cleaned ready for use – clean brushes in warm, soapy water and rinse well. Allow the brushes to dry naturally if possible, so that the shape of the brush is not distorted.

Disposing of waste materials

Contaminated waste should be disposed of according to legislative requirements. Any other waste products can be put with the normal rubbish, but remember to abide by COSHH guidelines for safe disposal of all products used within the salon. If carrying out a make-up service and applying false lashes, read the manufacturers' guidelines for disposal of adhesive or solvent products.

If you are carrying out a demonstration outside the salon, ensure that all waste is disposed of in accordance to the law.

Ensuring the client's records are up to date and accurate

Ensure that all records are kept up to date. For a make-up service this should include all products and shades used; any recommendations you have made; and products that have been purchased, so that you can follow up this information on subsequent visits. Skincare products should be recorded in the same way – remember that it would be worth making a note on the record card of any samples that you have given to the client. This will allow you to follow up their success at the next client visit.

TREATMENT SHEET (make-up) | Date: 18/5/2010 Client ref no. 789

Any factors which need to be considered today: Client going to wedding in June (mother of the bride). Outfit – gold hat, black & gold dress and jacket. Wedding in early evening not day; client doesn't want to look 'overdone'

Client's treatments:

Skin:	Colour:	Texture:	Type:	Sensitivity:		Problems:
Products used by client:	Cleanser:	Toner:	Moisturiser:	Mask:		Night/day creams:
Recommended products:	Cleanser:	Toner:	Moisturiser:	Mask:		Night/day creams:
	Serums:	Make-up base:	Corrective moisturiser:	Corrective treatments recommended (i.e eyebrow shape):		
Face:	Shape:	Bone structure:	Eye colour and shape:	Hair colour:		Brow colour and shape:
Make-up products used:	Foundation:	Concealer:	Powder:	Blusher:		Highlighter:
	Eye shadows:	Liners:	Mascara:	Lash curlers used:		Brow pencil:
	Lip liner:	Lipstick:	Other:			

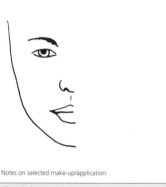
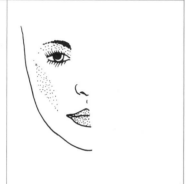

Notes on selected make-up/application:

Client declaration: *I declare the information is true and correct and that, as far as I am aware, I can undertake treatment with this establishment without any adverse effects. I am fully aware of any contra-indications: I am therefore willing to proceed and accept this treatment.*

Client signature*:	**Without signature, the treatment cannot proceed*	**Date:**
Therapist signature:		**Date:**

A partially completed make-up record card

TREATMENT SHEET (facials) | Date: 11/5/2010 Client ref no. 675

Any factors which need to be considered today: Client new to salon – 1st facial (present from husband for 30th bday on 15.05). Would like to buy products too.

Client's treatments:

Client: *Male*   Female ✓

Skin type: (Oily)/Dry/Combination/Mature/Young   **Massage medium:** oil/(cream)

Muscle tone: Good/(Average)/Poor

Age: under 21 (30s) 40s 50s 60s over 70

Client's health: good /(average)/ poor

Comments: Two small children/disturbed nights; complains of low energy sometimes (and feeling tired and irritable)

Medication taken: Occasional pain killers for period pain

Skin condition: *good/average/poor specific problems/conditions to be avoided:* Skin oily & a little congested, black heads along T zone. Showing as a combination skin but no dryness on cheeks. Face looking tired & a little drawn, poor colour, sallow look – could be caused by lack of sleep and wrong products

Client's lifestyle:

Sleep: Approx 4-5 hrs a night (see above) – disturbed sleep pattern	**Relaxation:** *good/poor*
Profession: Works from home (writer) often late pm/early am to fit round kids	**Fluid intake:** *eight glasses of water taken daily? No Other drinks: Tea*
Family life: Married with two children	**Smoking/drugs:** No
Exercise: None - no time & would have to organise child care	**Emotional balance:** 1-10 rating 1 being low 10 being highest:
Energy levels: 1-10 rating 1 being low 10 being highest: 1-2 (see above)	**Other:** *regular mealtimes / shift work / supplements / allergies: –*

Client's treatment:

Treatment chosen (and reasons):

Contra indication present: yes/no
Details:

Was client encouraged to seek medical advice? yes/no
Does treatment need adapting due to minor contra indication?: yes/no
Details:

Modifications to treatment: yes/no
Details:

Massage techniques used: *Effleurage / Petrissage / Tapotement / Vibrations*

Aftercare/homecare advice given (including details of recommended products):

Client declaration: *I declare the information is true and correct and that, as far as I am aware, I can undertake treatment with this establishment without any adverse effects. I am fully aware of any contra-indications: I am therefore willing to proceed and accept this treatment.*

Client signature*:	**Without signature, the treatment cannot proceed*	**Date:**
Therapist signature:		**Date:**

A partially completed skincare record card

Unit B8/B9

Provide make-up services and instruct clients in the use and application of skincare products and make-up

Obtain potential client information

Whenever you give a group demonstration, it is a good idea to ask potential clients if they would be happy to give you their personal details to be included in a mailing list for special offers and promotions. (Refer to Professional basics, page 63, for the correct storage of data under the Data Protection Act.)

For your portfolio

Devise a record card or information sheet that you could use for a group demonstration.

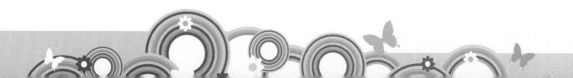

Consult, plan and prepare for make-up and skincare and make-up instruction

In this outcome you will learn about:

- using consultation techniques in a polite and friendly manner to determine the client's needs and preferences within the limits of your responsibility
- ensuring that informed and signed parental or guardian consent is obtained for minors prior to any service
- ensuring that a parent or guardian is present throughout the services for minors under the age of 16
- obtaining signed, written informed consent from the client prior to carrying out the service
- asking your client appropriate questions to establish their current skincare and make-up regime and ability level
- asking your client appropriate questions to identify if they have any contra-indications to skincare and make-up products
- accurately recording your client's responses to questioning
- ensuring the client is comfortable and correctly seated in a relaxed position, with a good view of the mirror
- ensuring the client's clothing, hair and accessories are effectively protected or removed
- ensuring the skin is clean, toned and suitably moisturised prior to the application of make-up
- accurately recognising and recording the client's skin type, age group and condition

- encouraging clients to ask questions to clarify any points
- taking the necessary action in response to any identified contra-indications
- ensuring client advice is given without reference to a specific medical condition and without causing undue alarm and concern
- agreeing the service and outcomes that are acceptable to the client and meet their needs
- ensuring the objectives of the skincare and make-up instruction are clear, realistic and agreed with the client
- selecting suitable make-up products to suit the client's age group, skin type, tone and condition, the occasion and their preferences
- ensuring the lighting conditions are appropriate to the type of make-up instruction
- providing a suitable range of skincare and make-up products for the client skin type, tone and condition and the type of instruction to be given
- ensuring that face charts and all necessary tools and equipment are available.

Recognising and recording the client's skin type

The knowledge you require to prepare the client for treatment is the same as that required for a full facial treatment as covered in Unit B4 Improve and maintain facial skin condition, pages 291–321.

Whatever the environment you are working in and whatever the treatment you are undertaking, you will need to carry out a skin analysis in order to ensure the correct products are selected. This will cover:

○ facial examination

○ skin types, e.g. normal, dry, oily or combination

○ record cards.

Refer to You and the skin, pages 184–88, for further detailed information on skin types and conditions. You should also refer to the risk assessment for facials that is included in Unit B4 on page 264.

Using consultation techniques to determine the client's needs and preferences and obtaining consent

Before a make-up application/instruction or skincare lesson can take place, a full consultation should be undertaken so that an accurate assessment of the client and her needs can be made. This should be both by visual assessment of the skin and by asking a series of questions.

Visual assessment

This should be carried out on a cleansed and toned dry face with the hair secured away from the face. The skin should not be moisturised at this stage because this will make the skin slightly greasy. A suitable moisturiser for the skin should be applied before the application of make-up. Refer to Unit B4, pages 277–91, for information on facial analysis, cleansing and toning routines.

You should analyse the client's skin type, facial features and bone structure in an upright position.

When carrying out an analysis for make-up the light should be falling directly onto the client's face. The light should be a combination of natural daylight and warm white fluorescent light.

Colour and shape of eyes and brows

Natural colour and shape of lips

Skin type and tone

Face shape

VISUAL ASSESSMENT OF THE AREA SHOULD INCLUDE

Skin blemishes and problems

Muscle tone

Bone structure and facial contours

Lines and wrinkles

Questioning the client

As well as the visual assessment, you should ask the client a few simple questions to help you both agree on a realistic service plan. Some useful questions to help you assess the client are listed below.

- How much make-up do you usually wear?
- What do you think are your best/worst features?
- Do you have any allergies or sensitivity to make-up or other related products?
- Is the make-up for a special occasion?
- Are there any colours you like/dislike?
- Are you trying to create a special look?
- What skincare regime do you use at present?
- Do you have any areas of particular concern/outcomes you would like to address/achieve? (This will encourage the client to ask any questions that she may have.)

> **Think about it**
>
> For every client, you will need their signed, written, informed consent before carrying out the service. Anyone under the age of 16 will require parent/guardian informed and signed consent for these services to go ahead, and the parent/guardian must be present throughout the service.

> **Think about it**
>
> The facial features look very different when the client is laid flat.

> **For your portfolio**
>
> In pairs, devise some more open questions that you could ask the client.

Unit B8/B9

Provide make-up services and instruct clients in the use and application of skincare products and make-up

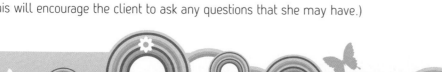

It is important to ask the client open questions so that you can gain maximum information. Always be positive, even if the client has no skincare regime.

When you have gathered all the information you can agree a suitable plan for your make-up and skincare instructional session or make-up application. You may have differing views from your client, so it is important to agree on a suitable and realistic plan. Remember, too, that the plan should reflect the client's level of ability. If she is a novice at applying skincare products and make-up, there is no point in giving her a complicated routine to follow.

Think about it

To carry out an effective make-up session, you will need to be able to identify and treat the client's individual skin type, so it is essential that you have sound knowledge of facial treatments and products.

Details of your analysis should be recorded on the client record card. This will support recommendation of skincare products and is a valuable tool when recording the make-up used. Recording your analysis is essential when doing a bridal make-up trial, as you would want to create the same result on the day.

Identifying if clients have contra-indications to make-up

Allergic reactions and sensitivity testing

European Union (EU) and US legislation requires that cosmetic companies conduct very strict safety tests on materials they use to formulate products. Nevertheless, there will always be some people who are allergic to a substance which other people can tolerate without a problem. It is therefore essential that you complete a **sensitivity** test if you are concerned that the client may react to a product. This can be done by testing a small sample of the product behind the client's ear or in the crook of the elbow. If a reaction occurs within 24 hours the product should not be used. A reaction could include:

- redness (erythema)
- swelling
- irritation to the area.

Treat with calamine lotion and a cold compress as necessary.

In some instances, medication can affect the condition of the skin and cause sensitivity to occur. Always carry out a thorough consultation and contra-indication check. If the client has an unidentified condition, recommend that she visits her GP for a diagnosis and treatment. Never diagnose yourself.

If the client has had **allergic reactions** to skincare products or make-up in the past, ensure that the products you select are **hypoallergenic**.

How long do cosmetics last?

The European Union Cosmetics Directive 1993 states that products which contain no preservatives and natural ingredients with a shelf life of less than six months have to be stamped with an expiry date. Cosmetics that have been tested and meet the European safety requirements are not required to be date stamped. The

Key terms

Sensitivity – the ability to react to a stimulus. This could be caused by an allergy such as hayfever or as a result of improper use of products over a period of time.

Allergic reaction – unpleasant reaction of the body when coming into contact with a particular ingredient, product, chemical or substance; symptoms may include sneezing, redness of the skin, skin rash, inflamed eyes and mucus membranes.

Hypoallergenic – designed to cause fewer allergic reactions.

EU gives a shelf life for cosmetics that is approximately 30 months from the time of manufacture, although this may vary depending on the product, so you could calculate how long you have had a product from the day that you opened it. The time after opening is denoted by a special symbol that looks like an open jar; inside the symbol will be a number that will reflect the number in months that the product can safely be used without harm.

Risk assessment for make-up application

Refer to Unit G20 Make sure your own actions reduce risks to health and safety, pages 73–85, for a complete discussion of risk assessment.

Hazard: only look for hazards that you could reasonably expect to result in significant harm under the conditions in your workplace. Use the following examples as a guide.

- **Allergies** (allergic reaction to make-up)
- **Cross-infections** (infections spread from tools)
- **Irritation** (caused by scratchy tools)
- **Contamination** (caused by ignoring contra-indications to service)

Many of the topics relating to both the application of skincare products and the application of make-up are covered in more depth in Unit B4, pages 261–325; Professional basics, pages 12–68; and Unit G20 Make sure your own actions reduce risks to health and safety, pages 71–103.

Think about it

In some instances allergic reactions can be severe and will require medical intervention. In the event of a client being allergic to a certain product or substance, ensure that you always read the ingredients and refer to the manufacturer's instructions. Always record details on the client record card.

Ensuring lighting is suitable for make-up application and instruction

It is important to work in good lighting when applying make-up to the client, carrying out make-up instruction and, where possible, for demonstrations. Always try to face natural light. Natural daylight is pure white light, but this light does not just fall on the face from above – it is reflected from any light coloured surface it hits. Natural daylight is the only light that shows true colours, but it is also the harshest form of light as it shows up imperfections. To achieve the best from your make-up, a combination of natural light and warm white fluorescent lighting gives the best effect.

Artificial lighting

Make-up colours tested in the wrong light can give the wrong effect when applied. It is therefore important to be aware of the differing effects of various types of lighting.

Standard light bulbs

These produce a yellowish colour which dulls blue tones and makes red tones appear darker. A light bulb cover with a shade directs the light down, creating unnatural shadows.

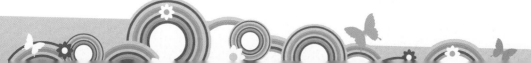

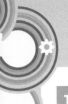

Think about it

Warm, white fluorescent light is the best substitute for natural lighting and the best for matching make-up colours.

Ingredients: Aqua (Water), Cetearyl Alcohol, Petrolatum, Caprylic/Capric Triglyceride, Ethylhexyl Palmitate, Vitis Vinifera, Stearate SE, Cera Alba (Beeswax), Stearic Acid, Cetearyl, Carbomer, Geranium Maculatum (Geranium Extract), Lavender, Extract), Camillia Sinensis (Green Tea), Theobroma Cacao, Chinensis (Jojoba) Seed Oil, Cocos Nucifera (Coconut Oil), Gel), Parfum (Fragrance), Linalool, Alpha-isomethyl Ionon, Methylpropional, Hydroxyisohexyl 3-Cyclohexene Carboxaldehyde, Limonene, Citronellol, BHT, Tetrasodium EDTA, Lauramine Oxide, Phenoxyethanol, Methylparaben, Butylparaben, Ethylparaben, Isobutylparaben, Propylparaben, CI 19140 (FD&C Yellow No.5).
salesinfo@pbs-beauty.com

12M   code - 077334

List of ingredients and shelf life of product

Fluorescent tubes

White tubes give out a harsh, blue-white light which makes colours appear cold. If the fluorescent tube is covered by a diffuser, this will soften the effect and create very little shadow. Warm white tubes with a diffuser will therefore be the best type of artificial light for matching make-up colours.

Preparing for a skincare or make-up service

The working area should be clean, tidy and well organised. Ensure you adhere to a professional standard regarding your appearance and that your working area complies with the health, safety and hygiene regulations. Consult your professional body for guidelines to prevent cross-infection. The main sources of infection during make-up are usually contaminated products, dirty tools and equipment, and applying make-up and skincare products over infected areas.

Make-up and skincare activities can be carried out individually or you may be asked to do a promotion or presentation to a group. Whichever method you are using it is important that you act in a professional manner. Whether you are in a cubicle with a client in a one-to-one setting or giving a presentation in a community centre, you should maintain the same high standards.

Recognising and recording the client's skin type, age group and condition

Before carrying out any make-up services, you need to ensure that you establish the client's skin type, age range and condition and select suitable skincare and make-up products for both the client's personal use and instruction. (Refer to Unit B4, pages 277–91, for more information on how to undertake a facial analysis and select appropriate products.)

Normal skin	Dry skin	Oily skin	Combination skin	Sensitive skin	Dehydrated skin	Mature skin
Eye make-up remover lotion Light cleansing lotion Facial wash if preferred 10–20 per cent alcohol toner Light moisturising lotion/cream Eye lotion/gel Gentle exfoliant Non-setting mask	Eye make-up remover – oil or cream based Cream cleanser 0 per cent alcohol toner Cream moisturiser Gentle exfoliant Eye cream Neck cream Non-setting mask	Eye make-up remover – lotion based Cleansing lotion or milk Facial wash or gel 2–50 per cent alcohol toner Cleansing grain or peel Moisturising milk Light eye gel Clay-based masks	Products to suit the variation in skin types – however, if the client has sensitive skin in the combinations, this should always take priority over other types of product	Treat as dry skin – consider using hypoallergenic products	As dry – recommend gentle exfoliation and facial treatments such as a galvanic facial to push moisture into the skin	Cream-based products that are suitable for drier skin and alcohol-free toners that prevent the skin from drying out, night, eye and neck creams should be recommended. Additional treatments such as non-surgical face lifts could also be discussed

At a glance – suitable skincare products for different skin types

The client should be shown how to use each of the recommended products, it is important for the therapist to let the client know the frequency of application, methods of application and any special equipment that should be used. This should be done by the use of demonstration and client application as a trial, diagrams, written home care leaflets as well as verbal instruction.

Think about it

If a product starts to smell, change colour or separate, it should be thrown away. Always refer to the manufacturer's instructions for use and storage and look at the symbol denoting the number of months the product can be used for once opened. If products are used incorrectly or not stored properly, then they will deteriorate more quickly than indicated on the symbol.

Think about it

You should have available a variety of products and equipment to suit all skin types and effects that you wish to create suitable for a varied range of clientele.

Basic trolley set-up for a skincare instructional session

○ Variety of cleansers, toners and moisturisers for each skin type
○ Exfoliants
○ Facial washes/scrubs
○ Eye creams
○ Neck creams
○ Lip balms
○ Masks
○ Magnifier lamp
○ Headband
○ Cotton wool/facial sponges
○ Tissues
○ Spatulas
○ Facial consultation charts

Basic trolley equipment for a make-up procedure

○ Towels or gown
○ Headband
○ Make-up sponges
○ Make-up brushes
○ Make-up products
○ Spatulas
○ Palette
○ Sharpener
○ Cotton buds
○ Mirror
○ Brush and comb

All brushes should preferably be disposable to prevent cross-infection.

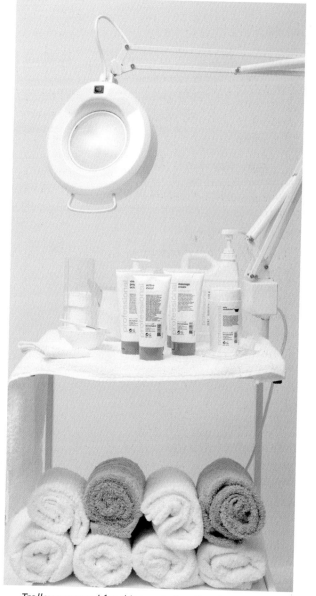

Trolley prepared for skincare instructional session

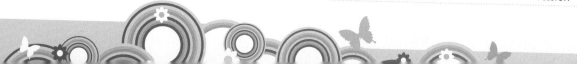

Unit B8/B9

Provide make-up services and instruct clients in the use and application of skincare products and make-up

Make-up brushes

A good set of brushes is essential in the application of any make-up. There are individual brushes available for each stage of the make-up application. For maximum benefit it is important to understand their usage.

Face-powder brush

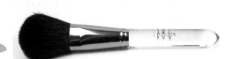

This is the largest brush as it covers the largest area. It is not restricted to defining shape, its primary purpose being to blend loosened face powder into the skin.

Blusher brush

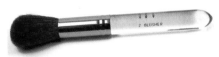

Used to apply blusher to the cheekbones. It looks similar to the powder brush but is slightly smaller in order to work on the cheekbone area.

Contour brush

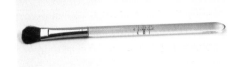

This brush has several uses: to apply contour powder under the cheekbones, to shade and highlight the face.

Eyebrow brush

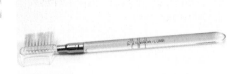

Used to shape the brows and to blend colour. It has short nylon bristles and may have a small comb on the other side to separate lashes.

Eyeliner brush

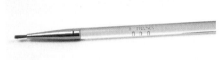

For the application of eyeliner or to blend in kohl pencils along the rim of the eye, a very thin, pointed brush is required.

Angled eyeshadow brush

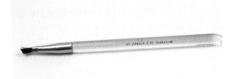

To apply and blend powder eyeshadow. The angle of the brush is important, it allows you to follow and blend into the socket area.

Eyeshadow brush

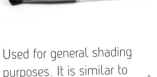

Used for general shading purposes. It is similar to the angle brush but with a straight edge.

Fluff brush

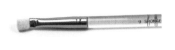

This brush is used to finish off the blending of the eye make-up. It is the largest of the eye brushes and it needs to be very soft, as it is used to soften the edges without disturbing the shape of the make-up.

Sponge applicator

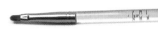

The sponge is good for applying both loose and powder eyeshadow. It is also used for blending and softening harsh pencil lines.

Lip brush

To apply lipstick, the brush must have short thin bristles to make it flat. This helps to give a clean outline to the lips.

One-to-one make-up and skincare sessions

A one-to-one make-up or skincare session usually takes place in a salon, in a well-lit cubicle or working area, and takes little organisation, except for clean tools, a good selection of products and the necessary accessories of tissues, cotton wool and cotton buds, as well as a large mirror. (Refer to basic trolley set-up above.)

When the client books in for a lesson, it is a good idea to suggest she brings her existing make-up — it might simply be that the client has excellent products and colours, but she just does not know how or where to use them, or she might be concerned about overusing them — or the range of skincare products she currently uses.

When using instructional techniques, whether for skincare products or the application of make-up, you are teaching the correct use and application in order for the client to gain the best results. With make-up application the best way to do this is to ask the client to follow your lead. You do one side of the face, and she matches the technique on the other.

For an individual skincare or make-up lesson you should:

○ seat the client in an upright or slightly reclined position in good light

○ discuss the client's requirements including any concerns

○ remove any accessories, and make sure hair is secured off the face

○ ask the client to remove her contact lenses if she has sensitive eyes

○ protect the client's clothing

○ check for contra-indications (refer to You and the skin, pages 199–203, for further information on contra-indications)

○ carry out a thorough skin analysis on cleansed skin.

Make-up consultation should include:

○ client preference

○ face shape

○ areas to be highlighted/shaded

○ any areas requiring corrective make-up

○ bone structure

○ shape of head

○ hair colour and texture

○ skin colour and tone

○ skin sensitivity

○ cultural and religious considerations.

Cultural and religious considerations

For some Asian women, facial adornment has religious significance that has its roots steeped in history. The application of facial and body adornment is a specialised art. If you treat people from several different cultures within your salon, it would be worth spending time researching this area. This would show excellent customer care to existing and prospective clients. You should also be aware of the ingredients in the make-up products and skincare range you use — some cultures and religions forbid the use of animal-based products.

> **Think about it**
>
> As a therapist, it is important to consider your posture as well as the client's when carrying out a service. When conducting a make-up application or demonstration you must be able to reach the client correctly. Positioning is important to prevent injury.

> **Think about it**
>
> When working one-on-one with a client, allow them to look in a mirror as you work with the products so they can see exactly what you are doing, and, if you are carrying out a make-up, how the effect can be achieved.

Provide make-up services and instruct clients in the use and application of skincare products **Unit BB7/B9**

- Agree a plan incorporating the above, taking into account the type of make-up required, the occasion, the colour of clothing to be worn, the client's clothing, and the client's skin type and tone, which should include both colour and muscle tone, condition and age group.
- Agree products with client.
- Apply the make-up and explain the procedure to the client.
- Assess the results with the client, entering the colours/products used on the record card.
- Recommend products for homecare use.
- Check client satisfaction.

Face shapes

It is useful to consider some general descriptions of face shapes and some hair styles that can **enhance** a make-up. This will help when you are analysing the client's face shape at the consultation stage. Remember when applying make-up to clients from different ethnic origins that characteristic facial features can differ.

Any corrective work on black or Asian clients should be approached in exactly the same way as for white Caucasian clients, using contouring products to enhance or reduce areas. Refer to skin characteristics in You and your skin, page 189.

Refer also to You and the skin, pages 198—99 for more information on face shapes.

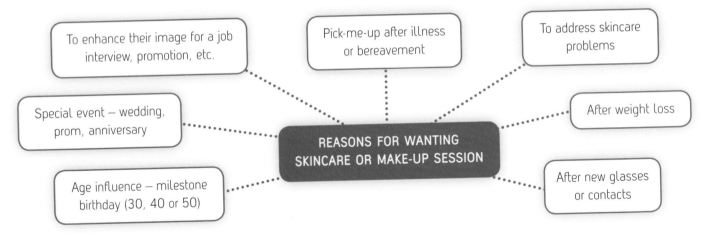

To enhance their image for a job interview, promotion, etc.

Pick-me-up after illness or bereavement

To address skincare problems

Special event — wedding, prom, anniversary

After weight loss

REASONS FOR WANTING SKINCARE OR MAKE-UP SESSION

Age influence — milestone birthday (30, 40 or 50)

After new glasses or contacts

Reasons why clients book a one-to-one make-up lesson

Group demonstrations

Local clubs and societies are often looking for opportunities to engage interesting speakers. You could offer to give a talk to the local Women's Institute (WI), mother and toddler group, slimming group or women's group, or your salon might be approached by one of these groups asking for a make-up or skincare demonstration. This is your opportunity to talk about the various treatments your salon offers or, if you are a mobile or independent home-based therapist, an opportunity for you to promote your business.

All of these groups are potential customers, so a professional, yet friendly, approach is essential. Your aim is to encourage them to come to you for the treatments and services you are demonstrating!

My story

Salon promotions

Hi, my name is Sam. I am manager of a large salon in Kent. Until recently, my therapists were all reluctant to take part in promotional events, so I devised an in-house training session to get them used to public speaking and doing demonstrations to larger groups. We invited family and friends along so that it was not so intimidating, and presented some of our latest treatments. We also did skin mapping. The session was a huge success, and it gave the therapists real confidence. We now do seasonal promotion evenings, and all the therapists enjoy taking part. It has increased our clientele and sales. It's also worth remembering that some product companies will provide a small amount of money for the organisation of a promotional event.

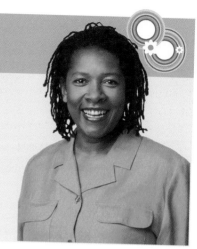

Meeting individual needs and interests

When organising a demonstration, you will need to consider:

○ the age group of the audience — this will impact on the type of skincare or make-up you focus on

○ the size of the group

○ the type of demonstration — face painting would interest a mother and toddler group but may not interest the WI, for example

○ the time of day when the event is to be held — day, evening or special interest, e.g. prom/ball/bridal

○ different product types, for example emphasis on products with sunscreens and protection from the environment — this could include
  - moisturisers and age-defying hand creams
  - products designed for sensitive skins/hypoallergenic products
  - suitable cosmetic make-up for treating skin disorders, port wine stains, etc.

If you are carrying out a group demonstration/instructional demonstration, there are a number of factors that you should consider to ensure that your audience is engaged.

Venue and format

Some points to bear in mind:

○ Where the event is to be held is very important. The venue can be anywhere, from the local village hall to a hotel (most commonly used for bridal fairs) to someone's home. Find out where and when, and then consider both the risk assessment aspect and health and safety implications.

○ You will need to check whether your insurance will cover you to do the demonstration. You should not assume that your public liability and indemnity insurances are valid when you are working away from your own premises (see Professional Basics, page 65). You also need to consider your car insurance: are you covered by business insurance and are your products insured when stored in and transported in your vehicle?

○ Accidents happen, and it is your responsibility to ensure that both you and your audience are adequately protected; both externally, for problems with the building, fire regulations, etc., for internal areas, such as safe seating and non-slip flooring.

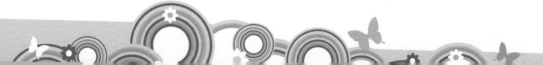

○ Ask the group's organiser if the premises have an up-to-date fire certificate, if there has been a recent risk assessment of the building and what access and exit facilities are available. Are there fire exits?

○ Will a first aider be present at the demonstration? What happens if a member of the group has an accident or is taken ill? This needs to be considered before the event so that contingency plans can be put in place – after the event is too late and may leave you and the organiser with serious issues of compensation or neglect charges.

○ If the demonstration is for people who have disabilities, then responsibility should be taken by the organisers to ensure that sufficient carers are present to support the audience. It should not be your responsibility to take guests to the toilet or deal with a medical emergency – you are not trained to do so. Find out if there are facilities for people with disabilities such as ramps and toilets.

○ For your own safety, ask the organiser about parking and how to get in to the building. A dark parking area may leave you vulnerable, and carrying your demonstration materials, make-up and stand up several flights of stairs because the lift is not working may not be very practical. Ideally, easy access on the ground floor is preferred, with well-lit parking available. You may need to enlist some help in setting up.

Budget and cost

The other important aspect of the group demonstration is who pays and for what. The issues of budget and cost should be sorted out at the planning stage. If your salon is approached by an organisation, the organiser will usually ask how much you charge for a make-up demonstration. Some salons would consider this an ideal opportunity to enhance their client base and a means of advertising, and would therefore agree to the demonstration for free. Other salons would look at the time involved, the wages of the member of staff to be covered and the cost of materials, and then calculate a set fee to cover their overheads. This is up to the individual salon – there is no right answer.

The timing of the demonstration may affect the issue of cost. If the therapist goes in her own time after work to an evening event, then she may expect to be paid for it. Often, bridal fairs are held over a weekend to allow people who work during the week to attend. This may mean the therapist is working on her only day off, Sunday, and she may wish to be paid. If she attends on Saturday, who will cover her clients in the salon? This could become expensive if a relief therapist has to be brought in or clients cancelled to allow the therapist time to attend a demonstration she is giving, with no charge.

However, often it is worth the investment for the publicity generated, and the profile of the salon can be raised enormously. Lots of business comes out of demonstrations, and further treatments and services can be linked into the make-up demonstration – facials, top-to-toe bridal treatments, skin improvement, and so on.

All of this needs discussing with the organisers and your line manager within the salon before you agree to the demonstration.

Products

The number of people attending the demonstration will affect how many products, testers and display materials you will need. This will also depend upon the type of demonstration you do. If it is a complete make-over, using one model, who you have brought along, to display your skills and entice people into the salon for treatments, then you will only need products for one. If you will be selecting a model from the audience, you will need one set of everything for each skin type.

If you are doing a demonstration en masse, where the audience actively participates, following your lead, applying their make-up as you go along, then many more products are required, unless everyone brings their own. As you are applying make-up to a clean skin, which has a make-up base or moisturiser on it, skincare products are essential, as well as a selection of make-up.

Active participation is a good idea, and encourages the audience to have the confidence to apply their own make-up. Make sure that everyone has a clear view of you and the step-by-step application.

Timing

It is important that you know how long you are expected to speak for and the length of time your full demonstration will take. If you are expected to take the whole meeting time, which may be several hours, you should have some activities which the audience can participate in, like a draw for a free treatment, to keep the interest high.

Have a dress rehearsal with a model before the day of the demonstration, so that you know how long the actual make-up application takes, and then add time for an introduction, and a question and answer session afterwards. This will allow you at the planning stage to tell the organiser that you will need a minimum of, say, an hour and a half, in which to work.

Setting up the room

The key to a successful demonstration is visibility. The audience needs to be able to see what you are doing, or they will lose interest and potential clients will have been lost. For good communication to take place, you also need to be heard, and a microphone may be needed for larger venues. A raised platform or stage is good for larger audiences, but it does not create an intimate, friendly feel, so it will depend upon the number of people and the facilities the venue has.

The best room set-up is a horse-shoe shape, with you and your model at the open end, with an eye-catching display behind you and all materials close at hand. This ensures everyone has a good view, you have command of the room and are able to make lots of eye contact to check that the audience understands your techniques and remains interested.

Try to be organised, so once you start and get into the swing of things, you do not have to return to your car for tissues, or stop the demonstration for any reason. This will break the attention span of your audience, and you will not appear to be professional.

Think through what you will need beforehand, and work logically so that nothing is missed.

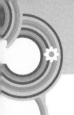

Deliver skincare and make-up instruction

In this outcome you will learn about:

- using instructional techniques which are clear, logical and delivered at a pace suitable for the client
- demonstrating skincare and make-up application in a way which promotes understanding
- guiding the client through application of the product(s) in a way which meets the needs of the client and the product(s) being used
- clearly explaining the use and purpose of make-up tools
- effectively using resources throughout the instructional activity
- adapting your instructional techniques to suit the client's needs
- using methods of communication that are suitable for the client
- allowing the client sufficient time to practise skincare and make-up application techniques on themselves

- encouraging the client to ask questions throughout the period of instruction
- responding clearly and positively to any questions and queries
- confirming that the client has a basic understanding of the basic techniques necessary to achieve their desired look
- providing the client with accurate information on the products, tools and equipment used and where to source them
- actively encouraging clients to take advantage of the products and services
- providing written instructions on how to apply skincare routine and make-up application to achieve their agreed look.

Introducing the demonstration

Once you have fully prepared your working area and the room is set up in a user-friendly manner so that everyone can see and hear you, you may begin.

It is important to consult with your model prior to starting — have a quiet word with her to ensure that your objectives marry up with her needs, and that she has no contra-indications present.

An introduction is always a good ice breaker, rather than just starting and hoping everyone will pay attention. It is a good idea to begin with something along the lines of 'Good afternoon, everyone — my name is Janine from Tranquillity salon, and I'd like to welcome you to Fern Hall for this demonstration.' Then tell the audience exactly what is going to happen and at what point they can ask questions. For example, 'I am going to give a make-up/skincare demonstration for about half an hour, talking you through the various stages, with some professional tips, and then there will be a question and answer session. After the tea break, we can talk about products and treatments.'

Using instructional techniques

For tips on general communication skills, refer to Professional basics, pages 16–21. Below are some specific tools for a short presentation. Remember, these tips would also apply in a one-on-one session with a client:

○ Pace your speech pattern — try to speak slowly and clearly, rather than very quickly, which is what often happens when you are nervous. Pace is literally the speed of the words. A calm, slow, measured speech reflects reassurance and confidence — the speaker is concentrating on getting across the message. Although interest and enthusiasm are important, these can sometimes lead to a more rapid delivery. Panic, anxiety and lack of confidence can produce fast, muddled speech.

○ Do not be afraid of short pauses or silence while you are either allowing the information to sink in, or you are concentrating on applying the make-up. Break up the silence if you think it has gone on too long by commentary such as 'Always apply foundation after the skin has been moisturised. Allow the moisturiser to be absorbed for a few seconds before continuing with the foundation ...'

○ Pauses can be either a comfortable silence, allowing reflection upon what has been said, or can be very awkward, even menacing. Judging a pause and knowing when to break it, takes a little patience and skill. Hesitation in speech patterns may indicate uncertainty or stress, or just tiredness, where the brain function is slowing down.

○ Varying the tone of your voice enlivens speech and helps retain the listeners' attention. Flat, boring tones will not engage the audience and will not help them understand what is being said to them.

○ Pitch is most noticeable when it is either high or low, and often reflects the emotional state of the person. Someone who is depressed often talks in a low, failing pitch, quite slowly, whereas a raised pitch conveys excitement, enthusiasm or anxiety. Voice coaches recommend to people in the public eye, who have to make a lot of speeches, to lower the pitch slightly and slow down their normal rate and rhythm of speech.

○ The use of graphics, a PowerPoint® display (if you have the technology and the facilities are available) or pictures of make-up products and skincare products along with demonstration samples add interest.

○ Make plenty of eye contact and try not to focus on one person as this may make them uncomfortable. Include everyone in your field of vision. Whether undertaking a group presentation or working with a client on a one-to-one basis, ensure that you give them your full attention. Focus on them when they are talking and be encouraging when they try out new techniques and products.

○ Respond kindly when asked questions. Listen carefully listen to the query, rather than interrupting the person, and nod to show you have understood. If you answer one person well, it encourages others to ask questions, too.

As well as talking through your demonstration, remember not to stand in front of the model as you are working – the audience will not be able to see. You need to perfect the art of working at the side so that your actions are plain to see, and you can stop at each stage to show the audience or client the type of effect. For example, 'After foundation and powder application, the skin tone is even and blemishes are well covered, but the colour comes with the application of blusher, lipstick and eye products, so don't expect too much colour in the face at this time.' Then show the audience your 'blank canvas', with just foundation and powder on.

These are just a few pointers to help you prepare and carry out a presentation and these techniques can be used when working with smaller groups and one to one. You may need to adapt your methods of communication to meet the needs of the client and the size of your audience to make sure that they fully understand. To aid your explanation you should also explain the purpose of the tools and products – a thorough explanation could boost your retail sales.

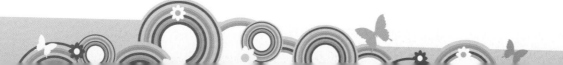

Apply make-up products

In this outcome you will learn about:

- using make-up products suitable for the client's age group, skin type, tone and condition and the occasion
- using equipment correctly following manufacturers' instructions
- using foundation that is suitable for the client's underlying skin tone
- applying any necessary foundations to create an even skin tone without demarcation lines
- ensuring any skin blemishes are effectively disguised using the correct colour and consistency of concealer
- using a suitable powder to achieve the desired finish
- using suitable eye products, when used, to define and shape the eyebrow
- using eyeshadows of a suitable texture, tone and colour for the client and the look required evenly blending eyeshadows and applying them in a way to enhance and balance the client's eye shape
- using eyeliners in a way that enhances the client's eye area and is suitable for the look required
- applying liquid eyeliners, when used, to leave a precise, clearly defined line with an even flow of colour
- leaving lashes evenly coated with mascara from base to tip, separated and without transfer to the surrounding skin
- using cheek products of a suitable texture, tone and colour for the client
- ensuring cheeks are left with an evenly blended finish with the product positioned to enhance the client's natural face shape and the look required
- using lip products in a way that enhances the client's lips and is suitable for the look required
- applying strong coloured lipsticks and lip liner, when used, to leave a clearly defined shape, with evenly balanced colour
- ensuring all elements of the make-up combine to complement each other to create the desired image in a way that flatters the client
- ensuring the finished result is to the client's satisfaction.

Refer to Unit B4 for the correct skin care products to suit the skin type of the client. You will need to take into account the client's age, texture and skin tone. A suitable product will provide the correct canvas to ensure that the make-up lasts throughout the day

To achieve a successful make-up application whatever the occasion, you need to understand how and when to apply make-up products. The following pages introduce you to the main kinds of make-up products before giving step-by-step guides to make-up application for various occasions and times of day.

Salon life

My story

My name is Yvette and I trained as a Beauty therapist six years ago. I knew from the start that make-up would be my passion and since qualifying I have developed my own business promoting skincare and make-up to a variety of people. I find the work very rewarding and diverse especially when presenting to groups. I also undertake wedding, prom and special event make-up which is great fun. When I first started I decided to keep a notebook of my ideas and thoughts and I still use it to this day. It helps me with inspiration for new ideas – I cut out and keep clippings of pictures that have inspired me and pictures of work that I have done. It is also useful for jotting down ideas prior to using them on clients or you could collect together the ideas as a book for your clients.

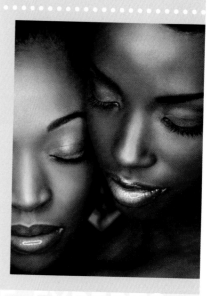

Benefits to client and therapist

Benefits of make-up application for the client:

- Effect of treatment is immediately visible
- Sessions can be tailored to meet individual requirements offering a more personalised service
- Hands-on opportunities for client within a make-up and skincare lesson to ensure correct procedure is used at home
- Clients can try different products and ask questions

Benefits of make-up application for the therapist:

- Can be offered individually or to larger groups
- Group work allows the therapist to capture more potential client data, therefore increasing revenue
- Allows therapist to link sell products and other treatments

ASK THE EXPERTS

Q *I sometimes struggle trying to find the correct shade of foundation. Do you have any tips that would help me?*

A Remember, if you can't find the correct shade of foundation then you can blend your own shades by mixing two or more colours together on a palette to obtain the right match. Use the colour wheel to help you remember which colours neutralise one another in order to get the right result.

Don't test foundation colour on the hand, as hands tend to be a completely different colour to the face. Test foundations on the jaw line for an accurate colour match. There is also nothing to stop you using different colour foundations for shading and highlighting purposes and to correct certain features.

Top tips

- For a flawless make-up application, a good base is essential and preparation is the key. A gentle daily exfoliant should be used after the cleanse to ensure the skin is smooth. This will prevent the foundation looking patchy.
- A great way to get the client to try a recommended product is to provide them with a small sample. This will allow them to try the product and see the results they get. Always write it on the client record so that you can follow up at the next visit.
- A small packet of shine paper is an excellent recommendation for a client who has an oily T–zone. Just press the paper over the oily area to remove excess grease and then finish with a pressed powder.

Unit B8/B9 Provide make-up services and instruct clients in the use and application of skincare products and make-up

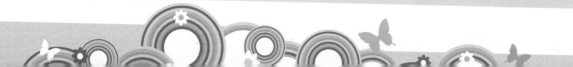

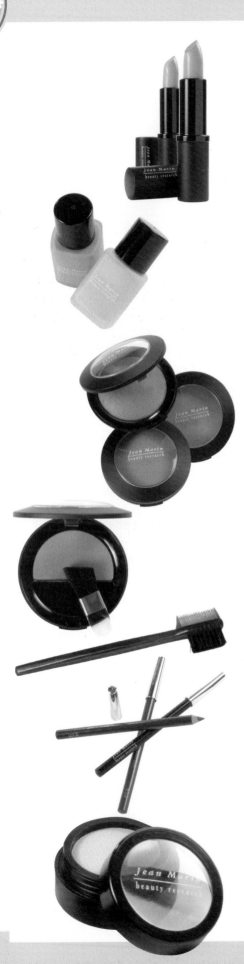

Sequence of make-up application

Concealer

This should be one or two shades lighter than the natural skin tone. Apply to the relevant area using a small brush or cotton bud. Press into the skin with a dry sponge. This applies both to the coverage of blemishes and to colour-corrective **concealer**. When using colour-corrective concealer (see page 380 for details) only apply to the areas that require it.

> ### Key terms
>
> **Concealer** – used to hide imperfections and to lighten and brighten areas. Available in many shades.

Foundation

The ideal shade will match the natural skin tone exactly – test the shade on the jawline. Work around the face using a damp sponge and fingertips, remembering to cover the eyelids and lips.

When you have finished, remove excess foundation from the hairline and eyebrows with some damp cotton wool.

Face powder

Tip a small amount of loose powder into a bowl. If using block powder, scrape a small amount off into a bowl and apply with dry cotton wool. Work downwards, covering the eyes and all of the face, and then blend with a powder brush.

Blusher and bronzing products

Remove a small amount of blusher or bronzer from the container and place on a make-up palette. Imagine a line from the centre of the eye to the cheekbones – blusher stops here. To apply, start at the hairline and follow the line to the cheekbones. Work down the face in the same direction as the facial hair. If corrective work needs to be carried out, apply according to the face shape. (See pages 384–87 for further information on contouring.)

Bronzers can be used to give the skin a sun-kissed look and can be applied to areas where the sun 'kisses' the face, such as the nose, chin and forehead.

Eyebrow pencil

Apply pencil if required. Brush brows to shape.

Eyeliner or kohl pencil

This can be applied to give definition to the eyes. A pencil creates a softer look, and can be used on the top and bottom lids. A liquid liner gives a more defined look, but is not always suitable for the more mature client (see page 390).

Eyeshadow

Place a folded tissue under the eyes – this will help to avoid shadow spillage on to the face. Apply individual eyeshadow colours. Blend on completion.

Mascara

Coat both sides of the lashes from base to tip using a disposable brush. Remove any specks with a cotton wool bud.

Lipliner

Apply to the outline of the lips. Ensure that colour is close to that of the lipstick, to avoid a harsh line.

Lipstick

Use a disposable lip brush. After the first coat, blot lightly and dust lips with face powder. Apply second coat.

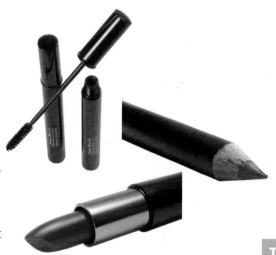

Moisturisers

These products come in many forms and your choice will depend on the skin type of the client. The purpose of a moisturiser when worn under make-up is to:

- even out the skin texture, and provide a smooth base for the foundation
- prolong the make-up by fixing it to the skin
- act as a barrier between the skin and the make-up by preventing pigmented products entering the pores, aiding cleansing.

Think about it

To minimise the risk of skin damage, you can use a moisturising product containing UVA and UVB sunscreens which protect against sunlight. These can be tinted to provide an alternative to foundation.

Concealing cosmetics

Concealer

Few people have a complexion without some imperfections or areas they wish to change – this can be done by using a concealer. Concealer should be applied on small areas where necessary before the application of foundation. Use a colour nearest to the natural skin colour. Concealers come in various forms.

Cream concealer (camouflage)

Usually containing talc and kaolin, these creams have a thick consistency which completely covers all blemishes – including pigmentation marks, red birthmarks and dark shadows under the eyes. These creams come in a variety of colours that can be blended to match the skin.

Stick cover

These come in various shades to match the skin tone and are used to mask minor blemishes and imperfections (spots, dark circles under the eyes). They can be either oil-based or water-based.

Medicated sticks

These are available for applying to minor spots and blemishes, containing antiseptic and drying agents. Never apply directly onto the skin as contamination or cross-infection may occur.

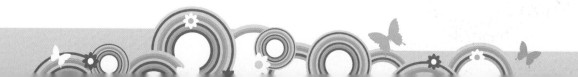

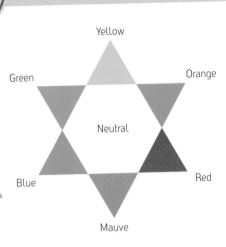

Key terms

Colour star – also known as colour wheel; a chart showing the relationship of colours to each other.

Think about it

When using colour corrector cream, only apply to the area of the face where it is required.

Apply foundation over it, using a tapping action to prevent the corrector cream spreading and to ensure you achieve a smooth finish.

Liquids

Liquid concealers are better for more mature skins where there are creases or wrinkles, as cream or stick concealers can clog in these areas, emphasising them. When covering crow's feet it may be best to use an anti-wrinkle product.

Correcting colour

Pigmentation creams can be used to help correct natural skin tone.

○ Green is used to counteract high colour (redness).

○ Lilac/pink brightens a sallow complexion.

○ Peach is used to conceal blue veins and pigmentation.

The colour star

The **colour star** shows how opposite colours neutralise – for a basic corrective colour. So, for sallow or yellow complexions, rather than applying corrective cream all over the face a tinted moisturiser containing lavender, lilac or mauve could be used.

Primary colours	Secondary colours
Red	Green
Yellow	Orange
Blue	Mauve

The range of colours for both Asian and African skins is vast. However, the skin may contain primary colours so a product should be selected with the same primary colour. The range includes:

○ pale olive

○ yellow

○ greeny olive

○ warm russet

○ warm brown/red

○ brown

○ grey brown

○ blue black.

A tinted product could be used if required and may be a more suitable alternative than a heavier foundation. Imperfections on darker skin types are often less obvious than on white skin. Therefore the make-up that is applied should be mainly to enhance facial features rather than to conceal imperfections.

If loss of pigmentation is present (seen as lighter patches – vitiligo), a camouflage product may be required to disguise the pigmentation loss and to provide an even skin tone and base for the application of the other products.

Choosing a suitable foundation

A good foundation is probably the most important product when carrying out a make-up. The depth, tone and colour can affect all the products used. Foundations also provide a barrier to protect the skin and many now incorporate a sunscreen. A foundation is therefore used to:

○ protect the skin

○ conceal minor blemishes and imperfections

○ provide a smooth finish

○ enhance the natural skin colour.

Choosing a foundation for the client's skin colour and tone

The foundation should match the facial skin, but this is not always the case when the hair has been dyed and the colour and tone have been altered.

The therapist should be aware of various tones that occur naturally in the skin. The tone of the skin is created by pigmentation in the epidermis. Skin is therefore described as:

○ light

○ medium (containing neutral, pink, red or blue tones)

○ dark.

You can match a foundation colour to any skin shade:

○ neutral tones (match or add warmth: honey, gold, tan)

○ pink/red tones (beige, olive)

○ yellow/blue (rose, gold, bronze)

○ dark tones (dark bronze, sun bronze, deep peach)

○ medium tones (cool beige, soft beige, tan).

It is important to get a good colour match when selecting your foundation — you do not want your client to look fake with an orange face or have a ghostly appearance. It is worth remembering that there are many different variations in skin tone, so choose carefully. This may take you a little time or may require you to mix two or more colours together to achieve the desired shade and tone.

To test a foundation on your client for the first time, apply to the angle of the jawline. If the colour becomes darker or has an orange tone, you will need to choose a paler or cooler shade of foundation for your client.

Types of foundation

Foundations are available in many forms:

○ cream

○ liquid

○ cake and pan cake

○ gel

○ medicated

○ mousse

○ mineral.

Most are oil-based or water-based with the addition of pigments for colouring and other ingredients to enhance and change their texture and aid the effectiveness of the product.

Cream foundations

This type of foundation blends easily on the skin because of the oil base, and contains wax, powder and a humectant (a product added to keep it moist), such as glycerol. This type of product gives medium coverage and is suitable for normal, dry, combination and mature skins. For a good finish this foundation should always be set with loose powder.

Unit B8/B9 Provide make-up services and instruct clients in the use and application of skincare products and make-up

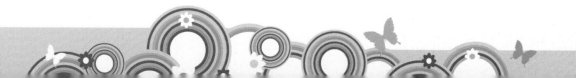

Liquid foundations

These foundations provide colour without being too heavy. They contain a higher proportion of water and give a light/medium coverage. In some products the oil is replaced with alcohol, which evaporates leaving only the powder and pigment. They are suitable for different skin types:

○ oil-based — normal, dry and mature skin types

○ water-based — combination greasy

○ alcohol — greasy.

The base of the foundation should be marked on the container.

Cake foundations

These foundations are usually applied with a damp sponge, thinly or thickly as required by adjusting the amount of water used on the sponge. Cake foundations usually contain compressed creams with extra powder for good coverage. Cake foundations give medium/heavy coverage suitable for:

○ normal skin

○ combination skin

○ blotchy, blemished, discoloured or scarred areas

○ dry or mature (cream-based)

○ greasy (powder-based).

Pan cake foundation

This product is used a lot in the Far East as it is suitable for humid climates. The colour that appears in the compact is the colour that will appear on the skin.

Gel foundations

A gel product will provide a thin, translucent colour that gives a natural look. Gels are produced like a liquid foundation but have an additional ingredient to produce a gel consistency, such as gum tragacanth.

Gels produce a natural tanned effect and are very popular in the summer; many now contain sunscreens. They are suitable for:

○ tanned skins   ○ smooth skin with no imperfections, requiring a natural effect.

Medicated foundations

This type of foundation is a liquid containing antiseptic ingredients, making it suitable for greasy, blemished skins. It can be used over mild acne, but care should be taken with hygiene. It is worth remembering that severe acne is a contra-indication to a make-up application.

Mousse foundations

This type of foundation is suitable for combination to normal skin. Most are made with mineral oils, although some are made with herbal extracts. This type of foundation can be slightly more expensive to buy. If you do apply this foundation to oily skin, be aware that it can be streaky if not carefully applied.

For your portfolio

Look at one range of cosmetics available locally and see what types of foundation they offer. Are you able to buy suitable products for all skin types and skin colours?

Mineral foundations

These products are derived from natural sources and give long-lasting colour. They are excellent for oily skin types as they help prevent comedomes and blemishes.

Skin type	Recognition	Suitable foundation
Normal	Small pores, fine texture Soft supple, flexible healthy	Cream/powder
Dry/dehydrated	Matt, uneven texture Lacks suppleness Lines and wrinkles Dilated capillaries common on nose and cheeks	Cream
Oily	Shiny, thick blackheads, papules, pustules Open pores	Medicated liquid foundation Mineral foundation Non oily block/cake
Combination	Any combination of skin types – most common: oily T-zone and dry cheeks	All-in-one fluid and powder combination Cream/powder combination
Sensitive/dry	Combination of dry cheeks and sensitivity Tight red appearance, broken capillaries	Hypoallergenic products
Sensitive/allergy prone	Reacts to products Skin flushes easily, which may appear as patches Dilated capillaries	Hypoallergenic products
Mature	Fine lines, crepey skin Poor muscle tone Broken capillaries Dry, thin and papery Pigmentation marks	Cream-based products

Summary of the most suitable foundations for the different skin types

Airbrush application

Many cosmetic houses and salons are now using airbrush applicators to apply foundation. The foundation is selected in the normal way to suit the client's skin colour and tones, and is then sprayed over the face. This form of application provides a flawless finish with no sponge or finger marks, and is excellent for bridal or photographic make-up.

Cautions when applying foundation

Apply with a clean sponge or flat brush — these help when applying to awkward areas such as nose or eyes. Thin coverage can be achieved by using a slightly damp, natural sponge. This type of sponge can, however, leave streaks because it is porous, so careful blending needs to take place. When a heavier coverage is required a latex sponge provides a smooth finish; a latex sponge is also less expensive.

Blend the foundation from the centre of the face to the hairline; this prevents clogging foundation in the hairline.

You need to work quickly or the foundation will streak. Cover eyes and lips as this will provide a good base for eyeshadow and lipstick. When applying foundation to a more mature client, who may have crepey skin around the neck and eyes, add a little moisturiser — this thins out the foundation and helps to prevent creases.

Check the application around the nose, hairline and chin to ensure smooth application and no visible lines.

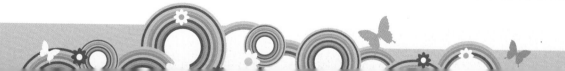

Face powder

For a really professional appearance, most cream-based, make-up products should be set with powder. Loose powder should be used for all professional make-up applications and the correct shade of pressed powder supplied for retail purchase by the client. A powder is applied to:

- 'fix' the foundation
- absorb grease
- give a smooth, matt finish
- protect the skin
- reduce shine
- help conceal minor blemishes.

Loose powder

Loose powders come in two different textures: heavy and fine.

Heavy powders are often pigmented to complement the foundation and give a good cover; they contain a high proportion of kaolin and chalk.

Fine powders contain talc and a majority are translucent, which allows the colour of the skin or foundation to show through.

Some powders contain metallic particles for a pearlised effect, suitable for evening wear. If you decide to use a pearlised powder, remember that it will accentuate lines and blemishes, so it will not be suitable for mature or blemished skins.

Loose powder should always be applied in a salon in preference to pressed powder because of hygiene. If, however, you apply pressed powder it should be decanted on to a palette before being applied, to prevent contamination.

Pressed powder

This is a product in a block that fits into a compact. The binding agent is usually gum or wax, which joins the particles together. Pressed powder is used for touching up the make-up during the day; however, this powder is not fine enough to produce an even finish on freshly applied foundation.

Always avoid areas with excessive hair growth as powder will collect there and draw attention to the area. Also avoid applying to dry flaking areas, because the area will dry out further and it will be accentuated.

Cautions when applying powder

- Dispense a small amount on to a palette.
- Firmly screw up a cotton wool pad and press into the powder, shake off excess in ro
movements, gently press into the foundation, covering all areas including eyes and
- Remove any excess with a brush — first against the hair growth and then down the f
to smooth the facial hairs and produce an even finish.
- Use a clean brush to remove any powder that has settled on the lashes or eyebrow

Contouring cosmetics

These are a range of products which are similar to foundations and powders, with the addition of coloured pigments. They come in powder, liquid, cream and gel. Contour cosmetics consist of:

- blushers
- **highlighters**
- shaders.

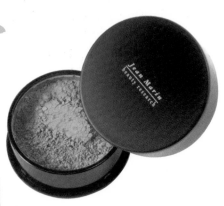

Loose powder should be used for all professional make-up applications

Blushers

Blushers add warmth to the make-up and give the skin a healthy glow to help define the facial features. They come in a wide range of colours. Pale colours can be used to soften and highlight areas. Bright colours can accentuate, and deep tawny colours and bronzes can shade areas. Blushers also come in a variety of forms, including mineral-based products, gels, creams and powders.

Gels

○ Best on clear skins.

○ Give cheeks a natural-looking, healthy glow.

○ Good for the summer.

○ Can be applied directly over moisturiser.

Creams

○ Give skins a moist, dewy finish.

○ Work best when applied over moisturisers and foundation.

○ Good for normal or dry skin types.

Powders

○ Matt or frosted finishes available.

○ Applied for best results over powder with a large brush.

○ Good on oily skins, but suitable for all skin types.

When choosing a blusher it should complement the foundation or natural skin tone. When applying a blusher it is best to build up the colour gradually to achieve the desired effect. It is the depth and tone of colour that needs to be selected carefully.

The use of blusher can help to alter the shape of the face. If you wish to reduce the width of the face, but give an illusion of length, keep the blusher to the side of the face, blending from just underneath the cheekbones to the temples. To create extra fullness, apply the blusher to the cheeks or blend from the angle of the cheekbones to the ears. If you do not wish to change the shape of the face, the blusher is usually placed on or near the cheekbones.

Highlighters

Highlighters are used to emphasise features and to create the illusion of extra length and width. The pale colours of highlighters reflect light, brighten and accentuate an area. Use white, ivory and cream on pale skins for a subtle effect. When using a highlighter on a dark foundation it should belong to the same tone family:

○ pale pink over rose shades

○ pale peach over warm foundations.

Pearlised products are effective as highlighters, but avoid these on mature skins or hairy areas as they will draw attention to the areas.

Shaders

Shading is used to create artificial shadows or to reduce the size of areas. The colours suitable for shading contain brown pigments, which range from medium beige to dark brown. Beige is dark enough to shade when used over a pale base.

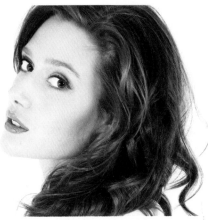

Blushers add warmth and give a healthy glow; highlighters emphasis features

> **Think about it**
>
> To check if the colour of the product is strong enough to show up effectively, take a small amount of the colour on to your finger – if the colour on your finger has the same depth as the compact, the colour is suitable.

> **Key terms**
>
> **Shader** – used to reduce the size of an area and to change the shape of the face.

Unit B8/B9

Provide make-up services and instruct clients in the use and application of skincare products and make-up

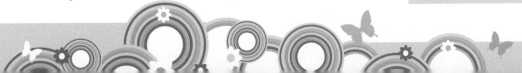

It is important to remember that the darker the foundation, the deeper the shade needs to be. Warm brown colours should be avoided as a shader as they tend to look orange when applied over foundation and then act as a blusher.

Cautions when applying contouring products

- Use soft, round-ended brushes that make blending easier.
- Tap any excess powder blusher on to a tissue or palette before applying, for a more subtle application. It is easier to build up colour in this way.
- When using a gel or cream apply with a damp sponge.
- Blusher application should start on the cheekbones level with the midpoint of the eye.
- Regularly check you are achieving a balanced effect.
- Keep blusher and highlighter away from the corners and the lines of the eye as they can accentuate fine lines.
- Ensure contouring is subtle for day wear for a natural appearance.
- Use corrective techniques to try to achieve a balance in the facial features. This helps emphasise the best areas and takes attention away from problem areas.

Corrective make-up

Contouring products can be used effectively to emphasise and diminish areas to achieve the desired face shape. The oval face shape with almond-shaped eyes is often admired, although trends change with fashion and very few people truly fall into that category. When carrying out your consultation, ensure that both you and your client have realistic expectations about what you can achieve.

Think about it

Light colours define areas.

Dark colours make areas **recede**.

Key terms

Recede – disappear.

Oval face shape

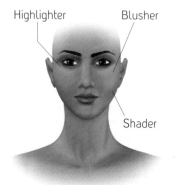

Highlighter

Blusher

Shader

The aim of any corrective make-up is to enhance bone structure and balance contours by blending blusher along the cheekbones towards the temples, applying shader below and highlighter above.

Round face shape

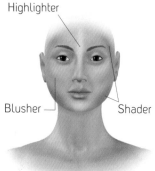

Highlighter

Blusher

Shader

The corrective work should create an illusion of length – to reduce the width from the sides of the face to the temples. To create length – subtle highlighter blended in a narrow strip down the centre of the face, apply blusher on the cheekbones up to the temples, shader over angles of the jaw and temple areas.

Square face shape

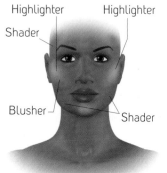

Highlighter

Highlighter

Shader

Blusher

Shader

The aim of the corrective work is to soften the jawline and reduce the width of the forehead and lower half of the face. Shader should be blended over the angles of the lower jaw and forehead. Blusher should be applied upwards from under the cheeks towards the temples or along the fullness of the cheeks.

Oblong face shape

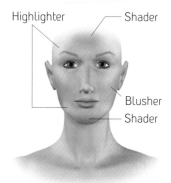

Highlighter

Shader

Blusher

Shader

The corrective make-up should reduce the length of the face, and create width and fullness. This can be achieved by applying shader to the tip of the chin and the narrowest part of the forehead. Apply highlighter to the temples and lower jaw and blusher to the cheeks to add fullness.

Heart face shape

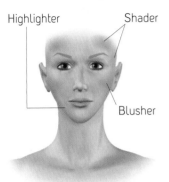

Highlighter   Shader

Blusher

The corrective work should aim to minimise the width of the forehead and widen the lower half of the face. This can be achieved by applying shader to the sides of the forehead and temples. Highlight the angles of the lower jaw. Apply blusher to the fullness of the cheeks.

Diamond face shape

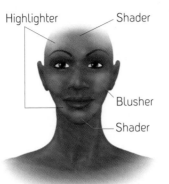

Highlighter   Shader

Blusher

Shader

The corrective work of this face shape is to reduce the length by applying shader to the tip of the chin and the narrowest part of the forehead. To give the illusion of width, apply highlighter to the sides of the temples and lower jaw. Apply blusher to the cheeks to create fullness in the centre of the face.

Pear face shape

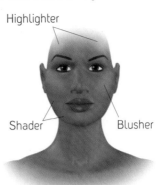

Highlighter

Shader   Blusher

The aim of this corrective make-up is to give width to the forehead by applying highlighter to the sides of the forehead and to reduce the width of the lower face through the application of shader on the side of the chin and angles of the lower jaw. Emphasise the cheekbones for a full appearance.

Triangular face shape

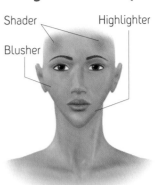

Shader   Highlighter

Blusher

This corrective make-up is similar to that used on a heart-shaped face. The relatively wide forehead and narrow jawline need to be balanced to prevent the face from looking top heavy. Use shader to minimise the forehead width and create the illusion of width along the jawline by applying highlighter. Use blusher on the cheeks to balance the centre of the face and even up the whole shape.

Eye cosmetics

The eyes are the focal point of the face. People often focus on the eye make-up as the eyes are used for communicating and expressing our feelings. The trick when applying make-up is to draw attention to the eyes and not to the make-up.

The use of colour can create illusions of depth, size and alter the shape. Always remember that lighter colours enhance, darker colours recede.

Care is always needed when working around the eyes, as the skin is very sensitive and thin and can be easily overstretched. The EC Cosmetics Directive of 1976 limits ingredients which may be contained in eye make-up products and only pigments which are known to be non-toxic and non-irritant are allowed.

Eyeshadow

Eyeshadows are used to emphasise the eyes and to coordinate the colour of the make-up and clothing. They are available as minerals, powder, liquid, gel and cream. Creamy, pressed powders are the most popular. Frosted products are available for highlighting and can be used to achieve a stunning effect when used for evening.

However, frosted and creamy products are not recommended for mature clients as they draw attention to lines and get trapped in crepey areas.

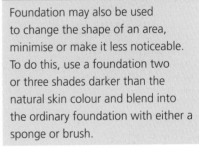

Think about it

Foundation may also be used to change the shape of an area, minimise or make it less noticeable. To do this, use a foundation two or three shades darker than the natural skin colour and blend into the ordinary foundation with either a sponge or brush.

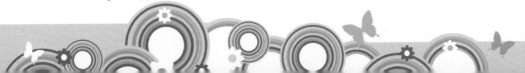

Powder shadows

These are talc-based with oil for a creamy texture, available in loose or pressed form.

Creams

Cream shadow contains wax and oil pigments, and is not so popular with mature clients as these products settle in the creases.

Gels

Gels give a natural appearance because they produce a translucent wash of colour.

Eyeshadow colours

- Dark, muted colours – use for defining and contouring. Effective on clients with dark hair and eyes. Applied with a fine brush, they can be used as a livening effect on people with light colouring.

- Pastel colours – produce soft effects, particularly on people with grey/blonde hair. They emphasise the colour of the eyes when applied in the same tone.

- Pale colours – have highlighting effects when contrasted with dark shadows. When applied near the brow makes the eyes appear bigger.

- Soft, muted shades – use when a more natural effect is required.

- Bright colours – use in young or fashion make-up. Some bright colours can be used as eyeliner to complement the eyeshadow, but be cautious when using bright colours on a mature client as they can give a hard and unattractive appearance.

Applying eyeshadow to a range of eye shapes

Small eyes

Lengthen small eyes by applying a soft eye pencil to the outer third of the bottom lid extending outward. Use a short stroke to join this line to the upper lash line, then smudge.

- Use light colours and iridescent shadows on the lid for an eye-opening effect.

- Highlight with a frosted shadow under the brow for evening sparkle.

- Curl the lashes or have them permed before applying the mascara to open the eyes even more.

- Try lining the inside of the lower lid with a soft, white pencil – this will also give the appearance of the eye being more open.

Prominent eyes

Use matt shadow on the lid and blend it into the crease. Apply a darker shade to the outer half of the lid, right over the first shade, and blend so the graduation looks natural and no harsh lines are visible. Highlight under the brow with a light or frosted shade.

If you wish to achieve a sultry look, which may be suitable for evening wear, line the inner rim of the eye with a soft eye pencil. Grey, navy, plum and black are excellent depending on the eye colour, but there are many more colours to choose from.

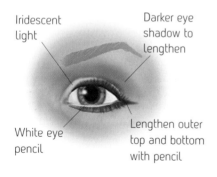

Iridescent light

Darker eye shadow to lengthen

White eye pencil

Lengthen outer top and bottom with pencil

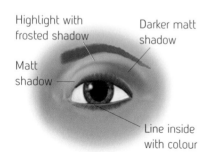

Highlight with frosted shadow

Darker matt shadow

Matt shadow

Line inside with colour

Round eyes

Elongate the eyes by using the deepest shades on the outer edge of the eye lid, and extend this to form a soft point. Lengthen the eyes even more by outlining the outer third of the top and bottom with a soft eye pencil, making sure that the outer point meets beyond the outer corner of the eye. Smudge for a softer effect. Narrow the eyes by lining the inner rim with a soft pencil.

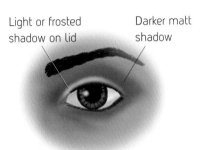

Matt shadow on lid

Darker matt shadow on outer 1/3 of eye

Line outer 1/3 top and bottom with pencil to elongate

Line with pencil

Deep-set eyes

Use light or frosted shadows on the lid if it is appropriate for the client and occasion. Apply a darker shade above the crease to recess this area. Apply a little shadow or soft eye pencil on the outer half of the bottom lid to balance the depth of the eyes.

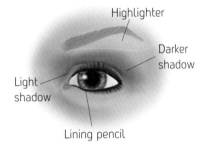

Light or frosted shadow on lid

Darker matt shadow

Oriental eyes

Divide the area beneath the brow in half vertically. Use a lighter shade on the inner half and a darker shade on the outer half and blend well together. The application of a darker shadow creates a socket line. Apply a highlighter under the brow and blend together.

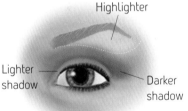

Highlight with frosted shadow

Light shade

Darker shade

Almond eyes

Unless the eyes are set too close together or too far apart, you will not need to undertake corrective techniques. Choose colours that complement the iris, and ensure the brows are groomed to make application of shadows easy.

Highlighter

Darker shadow

Light shadow

Lining pencil

Close-set eyes

Keep all medium or dark colours on the outer half of the eye. This will draw attention outward and the eyes will seem further apart. Ensure that the brows have been correctly shaped to maximise the space between the eyes.

Highlighter

Lighter shadow

Darker shadow

Wide-set eyes

Extend the shadows to the inner corner of the eye and blend inwards to the bridge of the nose to minimise the space. Also ensure the brows are correctly shaped.

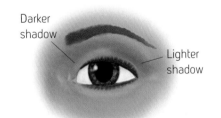

Darker shadow

Lighter shadow

Unit B8/B9

Provide make-up services and instruct clients in the use and application of skincare products and make-up

Cautions when applying eyeshadow

- Always use clean brushes and applicators. Do not overload the applicator with shadow as excess powder could fall into the eyes or on to the face — spoiling the other make-up. It is also not cost-effective to overload the applicator.
- Support the skin and protect the surrounding make-up with a tissue. Remember that the skin around the eye is very delicate, so do not be heavy handed and over-stretch the skin.
- Ensure your client keeps her eyes closed when applying the shadow and always keep the client informed of what you are about to do. Check the shadow is balanced on both eyes and evenly blended. If applying shadow beneath the eyes, ask the client to look away from the brush to prevent blinking or the eyes watering.

Eyeliner

This product is used for emphasising the shape of the eyelid and strengthening the colour of the lash line. It is good to use when strip lashes have been applied to give a more natural appearance. Liners are available in a number of colours and types. Like all make-up, eyeliner follows fashion trends. It was very popular in the 1950s and 1960s, and is currently enjoying a revival.

Cake eyeliner

This is the most versatile product but the most difficult to apply. It is applied with a fine brush that is dampened before applying to the eyes.

Liquid eyeliner

This is a gum solution containing pigments, which gives a heavier effect. It will provide a clearly defined line if correctly applied.

Pencils

These are available in a range of colours, usually soft enough to blend with the shadows because of their wax formulation, and should be used to complement the look that is required. Ensure they are sharpened between each eye to get an even application and to prevent cross-infection.

Kohl

This is a soft, waxy, black pencil which is applied to the inner rim of the lower eyelid to enhance the white of the eye. A kohl pencil is not recommended for use on a mature client as the effect can be harsh and can accentuate fine lines.

Cautions when applying eyeliner

- Gently lift the skin from beneath the brow so the line is drawn up to the base of the lashes.
- Ensure the client keeps the eyes shut when liner is applied to the upper lid.
- Always apply liner outwards towards the corner of the eye.
- Check that the thickness and angle of the eyeliner are the same for both eyes.

Mascara

Mascaras are available in a variety of colours — including clear mascara. Mascara is used to accentuate the eyes by darkening and thickening the lashes. Many now contain moisturisers and lash-building ingredients which include filaments of nylon and rayon. These fibres temporarily lengthen the lashes. Clear mascara enhances the natural features of darkened lashes and is especially useful after the lashes have been tinted.

When applying mascara with lash-building filaments be aware that the filaments can sometimes shed. If these enter the eye, they can cause irritation and this can especially aggravate the eyes of contact lens wearers.

Cake mascara

Cake mascara is made up of a mixture of waxes and pigments in a soap base, and is applied with a brush. This type of mascara is gaining popularity again in salons as the brush applicator can easily be cleaned and sterilised.

Liquid mascara

Applied with a brush or wand, this type of mascara is contained in a water or alcohol and water base with extra features: for example, waterproof, thickening, and protein enriched. Read the packaging to find out what the mascara contains. When applying this type of mascara to a client, disposable brushes should be used for each eye to prevent any contamination of the product.

Cautions when applying mascara

- Ensure that the client is relaxed as this makes the application of mascara easier — especially to the upper lashes.
- Apply mascara downwards on upper lashes and then upwards for maximum coverage.
- Place tissue under lower lashes, before applying, to prevent mascara marking the skin.
- Instruct the client to look away from the wand when applying the mascara to the lower lashes.
- Build up the mascara in fine coats to prevent clogging. Allow to dry between applications.

Eyebrow pencils

These pencils are used to strengthen the colour of the brows and define shape. They should be applied to the brow in light, feathery strokes for a natural look. The use of an eyebrow pencil is good for filling in bare areas if the brows are sparse. Use short strokes in the direction of the hair growth and blend into the natural brow shape with the aid of a brow brush.

Eyebrow pencils are produced in a limited range of colours to complement the natural brow colour. As with other pencils they should be sharpened after each eye to prevent cross-contamination occurring.

Cautions when using eyebrow pencils

- Brush brows into shape.
- Check the colour tone and shade of the pencil – this should look natural and complement the rest of the make-up.
- Ensure the pencils are sharpened after doing each brow, to prevent cross-contamination, and ensure feathery strokes are used rather than one harsh line for a natural look.

Think about it

Always check to see if your client wears contact lenses, even if they arrive at the salon wearing glasses. Lash tinting may be a preferred option for spectacle and contact lens wearers.

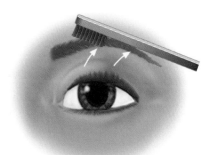

a Separate brow hairs

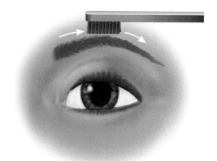

b Smooth them into shape

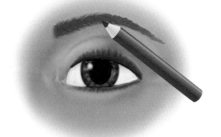

c Fill in the gaps and extend the length of the brow by using fine strokes that follow the natural hair growth

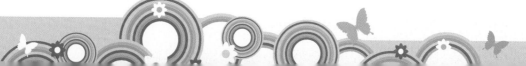

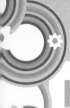

For your portfolio

Research one high street and one professional brand of cosmetics to compare the cost of the products and the variety of colour choice. Consider factors such as skin type and age range.

Lip cosmetics

There is a variety of cosmetics on the market for lips, in a range of colours and forms. There are lipsticks, glosses and pencils. These are used to define the mouth, by adding colour, and to protect the lips from the environment. Lip cosmetics can, as with other forms of make-up, be used as corrective make-up to enhance shape. All lip products contain the same ingredients of oils, fats and waxes, with the addition of safe pigments for colour.

Lipsticks

These contain a high wax content that makes them hard. Some products also contain sunscreens to protect the delicate skin of the lips from ultraviolet light. Lipstick should be applied with a brush to outline the mouth and spread colour over the lips evenly.

Lip gloss

This product can be used over lipstick or on its own for a natural look. It is usually of a gel consistency and is available in either lipstick form or as a gel.

Lip pencil

This is used for outlining the lips before applying lipstick and contains a high proportion of wax, which means it is less likely to smudge. It is useful to prevent lipstick colour from 'bleeding' into the fine lines around the mouth. It is also helpful for correcting lip shapes.

Lipstick sealer

Usually produced as a liquid, this is a colourless sealer, designed to prevent lipstick fading and to keep it in place. It should be applied with a brush.

Lip primer

This is used mainly for mature clients to prevent 'lipstick bleeding'.

Choosing a suitable lipstick

When selecting a lipstick it should be used to balance the colour scheme and coordinate with the clothing. Strong and vibrant colours draw attention to the mouth, so avoid them if you are trying to take the emphasis away from the mouth or jaw area. Strong colours look best with subtle and muted eye make-up colours.

Deep-colour lipstick or pencil should be used when outlining a corrective lip make-up. Pale, pearlised lipstick or lip gloss give lips a fuller appearance.

To reduce fullness, bronze, purplish pinks and blue-toned reds are useful.

Cautions when applying lip cosmetics

- Apply foundation and powder to the lips before applying lip cosmetics. This gives a good base and makes lip cosmetics last longer.
- Outline the mouth first and then fill in the colour.
- Blot the first application with a tissue as this helps to fix the colour.
- Apply a second coat for a final finish.
- Never apply lip cosmetics to any infected area or if the lips are excessively chapped or cracked.

Corrective lip make-up

Thin lips

The thickness of the lips can be increased by drawing a line slightly outside the natural lip shape.

Full or thick lips

Use dark colours to make the lips recede and create a new lip line inside the natural one by blotting out the natural line with foundation and powder.

Thin or straight upper lip

Create a new bow to the upper lip by pencilling just above the natural line to add fullness.

Thin lower lip

Create a new lower lip line slightly below the natural lip to give balance to the mouth.

Asymmetric lips

These lips are unbalanced so create a lip line where required to achieve balance.

Droopy mouth

Build up the corners of the lower lip, slightly extending upwards at the corners to meet the upper lip line.

Facial problem areas

Jawline shapes

Broad jaw

A broad jaw can be minimised by the use of a darker shader, starting from the temple area down and over either side of the angle of the mandible (refer to Related anatomy and physiology, page 225), bringing the centre of the face into sharper focus and so creating a more balanced width.

Narrow jaw

Narrow jaws are highlighted to create an illusion of width.

Square jaws

These can be shaded with a darker foundation applied to the width, to appear more rounded.

Chin and neck shapes

Prominent chin

A dark foundation or shader should be used on the chin, and sometimes a touch of blusher can be just as effective.

Receding chin

A lighter foundation or a highlighter will make a receding chin appear more prominent.

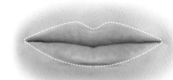

Thin lips

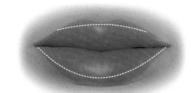

Full or thick lips

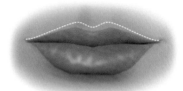

Thin or straight upper lip

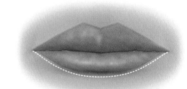

Thin lower lip

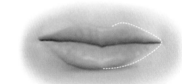

Asymmetric lips

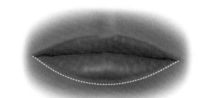

Droopy mouth

Double chin

A double chin or loose skin should be shadowed, with a dark foundation or shader.

Thin neck

This should be highlighted to create the illusion of roundness and prominence.

Thick neck

This requires shading to make it appear smaller.

Nose shapes

Large or protruding nose

This is made smaller by applying a dark foundation or shader, blending it smoothly into a lighter foundation on the sides of the cheeks. Blusher should be kept away from the nose.

Short nose

This is made narrower by shading the sides of the nostrils.

Long, thin nose

This can be broadened by applying a highlighter foundation down its centre to above the tip, which is to be shaded.

Colour and skin pigmentation

Freckles and moles

These can be faded with the use of a good foundation or cream which is slightly thicker. It must be toned into the rest of the foundation, otherwise it will stand out.

Age lines

Creases round the mouth and crow's feet around the eyes can be softened by making the eyes appear fuller. This is achieved by the use of a lighter coloured foundation applied over the area. The crevices appear to be lifted out and less noticeable, but do not apply too heavily or you will make the areas more noticeable.

Clients with contact lenses or glasses

The effects that glasses have on the appearance of the face and make-up will vary according to the colour of frame, frame size and lenses.

Frames

○ Heavy frames – can take strong lip colour and eye make-up to help balance the facial features.

○ Lightweight frames – ensure the colours are soft, using liner or mascara. Eyebrow pencil to define the brows and lashes will look more subtle with this type of frame. Bold colours will make light frames recede.

○ Coloured frames – make-up should complement them. Muted shades should be used if the frames are very bright.

Lenses

- Short sighted – these make the eyes appear smaller.
- Long sighted – these lenses make the eyes look larger.
- Tinted lenses – these lenses may change the colours of the make-up.

Contact lenses

Some clients are quite happy to have their lenses in place when the make-up takes place, but you should always take the following precautions to prevent irritating the eyes.

- Work gently.
- Avoid heavy creams that could smear the lenses.
- Avoid creating dust that could land on the contact lenses and irritate the eye, and always ensure the client keeps the eyes closed when applying powder shadow.
- Use eye make-up shadows with a creamy pressed texture.
- Use mascara without alcohol and added fibre filaments.

Make-up for day, evening and special occasions

Bridal make-up

Many brides have their make-up applied professionally so that they can be confident of looking their best. Therefore, to ensure you give the best advice, a preliminary consultation is essential. During the consultation you need to find out the following details.

- The date and time of the wedding. The final appointment must be scheduled within the overall preparations, as ideally make-up should be applied before the hair is dressed and the dress put on.
- Details of the dress – design, colour and material. Colours will look stronger if the dress is white. Lightweight fabrics need softer make-up than heavier fabrics.
- Hair style and headdress – this can affect the facial features.

Remember that lipstick and nail colours need to tone with the colour scheme of the dress and flowers. Pearlised products will emphasise flaws and defects and eye make-up will lose definition in photographs.

When carrying out a wedding make-up, avoid stimulating the skin for 48 hours before the wedding. Shape eyebrows and apply individual lashes one or two days prior to the wedding. Apply fake tan one or two days prior to the wedding if the dress is low cut and reveals paler areas of the body.

It is important to promote waxing, manicure and pedicure treatments before the wedding for a truly well-groomed appearance and for honeymoon preparation. Many salons include wedding packages in their price lists that include these treatments.

Photographic make-up

Many large photographic studios now employ a make-up artist to help clients get the best from their photographs. This service is included in the cost of the photographic package. You need to consider the following points.

- Lighting can be hot and make-up may melt, so do not apply a heavy make-up, and cool the skin if possible during application.

> **Think about it**
>
> The bride wants to look beautiful and radiant, but she also wants to be recognized – it is not the time for a dramatic change.

> **Think about it**
>
> When carrying out a bridal make-up, a practice should always be carried out in daylight to ensure true colouring in order to make certain all parties are satisfied.

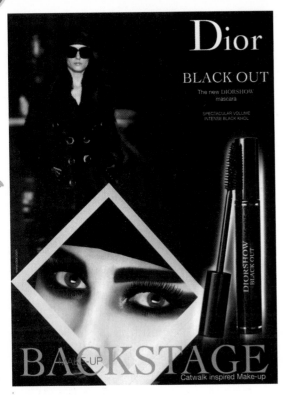

Photographic make-up can use dramatic effects

- Avoid greasy products and creamy, textured products as these emphasise shine, creases and open pores.
- Reapply translucent powder to achieve a matt finish.
- Pearlised products can cause glare and emphasise flaws.
- Ensure that all products are well blended. This is particularly important around the jaw and hair lines.
- Highlight under the eyes, chin and sides of the nostrils before applying foundation, to prevent discoloration and shadow created by skin folds.
- Use highlight and shadow techniques to create facial contours and define bone structure. Foundation should be as light as possible to enhance the contour cosmetics.

Creating mood

Colour can create the correct mood when taking photographs.

- Strong, rich colours create vibrant, active moods.
- Pale colours give a calming feel.
- Oranges and yellows give a feeling of warmth.
- Blues and greens have a cooling effect.

Contrasting colours

Red will bring the subject towards you or expand an area when taking a photograph. Blue allows the area to blend into the surroundings. Therefore, when selecting shades of make-up, it is important to look at the surroundings as well as the clothing or the effect you are trying to create may be lost. Using strongly contrasting primary colours could add emphasis to certain areas.

Lighting

If the photograph is to be taken outside, you need to be aware that the light will constantly change. It is for this reason that professional photographers use lighting when working outside to get controlled and better results. If, however, you have to work with natural light, remember:

- early mornings — when the sun is low, photographs will have more depth
- midday — natural light is flatter so little emphasis and depth are achieved
- strong sunlight — this will create hard outlines
- cloud — photographs taken when the light is diffused by light cloud gives a less harsh appearance of soft shadows and subtle highlighting.

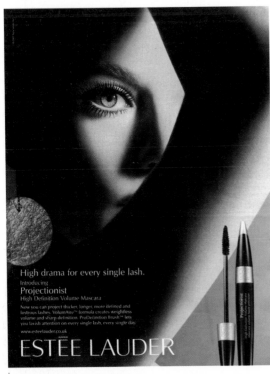

Lighting effects can have strong impact on the finished look

Step-by-step daytime make-up, converted to an evening look

1 Prepare the client, in an upright position, fully covered and the skin lightly moisturised. Headband and tissues protect the hair. It is best to apply daytime make-up in natural daylight.

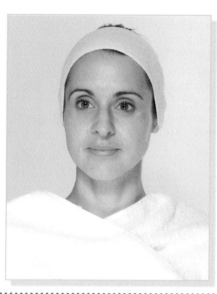

2 Apply concealer/colour corrector, if needed, followed by suitable foundation for the skin type.

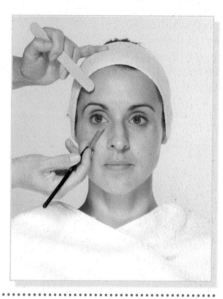

3 Apply foundation with a damp sponge or clean fingertips. Work from the centre of the face outwards using light movements.

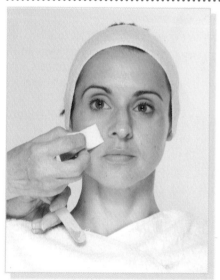

4 Using dry cotton wool, lightly pat on loose powder to set the foundation. Remember eyelids and lips. Using a large round brush, remove any excess powder, using downward strokes.

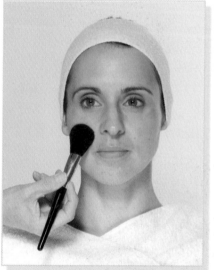

5 Shader, blusher and highlighter can now be applied to contour the face, as discussed in the treatment plan. Always decant products.

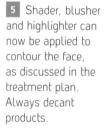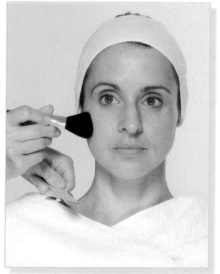

6 Apply eyeshadows, remembering to use disposable applicators and to decant the colours on to a pallet, to avoid contaminating the remaining eyeshadow.

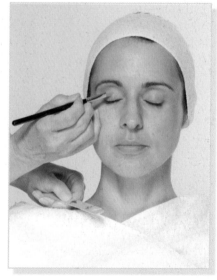

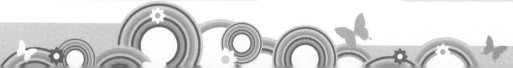

Unit BB8/B9

Provide make-up services and instruct clients in the use

397

7 Apply eyeliner or pencil, without dragging on the eye, and remember to sharpen the pencil between clients, for hygiene.

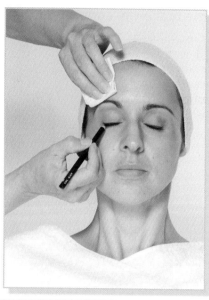

8 When applying mascara, remember to support the eye with a tissue, ask the client to look down, and stroke upwards, with the eyelash growth. A disposable wand is always used.

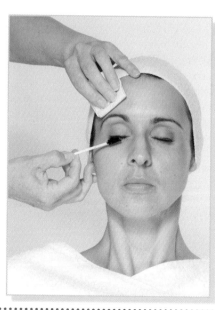

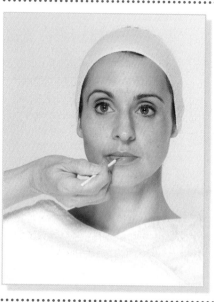

9 Lip liner and lipstick are next. Remember to sharpen the lip pencil, and to decant the lipstick onto a pallet, applying it with a clean brush.

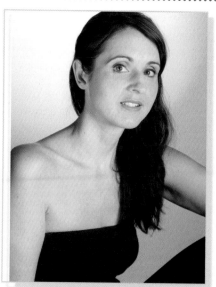

10 Show the client the finished result with all covering removed. Her own hair and clothes will give a natural look. Hold the mirror upwards for a flattering result. Ensure that the make-up effects combine and complement the client's look to create the image that she desires, and check that she is pleased with the result.

11 To convert the make-up for an evening look select complimentary colours. These may contain a shimmer.

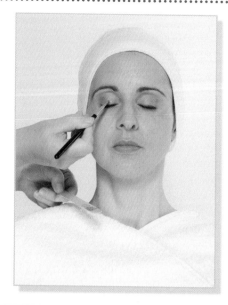

12 Additional eyeliner and mascara can be used to enhance the eyes and give lashes a more defined appearance.

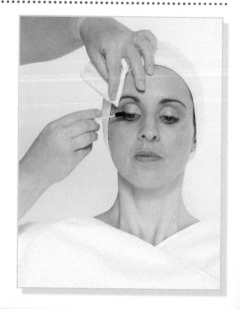

13 Apply blusher or bronzer to the cheekbones. These products may contain luminescent particles to enhance the cheeks.

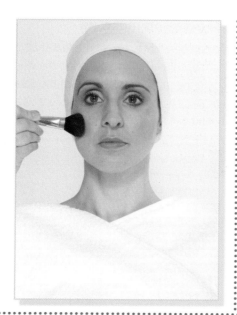

14 Lip products are usually darker for evening wear. A gloss may be applied over the lipstick for added sheen.

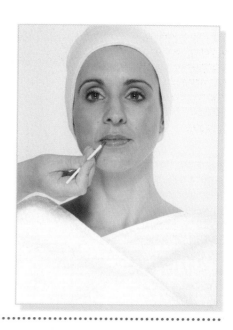

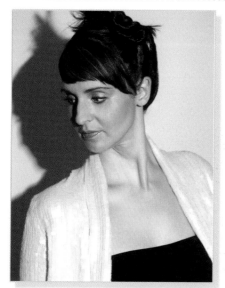

15 Evening make-up is more dynamic so false lashes could be applied to add impact. These should be applied prior to additional eye make-up.

Think about it

Application time should be approximately 45 minutes for a make-over. A lesson in skincare or make-up application should be approximately one hour. If you are demonstrating to a larger group, your time may be adjusted according to the service that you are presenting.

Think about it

To carry out an effective make-up service, you need to be able to identify and treat the client's individual skin type. Therefore, it is essential to have prior knowledge to ensure the best results.

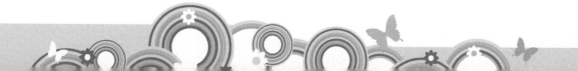

Step-by-step special occasion make-up

Special occasion make-up can be a little more individual than day make-up, but not quite as heavy as evening make-up. The key to making the whole look glamorous but not overdone is to coordinate the make-up colours with the outfit and add a touch of sparkle, with a lip gloss or shiny eyeshadow. Ask the client what she will be wearing; see the outfit, if possible, and definitely have a trial run before the event.

1 Study the client's natural skin and hair colouring, to avoid choosing make-up colours that clash. Research the type of special occasion and what the client will be wearing.

2 Decant and apply concealer/ colour corrector, if required. Take into account that your client may or may not be used to wearing much make-up. Keep application and colour light, particularly when applying make-up to mature skin.

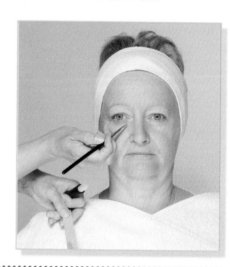

3 Apply foundation with a sponge or clean fingertips, blending from the centre of the face, outwards. Ensure foundation chosen is suitable for skin type — foundation for mature skin should be light in texture and colour.

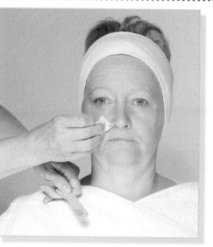

4 With a dry piece of cotton wool, pat loose powder all over the face, remembering eyelids and lips. Translucent powder is suitable for mature skin.

5 A light stroke with a large blusher brush will remove any excess powder. Stroke the brush all over the face, in a downward motion, to avoid a powdery look to the face.

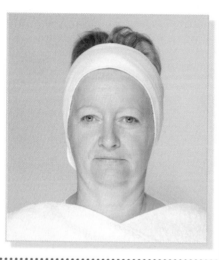

6 Eyeshadow is decanted and applied lightly over the lids. If the client wears glasses, or has quite lined eyelids, make the colour and application fairly light.

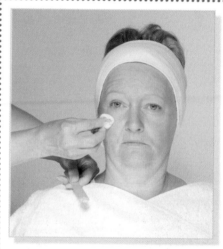

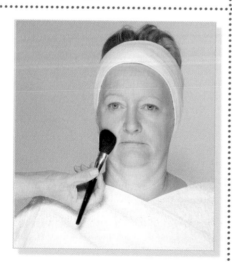

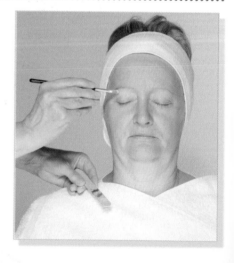

7 Apply a light application of mascara using a disposable wand. Soft shades of navy, grey or brown mascara are less harsh than black on mature skin.

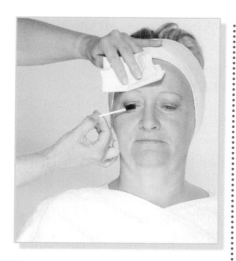

8 Decant the blusher on to the wooden spatula and apply lightly to the cheeks. Soft corals, peaches or pinks usually suit mature skin.

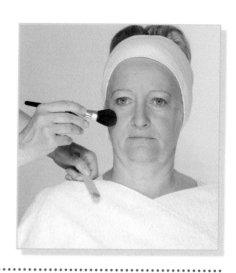

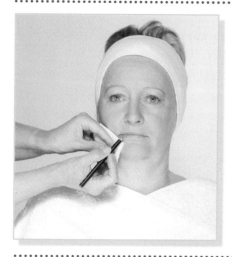

9 Sharpen the pencil and apply a light lip liner, which prevents the lipstick bleeding into the lines around the mouth.

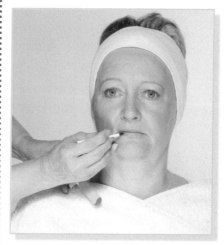

10 Choose a complementary lipstick and decant, then apply.

11 You gain the whole effect for special occasion make-up if you have a complete dress rehearsal – including the hat!

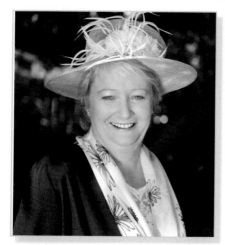

Children's face painting

Although not strictly a salon treatment, from time to time clients may request children's face painting for parties and birthday treats. No special skill is required – you just need some water-based face paints (child friendly for easy removal) and a flair for invention.

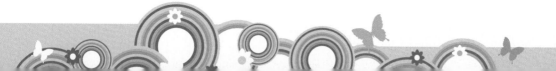

Carry out a consultation, checking for contra-indications, and skin analysis to determine which products to use

⬇

Ensure all products and equipment are close to hand

⬇

Apply moisturiser

⬇

Apply concealer and colour corrector if required

⬇

Apply foundation, check the colour on the jawline.

⬇

Apply powder to set the foundation

⬇

Apply shaders and highlighters to minimise or emphasise areas as discussed with the client

⬇

Apply eye shadow (hold a tissue under the eye to prevent flaking shadow)

⬇

Apply eyeliner or pencil (sharpen after each eye)

⬇

Apply mascara (using disposable mascara wands)

⬇

Apply lip pencil or liner

⬇

Apply lipstick

⬇

Show client the finished result and check she is happy

⬇

Record details, including products used and where applied, skin care products used and recommended

⬇

Products purchased

⬇

Show client the finished result. Record details, including products used and where applied, on client record

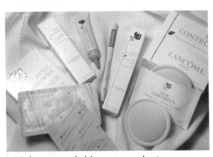

Make-up and skincare products can be purchased for the client to use at home

Provide aftercare advice

In this outcome you will learn about:

- giving advice and recommendations accurately and constructively
- giving the clients suitable advice specific to their individual needs.

Giving advice and recommendations to suit the client's needs

To enable the client to gain the most from the skincare and make-up instruction or make-up application, the client should be given the following information.

○ Correct preparation for applying skincare products and make-up suitable for the client's skin type.

○ Correct choice and application of cosmetics – colours, textures and types suitable for the features of the client and her skin type.

○ Effective and hygienic use of products and equipment.

○ How to keep make-up fresh by: applying pressed powder; applying a fine spray of water to keep the make-up from drying and cracking; applying more lipstick.

○ Removal of make-up with products suitable for the client's skin type.

○ In the event of an allergic reaction, remove all make-up, soothe with damp cotton wool and apply a soothing substance, e.g. calamine lotion.

All details should be recorded on the client record card.

Link selling and retail products

Many therapists work on a commission basis for the sale of retail products, and skincare tuition and make-up application provide the perfect opportunities to promote additional treatments and retail products to ensure the client gains the most from her visit to the salon.

Treatments could include:

○ application of false lashes for special occasions

○ regular facial treatment

○ eyebrow treatments including brow shaping and tinting

○ manicure and pedicure treatments

○ waxing.

Retail products could include:

○ cleanser, toner and moisturiser to suit skin type

○ foundation and powder

○ matching lipstick and varnish

○ make-up brushes and applicator

○ throat/neck cream, eye cream.

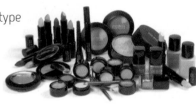

It is therefore important that you have a good knowledge of the products that you are recommending for home use and can demonstrate how to use these effectively. This will give the client confidence in you as a therapist. If the client purchases products, it is a good idea to record these sales on the record card, so you can assist the client on future visits if she wishes to repurchase.

Selling skills

Unit G18 Promote additional products or services to clients, pages 115–21, covers selling skills, including using open questions to aid the sale, and how to close when interest is shown.

Features and benefits of products

Many of the new age-smart products employ the latest technology, which introduces vitamins to the skin and removes dead skin cells. They have become big sellers and are directed not just at mature clientele but at all clients as preventative products.

A feature is an aspect of the product which is useful, but not necessarily part of the action of the product, such as a plastic, unbreakable bottle for travelling, or a pump action for easy dispensing. For example:

> Features of a one-to-one skincare and make-up instruction may be that it can be performed privately in the salon, and the client may not have to travel too far.

> Features of a group session are that it can be sociable and fun, and for the client who is shy, there is safety in numbers!

A benefit is the key selling point of the product to the client's advantage, such as a cream moisturising cleanser which helps keep the moisture in the skin, or a cream foundation which has a high moisture content to help a dry skin. For example:

> Benefits of a one-to-one skincare and make-up instruction may be that it can be tailor-made to suit the client's needs, and that a greater amount of understanding may take place because of the intimacy of just client and therapist.

> Benefits of a group session are that the therapist reaches a wider audience, the client may interact with friends within the audience and it provides a good opportunity for discussion with others.

My story

A satisfied client!

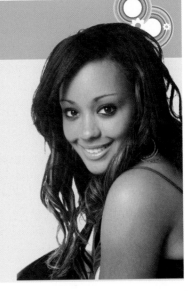

Hi, I'm Sienna. For a number of years my skin had been looking dry and sallow. A friend bought me a skincare and make-up session for my birthday and although I was very nervous I went along. My therapist Amitia was lovely, and after cleansing and analysing my skin and asking me a number of questions, she began selecting and demonstrating the products on me. She seated me in front of a mirror, showed me how to use the products and let me have a go. It was great fun and I learnt a lot. After selecting the correct skincare products for my skin type and condition, she showed me some very simple but effective day make-up techniques. The effects were stunning but not difficult to recreate. Amitia wrote down all of the products she recommended on a treatment planner, and although I could not afford to purchase all of the products in one visit I have now bought the range of products — and my skin and make-up application looks wonderful. I now regularly go to the salon for facials.

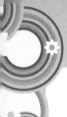

Evaluate the success of instruction

When you have carried out an individualised session or a group session you will need to evaluate the effectiveness of your treatment session with the client(s). This will enable you to work on your presentation and delivery techniques.

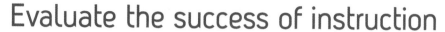

In this outcome you will learn about:

- asking the client to make an evaluation of their own learning and then providing additional support to meet their needs
- asking the client suitable questions on the effectiveness of the instruction process and recording their feedback.

Asking the client to evaluate their own learning and provide support

You could ask the client what she has enjoyed and what she found difficult to master. You may need to re-cap areas and give her product samples that she can take away and practise with at home.

Asking questions and using feedback

It may be that you have devised a treatment/evaluation card specifically for skincare/make-up lessons or demonstrations, or simply added notes to client record cards. Always make a note of products used and recommended so you can follow this up with the client in the future. This feedback will allow you to make improvements to your own skincare and make-up instructional techniques, if necessary.

After the skincare and make-up instruction — whether a one-to-one session, demonstration or group session — has been completed, hold a question and answer session. Have you:

○ met the objectives

○ checked the finished result with the client

○ been cost-effective, both with time and product use

○ carried out the service in a commercially acceptable time

○ filled in a client record card

○ obtained the audience's details for a promotional mailing (if group demonstration)

○ tidied away and left the area immaculate

○ enough products for other demonstrations, or will more need to be ordered?

After the event, it is important to look at your performance and judge if you were happy with all aspects of it. Ask yourself:

○ How do I think it went?

○ What would I change if I could?

○ Was I fully prepared?

○ What would I do differently next time?

○ What sort of feedback did I get from the audience? Were they interested and attentive? If not, why not?

○ Did the client(s) show full understanding of my instructions, and did she (they) show interest in purchasing a product, or booking a service or treatment?

Frequently asked questions

Q	Why is it important to ensure a client has the correct skincare products?
A	Having the correct products for the client's skin will ensure damage does not occur and enables the client to get the maximum benefit from any other services offered. Correct products also ensure make-up that is applied looks the best.
Q	What is the benefit of regularly using an exfoliator?
A	An exfoliator removes dead skin cells that can clog the surface of the skin making it appear dull and lifeless. Dry, dehydrated patches also cause foundation to look patchy.
Q	Why is giving samples of skincare products important as part of a good salon service?
A	Samples allow the client to try the recommended products for a few days to see how they get on with the application. Also, however good the products are, some clients will still react to some products and this can prevent costly mistakes. This will give the clients faith in your treatment planning and professionalism.
Q	Why is it important to do a skin analysis prior to carrying out a make-up application?
A	It is important so that you can fully assess the client's skin type and select suitable products. This should be carried out on cleansed, dry skin.
Q	What action should be taken if the foundations are not the correct shade?
A	You can blend your own shades by mixing two or more colours together on a palette to obtain the correct shade.
Q	Do I have to use a colour corrector if a concealer has been used?
A	Colour correctors do just what they say — they neutralise the colour to make a more even shade — so they should only be applied where they are needed.
Q	Is the lighting really that important when applying make-up?
A	The more natural the lighting and the closer to daylight, the better the finished results will look. Different coloured light bulbs and shades on light fittings can give a false appearance and you may find that that the application is too sparing or too heavy handed.
Q	Why is it important to use the correct products on black/Asian skins?
A	Because of the different colours and pigmentation of the skin, specialist products should be used so the correct skin tones and a natural look can be achieved.

Unit B8/B9 Provide make-up services and instruct clients in the use and application of skincare products and make-up

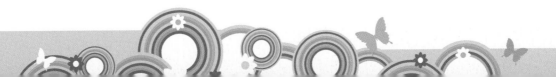

Check your knowledge

1   On which bone would you try the colour of foundation?
2   Which skin type would benefit from the use of a mineral foundation?
3   On the colour star, which colour would neutralise red colouring?
4   When applying eye make-up to more mature clients, what type of product should be avoided?
5   What aspects should you consider when undertaking a special occasion make-up?
6   What should you do between each eye when using a pencil to line the eyes?
7   Why is the position of the client important when applying make-up?
8   What type of mascara is best to use on a client who wears contact lenses?
9   How would you contour a client with a round face shape?
10 Does a highlighter enhance an area or make it recede?
11 Name two benefits of a one-to-one skincare and make-up instruction session.
12 Name two benefits of a group skin-care presentation.
13 When talking to clients why is it important to vary your tone and speech patterns?
14 Name three resources that you could use when carrying out a skincare instruction session.
15 Why is it important to demonstrate skincare products to clients?

Getting ready for assessment

You cannot do any simulation within this unit, but the evidence can be gained quite easily. Remember to keep all paper evidence of any actions, feedback or witness statements that you have been given to support this work.

Your assessor will observe your performance on at least three occasions, working with a variety of skin types and conditions involving different client groups and products as listed in the range to show day, evening and special occasion make-up techniques, and skincare choice and application.

For B8/B9 ranges:

*   Use all consultation techniques.
*   Identify skin types.
*   Use all the products listed in the range.
*   Apply make-up for all occasions as listed in the range.
*   Select skincare products that will suit the client's skin type.
*   Maintain environmental conditions (ventilation, heat, etc.).
*   Prepare the client to suit the treatment.
*   Deal with contra-indications that may prevent or restrict the treatment.
*   Deal with contra-actions.
*   Provide treatment advice.

Evidence of these can be provided for observation by your assessor but also by written work, projects, witness statements, photographic and video evidence, and APL (accredited prior learning) statements.

You must prove to your assessor that you have the necessary knowledge, understanding and skills to perform competently on all ranges within the criteria from this unit.

For B9, your assessor will be expecting you to provide skincare and make-up instruction, giving product advice to individual clients from a variety of age groups, as specified in the range, covering oily, dry and combination skins.

The instructions and demonstration should cover use of skincare products and make-up for day, evening and special occasion. You should use a variety of instructional techniques including skills demonstrations, diagrams, verbal explanation and written instructions. You will need to evaluate your skincare/make-up advice.

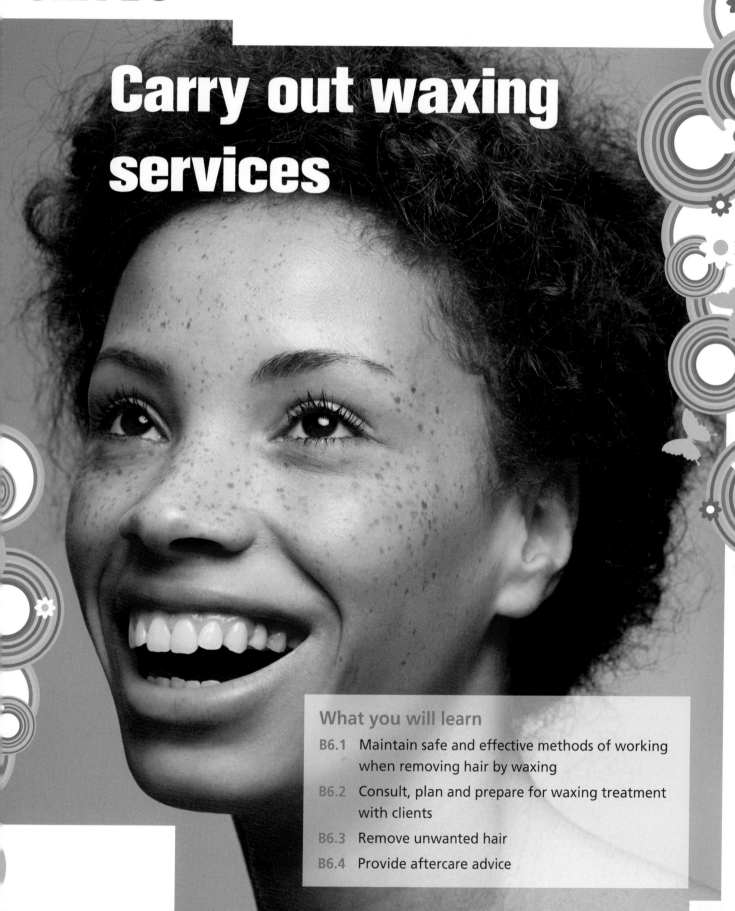

Unit B6

Carry out waxing services

What you will learn

B6.1 Maintain safe and effective methods of working when removing hair by waxing

B6.2 Consult, plan and prepare for waxing treatment with clients

B6.3 Remove unwanted hair

B6.4 Provide aftercare advice

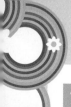
Unit B6 Carry out waxing services

Introduction

Waxing is the temporary removal of body hair by pulling it out of the skin by the roots, using some form of bond. A hot, warm or cold wax product is spread over the hairy area, and a cotton or paper strip is used to make the hair bond or stick to it. The strip is then removed in a quick, single movement. It should leave the area clean and hair-free. Hygiene, client care and lots of practice are necessary, which may mean this unit takes some patience to learn, but it is very rewarding for you and the client.

Waxing treatments always form a large part of any salon's business, as many women in western society dislike body hair. However, some cultures, such as eastern Europeans, do not dislike it. Waxing tends to be a steady source of income, with peaks at certain times of the year. With the first rays of sunshine, clients wish to shed their tights and show off hair-free legs, so spring is always busy. Christmas is another busy time, when more revealing party outfits are worn and bodies need tender loving care and that extra bit of maintenance.

Before you can give the client a full consultation, then plan and prepare for the treatment, you need to understand:

- hair facts
- wax facts
- other methods of hair removal.

This knowledge will allow you to make the best treatment decision for your client, based upon a sound understanding of the choices available to suit her needs.

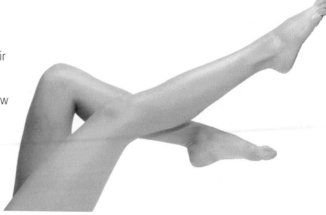

Benefits for the client:

- quick and effective method of removing **superfluous hair** to all areas of the body
- immediate result
- lasts 4–6 weeks depending on hair growth and colour of hair
- minimal pain.

Benefits for the therapist:

- mainstay salon treatment
- treatments can often be slotted in among other longer services, therefore saving salon time
- can be offered as a promotion, e.g. summer holiday package, to increase revenue.

Maintain safe and effective methods of working

In this outcome you will learn about:

- preparing the work environment to meet legal, hygiene and industry Code of Practice for Waxing Services requirements
- ensuring your personal appearance meets accepted industry Code of Practice for Waxing Services and organisational requirements
- wearing suitable personal protective equipment for the work that conforms to the industry Code of Practice for Waxing Services
- preparing the client and providing suitable personal protective equipment to conform to the industry Code of Practice for Waxing Services
- making sure that environmental conditions are suitable for the client and the treatment
- ensuring all tools and equipment are cleaned using the correct methods
- effectively disinfecting your hands prior to waxing treatments
- maintaining accepted industry hygiene and safety practices throughout the treatment
- selecting and correctly positioning suitable equipment, materials, applicators and products for the waxing treatment
- ensuring your own posture and position minimises fatigue and the risk of injury while working
- minimising wastage of product during application
- disposing of hazardous waste correctly to meet local authority requirements
- ensuring that the treatment is cost-effective and is carried out within a commercially viable time
- leaving the work area and equipment in a condition suitable for further waxing treatments
- ensuring the client's records are up to date, accurate, easy to read and signed by the client and practitioner.

Some of the topics in this outcome are also covered elsewhere:

The work environment and legal, hygienic and treatment requirements	pages 70–104
Personal appearance	pages 12–15
Cleaning tools and equipment	pages 41–45
Environmental conditions	pages 70–104
Hygiene	pages 39–45
Personal protective work wear	page 53

Learning about these topics will help you form a professional assessment and give the best treatment that is tailor-made to your client's requirements. Ensure that you refer to the Habia Code of Practice for Waxing Services and follow the guidelines that are set.

Preparing the work environment

Preparation for waxing is an essential part of the beauty therapist's role regardless of the treatment being carried out. Good preparation sets the whole atmosphere of any treatment, creating a calm and efficient impression. If the therapist and work area are not prepared, the client will be aware of this, which can detract from the benefits of the treatment.

In the case of waxing, preparation is vital. Most wax needs preheating so that the client is not kept waiting. All equipment and materials should be in place to avoid leaving the client alone.

Unit B6 Carry out waxing services

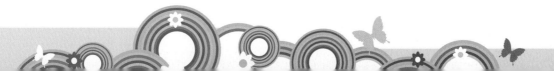

Preparation of the working area

Many salons have designated rooms or areas that are permanently prepared for waxing, with heaters and all necessary products never leaving the room.

The golden rule here is to leave everything fully prepared for the next therapist to use. This means replenishing anything that has run low, cleaning and being tidy during the treatment. It would be most off-putting for a new client to find the remains of the previous client's treatment.

The preparation of the working area should include the following.

○ Protective covering for the couch, so that any spillage or residue is easily removed and will not cause permanent damage.

○ Where plastic sheeting is used, paper couch roll should be placed over the top. This prevents cross-infection, as the paper can be replaced easily; it also provides client comfort.

○ Two waste bins, both with inner liners, should be placed behind or under the couch: one for general waste; one for wax waste — this is for contaminated materials, which will be put into a designated bin for collection by a licensed removal firm for incineration.

○ The chosen heating unit for the wax type to suit the client's needs and enough wax product for the area to be treated. Obviously, a lip wax requires a small amount of product, but a full leg wax will mean the heater needs to be quite full. Remember that it may take a full half-hour to heat the wax to a working temperature, so that needs to be the first job of the day. (Many salons keep a heater on all day, in anticipation of clients dropping in without appointments.)

○ Antiseptic cleaner for the skin, or the manufacturer's recommended skin cleanser.

○ Talc-free powder.

○ Fabric or paper strips which are compatible with the manufacturer's requirements for the wax chosen.

○ Disposable gloves, usually vinyl with a talc-impregnated lining so they are easy to put on — refer to your individual professional body's guidelines for use. Wearing gloves may help to prevent contact dermatitis.

○ Disposable wooden spatulas or a suitable applicator — again refer to your professional body's guidelines (there are no spatula requirements for roller waxing, of course).

○ Tissues, cotton wool and a jewellery bowl for the client.

○ A pair of scissors and tweezers in a container soaking in suitable disinfectant to sterilise — the scissors may be required to trim the hair length prior to treatment, and the tweezers to remove the odd stray hair which has escaped the wax.

○ After-wax lotion or oil.

○ Aftercare leaflets for the client to take away.

Wearing suitable personal protective equipment

The personal protective equipment a therapist should wear when waxing is a disposable apron and gloves.

Think about it

Check to ensure that the client does not have a latex allergy before putting on gloves. Alternative gloves are available, including vinyl or nitrile powder-free gloves. These should be used if either the client or the therapist has an allergy.

Think about it

The talc product you use should be labelled 'talc free' to prevent aggravating respiratory problems. Talc-free products work in the same way as talc when waxing to lift the hairs and absorb moisture. Talc-free products contain natural ingredients such as cornstarch and kaolin.

Checking your position and posture

When waxing, you may find that you get very close to the skin to inspect every pore and hair to make sure you have missed nothing. It is important to remember your posture to prevent back stain and repetitive strain injury. Remember to bend at the knees and keep a straight back.

Ensuring the treatment is cost-effective and minimising wastage

Cost is the price paid for something. It is measured in time, money or energy. Effectiveness means producing a result.

So how does this apply to hair removing? Imagine you own your own business and you have to pay for all outgoings, equipment, overheads, stock and products, along with staffing and wages.

How can a therapist be economical?

- Only use the amount of product needed. Do not be too quick to do a heavy application of wax — it does not give the best results.

- Do not be wasteful with disposable items. Couch roll can be split in half, cotton wool pads can be split, and smaller tissues can be used rather than 'man-sized' ones.

- Give time careful consideration. Time is money and if the treatment times are not planned carefully through the day, there may be a gap of 15 minutes per client. This adds up to an extra hour at the end of the day that could be put to good use, either with vital chores or another cash-paying client.

- Be organised and prepared. Time spent preparing the working area not only gives a professional appearance, it also saves time.

- Do not indulge in false economies. Paying to have equipment maintained and repaired makes good financial sense. If the equipment starts failing and the therapist is unable to offer some treatments because of it, revenue may be lost. Bad advertising through word of mouth will also mean lost revenue.

- Invest in good labour-saving equipment. For example, borrowing an old machine to wash all the towels may seem to cut costs, but an industrial washing machine will have low maintenance costs.

- Work out overhead costs on a realistic basis, and try to gear your prices to that figure. Work out how many hours you work a week.

- Be wary of both consultation and aftercare times. Some clients love to chat, and while the therapist wants to give a quality treatment, time can slip away, and that is expensive. Giving the client a leaflet is a good time-saving technique, and the client can take it away to refer to.

- Do some research and find out what sort of prices the competition asks for waxing treatments. The salon may offer both warm and hot wax. Adjust your prices so they are about the same — they should be not so expensive that custom is lost but not so cheap that clients think there is a catch.

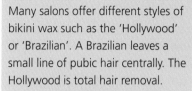

Think about it

Many salons offer different styles of bikini wax such as the 'Hollywood' or 'Brazilian'. A Brazilian leaves a small line of pubic hair centrally. The Hollywood is total hair removal.

You should be fully trained in intimate wax techniques before undertaking these treatments. If an accident occurs when waxing in this delicate area, you may find that your insurance is invalid.

Unit B6 Carry out waxing services

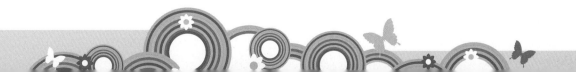

Think about it

It is vital that the waxing waste is not mixed with ordinary rubbish or waste from other treatments. If it is not separated, health inspectors could close down your salon as a health hazard.

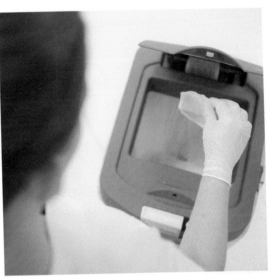

Dispose of waste such as wax strips in the correct way.

Disposing of hazardous waste

The disposal of waste is covered in Unit B4 Provide facial skincare treatment, page 265. However, it is an important topic. When waxing, you will be dealing with contaminated skin waste products from many different clients.

The following Acts require all clinical waste to be kept apart from general waste and to be disposed of to a licensed incinerator or landfill site by a licensed company:

○ Environmental Protection Act, 1990

○ The Controlled Waste Regulations, 1992 (as amended)

○ Special Waste Regulations, 1996 (as amended).

Clinical waste includes:

○ waste which consists wholly or partly of animal or human tissue

○ blood or other body fluids

○ swabs or dressings

○ syringes or needles.

Refer to 'You, your client and the law' in Professional basics, page 58, for further information.

All waste products from a waxing treatment must be classed as contaminated waste: there is a possibility that blood spotting will have occurred, especially when carrying out a bikini or underarm wax, and some skin cells will be caught up in the wax. You only need to perform a wax treatment on a tanned skin to see how much of the darker skin is removed along with the hairs.

Put all your used strips into a lined small bin, tie the bag up and put it into the larger, lined clinical waste bin that is provided by the salon. A contractor will empty this weekly, but if a salon is a busy wax centre, then twice weekly emptying stops the bin from becoming a health hazard.

The person who empties the clinical waste bins should wear industrial gloves as added protection. The bins are usually taken to the council incinerator for burning. Large hospitals often lease out one of their own incinerators to companies.

While it would be very unlikely that your waxing waste would contain any infections, as you thoroughly check for contra-indications before treatment begins, you must follow the procedures laid down by the law and by your own professional code of ethics to protect yourself and your clients.

Leaving the work area and equipment suitable for further treatments

After the client has left the salon, it is time to go back to your workstation to clear up. Waxing is a notoriously messy business, especially in your early training. You will probably have dripped wax down the side of the pot and on to the floor while trying to get it from the pot to the area to be waxed. You may also have flicked some of it on to yourself. Some of this is to be expected when you first start, but your technique must get cleaner as you progress.

To avoid dripping wax on to the floor, fold up a tissue in your free hand and hold it underneath the hand holding the spatula to catch any drips. This is much easier than trying to pick wax off the floor – it never comes off completely once it has set.

Always wear a protective apron – it is much easier to throw away a plastic apron than to get wax off a new overall.

Think about your method of work. Could you have been tidier as you went along? Unless the client is the last one of the day, you will not have the luxury of plenty of time to clean and tidy the area. Get into the habit of putting all waste straight into the bin, which should be beside you. Bad habits soon form, so do not put bits and pieces on the side of the trolley, or worse still, on the couch. If your next client is in straight away, you could be in trouble with treatment timing if you have to spend a long time tidying and preparing for your next treatment.

Good habits for keeping tidy

Organise the layout of the trolley in an ordered fashion. Arrange all the products in order of use with the labels facing you, so you can easily find the one you need. Replace them into their slot when you have finished with them. They will always then be at hand, and you will look tidy and in control.

Have a space for everything. Have a system whereby all necessary tools are in a jar or pot (even a plastic beaker is easy to clean), and the tissues and cotton wool are in their own plastic bowl or tub.

Tidy as you go along – put used tissues and cotton wool into a small pedal bin (lined with a bin liner) as you finish with them, rather than leaving them on the trolley.

Have gloves and strips at the ready. Wash your hands in front of the client, although this may not be possible if you do not have a sink near the workstation – but try not to leave the client unattended.

Minimise waste by using only the amount of product required. This is not only cost-effective, it also means there is very little product left over to have to clear up.

Mop up spills as they occur and do not allow them to endanger others.

After each treatment, cover the couch with clean couch roll. The trolley should be as you would wish to find it. Do not leave a wax pot with a tiny amount of wax in it that is not enough for the next client to have a treatment. Ask the receptionist or a junior therapist to put on a second pot, or ask your technician to add some more wax pellets or sugar, so it can be heating while you clear up.

These hints prevent a major clean-up being necessary at the end of your treatment. Becoming tidy is a skill that comes with experience.

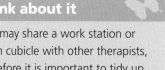

Think about it

You may share a work station or salon cubicle with other therapists, therefore it is important to tidy up after treatments to ensure you are effective with your time and do not annoy colleagues.

Ensuring the client's records are up to date and accurate

If the client is a regular visitor to the salon, a record card will be held. Each treatment will be recorded along with the area treated and any reaction to treatment.

With a new client a full consultation will take place and a patch test will be carried out prior to treatment, to make sure the client does not have an allergic reaction to the wax (see page 435).

A treatment plan will be needed that is mutually agreeable to both client and therapist. It will include:

○ type of hair growth (coarse, thick, thin, light, short or long)
○ the area to be treated
○ whether it is the first or a subsequent treatment
○ skin type and sensitivity
○ any reaction to a previous treatment
○ result of the sensitivity test
○ any contra-indications present.

A record card could look something like the one shown below.

Waxing and record of treatment client file copy

Client reference:

Initial consultation date:	Therapist:

First treatment: Yes ☐   No ☐

Contra-indications checked: Yes ☐   No ☐

Contra-indications noted: _____ None ☐

Allergies:	Disorders:
Skin conditions:	Wax used:

Date and treatment no.	Area	Contra-action	Special notes Contra-indications or adaptations	Therapist	Patch test
1					
2					
3					
4					
5					
6					

NB After 6 treatments client requires new consultation and analysis

Leaflet given: Yes ☐

Aftercare – for a period of 24 hours:

◆ No sunbathing or sunbeds
◆ Avoid bathing in sea or swimming pool
◆ Do not take a *hot* bath or shower
◆ Do not use deodorant / anti-perspirant

◆ Avoid tight clothing
◆ Do not use perfumed products on the area
◆ No make-up or self-tanning preparations
◆ Do not keep touching or picking at the area

Waxing treatment record card

Complete the client record card accurately. Refer to Professional basics (pages 29–31) for client record keeping.

It is important, both for the client and yourself, that you fill out the waxing sheet details accurately to avoid any health and safety problems and to protect your professional reputation. Do not return the record card to be filed incomplete, thinking you can do it later: you will not remember and vital information may not be recorded.

Be constructive when filling out the card. Be positive and helpful in what you write, and avoid making any negative comments or personal observations about the client. Clients are entitled to view their own records under the Data Protection Act. Also avoid leaving the card lying around for anyone to read. Once you have completed the write-up, give it to the person who is responsible for filing.

Consult, prepare and plan for waxing treatments with clients

In this outcome you will learn about:

- using suitable consultation techniques in a polite and friendly manner to determine the client's treatment
- obtaining signed, written informed consent from the client prior to carrying out the treatment
- ensuring that informed and signed parental or guardian consent is obtained for minors prior to any treatment
- ensuring that a parent or guardian is present throughout the treatment for minors under the age of 16
- asking the client appropriate questions to identify if they have any contra-indications to waxing treatments
- accurately recording the client's responses to questions
- encouraging clients to ask questions to clarify any points

- ensuring client advice is given without reference to a specific medical condition and without causing undue alarm and concern
- taking the necessary action in response to any identified contra-indications and the client's suitability for waxing treatments
- clearly explaining the possible contra-actions to the client prior to agreeing to the waxing treatment
- agreeing the waxing treatment and outcomes that are acceptable to the client and meet their needs
- ensuring the client is in a suitable position for the area to be treated during the waxing treatment
- ensuring your client's clothing, hair and accessories are effectively protected or removed.

Before you can effectively consult with the client and decide on her waxing needs and draw up a treatment plan, you need to have thorough background knowledge of all the products. So, look closely at hair facts (page 422) and wax facts (page 423) before deciding on your recommendations.

It is important to ensure that you treat every client equally and in line with current legislation (Disability Discrimination Act, 2005 and Equality Act, 2006 – refer to Professional basics, page 62). The service and standard of care you provide should be the same for everyone.

Some of the topics in this outcome are also covered elsewhere:

Consultation techniques	pages 31–35
Agreeing the treatment and outcomes	pages 47–48
Contra-indications (general)	pages 35–39
The client's position and safety	pages 46–47
Discussing and establishing treatment plans	pages 25–28, 34–35

Think about it

Regardless of treatment chosen, all under-16s require their parent/guardian's written consent for a treatment to be carried out, and hair removal is no exception. A parent/guardian should also be present at the treatment.

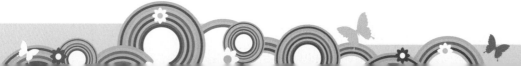

Using consultation techniques

You should use appropriate consultation techniques, including visual, questioning and manual checks, to establish the treatment plan for the client. Remember that you should record all details on the client record card and that clients must give their signed consent before the waxing treatment is carried out.

Remember that your consultation should be carried out with sensitivity and tact to give the client confidence. You should conduct the consultation in a polite and friendly manner to find out what the client's particular needs are.

Once you have conducted the consultation, you will be able to decide on the best treatment plan to meet the needs of the client. You should always agree your approach with the client before you begin.

Identifying contra-indications to waxing

The questions that you ask need to establish if the client has a contra-indication – that is, a condition that will prevent the treatment taking place, or mean that the treatment needs adapting. (Refer to You and the skin, pages 200–01, for photographs of the different types of infection.) It may be that an area has to be protected or avoided, for example where a mole or skin tag is present. Accurately record the client's answers and encourage them to ask questions so that you can establish any problems and take any necessary action if required.

The areas to be treated should be examined in good lighting to judge if any of the following conditions are present:

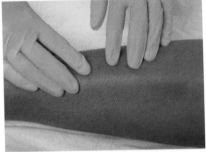

Look out for moles and skin tags which may restrict the treatment in the area

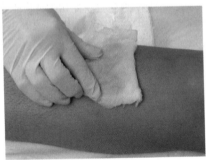

Use a pre-wax cleanser from a manufacturer to cleanse the area

- skin diseases or disorders
- open skin, infection, inflammation or healing skin (scabs present)
- bruising
- very thin or papery skin (diabetics have thin skin that does not heal very well because of poor circulation; also long-term use of steroid creams or medication can cause the skin to thin, which could cause tearing if the area is waxed over)
- sunburn – after a sunbed or natural tanning
- recent scar tissue
- moles, warts or any unidentified skin problems
- varicose veins or broken capillaries on the legs
- cold sores, eye infections, styes or colds when treating the face
- unidentified lumps, breast-feeding and mastitis when treating under the arm
- previous reactions to treatment
- excessive ingrown hairs from previous treatments.

The client would also not be suitable for treatment if she had just had heat treatment, such as infrared treatment or a sauna or steam bath.

Prior to or during menstruation, clients may have a lower pain threshold and the skin may be more sensitive and react unpredictably. You can suggest clients take an over-the-counter painkiller to help, but only if they have used them before with no adverse reactions.

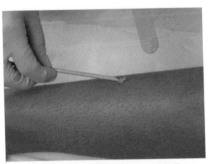

Cover the mole with petroleum jelly to prevent the wax from adhering to it – this will ensure you do not cause any damage to the mole

Explaining possible contra-actions

Even when you have been faultless in hygiene, safety and product use, your client may react to the wax – even if she has had the same treatment for years. It could be a reaction caused by medication being taken or the result of fluctuating hormones, or it could be that an allergic reaction has developed.

Possible **contra-actions** to waxing may be immediately visible, either during or after the treatment. They may also appear when the client goes home or back to work. Either way you should act responsibly and make your client aware of what action to take.

Unfavourable skin reaction

Recognised as redness or soreness to the area, this could be caused by the wax being too hot on the skin, by an allergic reaction or from too vigorous scraping of the spatula on the skin during application. Stop the treatment, apply a cold compress to the area, and apply and give aftercare cooling lotion for the client to continue applying.

Burning or blistering

Recognised as a burning sensation, this is caused by the wax being too hot. Was it tested on the therapist, and a little applied to the area prior to treatment?

Refer to the individual waxes for first aid recommendations (pages 426–32).

Swelling in the area

Recognised as the area being tender and the skin having a puffy appearance, swelling is caused by the wax having too high a temperature or by the strips being lifted off in an upward motion rather than back on themselves.

Refer to the individual waxes for first aid recommendations.

It is also advisable to give your client an aftercare leaflet to take away and refer to, so that any potential contra-action can be avoided and maximum benefit is gained from the treatment.

Agreeing the waxing treatment and outcomes to meet the client's needs

During the consultation the therapist needs to discuss the realistic outcomes of a waxing treatment.

Unrealistic aims of waxing

It would be unrealistic for the client to believe that:

- waxing is permanent hair removal
- waxing makes the hair growth weaken
- all the hairs grow back at the same time
- waxing lightens the hair colour
- the hairs grow back with a sharp, spiky feel to them
- waxing is painless.

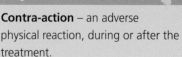

Key terms

Contra-action – an adverse physical reaction, during or after the treatment.

Think about it

All contra-indications that are present and contra-actions that have occurred as a result of the treatment should be recorded on the client's record card. There is usually a slight reaction to hair removal but a strong reaction should not occur.

Think about it

The golden rule is: 'If in doubt, don't treat!' Ask the client to provide a GP's written approval where appropriate and keep it with the record card along with the client's signature that the treatment can go ahead. Never try to diagnose a condition – you are not trained to do so – and remember to explain possible contra-actions prior to the treatment.

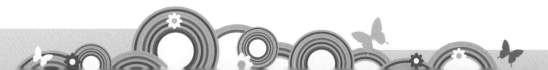

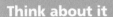

> **Think about it**
>
> It is important to be honest with the clients, so they know what to expect. Honesty between therapist and client is part of the ethical conduct that maintains high professional standards for all beauty therapists

Realistic aims of waxing

○ Waxing lasts 3–6 weeks depending on hair growth.

○ As the blood supply to the hairs is increased with waxing, the hairs may grow back slightly thicker and coarser.

○ The hairs grow back spasmodically as the hair growth cycle for each follicle is different.

○ Waxing does not change the hair colour.

○ Shaving and cutting blunt the ends of the hair, making them feel spiky; after waxing the hair grows back with its natural tapered end, feeling smooth to the touch.

○ Waxing feels like a plaster being taken from the skin. Pain thresholds will vary and some clients will feel more than others.

Ensuring the client is in a suitable position to be treated

○ The couch should initially be placed in an upright position to allow the client to be comfortably seated, and then placed into the appropriate position for the area to be treated. A pillow covered with a towel and protected with couch roll should be used. It is vital that the client is in the right position not only for their comfort and ease but to ensure that as the therapist you don't suffer any injuries when undertaking the treatment

○ Help the client into a comfortable and relaxed position. Offer a covered towel as a prop, should she or he require extra support under the knees or in the small of the back.

○ Ask the client to place protective couch roll around the panty line if doing a bikini wax, or around the bra if doing an underarm wax, rather than just assuming the client would be comfortable for you to touch those areas.

○ Remember when the couch is in a semi-reclining position and the client is having the front of the legs waxed, it is very comfortable. However, you must lower the couch head so it is flat again before you ask her to turn over, otherwise she will be in a very awkward position.

> **Think about it**
>
> Advise the client not to wear expensive underwear when having a wax. Protect the client's clothing with towels and tissues. If the client is having a bikini wax prior to a holiday, she should wear her swimsuit or bikini bottom for waxing to ensure the line is right. If not, an old pair of briefs with the same leg shape will give the correct line.

Salon life

My story

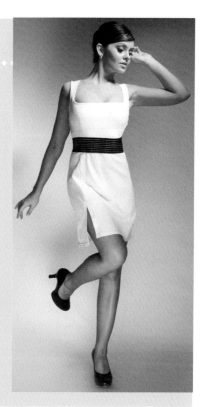

My name is Nikita. When I first left college I was not very quick or confident with my waxing skills. On my first day, my manager asked me about my favourite and least favourite treatments. I had to say that waxing was my least favourite. So instead of giving me a few wax clients during my first month, my manager made sure I had mostly waxing treatments in my column. My manager was always around to give me support and guidance and although I was nervous at first, my confidence and speed quickly grew. I'm really glad I faced up to my fears and worked hard on my weakest treatment. I now enjoy waxing and have many regular clients.

Benefits to client and therapist

Benefits of waxing for the client:

- Quick and visual treatment
- Areas stay hair free for longer
- All parts of the body can be covered
- Treatment available to male and female clientele
- After a number of treatments hair growth usually becomes sparser

Benefits of waxing for the therapist:

- Quick treatment to carry out
- Staple salon treatment that provides regular income
- Can be performed as a mobile treatment
- Good treatment to link with promotions; for example, leg wax and pedicure for the summer

ASK THE EXPERTS

Q *Do you have any tips for advice that I should give to clients to reduce the pain?*

A Firstly, remind the client that her pain threshold is at its lowest around her period and to avoid treatment at this time. Secondly, a client's pain threshold is also at its lowest if they are feeling under the weather or tired. Thirdly, suggest the application of an after-wax lotion following treatment to reduce redness and aid healing.

Q *I worry about causing bleeding when carrying out underarm and bikini-line waxing.*

A Make the client aware that as the hair in these areas is strong terminal hair there may be some blood spotting and that bleeding or spotting is a normal reaction. Use an after wax lotion which is formulated to deal with spotting.

Top tips

- It is important to make sure you are confident in your own abilities as this is reassuring for the client. If you feel weak in a particular skill or treatment, make sure that you keep practising it. Practice makes perfect and treatment times will improve with experience.

Unit B6 Carry out waxing services

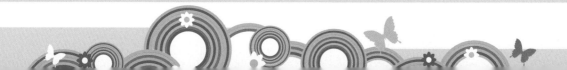

Remove unwanted hair

In this outcome you will learn about:

- using the correct pre-wax products prior to waxing following manufacturers' instructions
- conducting a test patch and skin sensitivity test immediately prior to the intended waxing treatment
- establishing the hair growth pattern prior to the application of the product
- using methods of application correctly and following manufacturers' instructions
- applying and removing the product in the treatment area according to the requirements of the hair removal method and hair growth pattern
- maintaining the client's modesty and privacy at all times
- providing clear instructions to the client on how and when to support their skin during the waxing treatment
- ensuring your work techniques minimise discomfort to the client
- checking the client's well-being throughout the waxing treatment
- stopping the waxing treatment and providing relevant advice if contra-actions occur
- ensuring the client's treatment area is left free of product and hair and treated with a suitable soothing product
- ensuring that the finished result is to the client's satisfaction.

Why is the human body hairy?

As the human body evolved it was extremely hairy all over for warmth; the body also laid down fat deposits to keep warm. Facial hair on men through the ages has been considered a sign of virility, strength and masculinity. Men only started shaving with razors during the twentieth century. In fact, most Edwardian gentlemen had handlebar moustaches or full beards. There has been a big change in fashion towards clean-shaven faces, except of course for the 'designer stubble' trend of celebrities.

We still retain hairs for the purpose of warmth and protection. Terminal hair (refer to Related anatomy and physiology, pages 245–47) grows long and is often coarse in texture:

- Scalp hair – protects the head and helps keep in the heat.
- Eyelashes – protect the eyes by catching particles that may fall into the eye.
- Underarm and pubic hair – protect the delicate skin and cushion against friction caused by movement.
- Body hair – protects against heat loss.

For the anatomy of the hair's structure and the hair growth cycle, refer to Related Anatomy and physiology, page 248.

Factors determining hair growth

Both men and women have terminal hair, but hair growth is determined by several factors.

The number of hair follicles

A large number of follicles equals lots of hair and the hair will look very thick. This tends to be genetic, which means it has been inherited from the parents. (If a man has baldness in his family, there is a strong possibility he will develop the same hair-growth pattern.)

Cultural influences

Hair-growth patterns as well as strength, texture and the amount of hair are also influenced by geography and ethnicity. There is a higher proportion of blonde and light-skinned people in countries such as Norway and Sweden. Face or body hair on these people is light and not noticeable. However, the nearer the Equator, and hence nearer the sun, that people live, the darker their skin and hair colour is likely to become. Italians, Spaniards and Greeks usually have dark hair and skin. Their facial hair or body hair may be more noticeable. British colouring can be a mixture of light and dark — Scottish and Irish people tend to have darker colouring. Generally, it is darker-haired clients who are more concerned with superfluous hair, mostly because it is more visible.

Hair strength and texture

Again, this tends to run in families. People with a thick, strong hair growth may also have lots of follicles and a really full head of hair. Others may have lots of follicles, but the hair itself may be very fine in texture. Some people have the combination of few follicles with fine hair texture. For these people body hairs are not noticeable and they may never need the services of **depilation**.

Illness

This can have a strong effect on hair growth, usually making the hair lank and lifeless, and could affect hair styling.

Medication

Some drugs have a strong effect on hair growth. They might produce coarse, thick hair, which can be depilated, with a doctor's permission, or the follicles might weaken and wither, causing the hair to fall out. Some forms of chemotherapy for the treatment of cancer cause baldness. Often this is only temporary and the hairs will regrow.

Hormones

Hormones can also have an effect on hair growth. Women going through the menopause, when hormone levels may be erratic, may find they develop 'whiskers' of coarse hair on the face.

Emotion

A sudden shock, accident or the death of a loved one can cause hair loss, which may regrow, or may not. This is called alopecia and can mean patches of hair loss or total baldness. It is unusual for alopecia to occur on a leg or an arm.

In our society some women dislike having hairy legs and body hair. Some men may also consider having hair removed from the body. For example, some professional sportsmen such as cyclists and swimmers may wish to enhance their performance by reducing body hair.

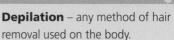

Key terms

Depilation – any method of hair removal used on the body.

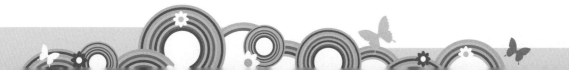

Hair facts

Superfluous hair

This term is used where hair growth is normal, but the client feels it to be unattractive. Dark-haired clients, especially, may feel that their growth is visible, for example on the upper lip.

Removal of unwanted hair, particularly by waxing and sugaring, is referred to as depilation. This is a popular salon treatment as it provides a quick and efficient way of removing unwanted hairs in both small and larger areas.

Some clients do not want the hair removed, but like it to be lightened by **bleaching**. Other clients wish to have their hair permanently removed using more advanced methods such as epilation or laser treatment.

Additional knowledge

Epilation is a specialist treatment at Level 3. It is permanent removal of the hair and requires considerable skill and training. A small needle is inserted into the hair follicle and a current is passed through the needle. If the hair is in the anagen start of hair growth, the dermal papilla has the blood supply sealed, preventing a new hair from growing. Epilation is a permanent method of hair removal if the hair is in the correct growth stage. The client will need to be aware that a number of treatments may be required before all the hair is permanently removed.

Laser hair removal is usually carried out in specialist clinics rather than local salons, and treatments can be costly. As with epilation a number of treatments may be required for successful hair removal, but unlike epilation larger areas can be treated in one session. The laser treatment involves a laser beam being passed down a handheld instrument; the laser energy is converted into heat, this heat destroys the hair follicle and dermal papilla preventing the hair from regrowing. The treatment causes a slight stinging sensation, especially in sensitive areas.

Many hair-removal creams can be bought over the counter, as well as electric shavers for women and disposable razors with adapted shaving foams. These ensure that the skin is kept soft and moisturised.

Hair removal is very much a matter of personal choice and the client should be given all the information available, so an informed decision can be made. The client needs to know the various methods of hair removal available, with the advantages and disadvantages of each, and to be given the therapist's professional advice for her particular problem area, with consideration of the cost and time involved.

Abnormal hair growth

Two terms are used when talking about abnormal hair growth:

- hirsutism
- hypertrichosis.

Hirsutism

This is when the hair growth of a woman develops male characteristics; it is seen as a strong growth of a beard-like formation, the development of chest hair, and more prominent back hair. The pubic hairline can grow upwards towards the navel – all the hair growth patterns of a male. It is caused by hormone imbalances, usually a sensitivity to androgens, which are one of a group of steroid hormones secreted by the adrenal cortex (above the kidneys) and in the ovaries in small amounts.

Hypertrichosis

This is the abnormal growth of terminal hair in an area not normally seen in either sex, such as along the forehead.

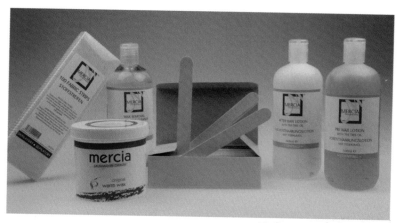

Various wax products

Key terms

Couperose – reddening of the skin associated with dilated or broken capillairies.

Wax facts

Advantages and disadvantages of the different methods of depilation and hair lightening

Method of hair removal	Advantages	Disadvantages
Warm wax	• Quick, cost-effective • Efficient over large areas • Once mastered, easy to apply	• Sticky • Can cause skin damage if reapplied over the same area • Can leave a residue, which if not fully removed can leave the client feeling sticky
Hot wax	• Good for strong hair growth • Suitable for ethnic hair types, which may have bent follicles (refer to anatomy section)	• Skilled technique of application may take some time to master • Because temperature control has to be accurate, application needs to be quick • Not suitable for some skin types, e.g. **couperose** skins • Can be messy when learning application
Impregnated cold wax strips	• Minimal skill needed • Less messy for home use • No specialist equipment needed • Quick	• Bruising or skin damage may occur as the strips stick to the skin and not to the hair • Painful to remove • Unsatisfactory results • Can be costly for large areas • If the hairs are not all the same length, this method may not be successful. The client would need to wait until the hairs were a similar length, as with hot or warm wax, for an effective result • If the client has bruised skin from waxing at home, this would contra-indicate a salon treatment
Strip sugaring	• As warm wax • Water soluble	• Can be less efficient than warm wax • Tricky technique to master
Manual sugaring	• Water soluble • Applied at body temperature, so less likely to burn skin • Cost-effective no paper/material strips necessary	• Difficult technique to master • More time-consuming to perform

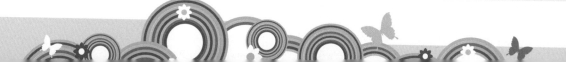

Method of hair removal	Advantages	Disadvantages and effects on waxing
Cutting	• Quick • No skill involved • Home treatment • No pain involved	• Short term only • Blunt regrowth, as hair removed only to skin level • Risk of cutting the skin *Effects on waxing:* Ensure that hairs are long enough to wax effectively
Shaving	• Quick • No skill involved • Home treatment • No pain • Equipment	• Suitable for all skin types • Blunt regrowth • Risk of skin damage • Not hygienic • Short term only • Only removes surface part of the hair *Effects on waxing:* Ensure that hairs are long enough to wax effectively
Tweezing	• Precise • Ideal for small areas, i.e. on the face • Equipment cheap to purchase	• Only suitable for small areas • Risk of skin damage (bruising or pinching the skin) • Breakage of hair may occur • Can be time-consuming • Not ideal as a DIY treatment for clients who wear glasses *Effects on waxing:* Can distort the hair follicle, which may cause the hair to twist and grow inwards. Also if the client wished to have epilation in the future, the hair follicle, where the needle is inserted, can become distorted, therefore epilation would not be a suitable treatment
Threading	• Cheap • No equipment needed • Suitable for Mediterranean and Asian clients as this is a common method used for many years in Asian countries • As effective as tweezing	• Skill needed to apply • Possible breakage of the hair *Effects on waxing:* Possible distortion of hair follicle, which may mean the area is unsuitable for epilation
Abrasives (mitts/pumice stones)	• No skill needed • No specialist equipment needed • Improves the skin texture as dead skin cells are shed (desquamation) • Cheap treatment for home use	• Hair breakage may occur • Hair is only removed at skin surface level • Could result in skin damage • Not terribly effective on strong dark hair growth *Effects on waxing:* Waxing should not be undertaken directly after using an abrasive glove as the skin could be sensitised; also the hairs should be of a similar length for the treatment to be effective
Electrical appliances (e.g. electric razors, etc.)	• No skill needed • Re-usable • Ideal for home use • Clean and quick	• Only removes surface hairs • May damage the skin • Some can be expensive • Regrowth produced is blunt and growth stubble *Effects on waxing:* Waxing should only be undertaken if the hairs are of the correct length. The use of electrical razors gives the same effect as shaving, where the hair is just cut off at skin level, whereas an epilator removes the hair from the root. As with all waxing treatments the result will depend on the length and the stage of hair growth

Method of hair removal	Advantages	Disadvantages and effects on waxing
Depilatory creams	• Cheap • Quick • Ideal for home use • No skill required	• Dissolves hairs by using a chemical reaction at skin level • Some products have an unpleasant fragrance • Not suitable for allergy-prone or sensitive clients – always carry out a patch test prior to use *Effects on waxing:* As with other methods, the hairs will need to grow to a suitable length if waxing is to be effective
Bleach	• Little skill involved in application • Quick results • Suitable for facial hairs • Suitable for clients having epilation	• Not suitable for all skin types • Sensitivity test required • Not suitable for large areas, e.g. the legs • Regrowth is more noticeable when it does come through • Skin irritation can occur *Effects on waxing:* This method could be used for clients who do not wish to have waxing but are concerned by the darker hair. It can also be used between epilation treatments if the client so wishes, as to wax or tweezer the hairs would be counter-productive to the treatment
Laser treatments (including intensive pulse light)	• Can be used for large or small areas • Precise application • Suitable for most skin types	• Costly • Specialist practitioner • More than one treatment may be required • Can be painful *Effects on waxing:* If a client is having laser treatments on an area, no other method should be used while the course of treatment is being carried out as it can affect the treatment and the skin can become over sensitised
Epilation	• Precise application • Salon treatment • More than one method available to suit client requirements	• More than one treatment required • Not for clients with a needle phobia • Can be costly to clear a large area *Effects on waxing:* Waxing could be used on a client at the commencement of the treatment to attempt to put all the hairs into the first stage of hair growth (anagen) to speed up the treatment process

For your portfolio

Research hot and warm waxing products and equipment. Look at manufacturers' websites and in salon supply magazines, and evaluate which you think are the most suitable and economic products to use.

Properties of wax treatments

There are many excellent types of wax available, with various ingredients and different effects. Wax is classed according to its working temperature. The temperatures below are supplied courtesy of Bellitas Ltd, beauty suppliers, known for their 'Strictly Professional' waxes. Manufacturers' instructions will vary with different products, so always refer to the recommended temperatures and heating units for maximum benefit and safety.

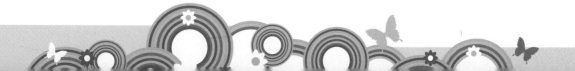

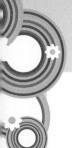

Type of wax	Working temperature
Hot hard depilatory wax	Works best at 48–68°C
Warm soft depilatory wax	Works best at 40–43°C
Cream depilatory wax	Works best at 35–43°C
Organic wax	Organic wax varies – refer to suppliers
Cold wax	Needs no heating

Bellitas Ltd

Type of wax and its working temperature

Key terms

Resin – a substance used in wax products; can be solid or semi-solid, natural or synthetic.

Beeswax – natural wax products produced by bees; used in wax preparations for its emollient properties.

Ingredients

The ingredients of a wax will determine its working temperature. The ingredients will vary from manufacturer to manufacturer, but the higher the proportion of good-quality **resin** in relation to **beeswax**, the more heat is required to get it to a manageable working consistency.

Resins are organic polymers that may be naturally occurring or synthetic. A polymer is a compound such as starch or Perspex. It forms the basis for all plastics and artificial fibres. Natural resins occur in certain plants and trees. The fluid that oozes out from a wound in the plant or tree hardens into a solid resin to protect the injured part. The balsam, pine, gum and rubber tree all produce resins. The gum tree produces chewing gum resin.

Resins are used in the making of perfume, waxing and some cosmetics. Chemists can now make synthetic resins to prevent the overexploitation of plants. Large quantities of resins are produced as a by-product of the petroleum oil business, and are extracted from crude oil after it has been pumped out of the ground.

EU directive 88/379 provides information on all precautions, correct handling, storage and first aid measures.

Latest ingredient developments

Companies are incorporating rich and natural ingredients into their wax formulas to help soften and moisturise the skin. Cannabis sativa is a drug-free hemp derivative that is rich in essential fatty acids to help lock in moisture. It also has anti-inflammatory properties. For sensitive skins, tea-tree wax is very soothing with antiseptic properties. Hemp wax is also very kind to a sensitive skin, and cream waxes moisturise.

Aloe vera wax has soothing, moisturising and healing properties, and is suitable for sensitive skin types. Some companies have started to add essential oils other than tea tree to their wax formulas — lavender, for example, has healing and soothing properties and has long been used to treat burns and irritations.

Types of wax

Hard depilatory wax

What is it?

It is a solid wax, sold in pellet form, which becomes molten when heated.

What is it made of?

It is a mixture of natural resins, beeswax and microcrystalline wax. Insoluble in cold water, this wax is quite soluble when hot. It has a low chemical reactivity and is stable

What are the hazards?

Hard wax is classed as non-hazardous if used in correct professional circumstances.

What are the first aid measures?

○ If used at the correct temperature and with the correct procedure for hair removal, this wax poses no hazard.

○ High temperatures should be avoided, as these will cause thermal burns.

○ If an overheated wax has solidified on the skin, leave it in place and consult a doctor.

○ If wax enters the eyes, they should be flushed immediately with water for 15 minutes and medical attention obtained.

What are the fire-fighting measures?

○ This wax is stable, but it has a flash point greater than 220°C. Make sure that the thermostat controlling the temperature on the heater is working!

○ Although not strictly classed as flammable, this wax will burn. Avoid contact with flammable fabrics, e.g. placing near the curtains.

○ In the event of a small fire, foam, carbon dioxide, dry chemical powder, sand or earth may be used to extinguish it. For a large fire, use foam or water spray.

What do I do in the event of an accident?

○ In the event of a large spillage, any wax entering the drains will solidify and cause blockages. The local health authority will need to be notified if this happens.

○ Allow spilt hot wax to cool and solidify, then scrape up for disposal.

How do I store it?

○ Hard depilatory waxes can be kept for up to six months in tightly closed jars in cool dry conditions, away from possible sources of contamination.

How do I handle it?

○ Adequate protective clothing must be worn when handling wax in a molten state.

○ It is recommended that advice be sought from the individual Awarding Body and professional organisation that is favoured by your training establishment.

○ To ignore their recommended guidelines may invalidate any assessments taking place, but more importantly may remove insurance protection. (Refer to 'You, your client and the law' in Professional basics, pages 48–68.)

Warm wax

What is it?

This is a soft, thick liquid. It may vary in colour from warm honey to amber or light brown.

Soft wax is supplied in a tin or plastic tub, which fits into a special heating unit.

There are many soft waxes on the market and it is recommended that the wax be heated only in the correct heater, following the manufacturer's instructions, as the temperatures for best performance may vary slightly.

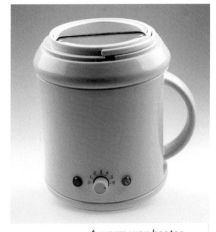

A warm wax heater

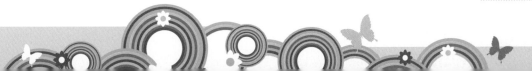

What is it made of?

It is composed mainly of refined gum resin and hydrocarbon tackifiers. This gives the wax its sticking properties.

What are the hazards?

Warm wax is classed as non-hazardous if used in correct professional circumstances.

What are the first aid measures?

○ If used at the correct temperature and with the correct procedure for hair removal, this wax poses no hazard.

○ High temperatures should be avoided, as this will cause thermal burns.

○ If overheated wax has solidified on the skin, leave it in place and consult a doctor.

○ If in contact with the eyes, irrigate immediately with large quantities of cold water for at least five minutes. Obtain medical attention.

○ If inhaled, move the person away from exposure to fumes from molten products. If irritation persists, obtain medical attention.

○ If ingested, no special treatment is necessary.

○ If accidental skin contact with the heated product occurs, cool the affected area by plunging it into cold running water for at least ten minutes. Do not remove the adhering material. Obtain medical attention. If a limb is completely surrounded by wax, the wax should be split to avoid a **tourniquet** effect.

○ If skin contact with the cold product occurs, wash thoroughly with soap and water.

What are the fire-fighting measures?

○ Although not strictly classed as flammable, soft wax will burn above 200°C. Avoid contact with flammable fabrics, e.g. placing near the curtains. Ensure that the thermostat on the heating unit is in working order by regularly maintaining the equipment.

○ In the event of a small fire, use carbon dioxide, dry powders or foam.

○ Do not use water on soft wax.

What do I do in the event of an accident?

○ When soft wax is molten, care must be taken to prevent burns by ensuring that application temperatures are kept to the minimum necessary for adequate product performance.

○ At no time is it necessary to heat the product above 60°C.

○ Ensure good ventilation in the working environment.

○ Where accidental overheating occurs the source of heat should be disconnected and the molten product left undisturbed until cool. Make sure that all persons are aware of the potential hazard.

How do I store it?

Soft wax may be maintained as a cool liquid within its own container, or heated within the unit on a daily basis. It may keep for up to six months in cool dry conditions.

Key terms

Tourniquet – tight bandage around a limb, which cuts off the blood supply to the area.

How do I handle it?

- Handle in the same way as for hard wax.
- Adequate protective clothing must be worn when handling wax in a molten state.
- It is recommended that advice be sought from the individual Awarding Body and professional organisation that is favoured by your training establishment.
- To ignore their recommended guidelines may invalidate any assessments taking place, but more importantly may remove insurance protection. (Refer to 'You, your client and the law' in Professional basics, pages 48–68.)
- Soft waxes are unlikely to cause any environmental hazards, but do remember that all waxes are generally non-biodegradable in the short term.

Cream waxes

Many manufacturers now produce a good quality cream wax. Cream wax contains ingredients such as moisturisers and azulene that help the skin's condition. Azulene is anti-inflammatory and soothing, and is suitable for more sensitive skin types. (Azulene is the ingredient that will turn the cream a blue colour.)

Cream wax also works on slightly lower melting and working temperatures, thereby enhancing client comfort during waxing.

Cream wax has enhanced sticking properties, which means that it can be spread thinly and is thus very economical to use.

Refer to the warm waxing information in the details above.

Organic waxes

Organic waxes are very popular as they contain natural ingredients such as honey as well as the chemical ingredients they need to keep them stable. Organic waxes do not set when cold but become very liquid when heated.

Cold waxes

Some cold waxes, such as pre-coated wax strips, are available over the counter; others are supplied to salons by the manufacturer.

Retail strips

- These can be purchased from most large chemists and come in packs of 6–10 strips.
- They are usually made by the companies that produce hair-removal creams.
- The pre-coated strips are double layered — one piece of wax paper is a non-stick backing strip from which the coated strip peels away to be placed on the skin.
- They contain hydrocarbon resins so are sticky, but as they are cold, the adhering properties are not as effective as warm or hot wax.
- Most manufacturers recommend the strips be warmed between the hands before splitting and applying.
- The wax coating is quite fine and may not be sufficient to grip strong hair growth, so the strips are only suitable for light growth. They are not normally recommended for facial use, elderly people, diabetics and people with skin irritations.

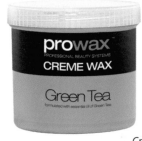

Cream wax

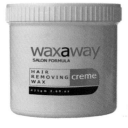

Cold wax

For your portfolio

Research products other than azulene that are often found in cream wax.

Carry out waxing services **Unit B6**

○ They can be used as a stopgap for quick removal of a light growth between waxing, and for special occasions should the client not be able to visit for warm waxing.

○ Follow instructions on the individual packaging.

Roller waxing

Many manufacturers provide complete systems with disposable roll-on heads. These are proving very popular in salons and with therapists offering a mobile beauty therapy service.

The applicators look a little like a roll-on deodorant stick, and come in various roller head sizes for different parts of the body. They can be disposed of after use. Alternatively, refill cartridges can be used and the head attachments taken off for cleaning and sterilisation.

Some salons favour the client purchasing the whole roller applicator, which the salon then keeps for that client to avoid cross-contamination.

Other products used in waxing

Pre-waxing lotion

What is it?

This is a cleansing lotion applied to the area before treatment to cleanse and remove any grease or dirt on the skin that may prevent good hair removal.

What is it made of?

The product usually contains ethanol and camphor oil in a cosmetic lotion. The ethanol is an alcohol for cleansing, and the camphor has antibacterial and anti-inflammatory properties as well as being antiviral. It is also a counter irritant.

What are the hazards?

If used properly, this product has no hazards.

What are the first aid measures?

○ If ingested, drink milk or water.

○ If it goes into the eyes, wash well with water. If irritation persists, seek medical advice.

What do I do in the event of an accident?

If spillage occurs, clean up with an absorbent material, then wash with detergent and water to avoid a slippery floor.

How do I store and handle it?

No special precautions are considered necessary.

Purified talc/or talc-free alternatives.

Purified talc or talc-free products are products that contain no additives or fragrance. They are used to prevent allergies and respiratory conditions when used regularly.

What is it?

It is a dry powder that is used as a light dusting over the area to be waxed. It ensures the hairs have a covering for the wax to adhere to and that the hairs stand away from the skin.

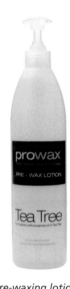

Pre-waxing lotion

What are the hazards?

All dry powders can give respiratory problems if precautions are ignored and they are inhaled. Avoid excessive use, especially near the nose and mouth.

This product is non-flammable.

What are the first aid measures?

- ◯ If ingested, drink milk or water.
- ◯ If inhaled, move the person to the fresh air and keep her warm.
- ◯ Avoid prolonged skin contact as this can lead to dry skin.
- ◯ If it goes into the eyes, wash well with water.

What do I do in the event of an accident?

Sweep or vacuum up the powder, avoiding dust.

How do I store and handle it?

Store in a cool, dry place, keeping containers tightly sealed.

After-wax lotion
What is it?

This is a soothing lotion used after treatment to help cool and calm the skin and prevent irritation.

What is it made of?

The product contains an emulsion of oils, waxes, water, water-soluble ingredients, emulsifiers, fragrance and preservatives.

What are the hazards?

If used properly, this product has no hazards.

What are the first aid measures?

- ◯ If ingested, drink milk or water.
- ◯ If it goes into the eyes, wash well with water. If irritation persists, seek medical advice

What do I do in the event of an accident?

If spillage occurs, clean up with an absorbent material, then wash with detergent and water to avoid a slippery floor.

How do I store and handle it?

No special precautions are considered necessary.

Wax equipment cleaner
What is it?

This is a liquid with a very strong smell!

What is it made of?

It is a hydrocarbon solvent and a very powerful cleaner.

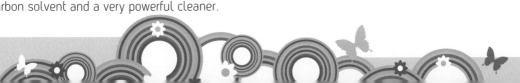

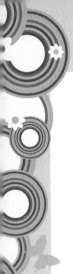

What are the hazards?

It is highly flammable and is hazardous. It should not be used in an enclosed space as the fumes are highly noxious.

What are the first aid measures?

- If it goes into the eyes, irrigate immediately with large quantities of cold water for at least five minutes. Obtain medical attention.
- Do not inhale as this may cause dizziness. If it is inhaled, move to fresh air.
- If ingested, drink plenty of milk or water.
- Avoid prolonged contact with the skin. If irritation occurs, seek medical advice.

What are the fire-fighting measures?

The cleaner is highly flammable. Evacuate the area and inform fire-fighters of the hazards.

What do I do in the event of an accident?

- Clean the contaminated area with lots of detergent and water to avoid slippery floors.
- Do not absorb on to combustible material such as a tissue.

How do I store it?

Store in a cool place away from direct sunlight. Large quantities should be kept in a fire-resistant store.

Benefits and effects of waxing

Type of wax	Benefits	Effects	Possible drawbacks
Hot wax	As hot wax needs to be heated to a high temperature it is extremely effective on strong hair growth.	The solid wax turns into a liquid when heated and when applied to the skin, it coats the hairs, gripping them firmly. The wax is applied with a disposable spatula in a thick layer. A lip of wax is then lifted to allow a firm hold to take the whole patch off.	Only really suitable on longer hair growth – results not good if the hair is shorter. Hot wax may cause a slight skin reaction, so not suitable for sensitive skin, or sensitive areas. Application is a skill that needs a lot of practice to master. The wax needs to be applied quite thickly, so it can be quite costly in materials. Wax should not be applied over the same area twice, as the skin may burn. Can be messy to apply so it is hard to keep the equipment clean. These considerations need to be thought about when choosing equipment.

Type of wax	Benefits	Effects	Possible drawbacks
Warm wax	More comfortable on sensitive skins than hot wax, and can be reapplied over the same area. Even short hairs can be successfully removed with warm wax. The equipment is easy to maintain and keep clean.	Warm wax is applied with a disposable spatula, in a very thin coating and a fabric or paper strip is applied over the top of the wax for easy removal – rather like a plaster coming off. The wax and hairs adhere to the strip. A single strip can be used over again until it reaches saturation point.	There is some risk of infection, as loose skin cells may also be lost during waxing, leaving hair follicles open to infection. As the wax is applied quite finely, it may not remove all strong growth in one go. Strips have to be used with warm wax, and may add to the cost of the treatment if not used economically.
Cold wax	This treatment can be done at home for a top-up treatment, and is therefore convenient.	Hairs are removed by an impregnated strip, with no heat.	Not very economical if using on large areas as lots of strips will have to be purchased. Not suitable on large areas of strong hair growth. As it can be applied to oneself, there is more pain and discomfort than when a trained therapist does it. For self-administration the angle of removal may not be correct for a swift, clean taking off, and that may be another reason for it to hurt.
Roller wax	Very little possibility of cross-contamination from the rollers. Very quick, clean and easy to use. Very economical. Safe – no possibility of spillage as the wax is contained within the cartridge.	Precise application of the wax can be achieved because there is a variety of roller head sizes, allowing more accuracy.	Very few, except that the initial outlay may be high for purchase of the heaters and cartridges. The units are specially made to fit each manufacturer's make of cartridge and therefore are not interchangeable if the type of wax proves to be unsuitable.

Suitability of hair removal products for different parts of the body

Method	Eyebrows	Facial hair	Legs	Bikini line	Forearms
Warm wax	✓	✓	✓	✓	✓
Hot wax	✓ Depends on skin sensitivity	✓ Depends on skin sensitivity	✓	✓	✓
Sugaring	✓	✓	✓	✓	✓
Hair removal creams	✓ Care required	✓	✓	✓	✓
Tweezing	✓	✓	✓ Only for stray hairs after depilation	✓ Only for stray hairs after depilation	✓ Only for stray hairs after depilation
Mechanical depilators	✗	✗	✓	✓	✓
Cutting/shaving	✗ Only to shorten brows	✓	✓	✓	✓
Shaving	✗	✗	✓	✓	✗

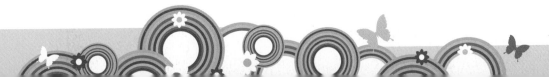

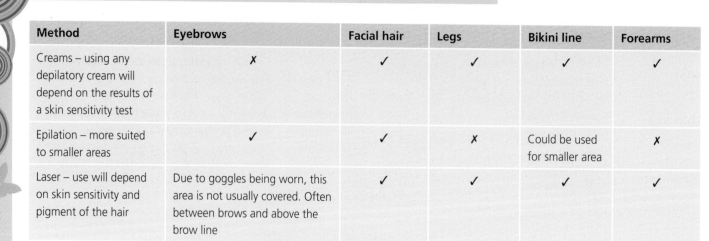

Method	Eyebrows	Facial hair	Legs	Bikini line	Forearms
Creams – using any depilatory cream will depend on the results of a skin sensitivity test	✗	✓	✓	✓	✓
Epilation – more suited to smaller areas	✓	✓	✗	Could be used for smaller area	✗
Laser – use will depend on skin sensitivity and pigment of the hair	Due to goggles being worn, this area is not usually covered. Often between brows and above the brow line	✓	✓	✓	✓

Waxing at a glance

	Legs	Eyebrows	Upper lip	Armpits	Brazilian	Bikini
Waxing facts	Waxing really does slow down the hair growth after several treatments.	Waxing gives a nice clean finish to the eyebrows – any stray hairs can be tweezed out.	A good way of getting a tidy upper lip with no shadow. It does hurt but the result is really clean.	Hot wax is still the favourite for underarm hair – several strips may be needed if the hair growth is circular or in different directions.	This does not render you completely bare between the legs (that's a Hollywood). A thin strip of hair is left, so thongs can be worn. Often called the landing strip.	You can keep underwear on for this as they become the guide line for your treatment.
How long it takes	Half leg 30 mins; full leg including bikini 45–60 mins	10 mins	5 mins	10 mins	15–20 mins	5 mins
How long it lasts	4–5 weeks depending on hair growth	3–4 weeks	About 3 weeks	2–3 weeks	4 weeks	4 weeks
Pain ratio	5/10	8/10	9/10	8/10	10/10	7/10

Other methods of hair removal

Hair removal creams

These creams use chemicals to break down the hair structure. The chemical is calcium thioglycollate and it attacks the hair keratin layer. The hair dissolves and can be scraped or washed away. Most over-the-counter preparations have a full list of instructions for use, and timings may vary. This type of product is not always suitable for young or sensitive skins and a reaction can occur. The regrowth is soft and with a tapered end, so the hair does not feel spiky and sharp.

Cutting or clipping

Scissors will trim the hair. They can be used in between treatments, as this does not distort the follicle. Scissors can obviously shorten long 'whiskers' but are not ideal for achieving a smooth finish. This is not a long-term solution to superfluous hair.

Shaving

Shaving is the chosen option for many people. It is a quick-fix option and can produce clean results providing care is taken, a clean razor is used, and a suitable lubricant is applied to the skin. Many razor companies have recognised the large female market and have designed razors, creams, shaving foams and after-shaving preparations in feminine colours and with attractive smells.

However, shaving is a double-edged sword! The ends of the hair are chopped at skin level and are very blunt, so the regrowth is spiky and gives stubble.

Shaving is not suitable for the face or arms, as once started it becomes quite a chore — if the hair growth is dark and thick, it could become a twice weekly job.

Tweezing

Tweezing of the eyebrows has always been done, but as the hairs are taken out individually tweezing is not suitable for removing hairs from large areas. The hair is pulled out of its follicle, and if the hair is taken out in the right stage of growth, regrowth can take some time. The hair grows back with its natural tapered end so does not feel spiky to the touch. Care must be taken to avoid infection. The tweezers should be clean and disinfected, and the skin cleaned and wiped with antiseptic. Avoid applying make-up straight away as the follicle is open and there is a risk of infection.

Threading

Threading is similar to tweezing. It is practised mostly in Asian communities and is sometimes seen in Mediterranean countries. A piece of cotton is entwined around the fingers and twisted over the hairs. The hair gets caught up in the thread and is plucked out of its follicle. This is quite a skill and requires practice.

Abrasives

An abrasive glove or pumice stone is rubbed over the skin and the hair is broken off at the skin's surface. There are many over-the-counter preparations that have this effect. They come in glove or mitt form and are sold as 'a sensible alternative to waxing and shaving'. They tend to resemble fine sandpaper in appearance.

For best results the skin must be dry, and the glove is rotated in a gentle circular fashion. Do rub gently. Do rub in circular motions. Do not rub up and down.

The fine powder that appears is an accumulation of skin **exfoliation**. This makes the product ideal on dry rough skin, provided that soothing body moisturising creams are applied after use.

Conducting a skin sensitivity test

A sensitivity test should be carried out on a clean, dry area of skin, usually on the forearm as this is hair free. Consult with your own Awarding Body and professional

Key terms

Exfoliation – shedding of dead skin cells.

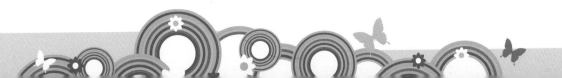

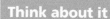

Unit B6 Carry out waxing services

Think about it

If a reaction occurs, it will be noticeable as redness in the area of the sensitivity test, which may also be itchy. This will indicate either that the wax type is unsuitable for the client, or that waxing cannot take place at all.

Think about it

Not all methods of hair removal are suitable for all clients. A full consultation will be needed to establish which method is suitable and agreeable to you both. Remember a sensitivity test would be advisable to people with sensitive skin.

a) front of legs   b) back of legs

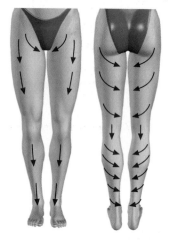

Direction of hair growth on the legs

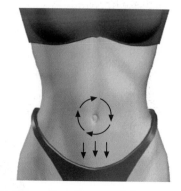

Hair growth pattern on abdomen

therapies federation, as they may insist you carry out a sensitivity test on the area you are treating. The test should always be carried out at least 24 hours prior to the treatment and recorded on the client record card.

Having heated the correct type of wax to be used for the client, test it on yourself for the correct temperature, then apply a small circle of wax to the client's forearm. Remove as for hair removal and note any immediate reaction on the skin.

Put the details on to the client's record card and ask her to monitor the result for the next 24–48 hours.

You must be tactful when informing the client that she is not suitable for treatment if there is an adverse reaction to the sensitivity test. Be discreet, too, and tell her somewhere private, rather than in the middle of reception where everyone can hear.

Warm wax and roller wax operate at much lower temperatures than hot wax, so an alternative product might prevent a reaction from occurring. Another sensitivity test will be required using the different product. If that proves satisfactory, and the client is happy, then the treatment can go ahead.

Think about it

A good tip to pass on to the client who has booked for a waxing treatment is to take a couple of over-the-counter pain killers prior to the treatment. This helps to block the pain killing nerve endings in the skin, therefore the treatment will be less painful. The pain killers must be ones the client has used before with no adverse reactions.

Establishing hair growth pattern before application

The direction of your wax application will depend upon the way the hair is growing, which varies in different areas of the body.

Closely examine the direction of the hair, from the point where it comes out of the skin to its tip. Always work in the direction of the hair growth and you will get great results.

The legs

Most hair on the front of the leg along the shins grows downwards towards the foot. However, the hair along the calf muscle (gastrocnemius) often starts to grow across the leg, going sideways and downwards. This is often dictated by the pressure of clothing on the hairs.

Along the top of the thigh the hair starts to grow inwards towards the inner thigh, but the bikini line tends to grow down and inwards.

The abdomen

The hair around the navel grows upwards from the pubic hairline, and then forms a circle around the navel. You may need several small strips to completely remove the circular pattern. Be careful if the client is menstruating – she may wish to avoid the area because of pressure. Do not wax a client on the abdomen if there is a possibility she may be pregnant.

The arm

The hair on the forearm tends to grow sideways across the arms, rather than downwards towards the hand and wrist. It usually grows from the inner to the outer sides.

Underarm hair varies — some clients have perfect circles of hair around the pit of the arm, some have downward hair and some have hair growing sideways. Very often more than one strip is required to remove underarm hair.

The face

Hair on the upper lip tends to grow in the male pattern of a moustache, that is downwards from the nose towards the upper lip, with some longer hairs growing down on the side of the lip.

Chin hairs often grow straight outward or down, depending on the strength of the hair.

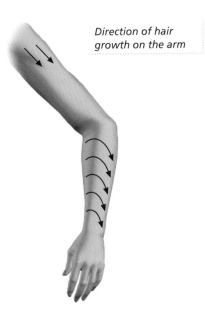

Direction of hair growth on the arm

Using methods of application correctly

Check this list before you apply the wax.

- ○ Is the working area fully prepared and the wax pre-heated?
- ○ Are you fully prepared with protective clothing and gloves?
- ○ Have all safety and hygiene precautions been observed?
- ○ Are the manufacturer's instructions being adhered to?
- ○ Has a full consultation been carried out?
- ○ Can the treatment proceed with no contra-indications present?
- ○ Has a sensitivity test been carried out before the treatment?
- ○ Has the client had a full explanation of the treatment so she knows what to expect?
- ○ Has the client been fully informed with regard to aftercare and home care?
- ○ Has a record card been filled out for the client, or the existing one updated?
- ○ Has the area for waxing been examined in a good light and the best method of waxing decided and agreed between the therapist and client?
- ○ Has the area to be waxed been cleaned so it is grease-free, has it been talced, and has pre-wax lotion been applied?

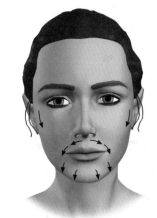

Direction of hair growth on the face

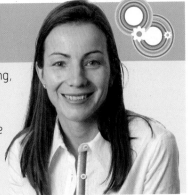

My story

The importance of good waxing techniques

Hi, my name is Martine. When I left college waxing was the treatment I really enjoyed doing, and the salon I worked for had a lot of regular waxing clients. As many of the clientele wanted intimate waxing, the manager sent me on a course to learn the correct techniques to use. It was a little strange at first, but I soon mastered the different methods. The course made me aware of what could occur when treating clients in this delicate area. I now feel confident and have many regular clients. It's worth remembering that if you are not properly trained, your insurance will be invalid.

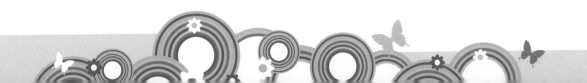

Unit B6 Carry out waxing services

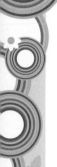

Health and safety

Health and safety information for the different types of waxes used in a salon is included on pages 426–32, along with potential hazards and first aid measures.

Refer to Professional basics, 'You, your client and the law', pages 48–68, for legislation affecting all beauty treatments.

Below are general precautions for safe practice when waxing.

○ Do not have any naked flame near waxing preparations or equipment as the ingredients make them very inflammable.

○ Do not have heating units near anything flammable, e.g. curtains, in case the thermostat breaks and the wax ignites.

○ Do not have the heater on a glass-topped trolley, in case the glass breaks and molten wax spills.

○ Do a thorough consultation, check for contra-indications and carry out a sensitivity test prior to treating the client.

○ Firmly stretch and support the skin in fleshy areas to avoid bruising, especially in the bikini and underarm areas.

○ Be aware of your own professional guidelines regarding insurance cover and the use of gloves and protective clothing.

○ Thorough moisturising after waxing can help to avoid the problems of ingrown hairs, which is when the hair grows back under the skin causing infection. This is always a problem with continual waxing.

○ When hot waxing, never allow the wax to become too cool on the skin as it will be too brittle to remove effectively, and may cause the client a great deal of discomfort.

○ With hot wax always test the temperature on yourself and carry out a small patch test on the client to avoid giving a burn.

○ With organic wax do not allow too much of a build-up on the muslin strip as this can cause undue lifting of the skin during removal.

○ With organic wax it is important to keep the angle of pull on the muslin strip horizontal to the skin's surface, as the hairs can break off at the skin's surface and bruising can occur in fleshy areas.

A thin layer of wax is more effective than a thick layer on a strip. Too much wax builds up on itself and does not coat the hairs. It is therefore less effective.

For maximum comfort and minimum embarrassment give the client lots of towels to protect her modesty, especially with a bikini wax. Plenty of protection will make the client feel more secure and means that the therapist can manoeuvre her into good positions for easy and effective removal. Ensure that the waxing area has adequate ventilation, especially with hot wax, which can give off fumes when first heated.

Risk assessment for hot and warm wax equipment

Refer to Unit G20, Make sure your own actions reduce risks to health and safety, pages 71–86, for a complete discussion of risk assessment.

Hazards: look for hazards that you would reasonably expect to result in significant harm under the conditions in your workplace. Use the following examples as a guide.

- **Fire** (e.g. from electrical flex or lead).
- **Burning of equipment** (through low wax level in the tank).
- **Burns to skin** (not testing wax temperature first on self).
- **Ejection of materials** (spitting hot wax).
- **Electricity** (e.g. poor wiring).
- **Manual handling** (spillage possible if moving when in liquid form).
- **Falling machinery** (if not securely positioned on a trolley).
- **Contamination** (poor waste disposal of contaminated wax strips).
- **Cross-infection** (ignoring possible contra-indications).

Many of the health and safety topics relevant to Unit B6 are covered in Professional basics, or in Unit G20, Make sure your own actions reduce risks to health and safety.

> **Think about it**
>
> Follow all electrical precautions: ensure there are no trailing wires to fall over, carry out regular maintenance checks for efficient and safe working of machines, follow manufacturers' instructions, follow health and safety guidelines.

Applying and removing the product

Leg wax

The lower leg is a simple area to treat as the hair growth can be seen easily. The hairs usually grow towards the ankle on the front of the leg but may go slightly sideways on the calf. Hair growth may be coarse if the client has shaved the area and results are usually good as the hair growth in the area is strong. Moving the leg around slightly will allow access to the ankle hair if the growth pattern is not straight down. The client may ask for the toes to be waxed too.

1 The client can be lying down, or sitting up for the front of the legs. Remember, though, to put the couch back into a flat position before the client is turned over for the backs of the legs.

2 It is important that the client's clothing is protected, so provide a towel for cover. Be aware of protecting the client's modesty if repositioning is required.

3 Cleanse the area and prepare for waxing following the usual sanitising procedure.

4 Start from the ankle and work up the leg systematically.

5 To keep the skin taut at the knee, ask the client to bend it.

6 Turn the client over (lowering the couch) and follow the same routine with the back of the leg. Pay special attention to the hair growth, which may be not straight down.

7 Do not apply wax to the back of the knee. There are usually no hairs present here, but if there are a few, then tweeze them.

8 If completing a full leg wax continue up the thigh at the front and then turn the client over, again paying attention to the direction of growth.

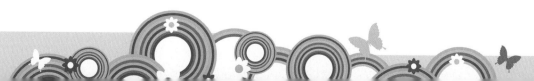

Unit B6 — Carry out waxing services

Step-by-step warm wax application for legs

1 Clean the whole area to be waxed with a suitable antiseptic cleanser on damp cotton wool.

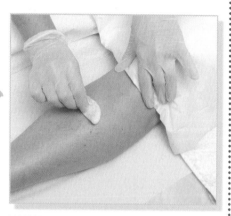

2 Blot the area with a tissue to ensure the skin is dry and grease-free.

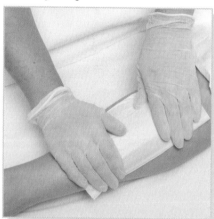

3 Test the wax on your inner arm to make certain you will not burn the client.

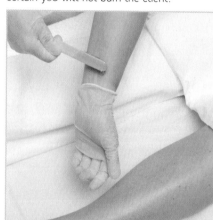

4 To avoid cross-infection drizzle the wax on to another spatula — it will also help you to check that the consistency is workable.

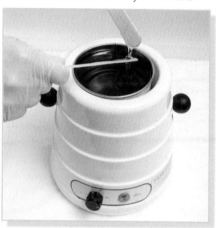

5 If temperature is acceptable to you, apply a small area on to the legs to check with the client that the temperature is tolerable for her.

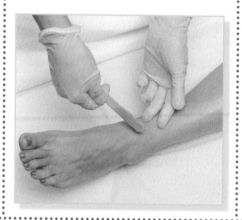

6 Following the hair growth, i.e. downward, apply a thin even strip of wax to the leg, approximately the width of the paper strip.

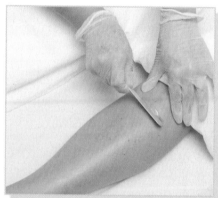

7 Press down firmly over the wax strip, to ensure all the hairs are fully attached to the strip.

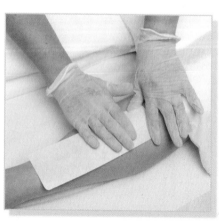

8 Peel back a small edge of the strip to hold on to.

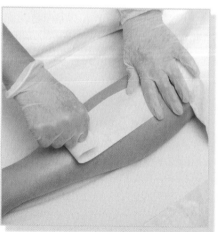

9 Holding the leg, grip the wax strip edge and pull the strip off. It is almost a peeling back of the strip, but it must be quick, to minimise pain.

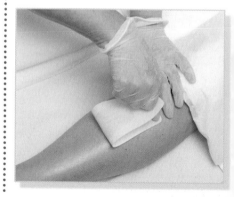

10 Any missed hairs, too short for the wax to pick, can be tweezed out. Sterilise the tweezers first.

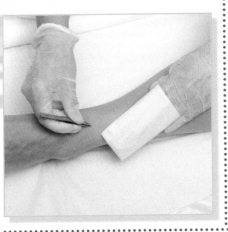

11 After-wax lotion will remove any wax residue.

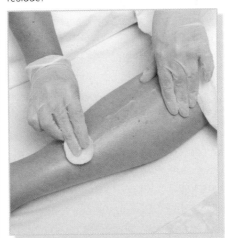

12 The finished result should be a moisturised, hair-free front of leg.

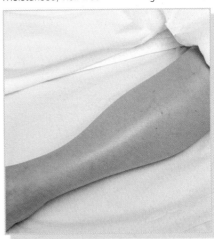

13 Ask the client to turn over — remember to ensure you put the back of the couch down first. Repeat the cleansing and blotting process.

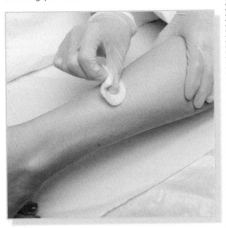

14 As the hairs grow in different directions, you will need to cut the wax strips into manageable sizes.

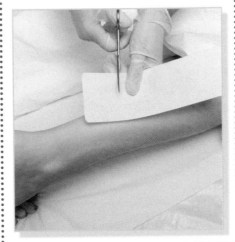

15 Check the direction of the hair growth, which may be diagonal as shown here. Remember to test the wax again — first on yourself and then on your client.

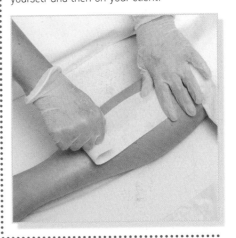

16 Apply a thin even strip of wax to the leg, following the hair growth, i.e. diagonally as shown here, and repeat the process as for front of leg

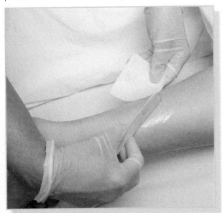

Think about it

Check with your own professional body with regard to the use of spatulas. Most state that once a spatula has come into contact with the skin, it has become contaminated and should be thrown away and a new one used for the next application. Refer to codes of practice for waxing.

Carry out waxing services Unit B6

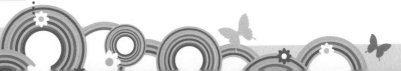

Note: Some Awarding Bodies only expect gloves to be worn if there is a danger of drawing bodily fluids, for example, underarm or bikini line. Therefore, it may be permissible to wax legs without gloves.

Warm wax is applied in a thin film using a spatula in the direction of hair growth with a firm press, without hurting the client.

1 Test the wax prior to use on the inside of the wrist. If it is at a comfortable temperature for the therapist, it should be fine for the client, but also test a small patch on the wrist or ankle of the client depending upon the area to be waxed.

2 Take up a manageable amount of wax on the spatula and twist it so that it stays on the end. Remove any excess on the side of the pot. In the other hand have a folded tissue covering the palm to catch any drips from the spatula and any spillage during the transfer from pot to client.

3 Transfer the wax onto the skin following the hair growth, holding the spatula at a 90-degree angle, and spread a strip-sized width of wax on to the hairs. (As skill levels increase and practice is gained, you will be able to apply and quickly remove longer strips.) Support the skin with the free hand.

4 Firmly press the fabric or paper strip and rub down several times to bond the wax to the hairs in the direction of the hair growth. Leave a small flap free at the end of the strip with which to grip the strip for removal.

5 Using the flap, grip firmly, stretch the skin slightly with the free hand and pull the strip away from the skin, going back against the hair growth, with the strip almost going back on itself, in one swift movement. Try not to lift upward as that may cause skin damage. The swiftness of the hand really does make a difference to the pain the client will feel. Do not hesitate, or stop halfway through, as that is just prolonging the agony.

6 Apply a little pressure to the area with your hand to help reduce the tingling and pain, which occurs after strip removal.

7 Work in a logical sequence over the whole area to be treated taking care not to miss any hairs, but avoid overlapping the strips as that will mean the skin may be sore in that area.

8 The strip will last for several removals before it becomes too laden with wax to pick up any more hairs. When that stage is reached, fold the wax strip in on itself so that the clean side is on the outside and place it in the bin with a liner that is designated for contaminated waste. Use a fresh strip for the next removal and continue.

9 After the waxing is complete, if any stubborn, stray hairs remain, they should be tweezed out with a sterile pair of tweezers. With warm wax it may be possible to reapply a strip over an area with lots of hairs remaining, as there is little skin reaction at low temperatures. This is not advisable with the higher temperature of hot wax.

10 Apply after-wax lotion liberally and go over aftercare with the client.

11 Clearing up can now take place. This is as important as the rest of the treatment as cross-infection can occur through the contaminated waste. Dispose of used spatulas, wax strips, gloves and couch roll in the appropriate bags (unless the strips are to be used again).

12 Clean the equipment with the recommended manufacturer's cleaner and clean the plastic couch covering. Wash hands and begin with the next client.

Step-by-step warm wax application for eyebrows

1 Cover the closed eye with a damp cotton wool round and cleanse the eyebrow area with suitable cleanser. Cut up some small pieces of paper or material strips.

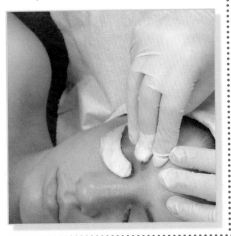

2 Decant petroleum jelly onto a spatula, using a covered orange stick; apply to hairs you do not want to remove. This barrier stops the wax sticking to the hairs.

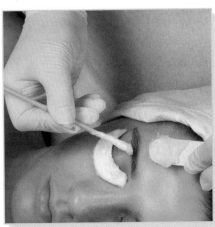

3 Remember to test the wax on your forearm, before applying to the client. You do not want to burn the delicate eye area.

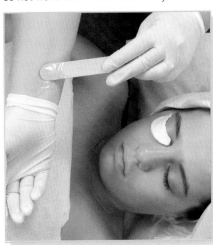

4 Apply a small amount of wax to the area under the eyebrow, working in the direction of the hair growth. Take care not to dribble wax on to the client's face.

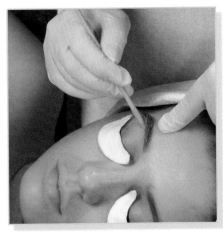

5 Using a small piece of wax strip, press on to the arch, under the eyebrow. Smooth over with your finger, to ensure all of the hairs are stuck to the strip.

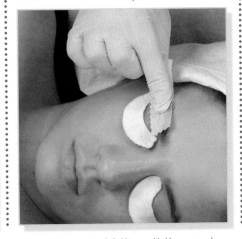

6 Stretch the eyebrow. Remove hairs against the hair growth, that is working inwards towards nose. The movement needs to be quick to avoid pain, and it is like peeling back on the strip. Apply after-wax lotion.

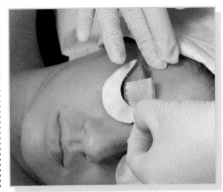

1 Cleanse the eyebrow area, having removed make-up, and follow all the usual sanitising procedures.

2 Cut a large wax strip into smaller manageable strips.

3 Discuss the shape required with the client taking into account face shape and the direction of hair growth.

4 Apply a suitable barrier cream to the eyebrows not being removed — this will prevent the wax adhering to them and avoid accidental total eyebrow removal.

5 Apply a small amount of wax to the hairs being removed, following the direction of hair growth (an orange stick may be a more suitably sized applicator than a spatula).

6 Press the small strip firmly to the skin.

7 Remove the strip against the hair growth and continue to shape the eyebrow as required.

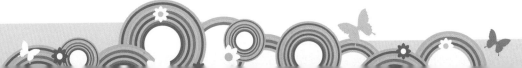

Unit B6 Carry out waxing services

8 Use a hand mirror to consult the client at every stage, and be flexible to client suggestions.

9 Follow aftercare and home care routines.

Step-by-step warm wax application for the lip and chin

1 Cleanse the upper lip area. The skin should be clean and grease-free. Blot if necessary.

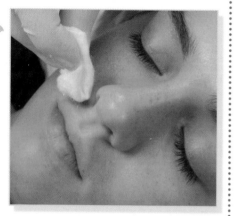

2 Decant petroleum jelly onto a spatula, using a covered orange stick, and cover the lip up to the lip line.

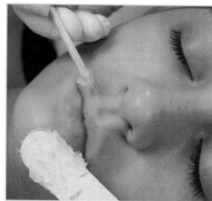

3 Remember to test the wax on your forearm, before applying to the client.

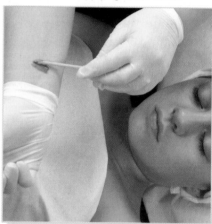

4 Carry out a sensitivity test. Use a small drop of wax near the area, to test the temperature is acceptable to the client.

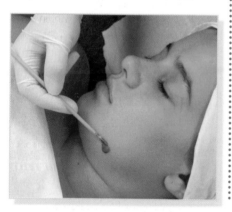

5 Build up a good layer of wax on upper lip. Ask the client to smile slightly to help stretch the skin. Remove as for all hot wax application and apply after-wax lotion.

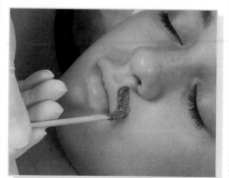

6 The finished result.

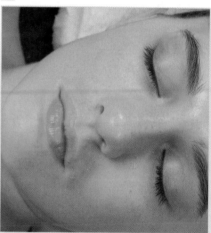

Think about it

Do not to press too hard on the jaw area, especially if the client is wearing dentures.

Lip wax

○ Cleanse the area and follow the usual sanitising procedures.

○ Protect the upper lip with barrier cream.

○ Apply wax to one side of the upper lip using a small spatula or orange stick and following the hair growth.

○ Apply and remove a small strip back on itself, pulling the skin as taut as possible but being careful of the nose.

○ Repeat on the other side.

○ Being careful not to re-wax the sides, apply wax to the centre panel working down to the centre of the lip.

○ Apply aftercare and discuss home care routines.

Chin wax

- Remove make-up and cleanse the area, following normal sanitising procedures.
- If the hairs are very long, trim with scissors, but not too short for waxing.
- Protect the lower lip with a barrier cream if going near the lip area.
- Apply the wax following the hair growth.
- Stretch the area and remove the hair with a small strip against the hair growth, keeping the skin as taut as possible. The client can help by jutting out the lower jaw and placing the tongue over the lower teeth.
- Repeat until all hairs are removed.

Step-by-step warm wax application for the bikini and thigh area

1 Clients should be in a reclined position with either a pillow for support or resting the leg on the couch.

2 Pay special attention to both client modesty (provide a towel) and protecting the client's undergarments with tissues or couch roll.

3 If the hair growth is long, trim with scissors, but not too short.

4 Hold the skin tight when applying the wax. If the area is fleshy, the client may help by stretching the leg as wide as possible.

5 Pay attention to hair growth patterns. Several directional strips may need to be applied rather than one big one.

> **Think about it**
>
> Make the client aware that as the hair in this area is strong terminal hair, there may be blood spotting, and that it is not unusual for this reaction to occur. Cold compresses can be applied and careful aftercare and home care must be adhered to.

1 Protect the edge of the client's underwear with couch roll. You can avoid embarrassment by asking the client to tuck the couch roll in.

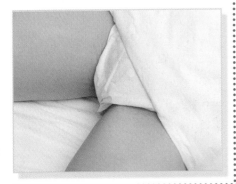

2 Clean the area with suitable cleanser, leaving the skin clean, dry and grease-free.

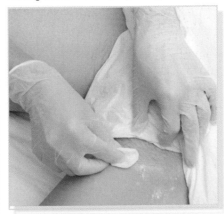

3 After testing temperature on yourself, apply the wax with the hair growth, in a firm pressing motion. Usually this is a downward direction towards the inner thigh.

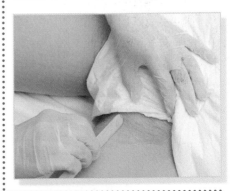

4 Apply the wax strip and press onto the hairs. Ask the client to help stretch the skin, to minimise pain, and remove the wax strip against the direction of hair growth.

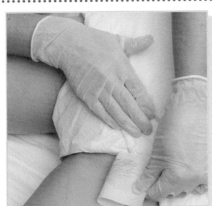

5 Should any blood spots appear, apply light pressure with a clean tissue and then wipe them away. Apply after wax-lotion.

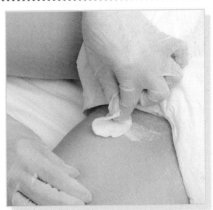

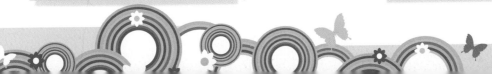

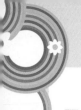

Forearm

1 Apply wax following the hair growth pattern

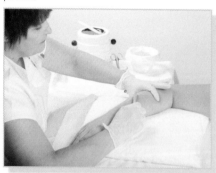

2 Press wax strip firmly onto arm, stretching skin

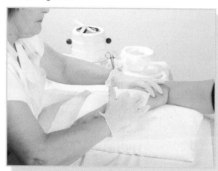

3 Remove against the hair growth, stretching the skin

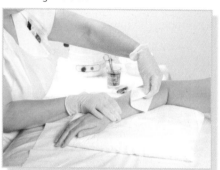

1 The client can be semi-reclined, or if this is the only area of the body to be waxed, the client could sit opposite the therapist across the couch.

2 If the client's sleeves are rolled up, remember to protect the clothing.

3 Follow the usual pre-wax preparation and cleansing routine.

4 Wax is applied in the same way as on other parts of the body; that is, following hair growth.

5 The skin can be kept taut by grasping the underside of the skin not being worked upon

6 Follow aftercare and home care routines.

Step-by-step warm wax application for underarms

1 Protect the client's clothing with couch roll and cleanse the area. A light dusting of talcum powder or talc-free product will absorb any residue perspiration and make the hair stand out from the skin.

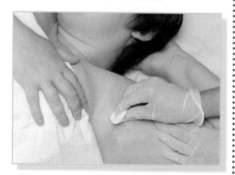

2 After testing on yourself, apply the wax, going with the hair growth. If hairs are diagonal, then go in that direction.

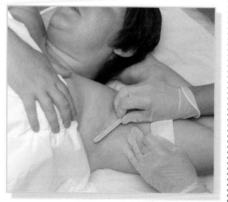

3 Firmly press the strip down to bond the hairs to it.

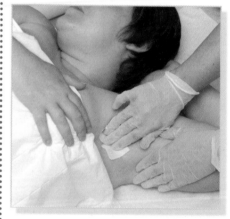

4 Stretch the armpit area and, if necessary, ask the client to help, with her free hand. Grip the edge of the strip and quickly and firmly remove the strip against the direction of hair growth.

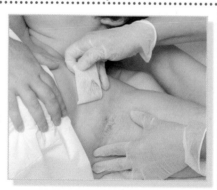

5 Should any blood spots appear, apply light pressure with a clean tissue and then wipe them away. Apply after-wax lotion.

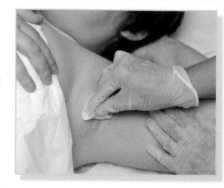

1 The client's armpit should be stretched and extended as far as possible.

2 The client should be in a semi-reclining position or flat down on the couch, depending upon client preference.

3 Follow the standard procedures for cleansing and hygiene.

4 Study the hair growth carefully as underarm hair can be very diverse in its growth, and some underarm hair can grow in circles.

5 Small strips should be used, and the hair may need trimming before treatment.

6 Remember to protect the bra with couch roll or tissues.

7 The skin can be extremely delicate and there is a danger that infection may occur, causing glands to swell.

8 Never treat the underarm if mastitis is suspected.

9 Aftercare and home care are extremely important for underarm treatment.

Area	Time
Eyebrows	10 minutes
Facial (lip and chin)	15 minutes
Full leg	45 minutes
Half leg (up to knee)	20–30 minutes
Underarm	15 minutes
Bikini	5 minutes
Forearm (wrist to elbow)	20 minutes

Treatment time guide for warm wax

The above is a guide only – the time it takes to complete a wax treatment will depend upon the amount of hair growth, how strong the growth is, and how experienced the therapist is. In time and with experience, timings can greatly improve as the confidence and judgement of the therapist improves.

However, it is important to remember to be cost-effective when waxing with both time and use of materials.

Hot wax application

Hot wax application is a skill that needs more practice than warm waxing, but many beauty therapists trained in hot wax prefer to use it. As the temperature is higher, the removal of strong, coarse hairs is very effective and it gives a nice clean finish.

Unlike warm wax, hot wax is applied as a thicker layer, which is built up by firstly going with the hair growth and then against the hair growth, until sufficient thickness for removal has been achieved. The procedure is as follows.

1 Test the wax on yourself on the inner wrist. Then, if the temperature is comfortable, test a small patch on the client on the area to be worked upon. If the client confirms that she is happy with the feel of it, commence the treatment.

2 Look closely at the hair growth in the area, as this affects both application and removal.

> ### Additional knowledge
>
> The abdomen is also suitable for warm wax hair removal, although it is not a range in this qualification. The same application techniques would apply.

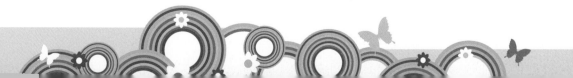

Step-by-step hot wax application for legs

1 Cleanse the area with a suitable cleanser, to make sure that the skin is dry and grease-free. Apply a light dusting of talcum powder or talc-free powder – this will make the hairs stand up.

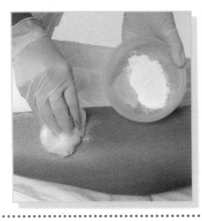

2 Test the hot wax on your forearm before applying any to the client.

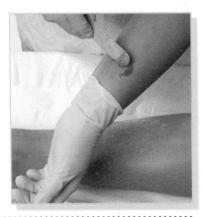

3 Decant a good amount of hot wax from the pot on to another spatula, to avoid contamination. The consistency of wax should be like soft treacle.

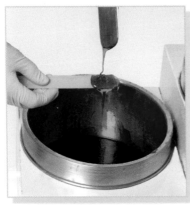

4 Test a small patch of wax on the client, to avoid burning the skin.

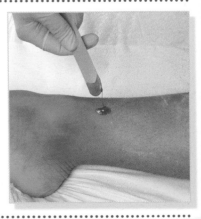

5 Working against the hair growth to begin with, apply the wax in a figure of eight shape. As you keep applying, you will build up a thick patch of wax.

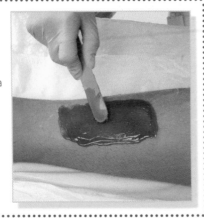

6 When the wax layer looks set, pressure from the knuckles will help bond the hot wax to the hairs. The wax takes on a matt finish as it cools.

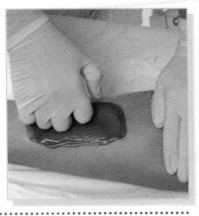

7 Using the same techniques as with a wax strip, flick a lip up, and gripping firmly, quickly remove the patch of wax – against the direction of hair growth.

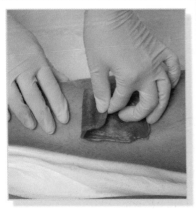

8 The hairs should be clearly visible, embedded in the wax strip you have removed.

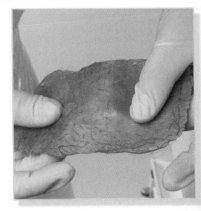

3 Gather a manageable amount of wax on to the spatula, and keep the spatula twisting to avoid drips, wiping any excess on to the edge of the heater. A tissue in the free hand, held underneath the spatula, will catch any drips on the way from heater to couch.

4 The wax should be the consistency of icing ready to go on a cake: spreadable but not too thick. Apply the wax, and build up several layers, working firstly against and then with the hair growth. Ensure that the edges are quite thick too, as when the wax is removed, the edges may break off if too thinly applied.

5 Try not to make the strips too large as this makes them difficult to remove. Two or three applications should give a covering about 3 mm thick. Avoid the temptation to apply too many layers, as the wax will just build up on itself and not adhere to the hairs.

6 The trick is to be quick, and apply several patches in one go. As the first patch is setting slightly, the second and third can be applied. Do not let any of them dry out totally on the skin, as they will become brittle and break off, and will hurt the client when removed.

7 A thick lip on the edges of each patch will allow a firm grip when removing.

8 As each strip starts to set slightly, press with the fingers. It should feel dry but still supple to the touch, and the lip can be flipped up.

9 Grip the lip you have created and with the other hand pull the skin slightly away from the wax patch to minimise client discomfort. Be quick and firm, and swiftly remove the wax against the direction of hair growth.

10 Immediately soothe the area by applying pressure to it. Quickly move on to the next patch as that will be setting.

11 Fold each wax strip in on itself, with the hairs inside, and put them into the lined bin for disposal into the collectable waste bin.

12 Should there be any small remains of wax, press the larger patch over the area and the remains should be picked up easily.

13 Work methodically all over the area to be waxed in a pattern, so that all hairs are removed, but avoid overlapping and therefore over-waxing.

14 Any hairs that have escaped may be tweezed away, and the result should be clean and clear. The skin will be slightly pinker than with warm waxing because of the higher temperature.

15 Aftercare and home care advice can be given. A soothing after-wax lotion can be applied, and a nice gesture is to provide the client with a sample-size aftercare lotion to take away and apply at home.

16 Clearing up can now take place. This is as important as the rest of the treatment, as cross-infection can occur through the contaminated waste. Dispose of used spatulas, wax, gloves and couch roll in the appropriate bags.

17 Clean the equipment with the manufacturer's recommended cleaner and clean the plastic couch covering. Wash hands and begin with the next client.

Area	Time
Eyebrows	10–15 minutes
Facial (lip and chin)	10–15 minutes
Full leg	45–60 minutes
Half leg (up to knee)	20–30 minutes
Underarm	15 minutes
Bikini	15–20 minutes
Forearm (wrist to elbow)	20 minutes

Treatment time guide for hot wax

Think about it

This treatment guide is dependent upon the skill of the therapist. Hot wax needs to be nurtured up to the correct working temperature and consistency, and then used. Temperature control is vital when using this method and this can affect the treatment timings. The application of hot wax requires more training and a higher skill level.

Unit B6 Carry out waxing services

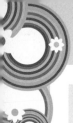

Preparation – you, your working area and the client.

Two waste bins with liners.

Choose wax most suitable for client and area. Heat it up half an hour before appointment.

On the trolley:
- antiseptic cleaner
  - talc
- fabric / paper strips
- disposable gloves
- wooden spatulas
- tissues and cotton wool
  - jewellery bowl
- scissors and tweezers
  - after-wax lotion
  - record card.

Consultation, with record card. Fully explain treatment.

Wash hands.

Test on self and patch test on client.

Area to be clean and grease-free. Commence treatment.

After wax – wash hands.

Aftercare and home care.

Dispose of used spatulas, etc. Clean working area.

Wash hands.

Start again with next client.

Waxing

Ensuring the client is satisfied with the finished result

The client will appreciate it if you discuss the finished result with her. You can make sure the client is satisfied, and that the agreed treatment plan has been met.

Carefully check the area over. If necessary, tweeze the odd hair away using sterilised tweezers.

Check the results before applying the aftercare lotion, as this makes the skin quite slippery so the odd hair is more difficult to pick up with the tweezers.

A mini-massage while applying the aftercare lotion is always very soothing to the nerve endings, and finishes the treatment with a pleasant feeling for the client. You do not have the time for a full massage routine, however.

Once you've completed the treatment, take time to fill out the client record card.

- ○ Were there any reactions during the treatment that will affect the future treatment plan? Remember, it may not be you doing the next treatment.
- ○ Did the client express any preferences or dislikes for waxing mediums?
- ○ Would you leave something out next time?
- ○ Did the client feel much pain? An over-the-counter painkiller could be taken prior to the next treatment.
- ○ Were products purchased?
- ○ How was the skin reaction? Were there contra-actions?

Provide aftercare advice

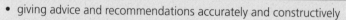

In this outcome you will learn about:

- giving advice and recommendations accurately and constructively
- giving the clients suitable advice specific to their individual needs.

Giving aftercare and home care advice

It is important that you discuss aftercare and home care with your client during the consultation, so that her skin reactions and contra-actions can be explained and understood.

A leaflet to take away is ideal for your client to refer to, as she may not take in all the information, especially if she finds the treatment painful.

Immediate aftercare

Your client should realise that the waxed area will be red and there may be some blood spots, especially where the hairs are strong, i.e. on the bikini line or underarm. The after-wax cleanser should be applied to remove any sticky remains on the skin followed by after-wax soothing lotion to help cool the skin and keep it moisturised.

Home care

Your salon may like to devise a home care card like the one below:

Aftercare – for a period of 24 hours:

- No sunbathing or sunbeds
- Avoid bathing in sea or swimming pool
- Do not take a *hot* bath or shower
- Do not use deodorant / anti-perspirant
- Avoid tight clothing
- Do not use perfumed products on the area
- No make-up or self-tanning preparations
- Do not keep touching or picking at the area

Waxing home care card

Long-term home care advice

○ Encourage your client to look after the skin on her body as she would the skin on her face.

○ Lots of moisturiser will stop the skin becoming too dry, especially in the winter months when legs are kept under trousers and tights.

○ Sloughing the skin with a loofah in the shower will help keep the blood circulation stimulated, bringing lots of oxygen and nutrients to the skin to keep it in good condition.

○ Massage will help remove the build-up of toxins in the skin and keep the area both nourished and smooth. Instruct your client to always work towards the lymph nodes to help the body's natural lymphatic drainage.

○ Exfoliating the skin will help to stop the hairs becoming ingrown.

○ Gentle exercise, regular sleeping patterns and eating plenty of fruit and vegetables, while cutting down on smoking and alcohol, and drinking lots of water really do work, and not just for the face.

Before leaving the salon, the client should be encouraged to make a repeat appointment, usually in 4–6 weeks. However, this will depend upon the colour and density of the hair and the area. It is important to stress to the client that for effective waxing the hairs should be at the correct length.

My story

Never ignore aftercare advice!

Hi, my name is Nicola. I won't forget my first leg wax! It was a lovely, sunny day and I was looking forward to going on holiday. I was telling the therapist all about it. She advised me not to sunbathe or to apply any products to the area for 24 hours after the treatment. When I got home, I wanted to show off my beautiful hair-free legs! So, forgetting the therapist's advice, I put on sunscreen and went and sat in the garden for a couple of hours. I really wish I hadn't – by early evening my legs were so painful. I learned my lesson the hard way and now always listen to the aftercare advice I'm given.

Think about it

For 24 hours after waxing, advise the client to avoid:

- tight clothing
- hot baths/showers, or swimming
- sunbeds, sunbathing or other heat-related treatments
- applying perfumed products, including deodorant, and make-up to the area.

Think about it

When giving treatment advice and recommendations for other treatments, be accurate and constructive. Consider what you and the client can realistically achieve.

For your portfolio

Devise an aftercare or information leaflet that you can give to a client following a waxing treatment. Consider both the short- and long-term aftercare that will be appropriate. Produce the leaflet on a computer.

Carry out waxing services **Unit B6**

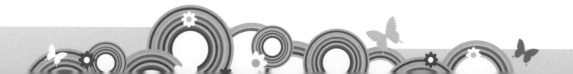

Frequently asked questions

Q	What would happen if grease is left on the skin?
A	The skin has a barrier of grease or oil on it which will prevent the wax getting a grip on the hairs. Always clean the skin thoroughly to prevent this barrier building up.
Q	Can waxing take place on any length of hairs?
A	If the hairs are too short, they will not stick to the wax.
Q	What would happen if the wax is not hot enough?
A	The removal of the hairs will not be effective and the wax could matt, making removal difficult.
Q	What would happen if the wax is applied too thickly?
A	The wax will not be able to get a grip on the hairs, and will congeal on itself.
Q	What would happen if the wax is applied or removed in the wrong direction?
A	The hairs will not be removed and this can cause pain and discomfort to the client.
Q	What would happen if the skin is not pulled taut when waxing?
A	The skin will be too slack, and the wax will set into the body's natural creases – very common when first attempting underarm waxing. Pull the skin so it is taut and ask the client to help. This makes it easier to apply the wax, and it is also less painful. This method should be adopted when waxing all areas.
Q	What would occur if the wax was not removed quickly enough?
A	This will result in an ineffective removal of hair, and pain for the client. Try not to lift upwards when removing the strip; always try to bring the strip back on itself. Be bold and confident, and it will be less painful and give a better result.
Q	What would occur if hairs are not trimmed when too long?
A	Hairs should be trimmed to prevent tangling and ineffective removal (especially on the bikini area).
Q	What should you do if the skin is red after the first strip is removed?
A	This could indicate that the wax is too hot. You should test it on yourself and the client before application. The pressure that has been applied with the spatula may also have dragged on the skin, so ensure that the wax is of the correct consistency before application.

Check your knowledge

1 Waxing is a:
   a) permanent method of hair removal
   b) temporary method of hair removal
   c) long-lasting method of hair removal
   d) short-term method of hair removal.

2 Hot wax is most suitable for use on:
   a) strong hair growth
   b) weak hair growth
   c) bent follicles.

3 Hair removal creams are:
   a) suitable for all skin types
   b) not suitable for all skin types
   c) a painless method of hair removal
   d) a permanent method of removal.

4 Warm wax is:
   a) most suitable for all areas
   b) easy to apply
   c) not easy to apply
   d) a temporary method of removal.

5 Hot wax works best at a temperature of:
   a) 48–68°C
   b) 20–30°C
   c) 60–80°C
   d) 15–20°C.

6 Warm wax works best at a temperature of:
   a) 48–68°C
   b) 20–30°C
   c) 60–80°C
   d) 15–20°C.

7 The main ingredients used in hair removal wax are:
   a) resins and beeswax
   b) starch and flour
   c) sugar and water
   d) crystals and polish.

8 Pre-wax lotion must be used to:
   a) dry up the skin
   b) cleanse the area
   c) make the area smell nice
   d) make the hairs stand on end.

9 Talc or talc-free products are used to:
   a) make the skin smell nice
   b) provide a coating for the wax to stick to
   c) make the hairs stand away from the skin
   d) make the skin white.

10 After-wax lotion helps:
   a) soothe the skin
   b) stop the area going pink
   c) make the skin smell nice
   d) calm the client down.

11 A patch test must always be carried out, to:
   a) try out the heat of the wax on the client
   b) see if the client is suitable for treatment (i.e. no reaction occurs)
   c) let the client know it hurts
   d) give the client a bald patch on her arm.

12 Aftercare is important, because:
   a) it prevents the client from irritating the area after the treatment
   b) it stops you from being sued for poor treatment
   c) it's just part of the job
   d) it stops the client from picking at the area.

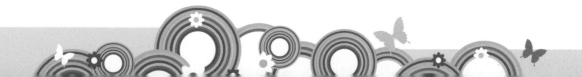

Getting ready for assessment

Once you have practised and feel fairly confident about all the skills in this unit, you can then think about how you can develop your techniques to meet employer expectations of a good therapist who can wax well. An employer or assessor would be looking for the following, especially if you were asked to perform a trade test for a job application.

- Minimise any wastage of product, strips or consumables you use during the treatment, including couch roll, tissues and cotton wool. Imagine you were paying for all of the items you used — you will soon realise that money is wasted if you throw away half-used products. When waxing, try not to end up with little bits of fabric or paper strips, or if you do, save them for small areas, such as when you do a lip wax or eyebrow wax. Split couch roll and tissues where possible and be economical with the amount of wax used.

- Minimise discomfort to the client by developing good techniques for the removal of wax — be firm, confident and quick. Remember to smooth the area afterwards — a soothing touch really does calm the nerve endings.

- Keep checking your client's well-being and be sympathetic. Even though some seasoned clients go to sleep when being waxed, it can be quite painful — it depends upon the pain threshold of the individual. Now is a good time to introduce other treatments, discuss possible enhancing treatments, and take the client's mind off the waxing process.

- Keep an eye out for any contra-actions which may arise, and follow the appropriate procedure. Give good immediate aftercare, and then home care advice. It may be that the treatment has to stop, and you invite the client to come in at a later date when the area has calmed down — or you might offer an alternative treatment if one is available.

- Work methodically in a logical sequence, so you do not miss any chunks of hair growth. In time, your own technique will develop and you will find yourself automatically working in a patchwork pattern, which works well for you. An employer does not often dictate how you achieve the end result, nor do many Awarding Bodies, but a good clean result is essential.

As this is a full practical unit, simulation is not allowed for any performance evidence within this unit.

The areas to be treated include the eyebrows, face to include lip and chin, full and half legs, underarm, bikini line in both hot and warm wax. You must be seen to treat at least four different clients on at least four occasions.

As well as performing the treatment and leaving a good clean result, the assessor will be checking that you have:

- used all consultation techniques

- carried out waxing treatments on all areas with hot and warm wax

- have dealt with at least one of the necessary actions in the range

- covered all the criteria for effective work techniques to ensure the client has a pain-free treatment

- provided suitable aftercare and home care advice.

Remember that waxing is a skill that requires a lot of practice to improve both your technique and cleanliness. Before attempting an assessment, make sure you have had sufficient practice to feel confident and self-assured in your knowledge of what to tell the client.

Although the areas of the body are specified, you may be able to cluster your assessments. One client may have several areas waxed in one treatment, and they all count.

Be careful that the length of hair is right. If the hairs are too short, the wax does not have enough of the hair shaft to adhere to, so the results will be patchy. If the hairs are too long, it will be advantageous to trim them down with scissors before starting. Otherwise the hair will become tangled and again the results will not be clean.

Be very careful to check the direction of hair growth, as that will dictate the direction for your wax strips. Show that you understand the relevance of hair growth even if it means using smaller strips, say for a circular direction of underarm hair growth.

Be clean and hygienic, and check with your professional body about when to use gloves. The best clean results on the skin will be spoilt by an unhygienic treatment approach and a messy workstation with wax on the floor.

Do not forget to test the wax on yourself and to carry out a small patch test on the client before you begin — burning the client's skin will not gain a competent assessment.

The assessor is looking at the whole approach, including client care, hygiene and a good result.

Unit N2/N3

Provide manicure and pedicure services

Key terms

Manicure – the care of hands and fingernails.

Pedicure – the professional treatment of feet, toes and nails.

Think about it

Remember health and illness can often be detected in the nails. Healthy nails require a balanced diet with essential vitamins A , B, and D, along with minerals calcium, zinc and iodine.

For your portfolio

Read the Code of Practice for Nail Services on the Habia website. If you are able to do so, you can print off a copy to keep as reference; if not make a note of the important points.

Introduction

The practices of improving the appearance of the natural nail and cuticle are known as **manicure** and **pedicure**.

This unit focuses on the treatment of natural nails and cuticles on hands and feet. Units N2 and N3 have been combined in the book as many techniques are common to both skill areas.

Manicure is a popular service in salons as smooth skin, well-shaped and varnished nails are vital in promoting a well-groomed appearance. As a therapist carrying out treatments in manicure and pedicure you need to be aware that there is a code of practice that should be followed when providing this service. The Code of Practice for Nail Services provides guidelines to protect both the therapist and the client, and it is important that you know what it says.

Regular professional attention will help prevent minor nail damage. This service is becoming increasingly popular with men who have regular treatments as part of their professional lives.

Pedicure is the professional treatment of feet, toes and nails. This service greatly enhances the appearance of feet and toenails, which are often a neglected part of the body. Professional attention to the nails and surrounding skin encourages nail growth, keeps cuticles pushed back and can prevent minor skin conditions.

Benefits for the client:

- improves the appearance of the nails
- softens the surrounding skin
- enhances overall appearance of grooming (important for men as well as women)
- immediate and visual effect.

Benefits for the therapist:

- mainstay salon service
- variety of treatments can be performed to enhance basic treatments and increase salon revenue
- can be used as part of a salon promotion, e.g. leg wax and pedicure for the summer.

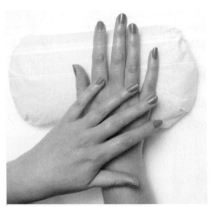 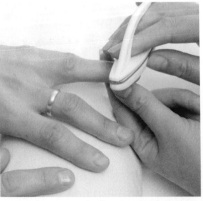 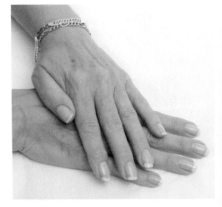

You will be required to create different looks to cover the ranges in the standards

As well as being able to successfully carry out a manicure or pedicure treatment, you will need to have an understanding of the structure of the nail and relate treatments to the bones, muscles and skin of the hands and feet. Refer to Related anatomy and physiology section and You and the skin for information on these areas.

Maintain safe and effective methods of working

In this outcome you will learn about:

- preparing the work area and environment to meet legal, hygiene and industry Code of Practice for Nail Services requirements
- ensuring your personal appearance meets accepted industry Code of Practice for Nail Services and organisational requirements
- wearing suitable personal protective equipment for the work that conforms to the industry Code of Practice for Nail Services
- ensuring all tools and equipment are cleaned using the correct methods
- effectively disinfecting your hands prior to nail services
- maintaining accepted industry hygiene and safety practices throughout the service
- selecting and correctly positioning suitable equipment, materials and products for the nail service

- ensuring your own posture and position minimises fatigue and the risk of injury while working
- ensuring the client is in a comfortable and relaxed position that permits access and minimises the risk of injury to you and the client
- disposing of waste correctly to meet local authority requirements and the industry Code of Practice for Nail Services
- ensuring that the service is cost-effective and is carried out within a commercially viable time
- leaving the work area and equipment in a condition suitable for further nail services
- ensuring the client's records are up to date, accurate, easy to read and signed by the client and technician.

Before beginning this section, many of the topics you need to know are addressed in earlier units, and you will need to refresh your memory by referring to the topics covered within Professional basics. Please refer to:

The unit	For topics on:
Professional basics – You and your client (pages 31–48)	Hygiene and avoiding cross-infection Salon requirements and presentation
Professional basics – You – the therapist (pages 11–31)	Personal appearance Personal safety
Professional basics – You, your client and the law (pages 48–68) Unit G20 Make sure your own actions reduce risks to health and safety (pages 71–103)	Risk assessment Preparing the working environment to meet legal, hygiene and treatment requirements
Professional basics – You – the therapist (pages 11–31) You and your client (pages 31–48) You – the therapist (pages 11–31) You, your client and the law (pages 48–68) and Unit G20 Make sure your own actions reduce risks to health and safety (pages 71–103)	Making effective use of your working time Ensuring the use of clean resources Ensuring your own posture and position minimises fatigue and risk of injury while working Disposing of waste materials safely and correctly

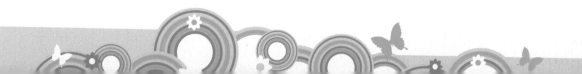

Preparing the work area and environment

Preparation is the key to being a professional beauty therapist regardless of the treatment being carried out.

Many salons have a designated working area for manicure and pedicure treatments. Sometimes this is in the reception area. Wherever you carry out a treatment you should ensure all materials, equipment and products are within easy reach.

The area required for manicure and pedicure varies greatly, with more versatility in manicure than pedicure.

Manicure	Pedicure
Client across a couch	Sitting only – can be combined with a manicure
Sitting across a table	
At a manicure station	
In a hair salon while having hair done	
Client lying on a beauty couch while having a facial	

Selecting equipment and materials for manicure and pedicure treatments

To ensure that no cross-infection or contamination occurs, the manicurist must make sure everything is clean.

Emery board

This has two sides: a coarse side for shortening nails and a fine side, which is used for shaping and bevelling. Emery boards are difficult to clean although some manufacturers have developed special cleansers for this purpose. If you cannot clean the file, it should be disposed of, or given to the client.

Orange stick

The two ends of the orange stick each have a different purpose. The pointed side is used to apply cuticle or buffing cream. The other side, when tipped with cotton wool, can be used to clean under the free edge, remove excess enamel and ease back the cuticle. When tipped with cotton wool this should be disposed of after each use. If not tipped, they are only for one use.

Think about it

Your salon will have correct work wear to conform to industry standards and this should always be worn when undertaking treatments.

Think about it

Some pieces of equipment are designed only for single use. The extra cost of these items should be reflected in the prices for manicure and pedicure treatments. Which items could be considered single use?

For your portfolio

Cost the price of single-use items. Find out the cost of buying in bulk and then work out the individual item price.

Do you think that the cost has been taken into account within your salon price list?

Think about it

When disposing of single-use items remember to put them in the appropriate waste bin.

Cuticle knife

This is used to mould back the cuticle and remove any excess attached to the nail plate.

Cuticle nipper

Used to remove hangnails and dead skin around the cuticle.

Nail scissors

Used to cut nails.

Toe nail clippers

Used to cut and shorten nails prior to filing.

Nail buffer

A pad covered with chamois leather and with a handle. Used in conjunction with buffing paste. Buffing adds sheen, stimulates circulation and growth at the matrix. Useful in pedicure, male manicure or when nail varnish is not going to be applied. To clean, wipe with a suitable cleansing solution.

3-way buffer

This is used to smooth the nail and to remove any longitudinal and horizontal lines. Wipe between uses with a suitable cleansing solution.

Nail brush

To brush the nails and clean them effectively. Also used to clean the therapist's nails. Wash in hot soapy water or sterilise in a chemical solution. Usually plastic, may be wooden, with a rubber end to ease back the cuticle. Pointed, and may be tipped with cotton wool to clean under free edge. When using from nail to nail, clean with a steriliser. On completion of treatment, sterilise in a cold sterilising solution.

Hoof stick

Usually plastic, may be wooden, with a rubber end to ease back the cuticle. Pointed, and may be tipped with cotton wool to clean under free edge. When using from nail to nail, clean with a steriliser. On completion of treatment, sterilise in a cold sterilising solution.

Hard skin rasp/file/grater

To be used after the feet have been soaked and can be used in conjunction with hard skin remover. Use on areas of hard skin in a rubbing action with light pressure. Wash after use in hot soapy water and remove debris; sterilise in chemical solution.

Pumice stone

As with hard skin rasp.

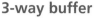

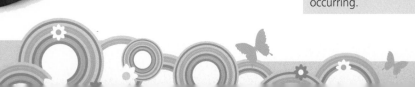

> **Think about it**
>
> Remember to sterilise all metal equipment: it should be placed in a chemical steriliser or autoclave. While performing the treatment, cleanse with a suitable sanitising solution. (Refer to Professional basics, pages 41–43, for information on sterilisation and sanitisation.)

> **Think about it**
>
> Some chemical solutions may dissolve the glue that attaches the rasp element or bristles in this equipment.
>
> All metal equipment should be regularly checked, e.g. hinges and springs on scissors and clippers. Also check that cutting surfaces are smooth and sharp. Once sterilised all equipment should be stored hygienically to prevent contamination occurring.

Unit N2/N3 Provide manicure and pedicure services

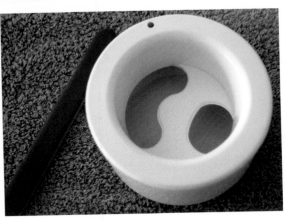

Manicure bowl

This contains warm soapy water and sometimes a few drops of oil or a soaking solution. This softens the cuticle ready for pushing back. To clean, wash in hot soapy water and dry thoroughly.

Towels

Use a clean towel for each client. It is useful to protect it with couch roll. Remember to have a separate towel for your personal use.

Couch roll

This is tissue that can be used to cover trolleys, and for drying hands and feet in the absence of towels. Dispose of after use.

Tissues/cotton wool

Use a different tissue or piece of cotton wool for each hand/foot.

Spatulas

Break wooden spatulas after use. Wipe clean plastic or metal spatulas with a suitable cleansing solution when using between different products. Sterilise in chemical solution after use.

Ensure that all products and equipment that cannot be sterilised are disposed of in the correct waste bin.

Selecting products for manicure and pedicure treatments

The following products are required for manicure and pedicure treatments:

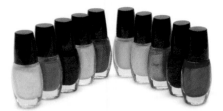

- cuticle cream
- buffing paste
- hard skin remover
- massage medium
- talcum powder
- nail varnish/enamel
- base and top coats
- nail hardeners
- nail strengtheners.

For all these products use the **cut-out system**, or pump action dispensers as these will prevent contamination of the product between uses. When using pump dispensers, do not allow the spout to come into contact with the client's hands or feet. Chemicals contained within varnishes will prevent infection spreading, but to avoid any infection use the client's own product or sell the product to the client.

Nail enamel/varnish remover

A solvent used to dissolve nail enamel. It is usually a mixture of acetone, glycerol and perfume. Acetone can have a drying effect on nails and surrounding skin. Some products also contain ethyl acetate (see below).

Nail enamel/varnish thinners

A solvent, usually ethyl acetate, used to thin down thick nail varnish/enamel. Nail enamel/varnish remover should not be used for this purpose due to the oil content contained in the remover. This may cause the varnish to discolour or separate.

Cuticle cream/oil

An emollient (softening, soothing) agent applied to the cuticle to make it pliable. Creams contain soft white paraffin, mineral oils and some also contain lanolin. Oils are a mixture of almond and jojoba and mineral oils.

Cuticle remover

A liquid or cream designed to dissolve and break down the cuticle to make removal easier. This contains potassium hydroxide (which is **caustic**), water and glycerol. As it is caustic, cuticle remover should be rinsed off the nails and skin directly after use. This product can be used as a nail bleach.

Nail hardeners

Used to strengthen fragile nails. It is a liquid which is painted on and allowed to soak into the nail plate. It acts as a binder to harden the nail.

Nail strengtheners

A mixture of powder acrylic and liquid plastic is painted on. Once set will reinforce the nail but still be flexible. This product is often combined in a base coat.

Rough skin remover/exfoliators

A cream or lotion containing abrasive particles, oils, emollients, perfume and water. Used to soften skin and aid removal of hard skin.

Buffing paste

An abrasive paste used in conjunction with a chamois buffer to smooth out ridges on the nail plate. The abrasive elements in the paste may be a mixture of kaolin, chalk, silica or talc.

Hand cream/massage cream

A cream that provides lubrication for massage and softens skin. It contains emollient, glycerol, lanolin, water, emulsifiers, colour and perfume.

Hand lotion

Contains the same elements as hand cream but has higher water content. It is therefore less sticky than cream.

Nail enamels and varnishes, base coat and topcoat

These products all have the same basic contents:

- ⚪ a film firming plastic, e.g. nitrocelluose
- ⚪ a plastic resin, e.g. aryl sufonamicide
- ⚪ a gloss, e.g. formaldehyde
- ⚪ a plasticiser, e.g. castor oil for flexibility
- ⚪ solvents to dissolve other substances causing the nail enamel to dry, e.g. ethyl acetate.

Coloured enamel/varnish

Colour is given by the addition of pigments, and a pearlised effect is made by adding, for example, bismuth oxychloride (for a metallic shine).

> **Key terms**
>
> **Caustic** – dissolves the skin; e.g. cuticle remover.

> **Think about it**
>
> Many of the products used in manicure and pedicure treatments are covered by COSHH regulations (refer to Professional basics, page 54). Always refer to the manufacturer's instructions prior to use.

Unit N2/N3 Provide manicure and pedicure services

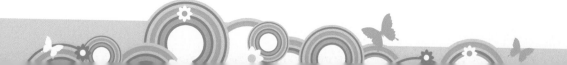

Base coat

Applied before colour, to prevent staining of the nail plate and to give a smooth surface for the coloured varnish to stick to.

Topcoat

Applied after colour, to give extra durability against knocks and wear for cream colours. Pearlised varnishes/enamels already have these additives to give this durability.

Nail bleach

Stains, such as dyes and nicotine, will discolour the free edge of the nail. Cuticle remover can lessen the staining as it may act as a mild bleach, but 20 per cent hydrogen peroxide will be most effective. This method is useful if the client wishes to have a natural finish or French varnish finish.

Nail white pencils

Used on the underside of the free edge when coloured varnish is not used. Use moistened.

Nail repair kit

Used for splits or tears in nails – comprised of fibrous tissue and liquid adhesive.

Quick dry spray

Contains solvents that evaporate and speed up the drying process.

Minimising the risk of injury

When setting up the work area make sure that your position and posture minimise the risk of harm to yourself, and prevent fatigue. Your trolley should have all the correct tools, materials and products on it, and be within easy reach to prevent strain.

The client should also be positioned so that she is comfortable and relaxed.

As a therapist, it is essential that you protect yourself from developing contact dermatitis, an inflammation of the skin caused by constant contact with harsh substances such as nail varnish remover. (Refer to You and the skin, page 202, for more information on dermatitis.) You should regularly check your hands, wash and dry them thoroughly, and apply moisturiser and barrier cream. Disposable gloves can be worn when dealing with harsh substances to prevent contact.

COSHH regulations for manicure and pedicure preparations

The Control of Substances Hazardous to Health (COSHH) Regulations control the safe use, disposal and storage of products (see Professional basics, page 54).

Many of the preparations used in manicure and pedicure treatments are governed by these rules. Therefore, as a manicurist, you have to know how to use these products correctly.

For your portfolio

Look at the Health and Safety Executive website for further information regarding dermatitis. If possible print off the information, or make notes for a group discussion.

Think about it

Contact dermatitis can stop a therapist from working, so hand care is very important as your livelihood could be at stake.

Think about it

If you don't effectively sanitise your hands and those of your client when checking for contra-indications, you could be open to infection. Remember your hands are your tools within beauty therapy – it is up to you to protect them.

Cuticle remover

Description

- A solution of sodium hydroxide in water with other cosmetic ingredients.
- Contains sodium hydroxide.

Ingredients

All ingredients are commonly used in cosmetic products and meet accepted standards of purity.

Hazards

Considered to be hazardous if precautions are ignored.

Flammability

Non-inflammable.

First aid procedures

- Ingestion: drink milk or water and seek medical attention.
- Inhalation: avoid. If prolonged inhalation occurs, remove to fresh air and keep warm.
- Skin contact: avoid. If prolonged contact occurs, wash well with water. If irritation persists, seek medical advice.
- Eye contact: wash well with water for a minimum of 15 minutes and always seek medical help immediately from a qualified doctor or hospital.

Spillage

Clean using liberal quantities of water.

Handling and storage

- Always wear gloves and avoid contact with skin and eyes.
- Store in a cool place away from direct sunlight. Keep closures tightly sealed.

Cuticle massage cream

Description

An emulsion of oils, waxes, water and water-soluble ingredients, emulsifiers, fragrance and preservatives.

Ingredients

All ingredients are commonly used in cosmetic preparations and meet acceptable standards of purity.

Hazards

Considered to be non-hazardous under normal conditions of use.

Flammability

Non-inflammable.

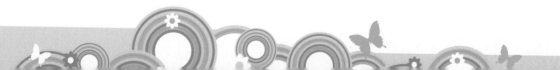

First aid procedures

- Ingestion: drink milk or water.
- Eye contact: wash well. If irritation persists, seek medical advice.

Spillage

Clean using absorbent material, wash with detergent and water.

Handling and storage

No special precautions are necessary.

Non-acetone nail polish remover

Description

A mixture of organic solvents.

Ingredients

All ingredients are commonly used in cosmetic products and meet accepted standards of purity.

Hazards

The product is considered hazardous if precautions are ignored.

Flammability

Inflammable.

First aid procedures

- Ingestion: drink milk or water and seek medical advice.
- Inhalation: avoid. If affected, remove to fresh air and keep warm.
- Skin contact: avoid. If prolonged contact occurs, wash well with water. If irritation persists, seek medical advice.
- Eye contact: wash well with water for a minimum of 15 minutes. If irritation persists, seek medical advice.

Spillage

Clean using liberal quantities of water.

Handling and storage

- Avoid contact with skin and eyes.
- Store in a cool place away from direct sunlight. Keep tightly sealed and store in a fire-resistant cupboard.
- Fire: advise fire service of storage quantities.

Acetone

Description

Dimethyl ketone or 2-propanone.

Ingredients

This product is commonly used in cosmetic products and meets accepted standards of purity.

Hazards

Considered to be hazardous unless normal safety procedures are followed.

Flammability

- Flammable.
- Flash point 17.2 = Highly flammable.

First aid procedures

- Ingestion: drink plenty of milk or water.
- Inhalation: may cause dizziness, remove to fresh air.
- Skin contact: avoid prolonged contact with the skin. If irritation persists, seek medical advice.
- Eye contact: rinse, seek medical advice.

Spillage

Clean contaminated area with lots of water, wash with detergent and water to avoid slippery floors. Do not absorb with combustible material, e.g. paper tissues.

Handling and storage

- Store in a cool place away from direct sunlight, in a fire-resistant store.
- Fire: contents are flammable. In case of fire evacuate areas known to contain products and inform fire-fighters of their presence.

Treatment timings

Your first manicure or pedicure treatments may take you some time, but once you have more experience, you should be able to perform treatments within a commercially acceptable time. It is important at the consultation stage, and when booking, to allocate enough time for the treatment. Always confirm the amount of time with clients — they may only have a lunch hour for treatment.

A salon will always want a service to be cost-effective. This will not only take into account the quantity of products and amount of heating and lighting a service uses but, more importantly, the time it takes, including the therapist's salary. If a service runs over time, this will impact on the rest of the day.

Here are some commercially acceptable times for these treatments

Treatment	Timings
Manicure without polish	25–30 minutes
Manicure with polish	35–40 minutes
File and re-polish	10 minutes
Pedicure without polish	40–45 minutes
Pedicure with polish	50–55 minutes
Pedicure soak, file and re-polish	15 minutes
Manicure and pedicure without polish	1 hour
Manicure and pedicure with polish	1 hour 15 minutes

Commercially acceptable timings. For a specialist treatment, 15 minutes will be added to the service

For a specialist treatment, another 15 minutes will be added to the service.

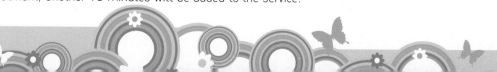

Think about it

If the client is having treatments using a specialist range of products, this should be taken into consideration and the correct time allowed, and agreed with the client. If nail extensions are to be removed, you will need to add an additional 30 minutes on to the service time for your treatments.

Think about it

Matching lipsticks could also be sold to colour coordinate with the nail varnish.

If the client requires treatment to improve both the condition and appearance of nails and the surrounding skin, the initial appearance at the consultation should identify that regular treatments are necessary, for example weekly over a six-week period, followed by a maintenance treatment every 4–6 weeks. This applies to both manicure and pedicure treatments.

How you decide on the appropriate timing and type of treatment must be mutually agreed with the client. The same treatment plan will not be suitable for all clients because of individual needs, such as:

- ○ work commitments
- ○ home life
- ○ leisure activities
- ○ money available
- ○ time available.

Consult, plan and prepare for the service with clients

In this outcome you will learn about:

- using suitable consultation techniques in a polite and friendly manner to record the service plan
- obtaining signed, written informed consent from the client prior to carrying out the service
- ensuring that informed and signed parental or guardian consent is obtained for minors prior to any service
- ensuring that a parent or guardian is present throughout the service for minors under the age of 16
- asking the client appropriate questions to identify if they have any contra-indications to manicure/pedicure services
- accurately recording the client's responses to questions
- encouraging clients to ask questions to clarify any points
- ensuring client advice is given without reference to a specific medical condition and without causing undue alarm and concern
- disinfecting the client's hands/feet and effectively removing any existing nail polish to restore the nails to a natural condition
- actively identifying the condition of the nails and skin
- explaining your assessment of the client's nail and skin condition in a clear way to help their understanding
- recommending suitable treatments and products for the client's skin type and nail condition
- taking the necessary action in response to any identified contra-indications
- agreeing the service and outcomes that are acceptable to your client and meet their needs.

Consultation techniques

In addition to the equipment you will use, ensure you always keep a client record card to hand to ensure a professional treatment. All client records are confidential and should be held in accordance with the Data Protection Act (refer to Professional basics, page 63).

These are the points you should cover during your consultation with the client:

- ○ contra-indications
- ○ skin and nail conditions (treatable)
- ○ nail shape
- ○ occasion (e.g. wedding)
- ○ products used
- ○ contra-actions
- ○ varnish used
- ○ home care advice
- ○ sales
- ○ next appointment/recommendations
- ○ therapist's name.

Encourage her to ask questions regarding the proposed treatment or service in order to ensure that both the client and therapist are in agreement and that, if required, the service is adapted to the client's individual needs.

Shaping the nail

At the consultation stage you will need to consider the shape that would most suit your client: discuss this with the client. It is important to remember that it is the client's choice, and, as a manicurist/therapist, you can only make recommendations. You will need to consider the client's working environment. Nail shapes should usually conform to the shape of the fingers for a more realistic and natural appearance. The following are shapes to be considered. Toe nails should always be filed straight across and not shaped, to prevent ingrowing toe nails.

Square
This shape is usually most suitable for manual workers or clients who do a lot of work with fingertips, e.g. typists, pianists.

Round
This is a good shape for clients who require a short neat style. It decreases the likelihood of breakage or injury. It is suitable for clients with large square hands.

Oval
This shape can appear to lengthen the fingers for a more elegant appearance. It is usually suitable for small hands.

Pointed
This shape is liable to breakage due to the exaggeration of the shape. It is therefore most suitable for special occasions.

Squoval
This is one of the most popular shapes used in manicure. The nail is slightly rounded in at the edges to prevent stress fractures of the nail plate and then filed straight across the top.

> **Think about it**
>
> Clients under the age of 16 should have signed parent or guardian consent before the service can take place, and a parent or guardian should be present throughout the service. Remember too that you need to obtain the signed consent of all clients before carrying out a manicure or pedicure service.

> **For your portfolio**
>
> What could happen if you do not correctly record the feedback that is given to you by the client? List some areas that you will need to consider, and then discuss them with your colleagues.

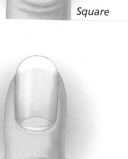
Square

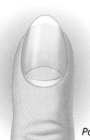
Round

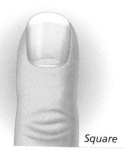
Oval

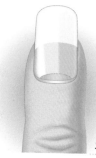
Pointed

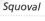
Squoval

Unit N2/N3 **Provide manicure and pedicure services**

Salon life

My story

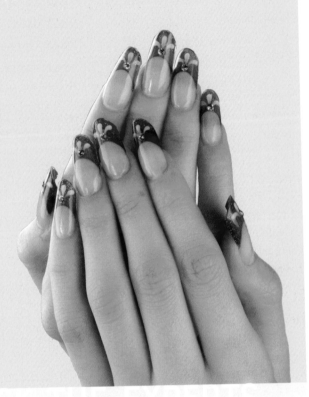

My name is Tanusha and I'm a therapist in a busy health spa. I spend a lot of my time giving clients' manicure and pedicure treatments. I really enjoy them as the result is instant and a hand or foot massage can be a great stress reliever for the client. There are so many finishes to choose from; no two treatments are exactly the same. You can choose from plain high buff right through to exotic paint and gem finishes. One of my clients had booked in for a pedicure as she was going on holiday and wanted her toes to look nice when she was wearing sandals. When she booked her appointment, the receptionist forgot to advise her to bring some open-toed sandals to go home in. Unfortunately the salon had run out of quick-dry spray and the client was in a rush to get back to work but didn't want to smudge her polish. One of my colleagues went and found the supply of disposable flip flops and we gave the client a pair to wear whilst her toes dried. The client went away happy, and her pedicure remained in tip top condition!

Benefits to client and therapist

Benefits of manicure/pedicure for client:

- Improves appearance of hands and nails
- Aids joint mobility
- Results are immediately visible
- Visually pleasing
- Treatment can be tailored to suit skin and nail condition

Benefits of manicure/pedicure for therapist:

- Staple salon treatment which increases revenue
- Can be offered as part of a promotion or treatment package; for example, bridal/summer holiday
- Excellent retail opportunity; for example, polish, files

Ask the experts

Q *When giving clients aftercare advice, how often should I suggest that they return for a further treatment?*

A This will vary from client to client – no two clients are the same. The initial consultation will identify the condition of the nails and their desired outcome for the treatment and it may be that regular treatments are necessary; for example, a weekly treatment for a period of six weeks followed by a maintenance treatment every 4-6 weeks. Other factors that need to be taken into consideration when devising a treatment plan include the client's work commitments and lifestyle and the amount of time and money they have available.

Top tips

- If you don't supply them in the salon, always get the client to bring flip flops for a pedicure treatment. Get the client to put the flip flops on before applying the varnish to prevent smudging.
- If the client does not have flip flops – or it's too cold to wear them! – and you have no quick-dry spray, apply massage oil over the toe nails and lightly wrap in cling film before the client puts on her shoes. This will prevent the nails from smudging on the way home.

Contra-indications to manicure and pedicure

It is important to establish during the consultation if contra-indications are present. A contra-indication means that the service cannot be carried out, as the client is unsuitable for this particular treatment, or that the service needs to be adapted. If an area with a contra-indication is treated, there is a risk of contamination and cross-infection occurring.

You need to assess not only the condition of the nails but also of the surrounding skin to establish if the treatment can be carried out. If a contra-indication is found it is important not to diagnose and refer the client to a medical practitioner for advice and treatment if required

The area to be treated should be examined in good light (refer to pages 184–197 and 236–239, for further information regarding skin and nail analysis). If natural daylight is not suitable and the salon lighting is inadequate, a magnifier lamp could be used to judge if any of the following conditions are present. Details should be recorded on the client record card. Here are the most common contra-indications that are found and associated with manicure and pedicure treatments. The term **onychosis** is used to describe any nail disease.

Fungal infections

Fungal infections spread very rapidly and often thrive in damp areas, and can appear soft and spongy. *Fungal infections should not be treated by manicure and pedicure.*

Onychomycosis (pronounced on-ee-ko-my-ko-sis) or ringworm

This is a fungal infection caused by the Tinea unguim fungus, otherwise known as ringworm. The infection invades beneath the free edge, spreading into the nail bed and then attacking the nail plate. The nail plate becomes brittle, rough and opaque, and separation starts to occur due to the build-up of scales between the nail bed and nail plate. This can also make the nail plate appear very thick. Yellow discoloration may also be present.

Ringworm of the hands is a highly contagious disease. The symptoms are papular, red lesions, which occur in patches or rings over the hands. Itching may be slight to severe.

Athlete's foot (ringworm of the foot) — in acute conditions deep, itchy, colourless blisters can appear, either singly, in groups, and sometimes on only one foot. They spread over the sole and between the toes, perhaps involving the nail fold and infecting the nail. When the blisters rupture they become red and ooze. The lesions dry as they heal. Fungus infection of the feet is likely to become chronic. Both the prevention of infection and beneficial treatment are accomplished by keeping the skin cool, dry and clean.

Bacterial infections

This type of infection is usually characterised by swelling, tenderness and redness in the area. Bacterial infection is a contra-indication to treatment.

> **Key terms**
>
> **Onychosis** – any nail disease.
> **Fungal infection** – an infection such as athlete's foot that thrives in damp moist conditions.

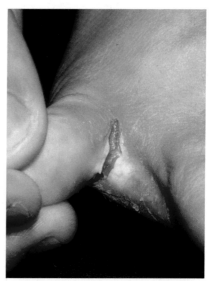

Athlete's foot (ringworm of the foot)

> **Think about it**
>
> Ringworm is a highly contagious disease and must not be treated. If in doubt, refer the client to her GP.

Unit N2/N3 Provide manicure and pedicure services

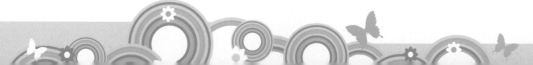

Paronychia (pronounced par-on-ik-ee-ah)

This is a bacterial infection of the nail fold, the two types of bacteria generally responsible being staphylococci and streptococci. In paronychia, the nail fold is damaged either from a bad manicure, or by the hands being constantly immersed in water and harsh detergents. The symptoms are **erythema**, swelling and tenderness around the nail fold. There may be signs of slight shrinkage of the nail plate, which is separated from the nail bed. If the condition is not treated, then the symptoms are accompanied by pus formation under the nail fold. After this, other types of bacteria set in, turning the nail plate a dark brown or black colour. Eventually, if the condition is not treated, a fungal infection known as Candida takes over. Candida is the worst form of paronychia and is hard to destroy. The more common form of paronychia is very often found among dental and nursing staff. *Paronychia should not be manicured.*

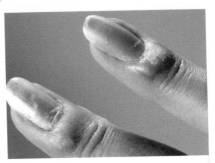
Paronychia

Key terms

Erythema – vasodilation of the blood capillaries, causing surface reddening of the skin.

Whitlows (Panaritium)

These are small abscesses at the side or base of nail. The skin around the nail becomes soft and open to infection by Herpes simplex virus or by bacteria, usually through a prick with a dirty pin or other sharp object. *Nails with this condition must not be manicured.*

Onychia (pronounced on-ee-kee-ah)

This is the inflammation of the nail matrix, accompanied by pus formation. Improper sanitisation of nail implements and bacterial infections may cause this disease. *Nails with this condition must not be manicured.*

Viral infections

These infections are very common and treatment can be adapted by using a waterproof dressing and avoiding the area. Gloves should be worn by the manicurist, as viral infections are highly contagious if touched, and disposed of after use.

Verruca vulgaris (common warts)

These are small and highly contagious. They are caused by a viral infection. They are rough and hard and can be darkish in colour or natural skin tone. They are found either singly or in groups and appear around the nail fold area. They create pressure above the matrix, which can lead to deformities appearing in the growing nail plate (dystrophy). Warts should be left alone or untouched since they tend to disappear of their own accord, as suddenly as they appear. *Area must not be manicured unless covered with a suitable waterproof dressing.*

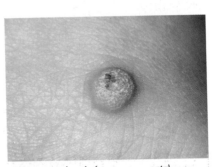
Verruca vulgaris (common warts)

Verruca plantaris (verruca of the foot)

This condition belongs to the same family as the common wart, but instead of being raised on the surface of the skin, verrucas tend to grow inwards, so until they get fairly large the client can be unaware of having a verruca. They are often caught in swimming pool areas and are highly contagious. The skin's surface can be smooth and the appearance can be like a circular piece of hard skin with a black dot or dots in the centre.

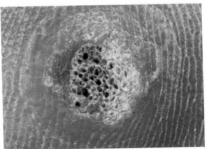
Verruca plantaris (verruca of the foot)

Parasitic infections

Scabies is a parasitic infection caused by a small mite that burrows into the skin, leaving tell-tale red tracking marks. This condition is highly contagious and *under no circumstances is the client to be treated*.

Other conditions

○ Eczema – clients who have eczema can be treated, providing the area is not open and weeping. Caution may be required when selecting products so they do not irritate or dry the skin.

○ Psoriasis – the same rules apply as with a client who has eczema.

○ Dermatitis – certain products could cause dermatitis to flare up, so caution should be used when selecting suitable products. Again, you should not treat if the area is open or infection is present.

Contra-indications that may restrict the service

There are also other conditions that may require an amendment in treatment but are not necessarily a reason for stopping treatment.

Onycholysis (pronounced on-ee-ko-lie-sis) or nail separation

This is a disorder where the nail separates from the nail bed (usually only part of and not the whole nail). It results from a build-up of debris found in the moist warm space between the digits, which attracts bacteria and fungal organisms, and in severe cases turns the nail plate a dark green or black colour. The infected nail plate grows faster than those that are uninfected. In feet, onycholysis occurs through wearing a tight-pinching shoe, poor general circulation and lack of attention to foot care.

Non-infectious nails can be manicured or pedicured as long there is no fungal or bacterial infection. However, severe separation should not be treated.

Onychocryptosis (or ingrowing nails)

This may affect either the fingers or toes. In this condition, the nail grows into the sides of the flesh and may cause infection. Filing the nails too much in the corners or over vigorous cutting is often responsible for ingrowing nails. If the area is open or infection is present, this would prevent the treatment from taking place.

Split nails, brittle nails (Defluvium unguinum)

Normally these are the result of abuse with drying agents, like those found in harsh detergents, cleaners, paint-strippers and film-developing fluids. Cotton-lined, rubber gloves are good protection. Since the nail begins forming at almost the last finger joint, sometimes injury to the finger or diseases like arthritis can result in split nails. If accompanied by an overall dryness of skin and hair, split nails could indicate poor circulation.

Treatment will increase the circulation, bringing more nutrients and oxygen to help with cell regeneration. Hydrate the nail plate and surrounding skin with hot oil or paraffin wax. The use of a cuticle cream or oil for home use will be effective between treatments. *Manicure should be given.*

Think about it

Although you must know what to look for, you must never attempt to diagnose fungal, bacterial, viral and parasitic conditions and disorders yourself as you are not medically trained to do so. Always refer clients to their own GP for treatment.

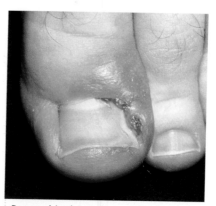

Paronychia due to in-growing toenail

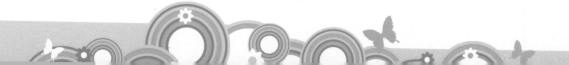

My story

Focus on manicure and pedicure

Hi, my name is Aisha. A client came into the salon for a manicure. She had brittle, ridged nails. I asked her how long she had worn nail extensions as her nails showed weakness often seen by clients who have worn nail extensions for a long period of time. The client said that she had never worn nail extensions, but when I carried out the consultation I realised that the nails were fragile due to the medical treatment she had been receiving. It was an important lesson for me to remember that health is reflected in the condition of the nail plate.

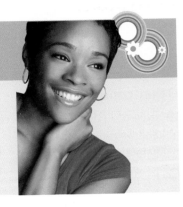

Blue nails

Usually a sign of bad circulation of blood or a heart condition, *manicures and pedicures may be given* and massage usually helps circulation.

Beau's line

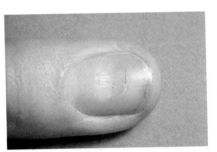

Beau's line

This is a disorder caused by an acute illness. As a result, the matrix temporarily stops producing new cells for the duration of the illness. When it once again begins to reproduce, the period of the illness is clearly marked by a definite furrow or series of furrows. This grows forward and eventually disappears as it is cut away as part of the free edge. *This disorder is non-infectious and can therefore be manicured.*

Nail biting/finger biting (onochophagy – pronounced on-o-ko-fag-ee)

This is a nervous habit where the individual bites and chews the free edge of the nail plate right down to expose the bulging nail bed below. The individual may also chew at the hardened cuticle and nail wall, causing a multitude of hangnails.

Nails should be regularly manicured. Massage and buffing will help to increase circulation and therefore stimulate growth. The use of special preparations to discourage nail biting may be recommended.

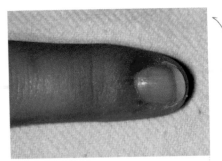

Finger biting

Hangnail

This is a condition whereby the cuticle around the nail plate splits leaving loose, flaky pieces of dry skin. It is caused by extreme dryness of the cuticle and from not keeping the cuticle free from the nail plate, so that it is stretched forward as the nail plate grows and eventually snaps leaving hangnails.

Splinter haemorrhages.

These appear as tiny streaks of blood under the nail plate, usually near the tip. Like nail separation, splinter haemorrhages can result from a traumatic blow to the nail. Sometimes, however, these red streaks can indicate a liver disease or possibly trichinosis (a ringworm infection caused by eating undercooked meat).

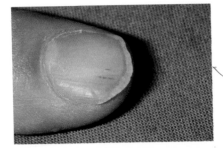

Splinter haemorrhages

Overgrown cuticles (Pterygium – pet-er-ee-gee-um)

This is caused by excessive cuticle growth that adheres to the base of the nail plate. Suggest that your client has a manicure or that she gently pushes the cuticle back with a soft towel after bathing and apply cuticle cream as often as possible. If the cuticles are very dry, a hot oil or paraffin wax manicure will help hydrate the area.

Pits and grooves
These are linked to both **dermatological** disease and systematic irregularities. However, many people who complain about pits and grooves in their nails have no apparent systematic diseases. It is very common and sometimes an unexplainable phenomenon, which can be dismissed with gentle buffing.

Flaking and breaking nails (Onychorrhexis – on-ee-ko-rex-is)
This is a very common complaint. The nail plate becomes dry and brittle and can be due to lack of vitamins A and B2, general ill-health, incorrect filing, excessive use of enamel remover, or excessive use of solvents and harsh detergents. Use of a nail strengthener may help this condition if applied regularly. It is also advisable to keep the nails fairly short to prevent them breaking.

Bruised nails
Bruising occurs when the nail receives a heavy blow. It is seen as a dark purple patch on the nail which will grow out with the nail. In severe cases the nail may detach itself from the nail base. Unless there is damage to the matrix, a new nail will grow normally to replace it. *Severely bruised nails should not be treated.*

Eggshell nails
These are recognised by the nail plate being noticeably thin, white and much more flexible than in normal nails. The nail plate separates from the nail bed and curves at the free edge. This disorder may be caused by chronic illness or may be of systemic or nervous origin.

Corrugations (or wavy ridges)
These are caused by uneven growth of nails, usually the result of illness or injury. When giving a manicure to a client with corrugations, buff to minimise ridges and use a ridge filler when painting for a smoother finish.

Furrows (depressions)
These may either run lengthwise or across the nail. They are usually the result of an illness or an injury to the nail cells, in or near the matrix. The nails are fragile, so care must be taken.

Leuconychia (pronounced loo-ko-nee-ee-kah) or white spots
These appear frequently in the nails but do not indicate disease. They may be caused by injury to the base of the nail or they might be air bubbles. As the nail continues to grow, these white spots eventually disappear. This is a very common disorder.

Other conditions of the feet
Callous
This is a hard build-up of skin that is often found in areas of friction or as a result of incorrectly fitting shoes. The skin over grows for protection.

Varicose veins
These are visible, distended veins which are often present in the legs (especially the lower legs). If serious, varicose veins will prevent massage taking place as this could be painful and cause extra blood to flow in the area.

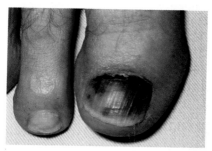
Bruised nail

Discoloured nails

This could be caused by the thickening of the nails due to age or fungal infection, or could be the result of staining from nail polish.

Dry nails

This condition often causes the nails to flake and become brittle. Dry nails would not contra-indicate treatment; a suitable service could be selected to help improve the condition.

Thickening of the nail.

This is often present in mature clients, and is usually more commonly seen on the big toe.

Bunions (Hallux valgus)

The term bunion refers to the swelling on the side of the big toe joint. The big toe leans towards the second toe and as the swelling is prominent, this is prone to rubbing from footwear. It can cause pain and inflammation. Bunions are often hereditary, but other causes are injury, arthritis and muscle imbalance. Unless there is severe pain or inflammation a bunion is not a contra-indication to a pedicure treatment.

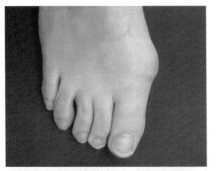

Bunions (Hallux valgus)

Corns

A corn is a small area of very thick skin; the overgrowth of skin penetrates the deeper layers of the skin and can be very painful. There are two types of corn: hard and soft. Hard corns are commonly found on the top or side of the little toe and are caused by footwear rubbing the area. Soft corns are usually found between the fourth and fifth toes and are soft as perspiration keeps them moist: these corns can become infected. Corns if infected or painful should be a contra-indication to a pedicure treatment and should be referred to a chiropodist. If there is no pain or infection, they can be treated.

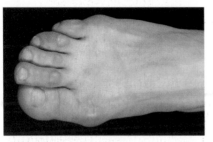

Corns

Nail shapes you might see

Koilonychia (spoon nails)

The nail plate is flat or concave giving a spoon-shaped appearance. This can be a hereditary condition, can be due to anaemia, or can be caused by the client's contact with oils, soaps or detergents. The nails of newborn babies are often spoon shaped, but this usually changes during their first year.

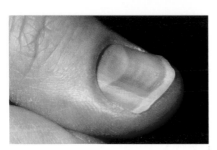

Koilonychia (spoon nails)

Onychogryphosis (claw or hook nails)

The nail plate of this condition is usually grainy and fibrous which gives it a thick, curved appearance. It is more common with toenails and is often caused by ill-fitting shoes. On the hands it is usually caused by trauma, although in some cases it can be caused by psoriasis of the nail. The nails should be kept short to prevent the nail looking too claw-like. However, care should be taken when cutting as this can cause bleeding.

Fan-shaped nails

The nail plate is narrower at the lunula and broadens out as the nail grows up to the free edge, a squoval shape for this nail or a gentle oval shape would help balance the proportions

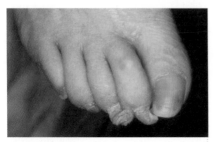

Onychogryphosis (claw or hook nails)

Selecting and adapting manicure and pedicure services to suit individual client needs

The condition of the skin and the nail need to be considered, along with the time that the client has for the treatment. Cost should always be established as a client needs to agree the treatment before it is started. Any adaptations need to be factored into the treatment plan as a result of the consultation and contra-indication check.

Male clients

The male grooming market is one of the largest growth markets within beauty therapy, so you should expect to treat men for both manicure and pedicure services. The timing for a manicure treatment will need to be adjusted as there will be no polish application but a high buff shine will be carried out on the client.

The shape that is good for all male clientele is square and all other services such as paraffin wax (see page 488) could be offered to enhance the condition of the nails and surrounding skin.

My story

Guys only!

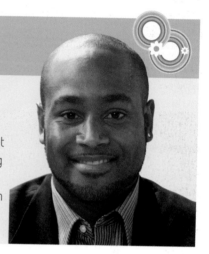

Hi, my name is Phillip. As an estate agent, I greet a lot of people, but as a nail-biter my hands and nails left a lot to be desired. My girlfriend goes to a salon that has a males-only night once a month, so she booked me an appointment for a manicure. As it was guys only, I didn't feel out of place going to the salon, and my therapist Jasmine soon put me at ease. She recommended a paraffin wax manicure which was pleasant and warming and helped to hydrate my skin and cuticles. My treatment was finished with a buff which made my nails shine and helps to stimulate nail growth. I enjoyed the treatment so much that I now go once a month, and although I have not completely stopped biting my nails the condition of my nails and hands is much improved.

Carry out manicure services

In this outcome you will learn about:

- confirming the desired nail length and shape with the client
- filing the nails correctly, ensuring that the nail free edge is left smoothed and shaped to the required length
- using the correct buffing technique for the service plan and the client's needs
- applying suitable cuticle products for the client
- using cuticle tools and products safely and effectively, ensuring that the cuticle and nail plate are undamaged
- using hand and nail treatments correctly to improve the appearance of the client's skin and nails
- using the correct quantity and type of massage medium to meet the service plan
- using massage techniques smoothly and evenly, at a pressure to the meet the client's needs
- leaving the hands and lower arms free of any excess massage medium
- ensuring the nail plate is dehydrated and the underside is clean and free of debris
- applying a suitable base coat relevant to the client's needs, if required
- applying sufficient polish coats and top coat for the desired finish, if required
- ensuring that the nail finish is left with a smooth even texture and with the cuticle and nail wall free of product and debris
- ensuring that the finished result is to the client's satisfaction and meets the agreed service plan.

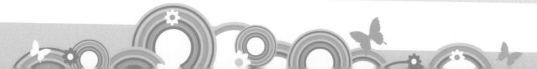

Suggested manicure procedure

If you do specialised manicures and pedicures at your salon using a particular brand of products, you will probably go on a course which shows you how to use these products and gives an order for the procedure that should be followed. You therefore need to adapt your treatments at all times according to the manufacturer's instructions. However, whichever products you use, the basic principles for manicure and pedicure are the same.

Before starting the treatment, always carry out the following steps.

○ Ensure equipment is sterile and all materials and products are easily accessible.

○ Complete a consultation form, check for contra-indications (see above) and discuss and agree with the client a service that meets their needs.

○ Remove all the client's jewellery, including watches, so that a thorough treatment can be carried out. Keep in a safe place.

Step-by-step manicure

1 During the consultation discuss the needs of the client and adapt the service to suit. You should cover preferred nail length and shape and the type of polish required. If there are no contra-indications present you are ready to begin.

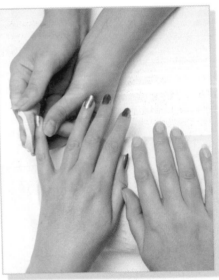

2 Ask the client to pick her choice of varnish – dark, plain, frosted or French manicure. You should recommend a nail finish suitable for the client. Remember, dark colours will make the nails appear shorter, so this may not be a suitable colour for short or bitten nails.

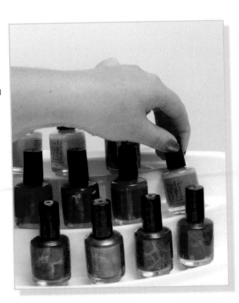

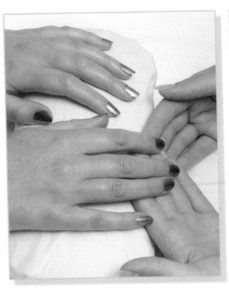

3 Remove the old varnish and check the nails for ridges and problems as you go. Removing the polish will allow the nail plate to be examined in a natural condition. Sanitise the hand to prevent cross-infection while you do a manual contra-indication check.

4 Cut the nails into shape if required, using sterilised scissors. Nail clippings need to be caught in a tissue and disposed of.

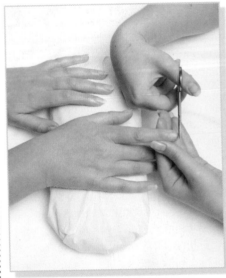

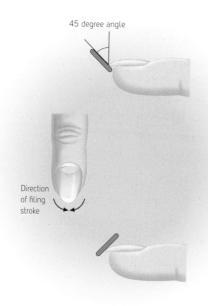

45 degree angle

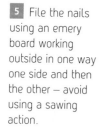

Direction of filing stroke

Think about it

When performing treatments on the cuticle never push back or nip beyond the eponychium or infection could occur.

Think about it

Do not use a sawing action as this can cause the layers of the nail plate to split and separate.

Bevelling seals the free edge layers to prevent water loss and damage.

5 File the nails using an emery board working outside in one way one side and then the other – avoid using a sawing action.

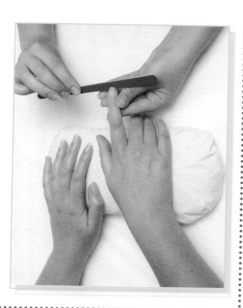

6 Bevelling seals the free edge layers to prevent water loss and damage.

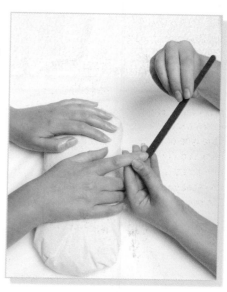

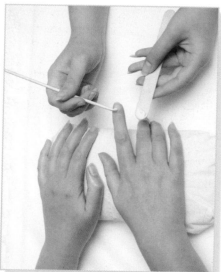

7 Using an orange stick decant and apply cuticle cream around the cuticles.

8 Gently massage the cream into the cuticles. This softens the skin, making removal easier.

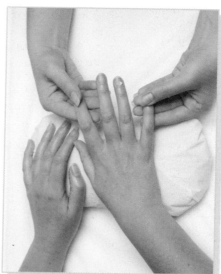

Unit N2/N3 Provide manicure and pedicure services

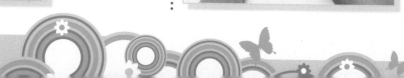

9 Soak the hands in warm water (tested by you first) to absorb the cuticle cream and to soften them.

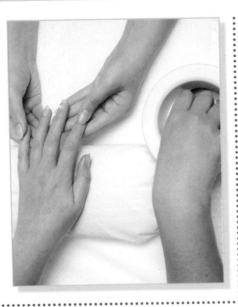

10 Remove one hand at a time and dry the hands thoroughly.

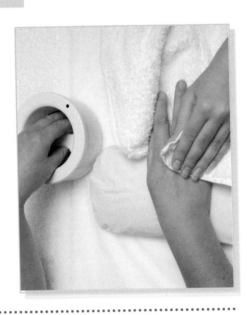

11 Apply cuticle remover with a cotton wool bud. It is caustic, so take care to apply sparingly and not on to the surrounding skin. Refer to COSHH regulations and the manufacturer's instructions.

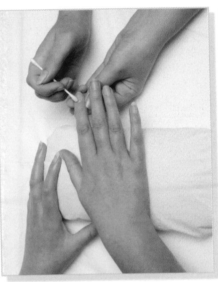

12 Using a hoof stick flat to the nail plate, gently push the cuticle back using circular motions.

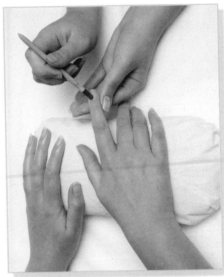

13 You may need to use the cuticle knife to ease the excess cutile away from the nail plate. This should be kept flat and the nail plate should be damp so that the nail plate is not scratched. The knife should also be kept flat to avoid cutting the cuticle.

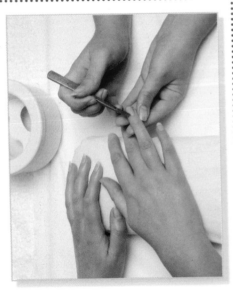

14 Cuticle nippers may be used to trim off the excess cuticle; use a tissue to dispose of the waste.

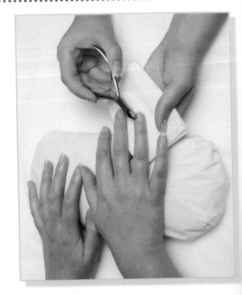

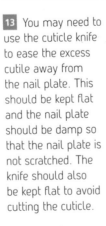

15 Bevel again, to give a smooth finish to the free edge.

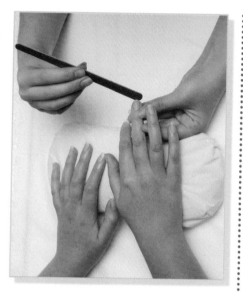

16 Using a suitable medium begin your hand massage with light effleurage movements. Support the hand and effleurage right up to the elbow.

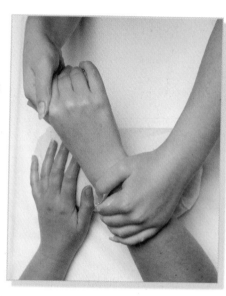

17 Circular thumb frictions get rid of tension in the flexors and extensors of the forearm.

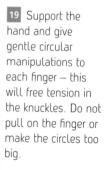

18 Do circular frictions over the back of the hand.

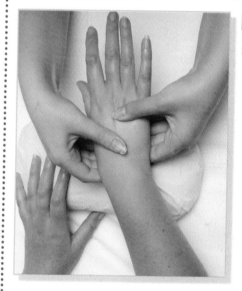

19 Support the hand and give gentle circular manipulations to each finger – this will free tension in the knuckles. Do not pull on the finger or make the circles too big.

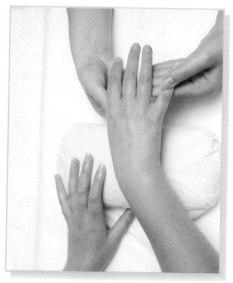

20 Grip the client's finger between your bent first and middle fingers and pull and twist gently down the length of the finger.

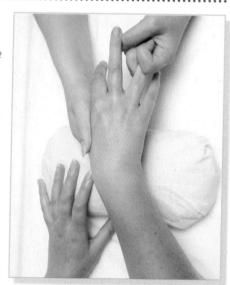

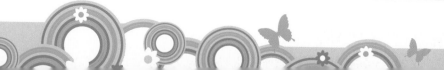

21 Interlock the client's fingers with your own and, supporting the forearm, gently manipulate the wrist backwards and then forwards, to loosen the wrist and get rid of tension.

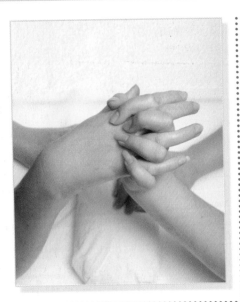

22 Apply circular thumb frictions to the palm. Stretch the palm out slightly.

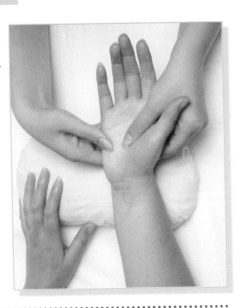

23 Finish your massage with effleurage up to the elbow.

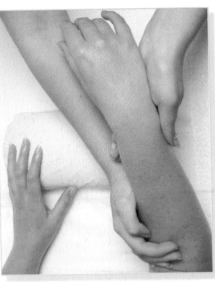

24 With warm soapy water, gently wash the nails with a soft brush to remove any grease from the massage medium. It is important to remove excess moisture, debris and product in order to prepare for the nail finish. Buffing can be carried out at this point if a natural finish is required. Buff from the matrix to the free edge to stimulate growth and promote shine. Buffing may also be carried out prior to polish, especially if the nail plate is ridged, as this could help to minimise the ridges. A ridge filler could be used here before a base coat is applied.

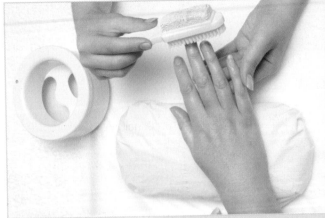

25 Apply a suitable base coat. Some nail systems have joint strengtheners or corrective properties within the base coat.

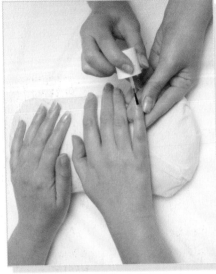

Think about it

There are some commercially prepared soaking preparations on the market, along with manicure bowls, to prevent spillage.

Think about it

The nail is made of three separate layers. 'Bevelling' holds the layers together and prevents splitting if the edge is traumatised.

26 Apply the varnish of the client's choice, with clean strokes, without flooding the cuticle area.

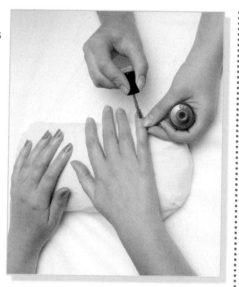

27 A topcoat will give a professional finish and the results should look good for some time.

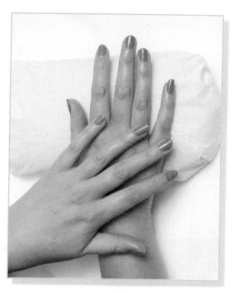

Nail finishes

Nail painting techniques

When painting nails, it is important to remember the following points.

- Try not to use more than four strokes per nail, as more strokes will make the paint finish look streaky.
- Hold nail enamel in non-working palm of hand and use finger to support nail being painted.
- Always allow coats to dry before reapplying. This prevents smudging and streaking.
- When painting large wide nails, leave a thin unvarnished line at each side of the nail to produce a slimming effect.
- Avoid flooding the cuticles with nail varnish, as this has a drying effect on the skin.
- Tidy up any flaws with a cotton wool bud soaked in varnish remover.

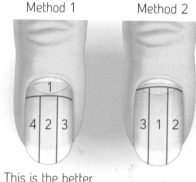

This is the better method for wide nails

Selecting a suitable colour

It is important that you recommend a nail finish that is suitable for the client. When selecting coloured enamel it may help your client if you remember these few rules.

- Very bright colours draw attention to hands or feet.
- Dark colours make nails look smaller.
- Small hands or feet usually suit a light colour.
- Oval-shaped nails suit most colours.
- Orange, peach or beige tones emphasise the bluish tinges to the skin often seen in clients with poor circulation.
- Pearlised nails reflect the light and will emphasise any flaws in the nails.
- Coloured enamel is not suitable for very short/bitten nails, or hands and nails that are in poor condition.

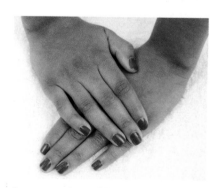

Recommend a nail finish that is suitable for the client

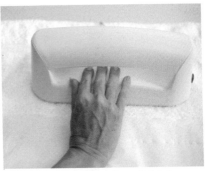

Nails can be dried under a light dryer

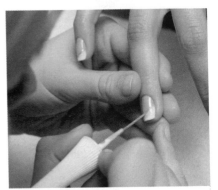

A nail art brush can be used to paint a neat free edge

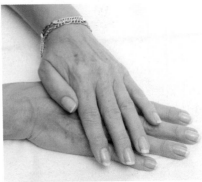

French varnish effect

For your portfolio

Why would it be important to ensure that the client is happy with the finished result before leaving the salon? Write a list of how it could impact on the salon.

Drying nail enamel

Nail enamel will dry quite well on its own, but on occasions it may be necessary to speed up the process. The application of either a topcoat dryer or quick dry spray can be used. Nail-drying preparations do not completely dry the varnish but form a barrier over the surface to prevent smudging. Always refer to the manufacturer's instructions and be aware of COSHH regulations when using these products. A light dryer can be used to speed up varnish drying.

Buffed nails

A buffer can be used to give a natural shine to the nail plate. Buffers come in many styles, such as chamois buffers to be used with an abrasive buffing paste, or three/four way buffers that have slightly different textures to each part to achieve the same effect as using an abrasive paste. Buffing is the required finish for a male treatment.

French manicure

This is a popular way of varnishing fingernails that gives a natural look. Kits that are sold usually contain white and flesh-coloured enamels. Always refer to the manufacturer's instructions for application. Below is a suggested method of application.

1 Apply base coat.

2 Apply white enamel to free edge only. Allow to dry.

3 Apply flesh-coloured varnish to entire nail.

4 Apply a topcoat.

Risk assessment for manicure and pedicure treatments

Refer to Unit G20, Make sure your own actions reduce risks to health and safety, pages 71–86, for a complete discussion of risk assessment.

Hazards: look for hazards that you would reasonably expect to result in significant harm under the conditions in your workplace. Use the following examples as a guide.

- **Allergies** (allergic reaction to chemicals used, nail enamel remover, nail polish, cotton wool).
- **Cross-infections** (infections spread from contaminated tools, or lack of sterilisation).
- **Skin breakage/bleeding** (caused by misuse of cuticle knife, or cutting of the skin with cuticle nippers, or cutting the skin when using nail clippers/scissors).
- **Irritation** (caused by scratchy tools, lack of lubricant when using knife on nail plate).
- **Contamination** (caused by ignoring contra-indications to treatment).

Massage

Hand/foot and arm/leg massage (to elbow or knee) is included in manicure and pedicure treatments. Refer to Related anatomy and physiology for information on the relevant bones, muscles and blood circulation, pages 224–229, 239–245 and 249–255. The effects of massage on blood circulation are described on pages 483–84.

Massage helps to:

- moisturise skin
- aid desquamation (shedding of skin cells)
- improve poor nail conditions
- stimulate blood supply, aiding cell regeneration
- relax tired muscles
- aid with the removal of waste products from the tissues
- aid client relaxation.

Massage mediums

There are number of different types of mediums that can be used to perform the massage: the most common is massage oil. Some clients prefer cream; if the client has an allergy, a hypoallergenic cream can be used.

Types of massage movements

Effleurage

These are gentle stroking movements that can often be used to link movements or to go from one part of the body to another.

Effleurage movements are used for:

- introducing massage medium to area
- introducing hands to area
- helping relaxation with long flowing moves
- soothing nerve endings.

Petrissage

Petrissage (kneading or friction) movements are used for:

- increasing the blood flow feeding the muscular tissue and cells
- desquamating cells from the surface of the skin
- increased removal of waste
- stimulating tissues, using deeper, more localised movements.

Tapotement

Tapotement movements, such as hacking and cupping where hands work briskly to stimulate the area, are used for breaking down areas of tension and nodules and adipose tissue.

This type of movement needs adaptation depending on the area being treated and tissue density, for example not over a bony area as it can be uncomfortable.

Step-by-step arm massage

1 With effleurage movement, apply oil or cream.

2 With your left hand, effleurage one side of arm 3 times from out to in.

3 With your right hand, effleurage the other side of arm 3 times in to out.

4 Carry out thumb rotaries up the arm in 4 lines (2 at front and 2 at back).

5 Petrissage side of arm with your left hand out and in, and repeat on the other side from in to out 3 times.

Ensure all equipment is to hand and sterilised

Consult to establish client requirements (discuss occupation to help with suitable nail shape)

Select nail colour

File/cut if required

Cuticle work

Apply specialist products according to manufacturers' instructions if required

Massage

Buff

Paint

Home care/aftercare advice

Record details on record card to include shape and varnish colour

Manicure

6   Thumb-flicks in between the metacarpals 2 times between digits.

7   Rotaries in between metacarpals 2 times between every digit.

8   Thumb-flicks again, in between the metacarpals 2 times between digits.

9   Rotaries to phalange joints, traction 2 times, full mobilisation – 3 in one direction (in towards your client), then repeat in the opposite direction away from your client.

10   Effleurage whole hand once.

11   Rotaries on carpals, traction of hand 2 times.

12   Full mobilisation of carpals, 3 times in one direction (in towards client).

13   Knead the palm with your thumbs.

14   Effleurage arms alternately 6 times and finish with pressure on the fingers.

Carry out pedicure services

In this outcome you will learn about:

- cleaning and drying the client's feet
- filing the nails correctly, ensuring that the nail free edge is left smoothed and shaped to the required length
- applying suitable cuticle products for the client
- using cuticle tools and products safely and effectively, ensuring that the cuticle and nail plate are undamaged
- removing any excessive hard skin using a foot rasp, without discomfort to the client, if required
- using foot and nail treatments correctly to improve the appearance of the client's skin and nails
- using the correct quantity and type of massage medium to meet the service plan
- using massage techniques smoothly and evenly, at a pressure to the meet the client's needs

- leaving the feet and lower legs free of any excess massage medium
- ensuring the nail plate is dehydrated and the underside is clean and free of debris
- applying a suitable base coat relevant to the client's needs, if required
- applying sufficient polish coats and top coat for the desired finish, if required
- ensuring that the nail finish is left with a smooth even texture and with the cuticle and nail wall free of product and debris
- ensuring that the finished result is to the client's satisfaction and meets the agreed service plan.

Suggested pedicure routine

Before starting the treatment, carry out the following steps.

○ Ensure equipment is sterile and all materials and products are easily accessible.

○ Check for contra-indications, specifically: athlete's foot, bunions, corns, verrucas, ingrowing toenails and nail disease, callouses and varicose veins.

○ The client should be seated comfortably with modesty towel over lap, and legs to knee exposed, to allow full pedicure with massage treatment.

○ Manicurist should have all materials to hand, be in a comfortable position with towel and single paper tissue roll on lap. Paper tissue to be replaced constantly through treatment to prevent cross-infection.

The client's feet should be washed and dried prior to commencement of treatment.

Step-by-step pedicure

1 During the consultation discuss the needs of the client and adapt the service to suit. You should cover their preferred nail shape, length and the type of polish required. After the consultation remove the nail enamel and soak the feet to soften and refresh them: this will sanitise the feet and you will be able to check for contra-indications.

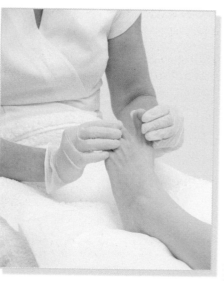

2 Using an emery board, file the toenails straight across – avoid any shaping, as it could cause ingrowing nails.

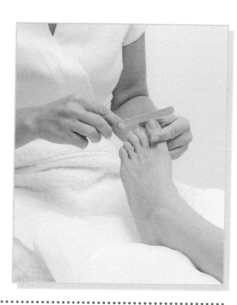

3 If the toenails are very long, use the clippers to get rid of the free edge, before filing.

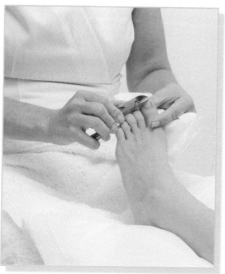

4 Apply cuticle cream.

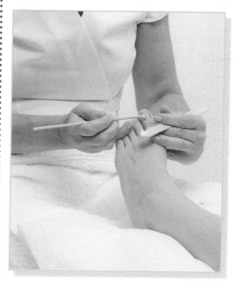

5 Soak the first foot in clean warm water, and repeat with the second foot.

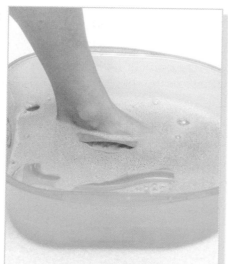

6 Apply cuticle remover with a cotton bud. It is caustic so be careful; only apply sparingly and not on the surrounding skin.

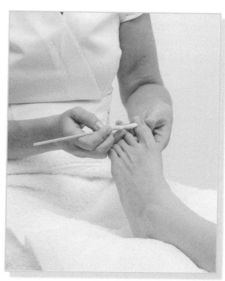

Unit N2/N3 Provide manicure and pedicure services

7 Using a hoof stick, flat to the nail plate, gently push the cuticle back, using circular motions.

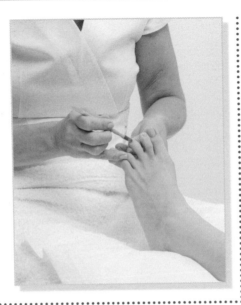

8 Depending on the amount of work to be done on the cuticle, you may need to use the cuticle knife to ease the excess away from the nail plate.

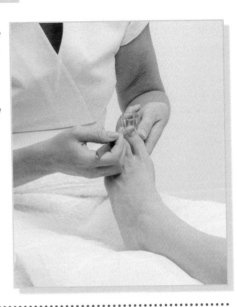

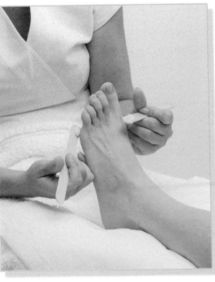

9 Rough skin remover may be applied to the areas that need attention, most commonly the ball of the foot, the heel and side of the big toe. You can use a foot rasp here if the skin is very hard.

10 Apply massage medium and begin with effleurage to the whole foot, and follow with thumb frictions to the upper foot.

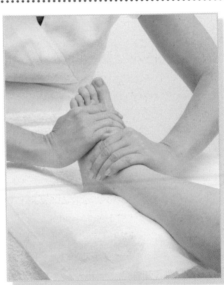

11 Follow the massage routine, as for manicure (see pages 482–84) – toe manipulations are really relaxing.

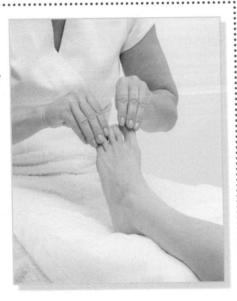

12 Finish with effleurage over the whole foot and lower leg. Remember, it is important to remove excess moisture, debris and product from the nail in order to prepare for the nail finish.

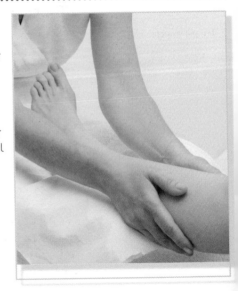

13 Paint toe nails to the client's choice of colour, using a base and topcoat for extra durability. Allow the varnish plenty of time to dry, before the client puts her shoes on.

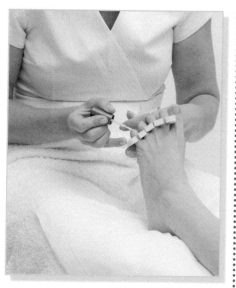

14 The end result.

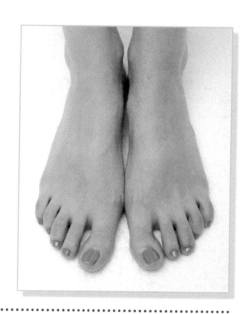

Think about it

Diabetes may not be considered a contra-indication to manicure and pedicure, but in some cases diabetes can cause limited sensation in the feet due to poor circulation. If this is the case, GP approval is required. In the case of varicose veins, avoid massage – a doctor's approval may be necessary.

Think about it

Do not file nails to shape into the nail grove – keep free edge straight (square) or slightly rounded, to avoid problems with ingrowing nails

Specialist treatments

In some cases, the condition of a client's hands or feet might mean that a standard manicure or pedicure is not enough, and so a specialist treatment would be recommended. These treatments include abrasive products (exfoliators) for hard skin and thermal mitts/boots for intensive moisturising. It is vital when using these products that you follow manufacturers' instructions. You may need to attend specialist training courses to use some of the products.

Product	What it does	Benefits
Abrasives and exfoliants	These products contain abrasive particles, which help remove (desquamate) excess skin. This type of product is especially useful for pedicure treatments.	Softens and removes hard skin while conditioning. For best results, feet should be soaked prior to application. A massage product should be applied to the area after use, to help replace lost moisture, making skin feel soft and smooth.
Thermal hand/foot masks	These products are usually wax- or oil-based, and are applied to a well-moisturised area in a heated liquid form. The treated area is usually wrapped in either foil or cling film to maintain the heat. The mask is usually left on for 15 minutes, but you should always check the manufacturer's instructions. An example of a thermal mask is paraffin wax.	Intensive rehydration and softening of skin and nail plate. Ideal for dry skin conditions. Increases circulation, promoting healthier growth. Decreases joint stiffness. Relaxes aching muscles. Increases absorption of moisturising products.

Step-by-step paraffin wax treatment for hands/feet

This can be used for both manicure and pedicure treatments. It is applied after the cuticle work and before the massage.

1 Prepare your working area and decant the melted paraffin wax into a bowl lined with tin foil.

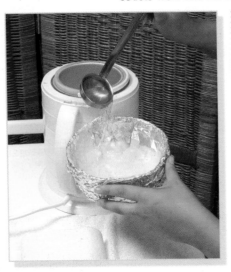

2 Test on self, prior to application on client, over a sheet of foil with a towel underneath it.

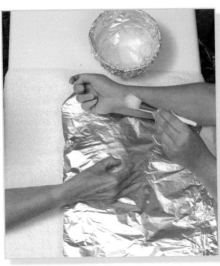

3 If the temperature is suitable, paint on a good even coating of wax, working quickly before it sets, turning the hand or foot to paint both sides.

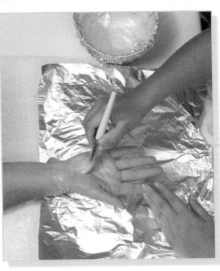

4 Wrap the hand or foot in tin foil, to retain the heat.

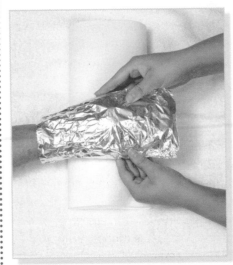

5 Wrap both hands or feet in the towels and allow the heat to soothe and soften.

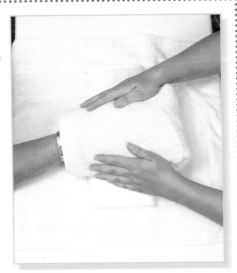

6 The wax cools and hardens, which makes removal easy – just peel it off. Any paraffin wax left in the bowl can be given to the client to use as a home treatment.

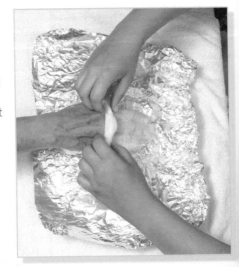

Risk assessment for paraffin wax equipment

Refer to Unit G20, Make sure your own actions reduce risks to health and safety pages, 71–86, for a complete discussion of risk assessment.

Hazards: look for hazards that you would reasonably expect to result in significant harm under the conditions in your workplace. Use the following examples as a guide.

- **Fire** (e.g. from electrical flex or lead).
- **Burning of equipment** (through low wax level in the tank).
- **Burns to skin** (not testing wax temperature first on self).
- **Ejection of materials** (spitting hot wax).
- **Electricity** (e.g. poor wiring).
- **Manual handling** (spillage possible if moving when in liquid form).
- **Falling machinery** (if not securely positioned on a trolley).

Warm oil treatment for hands

This treatment can also be offered in a salon. It is useful when treating dry hands/cuticles and flaky nails.

The oil used should always be vegetable-based such as sweet almond oil, olive oil or coconut oil.

Step-by-step warm oil treatment

1 Warm oil, either by immersing a suitable container in hot water or by using an infrared lamp.

2 Proceed with treatment – do not apply cuticle massage oil at this stage. Soak fingers in warmed oil for 5 minutes.

3 Massage in oil and wipe off any excess with a tissue.

4 Continue with routine.

Note: It is not necessary to carry out a massage with this treatment.

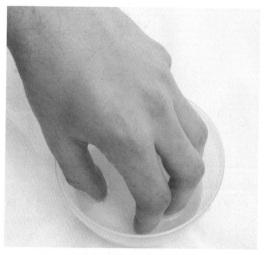

Soak the cuticles in warm oil to help soften, and massage

Risk assessment for warm oil equipment

Refer to Unit G20, Make sure your own actions reduce risks to health and safety, pages 71–86, for a complete discussion of risk assessment.

Hazards: look for hazards that you would reasonably expect to result in significant harm under the conditions in your workplace. Use the following examples as a guide.

- **Fire** (e.g. from electrical flex or lead).
- **Burning** of equipment (through light bulb burning out).
- **Ejection of bulb** (hot bulb falling on to skin, not screwed in properly, lamp should not be directed over the skin).
- **Electricity** (e.g. poor wiring, trailing leads).
- **Manual handling** (outer casing is hot and will burn if towel is not used for protection).
- **Falling machinery** (if supporting arm is not screwed in properly).
- **Contamination** (from brushes).
- **Cross-infection** (ignoring possible contra-indications).

Thermal mitts and boots

These are electrically heated items of equipment that are used on the same principle as thermal masks, with the added advantage of:

○ maintaining heat more effectively

○ being easy and less messy to use

○ being more cost-effective over a period of time, as no special product is required.

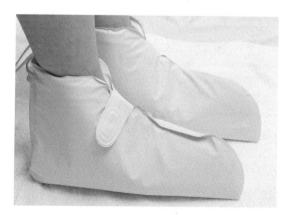

Thermal boots

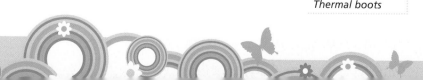

Step-by-step thermal treatments

1 Apply a moisturising product to the area.

2 Apply cling film to improve the rehydration process.

3 Place hands/feet in mitts/boots for 10–15 minutes.

4 After that time, continue with cuticle work and the rest of the treatment.

Provide aftercare advice

In this outcome you will learn about:

- giving advice and recommendations accurately and constructively
- giving the clients suitable advice specific to their individual needs.

Giving advice and recommendations to suit the client's needs

To ensure that your client gains maximum benefit from the treatment, you need to give advice that is both practical and achievable.

Wherever possible, it is advisable to show the client how to use the products that would be suitable for them to purchase. Many of the items and products listed below are sold through salons. It is worth remembering that many therapists/manicurists work on commission, so good product knowledge could earn you extra money.

Contra-actions that could occur after nail services

To protect the client's hands and nails from damage, it should be suggested that suitable gloves or a special barrier cream are used when completing tasks involving any dirty work, or other work involving the use of water or chemicals. Examples of these types of work include:

- gardening
- washing up
- hairdressing
- car maintenance.

The client should also be advised:

- not to bite nails or surrounding skin and to keep an emery board available to deal with ragged free edges to the nails, so that the temptation to bite is removed
- to use a moisturising hand cream or lotion regularly
- to avoid using the nails as tools (e.g. undoing screws, removing tight lids from containers and opening tightly sealed letters and parcels)
- to stop using a product immediately in the event of contra-actions occurring, such as a reaction to products in the form of extreme redness, rashes, irritation or swelling – advise the client to cool the area with cold water and visit the GP if treatment is required.

Think about it

Contra-indications to paraffin wax treatment:

- skin infections
- varicose veins
- nail diseases
- hypersensitivity.

Retail products

Retail products that may be stocked by your salon for care of the feet and hands to sell to clients are important income boosters, and many therapists earn commission from these sales. It is therefore important to have excellent knowledge of the products your salon retails, which could include the following.

Nail varnish remover

This is used to remove old varnish. Avoid using too frequently, as it can have a drying effect on the nails and surrounding skin. Always wash hands after use.

Base coat, nail varnish, topcoat

It is advisable to sell a selection of varnishes, and ensure your client realises the importance of wearing a base coat to prevent staining the nail plate.

Nail strengthener

Use these products according to manufacturers' instructions. Strengthener is often built into base coat varnishes, to improve the condition of the nails.

Cuticle cream

This product can be massaged around the cuticles daily to keep them soft and smooth. The massaging action will help stimulate the growth of the nail.

Emery boards

Recommend the fine side for shaping finger nails and the coarse side for hard nails and reducing the length of the nails. Show the client how to file correctly. Avoid sawing.

Buffers

These can be used to smooth out ridges and to give the nails a natural sheen. Show the client how to use them correctly, going from the base of the nail to the free edge. Buffing will stimulate growth, so this can be an incentive for nail biters.

Foot care

Clients should be advised of the importance of ensuring that all footwear is well fitting, so that the feet are not restricted, which may result in damage, discomfort and foot problems.

Rough skin remover

This is a slightly abrasive product that is effective against hard skin. Massage on to affected areas firmly in circular movements for softer feet.

Foot powder

This is a deodorised powder that can be applied regularly to keep feet fresh and dry. This product is worth recommending to clients who suffer with odour problems, or have a tendency to athlete's foot (this condition thrives in damp conditions).

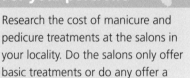

Think about it

All portable electrical equipment must be tested, so ensure thermal mitts and boots are tested, and check the flex and plug before every use. (For information on portable appliance testing, refer to Professional basics, page 57, and G20 Make sure your own actions reduce risks to health and safety, page 89.)

For your portfolio

Research the cost of manicure and pedicure treatments at the salons in your locality. Do the salons only offer basic treatments or do any offer a variety of specialist treatments?

For your portfolio

A client comes into the salon with dry nails and overgrown cuticles. What intensive treatment could you carry out for these conditions and what additional aftercare advice could you give?

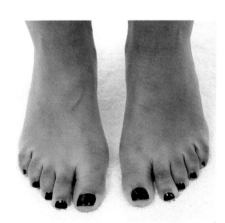

The right products will help to ensure your client gains maximum benefit from their treatment

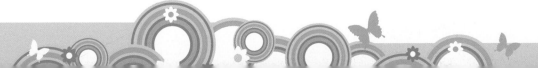

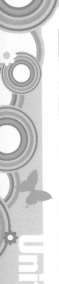

Frequently asked questions

Q	What will happen if I don't check for contra-indications?
A	Infections of the hands and feet can be spread very easily — especially warts and verrucas.
Q	Can I use a dark-coloured varnish on short or bitten nails?
A	Lighter colours will make the nails appear longer; a dark colour will draw attention to bitten and badly kept nails.
Q	What happens if I don't keep the cuticle knife flat and wet?
A	Keeping the knife flat helps prevent cutting the skin, and wetting the knife prevents scratching the nail plate.
Q	Why can't I use foam toe separators between the toes when painting the toe nails?
A	Tissues are used because they are disposable. Foam separators may harbour germs and cause infections to be passed from client to client. If you do use these in your salon they should be costed into the treatment price and given to the client to take home.
Q	Do I have to buff with every treatment?
A	Buffing stimulates nail growth and gives the nail a nice natural sheen, a must for natural looking nails. In a treatment that has colour applied to the nail plate it will help to even out the minor ridges as well as stimulating growth. Ridges are often more apparent on toe nails and buffing should be carried out.
Q	Do I really have to cut toe nails straight across?
A	Yes, this will prevent ingrowing toe nails, a condition which can cause pain and infection if left untreated and which, in severe cases, may require an operation.

Check your knowledge

1   How would you recognise a verucca?

2   Is athlete's foot a virus, fungus, or bacteria?

3   How should you cut toenails?

4   What is the purpose of a hoof stick?

5   If the nails are stained what could be the cause(s)?

6   What salon treatment could you recommend for a client with very dry skin or cuticles?

7   What is leuconychia?

8   Why do you bevel the nail when filing?

9   What are finger and toenails made from?

10   What nail shape suits most colours of varnish?

11   List five things that you should include in a consultation.

12   How should you store acetone and what legislation should you follow when storing it?

13   If the nails have corrugations, what treatments could you offer to minimise this?

14   What could incorrect filing do to the nails?

15   What is the purpose of cuticle cream?
   a)   To soften the skin on the hands and the feet
   b)   To massage hands and feet
   c)   To soften cuticles before soaking

16   What condition would a nail have if it flaked and broke easily?
   a)   Ridges
   b)   Overgrown cuticles
   c)   Dry brittle nails

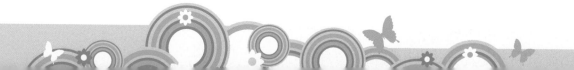

Getting ready for assessment

You cannot do any simulation within this unit, but the evidence can be gained quite easily. Remember to keep all paper evidence of any actions, feedback or witness statements that you have been given to support this work.

Your assessor will observe your performance on at least three occasions for both manicure and pedicure treatments (a minimum of six treatments for both the units).

* Treat a range of clients for both manicure and pedicure — although the range does not stipulate treatment on men, male treatments are becoming increasingly popular in both salon and spa.

* Use all consultation techniques.

* Use all the equipment and materials: files, scissors, nippers, clippers, cuticle tools and foot rasp.

* Apply all types of hand and foot treatments: paraffin wax, hand and foot masks, thermal mitts and boots and exfoliators.

* Apply all massage mediums.

* Apply all types of nail finish, including dark colour, French, high shine buff (manicure only).

* Maintain suitable environmental conditions (ventilation, heat, etc.).

* Prepare the client to suit the treatment.

* Deal with contra-indications that may prevent or restrict the treatment.

* Deal with contra-actions.

* Provide treatment advice: includes suitable aftercare products, home care routines, e.g. avoidance of activities that may damage the nails and surrounding skin, as well as recommended intervals between treatments.

Evidence of these can be provided by the observation of your assessor, but also by written work, projects, witness statements, photographic and video evidence and APL statements.

You must prove to your assessor that you have the necessary knowledge, understanding and skills to perform competently on all ranges within the criteria for this unit.

Unit B10

Enhance appearance using skin camouflage

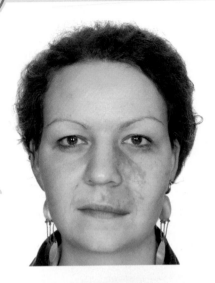

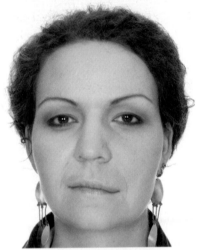

Unit B10 Enhance appearance using skin camouflage

Introduction

This unit is about providing suitable camouflage for the face and body, using make-up to cover tattoos, erythema and hyper/hypopigmentation disorders.

The application of remedial cosmetics can be used in a variety of ways, both in the salon and in more specialist environments such as hospital clinics. The skilled use of remedial camouflage make-up can be used to disguise a tattoo, scar tissue or pigmentation marks.

It is important to consider that clients requiring remedial work may be suffering from trauma and this can have psychological effects. The use therefore of skilled remedial cosmetic camouflage make-up can restore the client's self-esteem and confidence.

Benefits for the client:

○ increases self-esteem and confidence

○ a one-off treatment for a special occasion or for more permanent coverage if desired

○ may be combined with an ordinary make-up or skincare lesson (refer to Unit B8/ B9 Provide make-up services and instruct clients in the use and application of skincare products and make-up)

○ camouflage is waterproof, and can be worn when swimming.

Benefits for the therapist:

○ an excellent skill for a therapist or salon to offer as this specialist area can attract clientele, thereby increasing revenue

○ enhancement courses available for more advanced practitioner work.

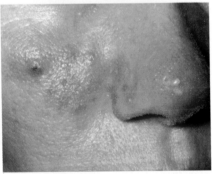

Acne rosacea – often seen as a red flush commonly over the nose and cheeks, sometimes accompanied by papules and pustules

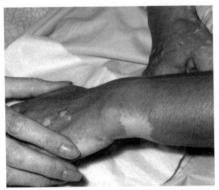

Vitiligo, or hypopigmentation. Light patches appear on the skin

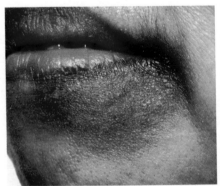

Chloasma, or hyperpigmentation. This is caused by the overproduction of melanocytes which produce melanin

Maintain safe and effective methods of working

In this outcome you will learn about:

- setting up and monitoring the treatment area to meet organisation procedures and manufacturers' instructions
- making sure that environmental conditions are suitable for the client and the skin camouflage
- ensuring your personal hygiene, protection and appearance meets accepted industry and organisational requirements
- effectively disinfecting your hands prior to treatment
- ensuring your own posture and position minimises fatigue and the risk of injury while working
- ensuring all tools are cleaned using the correct methods
- positioning skin camouflage products and application tools for ease and safety of use
- ensuring the client is in a comfortable and relaxed position suitable for the skin camouflage

- maintaining accepted industry hygiene and safety practices throughout the skin camouflage application
- adopting a positive, polite and reassuring manner towards the client throughout the treatment
- respecting the client's modesty, privacy and any sensitivities to their personal appearance
- checking the client's well-being at regular intervals according to organisational policy
- disposing of waste materials safely and correctly
- ensuring the skin camouflage is cost-effective and is carried out within a commercially viable time
- ensuring client record cards are up to date, accurate, complete, legible and signed by the client and practitioner
- leaving the treatment area in a condition suitable for further treatments.

Your personal hygiene, protection and appearance

As with any treatment it is important to maintain a professional appearance and to adopt hygienic and safe working practices to ensure no cross-infection occurs.

The main sources of infection during a camouflage session are caused by contaminated products, dirty tools and equipment. Consult your professional body for guidelines to prevent cross-infection.

Refer to Units B4, B8/9, G20 and the general Units Professional basics and You and the skin to ensure that you adhere to the correct health and safety protocols and can identify contra-indications and conditions that may affect the treatment, or that could potentially contaminate products or equipment.

Performance criteria

Setting up and monitoring the treatment area to meet organisation procedures and manufacturers' instructions

Making sure that environmental conditions are suitable for the client and the skin camouflage

Ensuring your personal hygiene, protection and appearance meets accepted industry and organisational requirements

Effectively disinfecting your hands prior to treatment

Ensuring your own posture and position minimises fatigue and the risk of injury while working

Ensuring all tools are cleaned using the correct methods

Positioning skin camouflage products and application tools for ease and safety of use

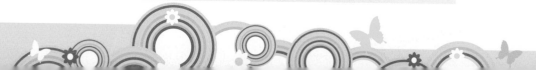

Performance criteria

Ensuring the client is in a comfortable and relaxed position suitable for the skin camouflage

Maintaining accepted industry hygiene and safety practices throughout the skin camouflage application

Adopting a positive, polite and reassuring manner towards the client throughout the treatment

Respecting the client's modesty, privacy and any sensitivities to their personal appearance

Checking the client's well-being at regular intervals according to organisational policy

Disposing of waste materials safely and correctly

Ensuring the skin camouflage is cost-effective and is carried out within a commercially viable time

Ensuring client record cards are up to date, accurate, complete, legible and signed by the client and practitioner

Leaving the treatment area in a condition suitable for further treatments

Organisational procedures and legal requirements

When providing skin camouflage it is essential to follow the legislation that is laid down with regard to the safe use, disposal and storage of products (COSHH) and follow manufacturers' instructions when using products. Products should be stored at the correct temperature and waste should also be disposed of according to manufacturer and salon guidelines.

Risks will be reduced to both the client and therapist, and safe running of the salon will be ensured, if skin care products are correctly selected and stored, contra-indications are checked at each visit and details accurately recorded. This will allow clients to agree to the treatment plan and an effective treatment to be carried out

If a client is sensitive it is important to carry out a sensitivity test before using a product and record the outcome on the client's record card. (Refer to Professional basics, page 29, for further information regarding legal requirements.)

Ensuring the client is comfortable and relaxed

Ensure that the client will be comfortable and that as a therapist you can carry out the treatment without damage to your posture. When working to blend camouflage make-up, it is important the lighting is correct. Make sure that the lighting is suitable natural daylight combined with warm white fluorescent light. This is the best light for matching make-up colours.

Your manner should be positive, polite and reassuring throughout the make-up service and you must respect any sensitivities the client may have about their personal appearance. Remember to check on the client's wellbeing at regular intervals during the service, according to your salon's policy.

Maintaining industry hygiene practices

Remember to carry out standard sanitisation and sterilisation procedures and to decant products to prevent contamination and cross-infection occurring (refer to Professional basics, page 39).

Therapist's hands	Wash hands before and after treatment using an appropriate cleanser.
Area to be treated	Check for contra-indications before treating and then cleanse area, blotting dry before applying camouflage product.
Trolley	Sanitise with suitable cleanser.
Brushes	Wash in warm soapy water and allow to dry naturally. Wipe with sanitiser while using, especially if you are using different coloured products.
Sponges	Wash in warm, soapy water and dry between clients.
Velour puffs	As for sponges.
Pallet	Wash with warm, soapy water and wipe with sanitiser prior to use.
Pump dispensers	Use where possible to dispense products to prevent contamination.
Disposable spatulas	Use spatulas for dispensing products on to pallet, and dispose after use.

Hygiene procedures

Consult, plan and prepare for skin camouflage

In this outcome you will learn about:

- using consultation techniques in a polite and friendly manner to determine the client's treatment needs
- ensuring that informed and signed parent or guardian consent is obtained for minors prior to any treatment
- ensuring that a parent or guardian is present throughout the treatment for minors under the age of 16
- obtaining signed, written informed consent from the client prior to carrying out the service
- clearly explaining to the client what the skin camouflage entails in a way they can understand
- asking your client appropriate questions to identify their skin camouflage needs
- encouraging clients to ask questions to clarify any points
- asking your client appropriate questions to identify if they have any contra-indications to the skin camouflage
- accurately recording your client's responses to questioning
- taking the necessary action in response to any identified contra-indications
- clearly identifying and agreeing the client's skin camouflage needs and the areas to be camouflaged.

The consultation and planning the treatment

With this particular treatment, the client may be very self-conscious about the problem area, and the consultation should be carried out with sensitivity and tact. This should take place away from others' view, and not in a public area. Remember, however small and insignificant you consider the problem, it is important to the client. In this way you will give the client confidence and boost her self-esteem.

The treatment plan and consultation should allow the therapist to clearly establish and identify the needs of the client, while encouraging the client to ask questions. This will allow the client and therapist to plan an achievable and realistic treatment plan.

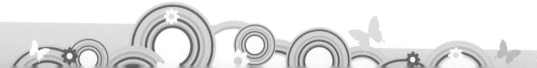

Identifying contra-indications

As with all treatments it is important to establish if the client is suitable for the treatment, so remember to check for contra-indications. Any open and infected areas will prevent the treatment as well as the contra-indications given in Unit B4, page 274, and Unit B8/B9, page 364.

Preparing for skin camouflage

The trolley set up for the treatment should be the same as for a routine make-up application with brushes, sponges and powder applicators. (Refer to Unit B8/B9 for trolley set-up and sterilisation, page 367.)

If you are combining camouflage application with traditional make-up, ensure that you have all products available.

Carry out skin camouflage

In this outcome you will learn about:

- ensuring empathy and sensitivity to the nature of the client's condition is shown throughout
- applying compatible skincare products when required before the skin camouflage application
- using application tools, techniques and camouflage products which are best suited to the skin camouflage needs
- ensuring camouflage products are applied in accordance with manufacturers' instructions to achieve required density, colour and effect
- establishing an acceptable colour match on the areas to be camouflaged to restore the skin colouration to the surrounding skin tone
- establishing and applying an appropriate complementary colour prior to the application of the acceptable skin colour match if required
- applying compatible cosmetic and skincare products when required after the skin camouflage application
- ensuring that the finished result is to the client's satisfaction and meets the agreed treatment plan.

Camouflage products

Camouflage make-up products have been developed to cover skin imperfections and disfigurements. They differ from ordinary concealers as they are designed to be worn for a long time without harming the skin.

Corrective products therefore need to have the following features:

- They are **opaque** (they do not transmit light).
- They have a light base.
- They have a matt finish.
- They are non-irritant.
- They are designed to even out skin tones.

- They can be easily mixed to produce the correct tone.
- They combine dense pigments.
- They allow the skin to breathe and perspire.
- They are waterproof.

Camouflage make-up can be purchased from some salons, chemists and wholesalers. The internet is also an excellent place for viewing the vast array of products on the market.

Selecting products suited to the client's camouflage needs

When selecting suitable camouflage products you should consider the following points:

- A cool environment will ensure the effectiveness of the make-up over a longer period.
- In a hot environment, due to perspiration, the oily consistency of the product will mean the make-up will loosen more quickly.
- Drier skins will find cover creams more effective.
- The sebum production of oily skins can cause thinning and lifting of products, therefore clients with oily skin should be told they may need more frequent applications.
- Facial camouflage should be removed and re-applied daily as natural perspirations and dirt could clog pores, causing spots.
- Clients should ensure that cleansing routines include the use of a cleansing cream which breaks down the camouflage product more effectively than regular cleansing products.
- If camouflage is applied to areas of the body other than the face, it can be left in place and clients may bathe/shower as long as soap is not used on the area as this can dislodge the cream. Swimming is permitted.
- Clients should always blot rather than rub the area dry to preserve the camouflage after a bath/shower.
- The client's skin tone.
- Any known allergies.

A number of companies produce camouflage products. It is important to think about the versatility of the product before purchasing a range to use, taking into account the area to be covered, the texture, colour range versatility and **blending**.

Some products may contain iron oxide, a colouring used in make-up, or titanium dioxide, a white matt powder. When manufacturers mix iron oxide or titanium oxide with zinc oxide the product will offer a degree of sun protection. However, it should not be used in place of SPF (sun protection factor) products. In certain conditions, such as under the flash of a camera, these products can alter the appearance of the skin. Professional photographers should be able to compensate for this when they take a light reading prior to the start of the shoot.

Key terms

Blending – ensuring that the product matches the natural skin tone using a variety of methods.

For your portfolio

Research companies that supply camouflage products, and compare the colours and the coverage that these products give. Do all of the products offer the same level of coverage?

Think about it

Although products are designed to be non-irritant, clients with sensitive skin should be given a patch test prior to application.

Enhance appearance using skin camouflage   Unit B10

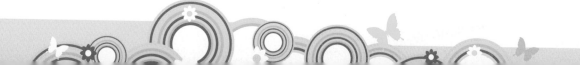

Some makes of product also contain lanolin, which can cause allergic reactions in a few clients, so always check for allergies when you are carrying out your consultation and refer to the manufacturer's list of ingredients and COSHH data if you are unsure. A sensitivity test should be undertaken if the client is known to suffer from allergies.

Features of camouflage products

Product/brand	Features
Dermablend	• Heavy texture • Wide range of colours from light to dark • Ideal for black skins • Good for covering tattoos
Veil	• Light texture • Ointment based • Excellent coverage • Wide range of shades available • Ideal for caucasian skin tones
Covermark	• Gives strong coverage • Ointment based • Includes grey shades • Ideal product for creating beard line effect on male clients
Dermacolour	• Fine texture • Good coverage • Ideal general purpose camouflage make-up • Wide range of colours • Long lasting • Ointment based • Yellow and dark tones good for blending
Keromask	• Thick texture • Excellent coverage • Variety of colours • Blends easily • Good for full facial concealment, e.g. acne scarring

Establishing an acceptable colour match

When using skin camouflage products you need to make sure the colour match to the client's skin is correct. The camouflaged skin should restore the skin colour to match the surrounding skin tone.

Camouflage make-up is usually selected by numbers and letters: the natural skin's colouring is given a letter and then the coverage cream within the selected range is chosen to match the skin colour.

Suitable skincare should be carried out prior to the application of the camouflage product such as using the appropriate cleanser and toner, and, if necessary, you should choose and apply an appropriate complementary colour before applying the skin colour match. You may need to neutralise a colour: for example, green concealer neutralises red.

Remember the colour star and the colours that help to neutralise each other: for example, green will diminish red. (Refer to concealing cosmetics in Unit B8/B9, pages 379–80.)

General rules for applying camouflage products

Following the few simple guidelines below will help to make the treatment result successful.

- Always follow manufacturers' instructions.
- Use less product than if applying ordinary make-up.
- Apply with clean brushes, sponges or finger to prevent cross-infection and build-up of products.
- Use green concealer with care — too much and the client will look ill!
- Always dispense products on to a palette for easy blending.
- Avoid using heavy concealer under the eyes or on crepey skin as this can emphasise lines and wrinkles — a little moisturiser added to the concealer for crepey skin gives a more natural look.
- Powder each layer to 'set' before applying another layer.
- Avoid over-blending — this may cause the make-up to **lift streak** or leave the skin **overstimulated**.

Refer to the risk assessment for make-up application found in Unit B8 Provide make-up services when undertaking any camouflage make-up treatments (see pages 364–65), ensuring that you follow salon procedures at all times.

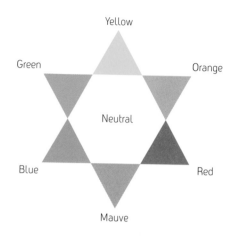

Think about it

If you use a variety of products, it is essential to remember that the shade, consistency and coverage may be different. Always refer to manufacturers' instructions.

Using tools and techniques to apply products

Brush

This method of application is used for marks that are small or thin. It is important to remember that the product should cover only the actual area, and a brush can be used to apply the product accurately.

After applying using the middle finger, tap to blur the edge of the cream and blend into the surrounding skin. If the area is tender, instead of **tapping** gently, press the area to blend the cream. When the cream is blended, apply setting powder and then blot with damp cotton wool.

Key terms

Lift streak – where the product is overworked and may lift and separate from the skin.

Overstimulated – where the skin is rubbed too much and may become red; to cause an erythema by overworking the area.

Key terms

Tapping – tapping with fingers to aid blending of the product.

Enhance appearance using skin camouflage **Unit B10**

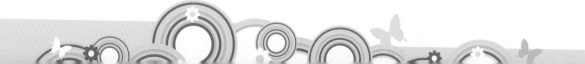

Sponge

This method is suitable for a light covering or toning down the skin. The use of natural sponges is better than synthetic sponges and the smaller the sponge, the better. Ensure that the sponge is damp as this will ensure the application is even.

To prevent contaminating the product decant onto a palette or the back of your hand and press the sponge into the product. Apply to area. If too much product has been applied, turn the sponge over and gently blot off excess.

Set and blot with damp cotton wool.

Velour puffs

These are used to apply the setting powder which seals the make-up.

If the therapist has a large area to cover, the puff can be used to rest on to prevent the previously applied make-up being disturbed.

Fingers

There are three ways to apply products with fingers and all methods produce good results.

1. Tapping – tap product in area to help with blending. This can only be done if there is no bruising or soreness.
2. Rubbing – a quick method of applying coverage to a large area.
3. Pressing – pressing the product on to the area. This is useful on tender areas.

Whichever method is used, a variety of blending and **setting** methods are required to make the effect last.

Setting

There are a few ways that the setting of make-up between layers of camouflage make-up can be carried out. The method given below takes account of salon time constraints and is the most cost-effective.

Apply concealer, set with powder, brush off excess and blot with damp cotton wool. Gradually build up the coverage until the desired effect has been achieved.

Applying camouflage products

Every client is different: the area to be covered, the effect the client wishes to achieve, and, with tattoo coverage, the density of the tattoo pigment will vary. Sensitivity and empathy should be adopted with each individual client.

> **Key terms**
>
> **Setting** – applying setting powder between the stages.

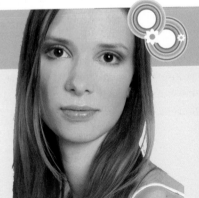

My story

Client satisfaction

Hi, my name is Sally. I have a tattoo on my left shoulder. When I was going to get married, I did not want it showing on my wedding day. Laser removal was not an option due to the cost, so a friend of mine recommended I go to a local salon where they do remedial make-up. The therapist, Helen, carried out a trial before the big day to ensure that the products and colours correctly matched my own skin tones. The process was painless but did take a little while as each layer needed to be built up gradually. The result was amazing and the photographs are proof!

Step-by-step tattoo camouflage

1 Discuss area to be covered with client and select suitable shade to match skin tone

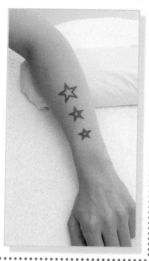

2 Use a white make-up to cover the darker tattoo outline. Set with powder between layers

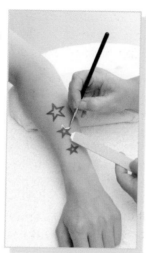

3 Cover with skin tone colour using brush, sponge, or fingers

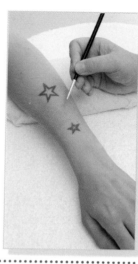

4 You may need to tap the product onto the skin to help blend the make-up

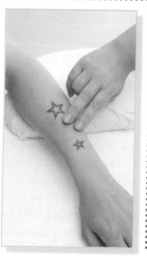

5 Use a puff to help set the make-up with powder

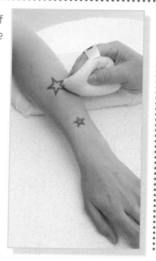

6 The covered tattoo

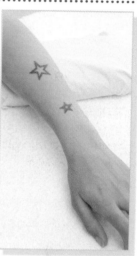

Depending on the depth of colour pigments in the tattoo, the dyes may show through the basic skin tone shade. The following colour shades are good for colouring these pigments:

○ Veil rose over blue shades

○ Veil olive over red shades.

Once the colour has been neutralised, proceed with selecting a suitable camouflage colour and follow procedure. Remember to follow the manufacturer's instructions.

Think about it

Due to the pigmentation in the inks used for tattoos, they can be very difficult to cover with camouflage products and the tattoo may start to appear through the make-up. It is therefore best to apply compatible make-up as late as possible to avoid this occurring.

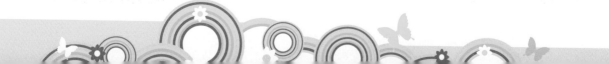

Salon life

My story

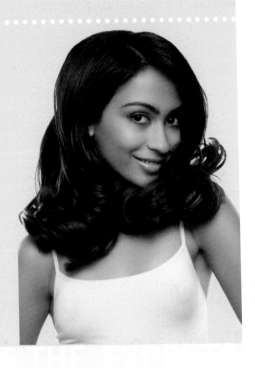

My name is Jessica. I have a sister who has vitiligo and was often teased at school because of her different-coloured skin. My parents learnt how to apply camouflage make-up from the Red Cross to help her cover the patches. When I left school I trained as a beauty therapist and have since specialised in camouflage make-up application as I know how my sister was affected by having pigmentation on her skin. Using camouflage techniques to help cover areas that a client is unhappy with is very rewarding as it gives them new-found confidence and self esteem. Remember that every client is different: the area to be covered, the effect the client wishes to achieve, and, with tattoo coverage, the density of the tattoo pigment will vary. Sensitivity and empathy should be adopted with each individual client.

Benefits to client and therapist

Benefits of camouflage make-up for the client:

- Increases confidence and self-esteem
- Can be worn in the bath or shower
- Can be applied at home if correct instruction given
- Colours are available to match the natural skin tone
- Can be used to cover tattoos for special occasions if the client requires; for example, weddings

Benefits of camouflage make-up for the therapist:

- Valuable service for vulnerable clientele
- Brings increased revenue to the salon
- Not all salons offer these specialist skills, so it will make your salon more unique
- Can be carried out in the client's own home — suitable for mobile therapists
- Advanced training courses are available

Q *Is there anyone that isn't suitable for skin camouflage?*

A Skin camouflage is suitable for men, women and children. However, clients who are under the age of 16 will need consent from their parent or guardian before treatment can commence and the parent/guardian will need to be present during the service. All other clients must sign a consent form prior to the service being carried out. Generally, it is not advisable to use skin camouflage on broken, dry or inflamed skin; for example, on skin with eczema.

Top tips

- Research the products that you wish to use before opting for a range to use in your work. Look at the colours and the coverage that the products offer. Many companies offer additional training to support their products.
- Keep different sets of brushes, sponges and puffs for applying your camouflage products. Do not use the same equipment as you do for general make-up application.

Hypo/hyperpigmentation camouflage

Hypopigmentation and **hyperpigmention** are both degrees of pigmentation that can be seen anywhere on the body.

Hypopigmentation or **vitiligo** is seen as pure white patches on the skin, where lack of the protective pigment melanin has left the skin sensitive to sunlight.

Hyperpigmentation or **chloasma** (sometimes referred to as melasma) is darker pigmentation. This is often seen around the eyes, mouth or cheeks, and may be as a result of pregnancy or seen in those taking the contraceptive pill.

Erythema camouflage

Erythema is caused by vasodilation of the small capillaries and can be seen as redness on the surface of the skin. Clients may wish to hide this redness.

Some clients may be suffering from the condition acne rosacea (see page 496), which often looks like a red butterfly running predominantly down the nose and across the cheeks. This will look like erythema.

Refer to You and the skin, pages 199–205, for skin conditions and pigmentation disorders.

Provide aftercare advice

In this outcome you will learn about:

- giving advice and recommendations accurately and constructively
- giving your clients suitable advice specific to their individual needs.

Giving clients advice and making recommendations

General rules for aftercare

- All aftercare should be directed to meet the individual needs of the client and aftercare should be appropriate to the area and the product used. The salon may consider selling colour concealers and some camouflage products to boost salon revenue.

- Make-up will need to be removed with a cream cleanser, and a suitable toner applied for the client's skin type.

- Products are designed to be worn when bathing, but soap should be avoided and only dab the area dry.

- Avoid extremely hot conditions as this can cause the make-up to separate.

- If irritation or swelling occurs, remove camouflage immediately and if required seek medical advice.

- Instruct the client in finger or brush application techniques for a touch up — ensure that the area is always grease-free prior to application.

Think about it

Ensure that the colour match and blending are as invisible as you can to meet the requirements of the client.

Key terms

Hypopigmentation – a condition of the skin, characterised by irregular patches of skin that are darker in colour.

Hyperpigmentation – a loss of skin colour caused by a lack of melanocytes.

Vitiligo – the appearance of single or multiple white areas of skin.

Chloasma – blotchy-brown pigmentation of the skin.

Erythema – vasodilation of the blood capillaries, causing surface reddening of the skin.

Enhance appearance using skin camouflage **Unit B10**

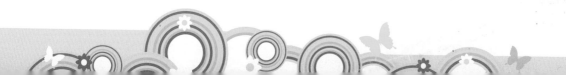

Frequently asked questions

Q Can any product be used for camouflage make-up?

A Only specialist products can be used which must be water resistant.

Q Why does the texture of products vary?

A This will depend on the coverage that the product gives, on the skin colour and tone, and the area where the product is to be applied.

Q Why should the outline of tattoos be covered first?

A Often the edges are darker and the colour can seep through. A white base colour is applied before the correct base shade is applied.

Check your knowledge

1 What is hyperpigmentation?
2 List three considerations when selecting suitable camouflage products.
3 What is erythema?
4 Describe vitiligo.
5 What is chloasma sometimes known as?
6 What colour powder is titanium dioxide?
7 What colour concealer will neutralise red?
8 Why are tattoos sometimes hard to cover?
9 What type of cleanser is recommended for removing camouflage products?
10 List three causes of over-blending camouflage products.

Getting ready for assessment

Carry out four treatments on four different clients on head or neck, chest or shoulders, limbs and back using brush, fingers, sponges and velour puffs while upholding health and safety requirements.

Show that you can successfully cover tattoos, pigmentation disorders and erythema, using creams, powders and setting products.

Carry out a full consultation remembering to ensure client confidentiality is maintained and a sensitive approach is used.

Provide full advice for home care and removal of the product.

Index

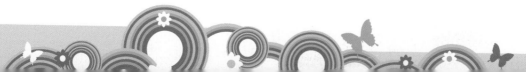